Fitness for Work

Fitness for Work
The Medical Aspects

SIXTH EDITION

Edited by

John Hobson
Julia Smedley

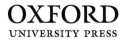
OXFORD
UNIVERSITY PRESS

Great Clarendon Street, Oxford, OX2 6DP,
United Kingdom

Oxford University Press is a department of the University of Oxford.
It furthers the University's objective of excellence in research, scholarship,
and education by publishing worldwide. Oxford is a registered trade mark of
Oxford University Press in the UK and in certain other countries

First Edition published in 1988
Second Edition published in 1995
Third Edition published in 2000
Fourth Edition published in 2007
Fifth Edition published in 2013
Sixth Edition published in 2019

Published in the United States of America by Oxford University Press
198 Madison Avenue, New York, NY 10016, United States of America

British Library Cataloguing in Publication Data
Data available

Library of Congress Control Number: 2018966723

ISBN 978-0-19-880865-7

Printed and bound by
CPI Group (UK) Ltd, Croydon, CR0 4YY

Oxford University Press makes no representation, express or implied, that the
drug dosages in this book are correct. Readers must therefore always check
the product information and clinical procedures with the most up-to-date
published product information and data sheets provided by the manufacturers
and the most recent codes of conduct and safety regulations. The authors and
the publishers do not accept responsibility or legal liability for any errors in the
text or for the misuse or misapplication of material in this work. Except where
otherwise stated, drug dosages and recommendations are for the non-pregnant
adult who is not breast-feeding

Links to third party websites are provided by Oxford in good faith and
for information only. Oxford disclaims any responsibility for the materials
contained in any third party website referenced in this work.

Foreword

Health problems can impact significantly upon people's ability to work, and influence their employment and career pathways. The assessment of fitness for work, a cornerstone of occupational medical practice, depends upon clinical evaluation and a knowledge of the workplace and its risks. It may depend upon collaboration with colleagues in other disciplines and an understanding of the advances in medical practice and treatment which can improve functional abilities. All clinicians across the healthcare landscape, in primary and secondary care, may also be called upon to give advice to their patients about work. They will be helped to do so by an understanding of the principles and legislative framework which underpin the health and work relationship.

The first edition of *Fitness for Work: The Medical Aspects*, was published thirty years ago in response to requests to the Royal College of Physicians and its fledgling Faculty of Occupational Medicine for authoritative guidance which would also provide a more rational approach to the employment of those with disabilities. The Faculty responded to the challenge and established a tradition of joint authorship by occupational physicians and specialists working in other fields of medical practice. This collaboration has been maintained throughout six editions and remains a striking example of the benefits of a cross specialty approach to the working population.

From the outset it was hoped that this book would be of use not only to doctors but also to occupational health nurses, workplace managers and others with an interest in employment. Today there is increasing recognition from health professionals and others that good work is good for health, and that work can itself be an outcome of excellence in clinical care.

We therefore commend the sixth edition of *Fitness for Work* to a wide multidisciplinary readership and thank the editors, John Hobson and Julia Smedley, for their enthusiasm and tireless commitment. With them we express our appreciation to all the authors who have given freely of their time and energy to produce this flagship publication of the Faculty of Occupational Medicine.

Dr Anne de Bono
President
Faculty of Occupational Medicine

Professor Andrew Goddard
President
Royal College of Physicians

Preface

Fitness for Work is the established and essential source of guidance to all those involved in the practice of occupational medicine, including occupational physicians, occupational health nurses, general practitioners, and hospital doctors. It has also become an important point of reference for non-medical professionals such as personnel managers, safety officers, trades union officials, lawyers, and careers advisers amongst others. The requirement for sound advice on fitness decisions in workers with health complaints ensures the book's enduring popularity.

Since the last edition the recognition that good working age health is essential has continued to increase at all levels of society. Various initiatives have been launched to try and facilitate those with health issues to return to the workplace, not all with success. The UK government has recently set out its long term vision of how it will prevent work loss due to health and support those with health problems to work or return to work. These initiatives recognise the enormous cost to society, the economy and individuals from worklessness. The importance of the right occupational health advice has never been higher and yet the number of trained professionals able to deliver that advice has never been under more pressure. As with every previous edition of this book, it can still be said that most employers and a large proportion of the workforce still do not have access to specialist occupational health advice. The existence of this book therefore remains an essential resource for those who are not specialist occupational health professionals to provide appropriate and accurate advice to employers.

The sixth edition follows the tried and trusted formula where most chapters are co-authored by a specialist occupational physician and a topic specialist. The persistence of this format is testimony to the excellence of the authors and editors who have gone before and mention must be made of Keith Palmer and Ian Brown who guided this book through a number of previous editions. Its ongoing success bears testimony to them.

Every chapter has been updated and a number of other significant changes have been made. The first part of the book now deals with occupational health specific topics and the second with specific medical specialities. The appendices from the fifth edition have been replaced with chapters including new chapters on transport, maritime, travel and vibration. A new chapter has been added on hidden impairments including autism spectrum disorder and attention deficit hyperactivity disorder. The musculoskeletal chapters have been reorganised and elsewhere overlap between chapters has been reduced. A revised chapter on blood borne viruses now includes viral hepatitis and HIV. Each chapter has been formatted to follow a similar template and includes key points and a useful websites resource. We hope these changes make sense and will make it easier for users of the book to find the information they need.

In total, some 29 new authors have contributed to this new edition. Most chapters have significant new content with the emphasis as before on evidence making particular use of consensus guidelines where these exist. Where this does not exist, *Fitness for Work* continues to provide a wealth of useful consensus guidance, codes of practice, and locally evolved standards with practical value to occupational health professionals.

Although Fitness For Work is aimed at the United Kingdom, we feel that most of the topics are covered in such a general way that it will also be a great help wherever in the world there is a need to make informed decisions about the medical aspects of fitness for work. In fact, this book will be invaluable to anyone practising occupational medicine.

To an extent, occupational medicine, like medicine as a whole, is an art that tailors advice to individual patients under specific and unique circumstances. As with any clinical judgement, the medical advice that is given remains the responsibility of the health professional concerned, and the general guidance contained in this book must always be interpreted in that light. None the less, we believe this book will underpin the considered opinions of clinicians and other professionals involved in the practice of occupational medicine.

Acknowledgements

A book of this size, complexity, and significance would not be possible without tremendous effort on the part of many people and the support of several bodies. We would particularly like to acknowledge the 63 contributors to this edition, who tread in the footsteps of previous authors making significant contributions to earlier editions of the work. These specialists have given freely of their time and shared their expertise and knowledge for the benefit of the health of working people and have helped to create this much revised sixth edition of the Faculty's flagship publication. They have also borne patiently the enquiries of editors and publishers and can take credit for their individual chapters as we the editors take pride in the final book. We would seek to dedicate this edition of Fitness For Work to Felicity Edwards OBE (1927–2018) editor of the first three editions of the textbook and Tar-Ching Aw (1948–2017) who contributed to the fourth, fifth and sixth editions. We also wish to thank the staff from Oxford University Press for their role in helping to co-ordinate this dauntingly large endeavour.

John Hobson
Julia Smedley

Contents

Abbreviations

ACJ	acromioclavicular joint
ACL	anterior cruciate ligament
ACR	albumin:creatinine ratio
ADHD	attention deficit hyperactivity disorder
AED	antiepileptic drug
AF	atrial fibrillation
AIHA	autoimmune haemolytic anaemia
ALT	alanine transaminase
AME	aeromedical examiner
AMED	Approved Medical Examiner of Divers
APD	automated peritoneal dialysis
ARDS	acute respiratory distress syndrome
ART	antiretroviral treatment
AS	ankylosing spondylitis
ASD	atrial septal defect; autism spectrum disorder
ATCO	air traffic controller
BAC	blood alcohol concentration
BCG	bacillus Calmette–Guérin
BGL	blood glucose level
BHIVA	British HIV Association
BMA	British Medical Association
BMI	body mass index
BNF	*British National Formulary*
BOFAS	British Orthopaedic Foot and Ankle Society
BP	blood pressure
BPPV	benign paroxysmal positional vertigo
CAA	Civil Aviation Authority
CABG	coronary artery bypass grafting
CAD	coronary artery disease
CAPD	continuous ambulatory peritoneal dialysis
CBT	cognitive behavioural therapy
CCS	Canadian Cardiovascular Society
CES	cauda equina syndrome
CHD	coronary heart disease
CI	confidence interval
CIPD	Chartered Institute of Personnel and Development
CJEU	Court of Justice of the European Union
CKD	chronic kidney disease

CMD	common mental disorder
CNS	central nervous system
CO	carbon monoxide
COPD	chronic obstructive pulmonary disease
COSHH	Control of Substances Hazardous to Health
CPAP	continuous positive airway pressure
CRPS	complex regional pain syndrome
CT	computed tomography
CTS	carpal tunnel syndrome
CVD	cardiovascular disease
DCD	developmental coordination disorder
DCI	decompression illness
DDA	Disability Discrimination Act 1995
DKA	diabetic ketoacidosis
DMAC	Diving Medical Advisory Committee
DMARD	disease-modifying antirheumatic drug
DOAC	direct oral anticoagulant
DSE	display screen equipment
DSM-5	*Diagnostic and Statistical Manual of Mental Disorders*, fifth edition
DVLA	Driver and Vehicle Licensing Agency
DVT	deep vein thrombosis
DWR	Diving at Work Regulations 1997
EAGA	Expert Advisory Group on AIDS
EASA	European Aviation Safety Agency
EAT	Employment Appeal Tribunal
EAV	exposure action value
ECG	electrocardiogram
EDSS	Expanded Disability Status Scale
EEG	electroencephalography
eGFR	estimated glomerular filtration rate
EPP	exposure-prone procedure
EqA	Equality Act 2010
ERT	emergency response team
ESA	Employment and Support Allowance
ESRD	end-stage renal disease
ESWT	extracorporeal shock-wave therapy
ET	Employment Tribunal
EU	European Union
FEV1	forced expiratory volume in 1 second
FMS	fibromyalgia syndrome
FOM	Faculty of Occupational Medicine
FVC	forced vital capacity
GDM	gestational diabetes mellitus
GFR	glomerular filtration rate

GHJ	glenohumeral joint
GMC	General Medical Council
GSL	general sale list
HASAWA	Health and Safety at Work etc. Act 1974
HAVS	hand–arm vibration syndrome
HbA1c	glycosylated haemoglobin
HBV	hepatitis B virus
HCV	hepatitis C virus
HCW	healthcare worker
HD	haemodialysis
HHS	hyperglycaemic hyperosmolar state
HIV	human immunodeficiency virus
HLA	human leucocyte antigen
HPV	human papillomavirus
HR	human resources
HSE	Health and Safety Executive
HSL	Health and Safety Laboratory
HTV	hand-transmitted vibration
ICD	implantable cardioverter defibrillator
ICD-10	International Classification of Diseases, tenth revision
ICOH	International Commission on Occupational Health
ICU	intensive care unit
Ig	immunoglobulin
IHD	ischaemic heart disease
IHR	ill health retirement
IIDB	Industrial Injuries Disablement Benefit
ILAE	International League Against Epilepsy
ILO	International Labour Organization
IMO	International Maritime Organization
INR	international normalized ratio
ISO	International Organization for Standardization
IT	information technology
ITP	idiopathic thrombocytopenia
IVF	*in vitro* fertilization
LASIK	laser-assisted *in situ* keratomilieusis
LR	likelihood ratio
LTD	long-term disability
MCA	Maritime and Coastguard Agency
MHRA	Medicines Healthcare products Regulatory Agency
MI	myocardial infarction
MPS	Medical Protection Society
MRC	Medical Research Council
MRI	magnetic resonance imaging
MRO	medical review officer

MRSA	methicillin-resistant *Staphylococcus aureus*
MS	multiple sclerosis
MSD	musculoskeletal disorder
MTP	metatarsophalangeal
MTPT	methyl-4-phenyl-1,2,3,6-tetrahydropyridine
NGPSE	National General Practice Study of Epilepsy
NHS	National Health Service
NICE	National Institute for Health and Care Excellence
NIHL	noise-induced hearing loss
NMC	Nursing and Midwifery Council
NPS	new psychoactive substances
NPV	negative predictive value
NSAID	non-steroidal anti-inflammatory drug
NYHA	New York Heart Association
OA	osteoarthritis
OGUK	Oil & Gas UK
OH	occupational health
OPITO	Offshore Petroleum Industry Training Organisation
OR	odds ratio
ORR	Office of Rail and Road
OSA	obstructive sleep apnoea
OTC	over-the-counter
PCI	percutaneous coronary intervention
PCOS	polycystic ovary syndrome
PCP	*Pneumocystis* (*carinii*) *jirovecii* pneumonia; provision, criterion, or practice
PCR	protein:creatinine ratio
PD	Parkinson's disease; peritoneal dialysis
PEF	peak expiratory flow
PEP	post-exposure prophylaxis
PFO	patent foramen ovale
PHI	permanent health insurance
PID	prolapsed intervertebral disc
PN	peripheral neuropathy
PO	Pensions Ombudsman
POAG	primary open-angle glaucoma
PoM	prescription-only medicine
PPE	personal protective equipment
PPV	positive predictive value
PTA	pure tone audiometry
PTSD	post-traumatic stress disorder
RA	rheumatoid arthritis
RCOG	Royal College of Obstetricians and Gynaecologists
RCS	Royal College of Surgeons of England
RCT	randomized controlled trial

ROC	receiver operating characteristic
RPS	Royal Pharmaceutical Society
RRT	renal replacement therapy
RSSB	Rail Standards and Safety Board
RV	residual volume
SAMHSA	Substance Abuse and Mental Health Services Administration
SCD	sickle cell disease
SCRA	synthetic cannabinoid receptor agonist
SCT	stem cell transplantation
SLD	specific learning disorder
SLE	systemic lupus erythematosus
SMI	serious mental illness
SNHL	sensorineural hearing loss
SNRI	serotonin–noradrenaline reuptake inhibitor
SSRI	selective serotonin re-uptake inhibitor
T1DM	type 1 diabetes mellitus
T2DM	type 2 diabetes mellitus
TB	tuberculosis
TIA	transient ischaemic attack
TKA	total knee arthroplasty
TLC	total lung capacity
TOC	train operating company
UK	United Kingdom
US	United States
UV	ultraviolet
VA	visual acuity
VTE	venous thromboembolism
VTEC	verocytotoxin-producing *Escherichia coli*
WBV	whole body vibration
WRLLD	work-related lower limb disorder
WRULD	work-related upper limb disorder

Contributors

Marios Adamou
Consultant Psychiatrist, South West
Yorkshire Partnership NHS Foundation
Trust, UK; Visiting Professor, School of
Human and Health Sciences, University of
Huddersfield, UK

Kaveh Asanati
Consultant Occupational Physician,
Epsom and St Helier University Hospitals
NHS Trust; Honorary Clinical Senior
Lecturer, National Heart and Lung
Institute, Imperial College London, UK

Tar-Ching Aw
Professor of Occupational Medicine
and Chair, Department of Community
Medicine, United Arab Emirates
University, United Arab Emirates

Birender Balain
Consultant Spine Surgeon, RJ&AH
Orthopaedic Hospital, Oswestry, UK

Sally Bell
Chief Medical Adviser, UK Maritime and
Coastguard Agency, UK

Blandina Blackburn
Consultant Occupational Physician,
NHS, UK

Julia Blackburn
Specialist Trainee in Trauma &
Orthopaedics, University Hospitals Bristol
NHS Foundation Trust, UK

Joseph De Bono
Cardiologist, Queen Elizabeth Hospital
Birmingham NHS Trust, UK

Steve Boorman
Director of Employee Health, Empactis, UK

Patrick Bose
Obstetric Consultant, The Royal Berkshire
NHS Foundation Trust, Reading, UK

David Brown
Consultant Occupational Physician,
Gloucester, UK

Edwina A. Brown
Consultant Nephrologist, Department
of Medicine, Imperial College London,
Hammersmith Hospital, London, UK

Ian Brown
Consultant Physician in Occupational
Health Medicine and Clinical Research
Fellow, Oxford Epilepsy Research
Group, Nuffield Department of Clinical
Neurology, Oxford University and Oxford
University Hospitals, Oxford, UK

Phil Bryson
Medical Director of Diving Services,
Abermed Intl, UK

Tim Carter
Professor Emeritus, Norwegian Centre of
Maritime and Diving Medicine, Bergen,
Norway

Rae-Wen Chang
Chief Medical Officer, Occupational &
Aviation Medicine, NATS Aeromedical
Centre, UK

Andrew Colvin
Consultant Occupational Physician, OH
Assist Limited, UK

Christopher Conlon
Reader in Infectious Diseases and Tropical Medicine, University of Oxford; Consultant in Infectious Diseases, Nuffield Department of Medicine, John Radcliffe Hospital, Oxford, UK

Roger Cooke
General Practitioner, Whitbourn, UK

Paul Cullinan
Professor in Occupational and Environmental Respiratory Disease, National Heart and Lung Institute, Imperial College, UK

Mike Doig
Consultant Occupational Physician, UK

John English
Consultant Dermatologist, Queen's Medical Centre, Nottingham, UK

Glyn Evans
Clinical Lead, Pensions, Medigold Health, UK

Julian Eyears
Consultant Specialist in Occupational Medicine, MFOM, UK

Neil Greenberg
Professor of Defence Mental Health, Kings College London, UK

Paul Grime
Consultant Occupational Physician and Honorary Clinical Senior Lecturer, Occupational Health Service, Guys and St Thomas' NHS Foundation Trust, The Education Centre, St Thomas' Hospital, London

Richard Hardie
Consultant Neurologist, Frenchay Hospital, Bristol, UK

Ali Hashtroudi
Clinical Director and Honorary Senior Lecturer, Guy's and St Thomas' NHS Foundation Trust, London, UK

Simon Hellier
Consultant Gastroenterologist, Gloucester Royal Hospital, UK

Robbert Hermanns
Honorary Senior Clinical Lecturer, Healthy Working Lives Group, University of Glasgow, UK; Consultant Physician in Occupational Medicine, Health Management Ltd., UK

Richard J.L. Heron
Vice President Health, BP International, UK

John Hobson
Honorary Senior Lecturer, College of Medical and Dental Sciences, University of Birmingham, UK

Gillian S. Howard
Employment lawyer, UK

Kristian Hutson
Specialist Registrar ENT Surgery, Sheffield Teaching Hospitals

Christopher W. Ide
Honorary Senior Clinical Lecturer, Healthy Working Lives Group, University of Glasgow; Consultant Physician in Occupational Medicine, Health Management Ltd., Altrincham, UK

Richard S. Kaczmarski
Consultant Haematologist, Hillingdon Hospital NHS Trust, The Hillingdon Hospital, Uxbridge, UK

Diana Kloss
Honorary President at Council for Work and Health, UK

David Koh
Distinguished Professor of Occupational Health and Medicine, PAPRSB Institute of Health Sciences, Universiti Brunei Darussalam, Brunei Darussalam; Professor, SSH School of Public Health and YLL School of Medicine, National University of Singapore, Singapore

Mark Landon
Partner, Employment, Pensions and Immigration Team, Weightmans LLP, UK

Ian Lawson
Specialist Advisor HAVS Rolls-Royce PLC, Derby, UK

Ira Madan
Reader in Occupational Health, Kings College London, UK

Peter McDowall
GP Partner and Occupational Medicine Trainee, Newcastle-upon-Tyne, UK

Stuart J. Mitchell
UK Civil Aviation Authority, UK

Elizabeth Murphy
Clinical director, NewcastleOHS, The Newcastle upon Tyne NHS Hospitals Foundation Trust, UK

Syed Nasir
Consultant, Occupational Health Group, Saudi Aramco, Saudi Arabia

Steven Nimmo
Occupational Physician, University Hospitals Plymouth NHS Trust, UK

Dipti Patel
Chief Medical Officer, Foreign and Commonwealth Office, UK and Director of the National Travel Health Network and Centre, UK

Mayank Patel
Consultant in Diabetes, University Hospital Southampton NHS Foundation Trust, UK

Neil Pearce
Gastrointestinal Surgeon, University Hospital Southampton NHS Foundation Trust, UK

John Pitts
Consultant Ophthalmologist to the Civil Aviation Authority, UK

Jon Poole
Consultant Occupational Physician, Sheffield Teaching Hospitals NHS Trust and the Health & Safety Executive, Buxton, UK

Richard Preece
Executive Lead for Quality of the Greater Manchester Health and Social Care Partnership, Manchester, UK

Martin C. Prevett
Consultant Neurologist, University Hospital Southampton NHS Foundation Trust, UK

David Rhinds
Consultant Psychiatrist in Substance Misuse/Clinical Stream Lead SMS, UK

Hanaa Sayed
Consultant, and Clinical Lead, Occupational Health and Wellbeing Services, Luton and Dunstable University Hospital NHS Foundation Trust, UK

Julia Smedley
Consultant in Occupational Medicine, Occupational Health, Southampton University Hospitals NHS Trust, UK

Caroline Swales
Consultant Occupational Physician for Roodlane, HCA Hospitals, UK

Sam Valanejad
Consultant Specialist in Occupational
Medicine, UK

Karen Walker-Bone
Professor, University of Southampton,
MRC Lifecourse Epidemiology Unit,
Southampton General Hospital, UK

Tony Williams
Consultant Occupational Physician, and
Medical Director, Working Fit Ltd., UK

Danny Wong
Senior Consultant Occupational
Physician, Occupational Health
Department, North Tyneside General
Hospital, UK

Philip Wynn
Occupational Health Service, Durham
County Council, UK

Anli Yue Zhou
Postgraduate Student, The University of
Manchester, UK

Chapter 1

A general framework for assessing fitness for work

John Hobson and Julia Smedley

Introduction

This book on fitness for work gathers together specialist advice on the medical aspects of employment and the majority of medical conditions likely to be encountered in the working population. It is primarily written for occupational health (OH) professionals and general practitioners (GPs) with an interest or qualification in OH. However, other professionals including hospital consultants, personnel managers, and health and safety professionals should also find it helpful. The aim is to inform the best OH advice to managers and others about the impact of a patient's health on work and how they can be supported to gain or remain in work. Although decisions on return to work or on placement depend on many factors, it is hoped that this book, which combines best current clinical and OH practice, will provide a reference to principles that can be applied to individual case management.

It must be emphasized that, alongside relieving suffering and prolonging life, an important objective of medical treatment in working-aged adults is to return the patient to good function, including work. Indeed, the importance of work as an outcome measure for health interventions in people of working age has been recognized by both the government and the health professions, and was emphasized in the recent UK government report *Improving Lives: The Future of Work, Health and Disability*.[1] Patients deserve good advice about the benefits to health and well-being from returning to work so that they can make appropriate life decisions and minimize the health inequalities that are associated with worklessness. A main objective of this book is to reduce inappropriate barriers to work for those who have overcome injury and disease or who live with chronic conditions.

The first half of the book deals with the general principles applying to fitness to work and OH practice. This includes the legal aspects, ethical principles, health promotion, health surveillance, and general principles of rehabilitation. There are also chapters dealing with topics such as sickness absence, ill health retirement, medication, transport, vibration, and travel. These are specific areas that most OH professionals will be required to advise about during their daily practice.

The second half of the book is arranged in chapters according to specialty or topic. Most chapters have been written jointly by two specialists, one of whom is an occupational physician. For each specialty, the chapter outlines the conditions covered, notes relevant statistics, discusses clinical aspects, including treatment that affects work capacity, notes rehabilitation requirements or special needs at the workplace, discusses problems that may arise at work and necessary work restrictions, notes any current advisory or statutory medical standards, and makes recommendations on employment aspects of the conditions covered.

Health problems and employment

Workers with disabilities are commonly found to be highly motivated, often with excellent work and attendance records. When medical fitness for work is assessed, what matters is often not the medical condition itself, but the associated loss of function, and any resulting disability. It should be borne in mind that a disability seen in the consulting room may be irrelevant to the performance of a particular job. The patient's condition should be interpreted in functional terms and in the context of the job requirements.

As traditionally used, impairment refers to a problem with a structure or organ of the body; disability is a functional limitation with regard to a particular activity; and handicap refers to a disadvantage in filling a role in life relative to a peer group (see Table 1.1).

Prevalence of disability and its impact on employment

Figures on the prevalence of disability in different populations vary according to the definitions and methods used and the groups sampled. There is no doubt that, however measured, disabling illness is common and an obstacle to gainful employment. Important information about the impact of long-term ill health on employment in the UK comes from the Labour Force Survey[2] and the related Annual Population Survey[3] (a locally boosted household survey). Data analyses from these and other sources informed a government green paper and public consultation on health, work, and disability in 2016.[4] In these reports, long-term health conditions were defined as illness lasting for 12 months or more, and the subgroup of

Table 1.1 Definitions

Term	Definition
Impairment	Any loss or abnormality of psychological, physiological, or anatomical structure or function
Disability	Any restriction or lack (resulting from an impairment) of ability to perform an activity in the manner or within the range considered normal for a human being
Handicap	A disadvantage for a given individual that limits or prevents the fulfilment of a role that is normal

Source: data from World Health Organization (1980). *The International Classification of Impairments, Disabilities, and Handicaps*. Geneva, Switzerland: World Health Organization. Copyright © 1980 WHO.

those who are disabled were defined as having reduced ability to carry out day-to-day activities (in line with the Equality Act 2010). The key conclusions were as follows:

- Among 11.9 million working-age people with a long-term health condition in 2016, 7.1 million were disabled.
- People in employment have better levels of well-being and lower risk of death than those who are out of work.
- Despite increasing rates of employment in the general population in recent years, fewer disabled people (48%) were employed compared with the non-disabled population (80% employed)—a gap of 32%.
- However, those with long-term health conditions that are not disabling have similar employment rates to people with no long-term health condition.
- There is a similar distribution of disabled people working across different industries and workplaces of various sizes, compared to non-disabled people.
- Disabled people are more likely to work part-time than non-disabled people.

In the UK, there are 3.4 million disabled people in work and 3.7 million out of work compared to 27 million non-disabled people in work and 6.7 million out of work. However, disabled people are twice as likely to leave work and nearly three times less likely to find work compared to non-disabled people.

With regard to common illnesses that affect those of working age:

- The overall cost of ill health among working-age people is around £100 billion annually.[4]
- Sickness absence is estimated to cost employers £9 billion annually.[5]
- About 14% of people with epilepsy are unemployed (compared to 9% of those with disability) but there is no evidence that those with epilepsy (or diabetes) are at increased risk of injury or absence.[6]
- A cohort study of 20,000 French electricity workers reported that diabetics were 1.6 times as likely as other workers to quit the labour force.[7]
- In England in 2014, 19% of people of working age had at least one common mental health condition. One in two people on out-of-work benefits had a mental health condition, compared to one in five of all working-age people and one in seven of those in full-time employment.[8]
- The Health and Safety Executive estimates that in 2014/2015, 1.3 million working-aged adults in Britain were suffering from an illness which they believed was caused or made worse by work, with 500,000 new cases each year. This caused 25.9 million lost working days and at a cost of £9.8 billion.[9,10]

The socioeconomic impact of working-age ill health is summarized in Box 1.1.[11]

Evidently, common as well as serious illness can prevent someone working, but many people who have a major illness *do* work with proper treatment and workplace support. Thus, the relation with unemployment is not as inevitable as these statistics suggest.

> ## Box 1.1 Socioeconomic impact of working-age ill health
>
> ◆ 131 million days lost due to sickness absences in the UK in 2013.
>
> ◆ Minor illness, 27 million days; musculoskeletal, 31 million days; mental health, 15 million days.
>
> ◆ 4.4–6.9 days lost/employee/year.
>
> ◆ Sickness absence rates of 2.1–3.0%.
>
> ◆ Overall median cost of absence per employee estimated to be £554 or 2–16% of payroll.
>
> ◆ £14.5 billion paid out as Employment and Support Allowance in 2015/2016.
>
> Source: data from Nicholson, PJ. *Occupational health: the value proposition.* London, UK: Society of Occupational Medicine. Copyright © Society of Occupational Medicine 2017.

Rather, the job prospects of people with common illnesses and disabilities can often be improved with thought, both about the work that *is* still possible and the reasonable changes that could be made to allow for their circumstances.

The relationship between work and health

Work forms a large part of most people's lives and allows full participation in society, boosting confidence and self-esteem. The way people work has changed over the years. More women work outside the home, there is more shift work, and greater use of flexible hours. People may choose or need to work for longer. Jobs are no longer for life and during a working lifetime an individual is likely to do a variety of jobs and may work either full-time or part-time at different stages. Work need not necessarily be for financial gain; voluntary or charitable work brings many non-financial benefits of employment.

While work and health are intimately related, health is not a necessary condition for work, and work is not normally a risk factor for health. The beneficial effects of work generally outweigh the risks and many people work despite severe illness or disability. This reinforces economic, social, and moral arguments that work is an effective way to improve the well-being of individuals, their families, and their communities. However, the preconditions are that jobs are available, there is a realistic chance of obtaining work, preferably locally, allowance is made for age, gender, and (lack of) qualifications, and there are 'good' jobs from the perspective of promoting health and well-being.

The adverse health effects of unemployment and worklessness are now recognized. Unemployment causes poor health and health inequalities, even after adjustment for social class, poverty, age, and pre-existing morbidity. A person signed off work who is sick for 6 months has only a 50% chance of returning to work, falling to 25% at 1 year and 10% at 2 years. Most importantly, regaining work may reverse these adverse health effects and re-entry into work leads to an improvement in health. Worklessness and the problems it can bring are now recognized as an important public health issue in the UK.[1]

However, despite the health consequences of worklessness and comprehensive health and safety legislation, too many people are still injured or made ill as a result of their work. Unsafe working conditions may be a direct cause of illness and poor health. Improvements in health and safety risk management could prevent much avoidable sickness and disability. Thus, a balanced view of the relationship between work and health is desirable. Safety is important, but a healthy working life is much more than this, it enables workers opportunity, independence, and the ability to maintain and improve their own health and well-being and that of their families—a broader and more positive concept.

There are, thus, implications for the provision of advice about work and for sick certification. Sick certification is a powerful therapeutic intervention, with potentially serious consequences if applied inappropriately, including in particular the slide into long-term incapacity (Box 1.2).

Box 1.2 Work versus worklessness

Work—the advantages

- Important in obtaining adequate resources for material well-being and to be able to participate in society.
- Work and resulting socioeconomic status are the main drivers of social gradients in physical health, mental health, and mortality.
- Central to individual identity, social roles, and status.
- Important for psychosocial needs where employment is the expected normal.
- Good work is therapeutic and promotes recovery and rehabilitation.
- Associated with better health outcomes and reduces the risk of long-term incapacity.
- Minimizes the harmful physical, mental, and social effects of long-term sickness absence.
- Promotes full participation in society, independence, and human rights.
- Reduces poverty.
- Improves quality of life and well-being.

Worklessness—the disadvantages

- Higher mortality—cardiovascular lung disease and suicide.
- Poorer general health, long-term illness—hypertension, hypercholesterolaemia, repeated respiratory infections.
- Poorer mental health, psychological/psychiatric morbidity.
- Higher medical consultation, medication usage, and hospital admission rates.
- Overall reduction in life expectancy due to the above factors.

The Equality Act 2010

The Equality Act 2010 and its forerunner, the Disability Discrimination Act 1995, have major significance both for the disabled and for OH professionals. In broad terms, and with certain important details of interpretation, the Act makes it unlawful for employers to discriminate against workers, including job applicants, on grounds of medical disability; rather, it requires that all reasonable steps are taken to accommodate their health problems. This is a form of positive discrimination in favour of preserving employment opportunities. It is also the legal embodiment of good OH values; long before the Act, OH professionals strove for the same outcome. However, employers are influenced strongly by legal mandate, so the Act is an instrument for good.

OH professionals need a good working knowledge of this legislation. Such is the Act's importance that a whole chapter (see Chapter 3) is devoted to its application and the recent development of case law, while references to the effects of the Act in clinical situations are made throughout the book. Here, only a few essential points are made.

In the Act, 'disability' is not defined in terms of working ability or capacity but in terms of 'a substantial and long-term adverse effect on the ability to carry out normal day-to-day activities'. Work itself does not, therefore, have to be considered in deciding whether an individual is disabled or not, but of course it does have to be considered when a disabled person is in a work situation. It is in this circumstance that the opinion of the OH professional will be required and they may be asked:

◆ whether an individual's disability falls within the definition of the Act?

◆ if it does, what adjustments may be needed to accommodate the disabled individual in the workplace?

Adjustments may be to the physical and psychological nature of the work or to the methods by which the work is accomplished. It is for management, not the OH professional, to decide in each individual case whether such adjustments are *reasonable*, although OH services may be well placed to *identify* potential adjustments. Before offering such opinions the OH professional must make an accurate determination of the individual's disability, not in medical but in functional terms. This requires a detailed understanding of the work and the workplace in question—another abiding principle of good OH practice.

Increasingly, many employers and their OH providers are not questioning whether the Act may or may not apply, but are focusing on whether reasonable adjustments have been made. Good employers will make adjustments whether or not the Act applies. This approach could be seen as sensible and represent good or best practice.

The 'fit note'

To raise awareness of the principle that many jobs can be performed adequately by people with health limitations, and to support its implementation, the UK government introduced a redesigned Statement of Fitness for Work ('fit note') in 2010 to replace the old 'sick note'. The form includes an option for the certifying doctor to indicate that, while not fit for normal work, the patient may be capable of working in a suitably modified job. In doing so, it supports the right to work of those with short- and long-term health problems, and recognizes that suitable work can bring tangible health benefits.[12] Advice on completing a fit note is provided in Chapter 10 and elsewhere.[13,14] The UK government plans to review the use of the fit note in their 10-year plan to transform work, health, and disability.[1]

The ageing worker

Increasing longevity, a growing shortfall in pension resources, and changes to employment law mean that more people will work past the traditional retirement age. This may be beneficial to individuals' wealth and health, though some will need modifications to their work or working time to accommodate impairments of ageing. Age, per se, can no longer be a blanket bar to gainful employment, though the advice contained in this book and the advice of an OH professional may be needed to integrate the older worker into employment effectively.

Some major issues surrounding practice in this area are aired in Chapter 7. Here, we stress the importance of the topic and its close relation to occupational medicine. Avoidance of ageist judgements about work fitness and greater flexibility in job deployment are increasingly commercially important but are already basic values in OH practice, while the underpinning medical advice will come from health professionals with experience in the occupational setting.

Occupational health services

All employees should have access to OH advice, whether this is provided from within a company or by external consultants. Ideally such advice should be provided by specialist OH professionals whether nurses or physicians. For some problems (e.g. in providing evidence for industrial tribunals or in other medico-legal cases), employers should be advised to seek advice from a specialist occupational physician where possible. The exact nature and size of the OH service to which any company needs access depends on the size of the company and the hazards of the activities in which it is engaged. Some companies find it advantageous to buy in or share OH services.

In the main, OH services advise on fitness for work, vocational placement, return to work after illness, ill health retirement, work-related illness, and the control of occupational hazards. Some of these functions are statutory (e.g. certain categories of health surveillance) or advisable in terms of meeting legal responsibilities (e.g. guidance on food safety, application of the Equality Act 2010). Some employers regard the main function being to control sickness absence. Although OH professionals can help managers to understand and possibly reduce sickness absence, its control is a management responsibility; OH practitioners should be careful to avoid the policing of employees who are absent for reasons attributed to sickness (see Chapter 9). Increasingly, OH plays a major part in supporting the wider health and being of employees, including promoting healthy lifestyles and behaviours.

Contacts between the patient's medical advisers and the workplace

The patient's own medical advisers have an important part to play. The importance of their contact with the workplace cannot be overemphasized. Consultants, as well as family practitioners, should ask the patient if there is an OH service at the workplace and obtain written consent to contact the OH adviser or service.

Where there is no OH service, early contact between the patient's doctor and management (usually the personnel manager) may be useful. It helps the employer to know when the patient is likely to return to work, and whether some work adjustment will be helpful, while family practitioners will be helped by having a better understanding of their patient's job and better equipped to complete a meaningful 'fit note'. Recognition of the importance of consistent advice about fitness for work from all health professionals in a patient's journey, and the improvement of access to specialized OH services were important features of *Improving Lives: The Future of Work, Health and Disability*.[1]

Confidentiality

Usually, any recommendations and advice on placement or return to work are based on the functional effects of the medical condition and its prognosis. Generally there is no requirement for an employer to know the diagnosis or receive clinical details. A simple statement that the patient is medically 'fit' or 'unfit' for a particular job, or requires additional adjustments, often suffices. However, sometimes further information may need to be disclosed using a fit note or in an OH report, particularly if limitations or modifications to work are being proposed. The certificated reason for any sickness absence is usually known by personnel departments, who maintain their own confidential records.

The patient's consent must be obtained before disclosure of confidential health information to third parties, including other doctors, nurses, employers, or other people such as staff of the careers services. It is recommended that all consent is in writing so this can be demonstrated if required. The purpose of the consent should be made clear to the patient, as it may be required to help with the finding of suitable safe work. A patient who is found to be medically unfit for certain employment should be given a full explanation of why the disclosure of unfitness is necessary. Further advice may be found in the Faculty of Occupational Medicine's *Guidance on Ethics for Occupational Physicians*[15] (see also Chapter 4).

Medical reports

When a medical report is requested on an individual, the person should be informed of the purpose for which the report is being sought. If a medical report is being sought from an employee's GP or specialist, then the employer is required to inform the employee of their rights under the Access to Medical Reports Act (AMRA) 1988 which include the right to see the report before it is sent to the employer and the right to refuse to allow the report to be sent to the employer. If the report is sought from an occupational physician it will also come under the AMRA if the occupational physician has had clinical care of the patient. OH nurses often follow these same ethical principles as a matter of good practice. Even if the OH professional has not cared for the patient, it is good ethical practice to follow the requirements of this Act. Employees are also entitled to see their medical records, including their OH records. The healthcare worker can withhold consent if they consider the contents to be possibly harmful to the employee but this may need to be justified in a court of law or tribunal.

Any doctor being asked for a medical report should insist that the originator of the request writes a referral letter containing full details of the individual, a description of their job, an outline of the problem, and the matters on which opinion is sought.

At the outset, the doctor should obtain the patient's consent, preferably in writing, to carry out a consultation and furnish the report. Even if the patient has given consent, the report should not contain clinical information, unless it is pertinent and absolutely essential. The contents should be confined to addressing the questions posed in the letter of referral and advising on interpreting the person's medical condition in terms of functional capability and their ability to meet the requirements of their employment. The employer is entitled to be sufficiently informed to make a clear decision about the individual's work ability, both currently and in the future, and any modifications, restrictions, or prohibitions that may be required. The doctor should express a clear opinion and offer the employee an opportunity to see the report before it is sent. The employee can then request correction of any factual errors but they are not entitled to require the doctor to modify the opinion expressed, even if they strongly disagree with it. A patient's return to work or continuation in work may depend on the receipt of a medical report from their GP, consultant, or OH adviser. It is in the patient's interest that such reports are furnished expeditiously.

When writing a medical report the OH professional should always remember that the document will be discoverable if litigation ensues. It should be clear from the report's content, letter heading, or the affiliation under the signature, why the doctor is qualified to address the subject in question.[16]

Assessing fitness for work: general considerations

The primary purpose of a medical assessment of fitness for work is to make sure that an individual is fit to perform the task involved effectively and without risk to their own or others' health and safety. It is not the intention to exclude from the job if at all possible, but to modify or adjust as necessary to allow the applicant to work efficiently and safely.

Why an assessment may be needed

1. The patient's condition may limit or prevent them from performing the job effectively (e.g. musculoskeletal conditions that limit mobility).
2. The patient's condition may be made worse by the job (e.g. physical exertion in cardio-respiratory illness; exposure to allergens in asthma).

3. The patient's condition may make certain jobs and work environments unsafe to them personally (e.g. liability to sudden unconsciousness in a hazardous situation; risk of damage to the remaining eye in a patient with monocular vision).

4. The patient's condition may make it unsafe both for themselves *and for others* in some roles (e.g. road or railway driving in someone who is liable to sudden unconsciousness or to behave abnormally).

5. The patient's condition may pose a risk to the community (e.g. for consumers of the product, if a food handler transmits infection).

There is usually a clear distinction between the first-party risks of points 2 and 3 and the third-party risks of point 5. In point 4, first- and third-party risks may be present.

Thus, when assessing a patient's fitness for work, the OH professional must consider:

◆ the level of skill, physical and mental capacity, sensory acuity, and so on needed for effective performance of the work

◆ any possible adverse effects of the work itself or of the work environment on the patient's health

◆ the possible health and safety implications of the patient's medical condition when undertaking the work in question, for colleagues, and/or the community.

For some jobs there may be an emergency component in addition to the routine job structure, and higher standards of fitness may be needed, on occasion.

When an assessment of medical fitness is needed

An assessment of medical fitness may be needed for those who are:

1. being recruited for the first time

2. being considered for transfer to a new job—transfer or promotion may bring new fitness requirements, such as more responsibility or overseas travel

3. returning to work after significant illness or injury, especially after prolonged absence

4. undergoing periodic review relating to specific requirements (e.g. regular assessment of visual acuity in some jobs, statutory health surveillance if working with respiratory sensitizers)

5. being reviewed for possible retirement on grounds of ill health (see Chapter 12)

6. unemployed and seeking work in training, but without a specific job in mind.

For points 1–5, the assessment will be related to a particular job or a defined range of alternative work in a given workplace. The assessment is needed to help both employer and employee, and should be directed at the job in question. In all of these situations, there is a legal requirement to consider 'reasonable adjustment' if the individual has a disability within the definition of the Equality Act 2010, and it is good practice to do so in any case.

After a pre-placement (pre-employment) medical examination (point 1 or 2), employers are entitled to know if there may be consequences from a medical condition that may curtail a potential employee's working life in the future.

For point 6, where there may be no specific job in view and the assessment must be more open-ended, health assessments may be required, for instance, by employment or careers services in their attempt to find suitable work for unemployed disabled people. It is important to avoid blanket medical restrictions and labels (such as 'epileptic') that may limit their future choice.

Recruitment medicals

Employers often use health questionnaires as part of their recruitment process. These should be marked 'medically confidential' and be read and interpreted only by a physician or nurse. A specific health questionnaire should not be returned to a non-medical person and to do otherwise could be seen as a breach of the Data Protection Act.

Some individuals may be reluctant to disclose a medical condition to a future employer (sometimes with their own doctor's support), for fear that this may lose them the job. It must be pointed out that should work capability be impaired or an accident arises due to the concealed condition, dismissal on medical grounds may follow. An employment tribunal could well support the dismissal if the employee had failed to disclose the relevant condition. It is not in the patient's interest to conceal any medical condition that could adversely affect their work, but it would be entirely reasonable for the applicant to request that the details be disclosed only to an OH professional.

For some jobs (e.g. driving) there are statutory medical standards and for others, employing organizations lay down their own advisory medical standards (e.g. food handling, work in the offshore oil and gas industry). For most jobs, however, no agreed advisory medical standards exist, and for many jobs there need be no special health requirements. Job application forms should be accompanied by a clear indication of any fitness standards that are required and of any medical conditions that would be a bar to particular jobs, but no questions about health or disabilities should be included on job application forms themselves. If health information is necessary, applicants should be asked to complete a separate health declaration form, which should be inspected and interpreted only by health professionals and only after the candidate has been selected, subject to satisfactory health.

The reason for a pre-placement health assessment should be confined to fitness for the proposed job and only medical questions relevant to that employment should be asked (Box 1.3).

Recruitment and the company pension scheme

There should not normally be health-related entry requirements to an occupational pension scheme and any such requirements could be in breach of the Equality Act 2010. Where this is not certain, enquiry should be made to the pension scheme or The Pensions Regulator (see 'Useful websites').

There may be modification in relation to death in service benefit as there would be for life insurance and in this case the individual should seek advice from the scheme or provider.

Box 1.3 The status of medical standards

Medical standards may be advisory or statutory. They may also be local and tailored to specific job circumstances. Standards are often laid down where work entails entering a new environment that may present a hazard to the individual, such as the increased or decreased atmospheric pressures encountered in compressed-air work, diving and flying, or work in the high temperatures of nuclear reactors. Standards are also laid down for work where there is a potential risk of a medical condition causing an accident, as in transport, or transmitting infection, as in food handling. For onerous or arduous work such as in mines rescue or in firefighting, very high standards of physical fitness are needed. Specific medical standards will need to be met in such types of work: where relevant, such advisory and/or statutory standards are noted in each speciality chapter.

Special groups

Young people

Medical advice on training given to a young person with a disability who has not yet started a career may be different from that given to an adult developing the same medical condition later in an established career. It is particularly important that young people entering employment are given appropriate medical advice when it is needed. A young person with atopic eczema may not wish to invest in training for hairdressing if advised that hairdressing typically aggravates hand eczema. A school-leaver with controlled epilepsy might be eligible for an ordinary driving licence at the time of recruitment but they and their employer may need to be advised if vocational driving is likely to become an essential requirement for career progression.

In general, young people, defined as under 18, are regarded as a vulnerable group by the Health and Safety Executive and may be at increased risk of injury or health problems in the workplace. This can be due to them working in an unfamiliar environment and lack of maturity among other factors. There may also be physical factors where they lack the strength to carry out manual handling activities as safely as older workers. They require additional training and supervision and there should be review of an employer's risk assessment (see 'Useful websites').

Supported employment

Supported employment is a model for supporting people with significant disabilities to secure and retain paid employment. It uses a partnership strategy to enable people with disabilities to achieve sustainable long-term employment and businesses to employ valuable workers. The same techniques are also being used to support other disadvantaged groups such as young people leaving care, ex-offenders, and people recovering from drug and alcohol misuse. Employment terms and conditions for people with disabilities should be the same as for everyone else including pay at the contracted rate, equal employee benefits, safe working conditions, and opportunities for career advancement.

Where a medical condition has significantly reduced an individual's employment abilities or potential then supported work should be considered as an alternative to medical retirement. Further information about supported work and a directory of organizations providing supported employment is available from the British Association for Supported Employment (see 'Useful websites').

The assessment of medical fitness for work

A general framework

As previously emphasized, the OH assessment should always be reported in terms of *functional capacity*; the actual diagnosis need not be given. Even so, an opinion on the medical fitness of an individual is being conveyed to others and the patient's written consent is needed for the information to be passed on, in confidence.

Each of the specialty chapters that follow outlines the main points to be considered when faced with specific health conditions. In this section we summarize a general framework, although not all of the points raised will be relevant to all individuals. The key outcome measure is the *patient's residual abilities relative to the likely requirements at the workplace*, so a proper assessment weighs functional status against job demands.

Functional assessment

To estimate the individual's level of function, assessments of all systems should be made with special attention both to those that are disordered and relevant to the work. This includes physical systems, sensory and perceptual abilities, psychological reactions, such as responsiveness and alertness, behaviour towards colleagues or customers, and other features of the general mental state. The effects of different treatment regimens on work suitability should also be considered such as the possible effects of some medication on alertness, or the optimal care of an arthrodesis. Any general evaluation of health forms the background to more specific inquiry. Assessment should also consider the results of relevant tests. The following factors may be material but are not exhaustive:

- *General*: stamina; ability to cope with full working day, or shift work; susceptibility to fatigue.
- *Mobility*: ability to get to work, and exit safety; to walk, climb, bend, stoop, crouch.
- *Locomotor*: general/specific joint function and range; reach; gait; back/spinal function.
- *Posture*: ability to stand or sit for certain periods; postural constraints; work in confined spaces.
- *Muscular*: specific palsies or weakness; tremor; ability to lift, push or pull, with weight/time abilities if known; strength tests.
- *Manual skills*: defects in dexterity, ability to grip, or grasp.
- *Coordination*: including hand–eye coordination if relevant.

- *Balance*: ability to work at heights; vertigo.
- *Cardiorespiratory limitations*, including exercise tolerance; respiratory function and reserve; submaximal exercise tests, aerobic work capacity, if relevant.
- *Liability to unconsciousness*, including nature of episodes, timing, warnings, precipitating factors.
- *Sensory aspects*: may be relevant for the actual work, or in navigating a hazardous environment safely.
  - *Vision*: capacity for fine/close work, distant vision, visual standards corrected or uncorrected, aids in use or needed. Visual fields. Colour vision defects may occasionally be relevant. Is the eyesight good enough to cope with a difficult working environment with possible hazards?
  - *Hearing*: level in each ear; can warning signals or instructions be heard? What is the effect of hearing protection if required?
  - For both *vision and hearing* it is important that if only one eye or one ear is functioning, this is noted and thought given to safeguarding the remaining organ from damage.
- *Communication/speech*: two-way communication; hearing or speech defects; reason for limitation; ability to behave and function constructively within teams.
- *Cerebral function* will be relevant after head injury, cerebrovascular accident, some neurological conditions, and in those with some intellectual deficit: presence of confusion; disorientation; impairment of memory, intellect, verbal, or numerical aptitudes.
- *Mental state*: psychiatric assessment may mention anxiety, relevant phobias, mood, withdrawal.
- *Motivation*: may well be the most important determinant of work capacity. With it, impairments may be surmounted; without it, difficulties may not be overcome. It can be difficult to assess by an OH professional who has not previously known the patient.
- *Treatment of the condition*: special effects of treatment may be relevant (e.g. drowsiness, inattention); implications of different types of treatment in one condition (e.g. insulin versus oral treatment for diabetes).
- *Further treatment*: if further treatment is planned (e.g. further orthopaedic or surgical procedures), these may need to be considered.
- *Prognosis*: if the clinical prognosis is likely to affect work placement (e.g. likely improvements in muscle strength, or decline in exercise tolerance), these should be indicated.
- *Special needs*: these may be various—dietary, need for a clean area for self-treatment (e.g. injection), frequent rest pauses, no paced or shift-work, etc.
- *Aids or appliances* in use or needed. Implanted artificial aids may be relevant in the working environment (pacemakers and artificial joints). Prostheses/orthoses should

be mentioned. Artificial aids or appliances that could help at the workplace (e.g. wheelchair) should be indicated.

◆ *Specific third-party risks* that could be conferred on other workers or members of the community (e.g. via the product such as infection in food handlers, etc.).

Functional assessment profiles

Many standard functional profiles of individual abilities are available. The PULHHEEMS is a system of grading physical and mental fitness used by Britain's armed forces. PULHHEEMS stands for physical capacity, upper limb, locomotion, hearing, eyesight, mental capacity, and stability (emotional). Its purpose is to determine the suitability of its employees for posting into military zones. It is not a fitness test as such but a test of suitability for purpose. The US uses a system called PULHES. PULSES is used in stroke rehabilitation to grade levels of disability and differs from the PULHHEEMS in that it also examines the digestive system. Other profiles have combined the evaluation of physical abilities with indications of the frequency with which certain activities may be undertaken. Although such profiles are relatively objective and systematic, and allow for consistent recordings on the same individual over a period of time, they take time to complete and much of the information may not be needed. They do not necessarily transfer to other work settings, for instance, when dealing with the complex practical problems affecting individual employees.

Requirements of the job

The requirements of work may relate not only to the individual's present job but also to their future career. Always considering the possibility of 'reasonable adjustment', some of the following aspects may be relevant:

◆ *Work demands*: physical (e.g. mobility needs; strength for certain activities; lifting/carrying; climbing/balancing; stooping/bending; postural constraints; reach requirements; dexterity/manipulative ability); intellectual/perceptual demands; types of skill involved in tasks.

◆ *Work environment*: physical aspects, risk factors (e.g. fumes/dust; chemical or biological hazards; working at heights).

◆ *Organizational/social aspects*: for example, working in small groups; intermittent or regular pressure of work; need for tact in public relations, etc.

◆ *Temporal aspects*: for example, need for early start; type of shift work; day or night work; arrangements for rest pauses or breaks, etc.

◆ *Ergonomic aspects*; workplace (e.g. need to climb stairs; distance from toilet facilities; access for wheelchairs); workstation (e.g. height of workbench; adequate lighting; type of equipment or controls used). Adaptations of equipment that could help at the workplace should be indicated.

◆ *Travel*: for example, need to work in areas remote from healthcare or where there are risks not found in the UK (see Chapter 17).

Box 1.4 The typical physical demands of work

1. Strength

Expressed in terms of sedentary, light, medium, heavy, and very heavy.

Measured by involvement of the worker with one or more of the following activities:

(a) Worker position(s):

    (i) Standing: remaining on one's feet in an upright position at a workstation without moving about.

    (ii) Walking: moving about on foot.

    (iii) Sitting: remaining in the normal seated position.

(b) Worker movement of objects (including extremities used):

    (i) Lifting: raising or lowering an object from one level to another.

    (ii) Carrying: transporting an object, usually in the hands or arms or on the shoulder.

    (iii) Pushing: exerting force upon an object so that it moves away (includes slapping, striking, kicking, and treadle actions).

    (iv) Pulling: exerting force upon an object so that it moves nearer (includes jerking).

The five degrees of physical demands are (estimated equivalents in Mets):

S Sedentary work (<2 Mets): lifting 10 lbs (4.5 kg) maximum and occasionally lifting and/or carrying such articles as dockets, ledgers, and small tools. Although a sedentary job is defined as one that involves sitting, a certain amount of walking and standing is often needed as well. Jobs are sedentary if walking and standing are required only occasionally and other sedentary criteria are met.

L Light work (2–3 Mets): lifting 20 lbs (9 kg) maximum with frequent lifting and/or carrying of objects weighing up to 10 lbs (4.5 kg). Even though the weight lifted may be only negligible, a job is in this category when it requires walking or standing to a significant degree, or sitting most of the time with some pushing and pulling of arm and/or leg controls.

M Medium work (4–5 Mets): lifting 50 lbs (23 kg) maximum with frequent lifting and/or carrying of objects weighing up to 25 lbs (11.5 kg).

H Heavy work (6–8 Mets): lifting 100 lbs (45 kg) maximum with frequent lifting and/or carrying of objects weighing up to 50 lbs (23 kg).

V Very heavy work (8 Mets) lifting objects in excess of 100 lbs (45 kg) with frequent lifting and/or carrying of objects weighing 50 lbs (23 kg) or more.

2. Climbing and/or balancing

(a) Climbing: ascending/descending ladders, stairs, scaffolding, ramps, poles, ropes, etc., using the feet and legs and/or hands and arms.

(continued)

Box 1.4 Continued

(b) Balancing: maintaining body equilibrium to prevent falling when walking, standing, crouching, or running on narrow, slippery, or erratically moving surfaces; or maintaining body equilibrium when performing gymnastic feats.

3. Stooping, kneeling, crouching, and/or crawling

(a) Stooping: bending the body downward and forward by bending the spine at the waist.

(b) Kneeling: bending the legs at the knees to come to rest on the knee or knees.

(c) Crouching: bending the body downward and forward by bending the legs and the spine.

(d) Crawling: moving about on the hands and knees or hands and feet.

4. Reaching, handling, fingering, and/or feeling

(a) Reaching: extending the hands and arms in any direction.

(b) Handling: seizing, holding, grasping, turning, or otherwise working with the hand or hands (fingering not involved).

(c) Fingering: picking, pinching, or otherwise working with the fingers primarily (rather than with the whole hand or arm as in handling).

(d) Feeling: perceiving such attributes of objects/materials as size, shape, temperature, texture, by means of receptors in the skin, particularly those of the fingertips.

5. Talking and/or hearing

(a) Talking: expressing or exchanging ideas by means of the spoken word.

(b) Hearing: perceiving the nature of sounds by the ear.

6. Seeing

Obtaining impressions through the eyes of the shape, size, distance, motion, colour, or other characteristics of objects. The major visual functions are defined as follows:

(a) Acuity:
Far—clarity of vision at 20 feet (6 m) or more.

Near—clarity of vision at 20 inches (50 cm) or less.

(b) Depth perception: three-dimensional vision: the ability to judge distance and space relationships so as to see objects where and as they actually are.

(c) Field of vision: the area that can be seen up and down or to the right or left while the eyes are fixed on a given point.

(d) Accommodation: adjustment of the lens of the eye to bring an object into sharp focus; especially important for doing near-point work at varying distances.

(e) Colour vision: the ability to identify and distinguish colours.

OH reports should avoid terms such as 'fit for light work only'. The dogmatic separation of work into 'light', 'medium', and 'heavy' often results in individuals being unduly limited in their choice of work. Jobs can be graded according to physical demands, environmental conditions, certain levels of skill and knowledge, and specific vocational preparation required, but OH practice requires more specific adjustment of the job to the individual. The O*NET Program provides a database of 1000 occupations and categorizes their demands, tasks, and activities (see 'Useful websites'). The database contains hundreds of standardized and occupation-specific descriptors on almost 1000 occupations covering the entire US economy. The database, which is available to the public at no cost, is continually updated from input by a broad range of workers in each occupation.

The physical demands listed in Box 1.4 express both the physical requirements of the job and capacities that a worker must have to meet those required by many jobs. For example, if the energy or metabolic requirements of a particular task are known, the individual's work capacity may be estimated and, if expressed in the same units, a comparison between the energy demands of the work and the physiological work capacity of the individual may be made. (See also Chapter 26.) Energy requirements of various tasks can be estimated and expressed in metabolic equivalents, or Mets. (The Met is the approximate energy expended while sitting at rest, defined as the rate of energy expenditure requiring an oxygen consumption of 3.5 mL per kilogram of body weight per minute.) The rough metabolic demands of many working activities have been published and the equivalents for the five grades of physical demands in terms of muscular strength adopted by the US Department of Labor are listed for information in Box 1.4. Work physiology assessments in occupational medicine provide a quantitative way of matching patients to their work and are commonly used in Scandinavia and the US.

Factors influencing work performance

Factors which may influence work performance, directly or indirectly, include:

◆ training or adaptation
◆ the general state of health of the individual
◆ gender (e.g. the maximal strength of women's leg muscles is 65–75% of that of men's)
◆ body size
◆ age (the maximal muscle strength of a 65-year-old man is about 75–80% of that when he was 20 years old and at his peak)
◆ nutritional state—particularly important when working in cold environments
◆ individual differences
◆ attitude and motivation
◆ sleep deprivation and fatigue

- stress
- nature of the work, workload, work schedules, work environment (heat, cold, humidity, air velocity, altitude, hyperbaric pressure, noise, vibration).

Objective tests

The result of any objective tests of function relevant to the working situation should be noted. For instance, the physical work capacity of an individual may be estimated using standard exercise tests, step tests, or different task simulations. Muscular strength and lifting ability can be assessed objectively by using either dynamic or static strength tests.

Matching the individual with the job

A functional assessment of the individual's capacities will be of most use when as much is known about the job as about the individual assessed. Sophisticated equipment is available to make a functional capacity assessment that will match an individual to a task. Less formally, the requirements of the task can be categorized, so that a match can be made with the individual's capacity.

There are wide variations in the practice of occupational medicine in different countries. In both France and Germany, job matching is used formally in some work settings, and in Finland, the Work Ability Index (a short questionnaire-based self-assessment of work capacity) has been developed.[17] Systematic job analysis and matching is less common in the UK but assessment of the disabled employee in their workplace together with appropriate discussion between managers, human resources, health and safety, and OH can bring about successful adjustment and placement. Practical assessments of a worker's ability to do their job can be invaluable if an impairment has been identified. Outside the workplace itself, more formal assessments may be made in medical rehabilitation or occupational therapy departments (see Chapter 10).

A comprehensive review of current approaches to the analysis of both the physical demands of jobs and the physical abilities of individuals, job matching, and functional capacity assessment has been published by Fraser.[18] Accommodation at the workplace is also discussed, and appendices include details of physiological and biomechanical techniques for work capacity measurement.

The OH professional who is assessing medical suitability for employment must have an intimate understanding of the job in question.

Presentation of the assessment

If a written report is needed, it should be typewritten, clearly laid out, signed, and dated. The report should mention any functional limitations and outline activities that may, or may not, be undertaken. Any health or safety implications should be noted and the assessment should aim at a positive statement about the patient's abilities. Any adaptations, ergonomic alterations, or 'reasonable adjustments' to the work that would be helpful or required by the Equality Act 2010 should be indicated. Recommendations on restriction or limitation of employment, particularly for health and/or safety reasons, should be unambiguous and precise, and should be made only if definitely indicated.

Recommendations following assessment

Recommendations following assessment depend on the circumstance of referral and the findings.

If the patient is employed, it should be possible to make a medical judgement on whether they are:

1. capable of performing the work without any ill effects
2. capable of performing the work but with reduced efficiency or effectiveness
3. capable of performing the work, although this may adversely affect their medical condition
4. capable of performing the work but not without risks to the health and safety of themselves, other workers, or the community
5. physically or mentally incapable of performing the work in question.

For the employed patient, where the judgement is options 2–5, the options of 'reasonable adjustment' may include work accommodation, alternative work on a temporary or permanent basis, sheltered work, or, in the last resort, retirement on medical grounds.

If the patient is unemployed but a pre-placement assessment is being carried out for recruitment to *a particular job*, options 1–5 will still be appropriate.

The return to work

Even if the patient is assessed as medically fit for a return to their previous job without modification, medical advice may still be needed on the timing of return to work. A clear indication to the patient, or employer, on when work may be resumed should be given wherever possible. Work should be resumed as soon as the individual is physically and mentally fit enough, having regard to their own and others' health and safety. Return to work at the right time can assist recovery, whereas undue delay can aggravate the sense of uselessness and isolation that so often accompanies incapacity due to illness, disability, or injury.

The contact between the patient's doctor and their employer or OH adviser, stressed earlier in this chapter, will ensure that preparations for the patient's return to work can be put in hand. Recommendations on when work may be resumed and on the patient's functional and work capacities should be clear and specific.

Patients who have been treated for cancer may have particular difficulties in integrating on their return to work, but, with modern treatment and suitable advice from an OH professional, many cancer patients return to full and productive employment (see Chapter 29).

Work accommodation

The patient's condition, which may or may not come within the Equality Act 2010, may be such that their previous work needs to be modified. Both physical and organizational aspects of the job must be considered. Simple features such as bench height, type of chair or stool, or lighting may need adjustment, or more sophisticated aids or adaptations may be required. The workplace environment may need to be adapted, for example, by building a ramp or widening a doorway to improve access for wheelchairs. Advice on work accommodation and financial assistance may be available through Jobcentre Plus whose Access to Work advisers can visit the workplace (see Chapter 10). Information on support available to those with disabilities is available from Disability Rights (see 'Useful websites').

Certain organizational features of the work may need adjustment—for instance, adjustment of objectives, more flexible working hours, more frequent rest pauses, job sharing, alterations to shift work or arrangements to avoid rush-hour travel. A short period of unpaced work may be necessary before resuming paced work. .

Alternative work

In many occupations, work accommodation or job restructuring is not possible and some type of suitable alternative work, possibly only temporary, may have to be recommended. This is usually judged on an individual basis by the OH professional who can keep the employee under regular review.

Medical retirement

Medical retirement should only be considered as a last resort and once all other options have been considered. For instance, where further treatment is impossible or ineffective, and if suitable alternative work cannot be provided. If the 'threshold of employability for a particular job' cannot be reached, either through recovery of fitness, or adjustment of work, retirement on medical grounds should be considered before employment is terminated. *A management decision on early retirement on grounds of ill health should never be made without a supporting medical opinion that has taken the requirements of the job fully into account.* Medical retirement is discussed in Chapter 12. Other aspects of early medical retirement in relation to the law are discussed in Chapter 2.

Recent developments and trends

Government initiatives

In recent times, there has been great emphasis on maximizing fitness for work and job retention. There have been several flagship policy documents, including *Working for a Healthier Tomorrow, Improving Health and Work: Changing Lives, Our Healthier Nation,*

A Framework for Vocational Rehabilitation, Securing Health Together, Pathways to Work, and the National Service Frameworks. The government's aspiration to tackle health inequalities produced by the disability employment gap is most recently described in *Improving Lives: the Future of Work, Health and Disability.*[1]

Increasingly, NHS and independent OH services are participating in a quality assurance accreditation scheme developed by the Faculty of Occupational Medicine (SEQOHS).

Finally, the new alignment of the Department for Work and Pensions and Department of Health with a joint Health and Work Unit has encouraged a more holistic approach to health problems in employment. Public Health England is taking a more active interest in workplace health. Local authorities are now responsible for having a health and well-being board that must produce a Joint Strategic Needs Assessment, essentially a plan for addressing the health of the local population that includes workplace health.

The important effort of controlling risks at work continues unchecked, but greater attention is being paid to rehabilitation and the common health problems that serve as barriers to job retention and job placement.

These initiatives are to be welcomed. The costs of making reasonable adjustments to retain an employee who develops a health condition or disability are likely to be far lower than the costs of recruiting and training anew. Moreover, work brings with it health benefits to the individual—it can be therapeutic, it is associated with lower morbidity and mortality, and it carries important social benefits and a sense of well-being and integration with society. Thus, in both financial and in human terms (as well as in terms of legal responsibilities), these efforts are important.

Maintaining fitness for work

From the viewpoint of the OH professional, fitness for work does not end with medical assessment. An employee must remain fit, which means attention to those factors that will prevent the deterioration of health. These may include policies or advice on smoking, exercise, diet, and alcohol consumption. The subject of health promotion is covered in Chapter 5, and that of health screening in Chapter 6. These activities are important ones in terms of the well-being of working-aged people. The prevention of vascular disease is particularly important as this disease takes a high toll on the working population and simple initiatives can be effective. Doctors also have a duty to support smoking bans and quit smoking initiatives. Finally, OH professionals should encourage employers to provide facilities for employees to take regular exercise and be prepared to advise on sensible eating and the food available in eating places at work. Recent guidance from the National Institute for Health and Clinical Excellence highlights workplace opportunities to combat physical inactivity, obesity, mental ill health, and smoking.[19-23] The long-term prevention of ill health, by whatever means, is as important to the prudent employer as ensuring that a new employee is fit for work.

Key points

♦ Medical fitness is relevant where illnesses or injuries reduce performance, or affect health and safety in the workplace; it may also be specifically relevant to certain onerous or hazardous tasks for which medical standards exist.

♦ Medical fitness has limited relevance in most employment situations: many medical conditions, and virtually all minor health problems, have minimal implications for work and should not debar from employment.

♦ When a manager requires OH advice, it should be sought with the full knowledge and consent of the individual and when providing advice, the OH professional should obtain sufficient knowledge about the work and the workplace.

♦ The OH report should advise the individual and their employer about fitness for work. It should contain relevant simple information that helps a manager to do their job without containing unnecessary medical detail.

♦ Medical fitness for employment is not an end in itself. It must be maintained.

Useful websites

The Pensions Regulator	http://www.thepensionsregulator.gov.uk/
British Association for Supported Employment	https://www.base-uk.org/
The Health and Safety Executive. Young people at work	http://www.hse.gov.uk/youngpeople/index.htm
The O*NET program. Database of job requirements	https://www.onetonline.org/
Disability Rights UK	https://www.disabilityrightsuk.org/

References

1. **Department for Work and Pensions and Department of Health**. *Improving Lives: The Future of Work, Health and Disability*. London: Department for Work and Pensions and Department of Health; 2017. Available at: https://www.gov.uk/government/uploads/system/uploads/attachment_data/file/663400/print-ready-improving-lives-the-future-of-work-health-and-disability.pdf.

2. **Office for National Statistics**. Labour Force Survey performance and quality monitoring reports. Available at: https://www.ons.gov.uk/employmentandlabourmarket/peopleinwork/employmentandemployeetypes/methodologies/labourforcesurveyperformanceandqualitymonitoringreports.

3. **Office for National Statistics**. Annual Population Survey. Available at: https://www.ons.gov.uk/employmentandlabourmarket/peopleinwork/employmentandemployeetypes/methodologies/annualpopulationsurveyapsqmi.

4. **Department for Work and Pensions and Department of Health**. Work, Health and Disability Green Paper Data Pack. 2016. Available at: https://www.gov.uk/government/uploads/system/uploads/attachment_data/file/644090/work-health-and-disability-green-paper-data-pack.pdf.

5. **Black C, Frost D.** *Health at Work – An Independent Review of Sickness Absence.* London: Department for Work and Pensions; 2011. Available at: https://assets.publishing.service.gov.uk/government/uploads/system/uploads/attachment_data/file/181060/health-at-work.pdf.

6. **Palmer KT, D'Angelo S, Harris EC, Linaker C, Coggon D.** Epilepsy, diabetes mellitus and accidental injury at work. *Occup Med* 2014;**64**:448–53.

7. **Herquelot E, Guéguen A, Bonenfant S, Dray-Spira R.** Impact of diabetes on work cessation: data from the GAZEL cohort study. *Diabet Care* 2011;**34**:1344–9.

8. **NHS Digital.** Adult Psychiatric Morbidity Survey. Survey of Mental Health and Wellbeing, England, 2014. 2016. Available at: https://digital.nhs.uk/data-and-information/publications/statistical/adult-psychiatric-morbidity-survey/adult-psychiatric-morbidity-survey-survey-of-mental-health-and-wellbeing-england-2014.

9. **Health and Safety Executive.** *Health and Safety at Work. Summary Statistics for Great Britain 2016.* Bootle: Health and Safety Executive; 2016.

10. **Health and Safety Executive.** *Health and Safety Statistics Annual Report for 2014/15.* Bootle: Health and Safety Executive; 2015.

11. **Nicholson PJ.** *Occupational Health: The Value Proposition.* London: Society of Occupational Medicine; 2017.

12. **Waddell G, Burton AK.** *Is Work Good for Your Health and Well-Being?* London: The Stationery Office; 2006.

13. **Department for Work and Pensions.** Statement of fitness for work; a guide for general practitioners and other doctors. Available at: http://www.dwp.gov.uk/docs/fitnote-gp-guide.pdf.

14. **Coggon D, Palmer KT.** Assessing fitness for work and writing a 'fit note'. *BMJ* 2010;**341**:c6305.

15. **Faculty of Occupational Medicine.** *Guidance on Ethics for Occupational Physicians*, 8th edn. London: Faculty of Occupational Medicine, Royal College of Physicians; 2018.

16. **Faculty of Occupational Medicine.** Good medical practice: guidance for occupational physicians. 2017. Available at: http://www.fom.ac.uk/professional-development/publications-policy-guidance-and-consultations/publications/faculty-publications.

17. **Ilmarinen J.** The Work Ability Index (WAI). *Occup Med* 2007;**57**:160.

18. **Fraser TM.** *Fitness for Work: The Role of Physical Demands Analysis and Physical Capacity Assessment.* London: Taylor & Francis; 1992. Available at: http://www.ssu.ac.ir/cms/fileadmin/user_upload/Daneshkadaha/dbehdasht/khatamat_behdashti/kotobe_latin/Fitness_for_work.pdf.

19. **National Institute for Health and Care Excellence.** Physical activity in the workplace. Public health guideline [PH13]. 2008. Available at: https://www.nice.org.uk/guidance/ph13.

20. **National Institute for Health and Care Excellence.** Smoking: workplace interventions. Public health guideline [PH5]. 2007. Available at: https://www.nice.org.uk/guidance/ph5.

21. **National Institute for Health and Care Excellence.** Obesity prevention. Clinical guideline [CG43]. 2006 (Last updated: March 2015). Available at: https://www.nice.org.uk/guidance/cg43.

22. **National Institute for Health and Care Excellence.** Workplace health: management practices. NICE guideline [NG13]. 2015 (Last updated: March 2016). Available at: https://www.nice.org.uk/guidance/ng13.

23. **National Institute for Health and Care Excellence.** Healthy workplaces: improving employee mental and physical health and wellbeing. Quality standard [QS147]. 2017. Available at: https://www.nice.org.uk/guidance/qs147.

Chapter 2

Legal aspects of fitness for work

Gillian S. Howard

Introduction

This chapter outlines some of the ways in which the law may affect the employment of people with health issues. There are three major legal sources relevant to employment in the UK—the common law, statute law, and (since the 1970s) European directives. Even though the UK has voted to leave the European Union (EU), our case law has been determined and decided upon by European Court decisions and they are now embedded as precedent in our law. Current domestic health and safety legislation enacting EU directives will remain in force until or unless they are amended or repealed. Therefore, neither statutory nor case law will change when we have left the EU.

Statutory employment protection in the form of unfair dismissal and disability discrimination legislation has transformed the rights and protection for employees who are injured or become ill at work and cannot work in the short or long term.

Common law

The English legal system is based on the common law. It has developed from the decisions of judges whose rulings over the centuries have created precedents for other courts to follow and these decisions were based on the 'custom and practice of the Realm'. The system of binding precedent means that any decision of the Supreme Court (formerly the House of Lords), the highest court in the UK, will bind all the lower courts. This applies unless the lower courts can argue that the previous binding decision(s) cannot apply because of differences in the facts of the two cases. The courts call these decisions 'fact-sensitive cases'.

When the UK joined the EU, the decisions of the Court of Justice of the European Union (CJEU) could supersede any decisions of the domestic courts and could require the UK national courts to follow its decisions. Scotland has a system based on Dutch Roman law, with some procedural differences although no fundamental differences in relation to employment law. Even though the UK has left the EU, nothing will change for a long time as EU law is embedded in our statutes and case law.

Common law duties of employers

At common law, employers have an implied duty to take *reasonable care* of all their employees and to guard against the risk of injury only if the risks were *reasonably foreseeable*.

These duties are judged in the light of the 'state of the art' of knowledge of the employer—what they either knew or ought to have known.

Standard of care of occupational health professionals

The common law requires a certain 'standard of care' from medical professionals. The standard of care expected of a medical professional is set out in a case that established the so-called *Bolam* test.[1] This held that a doctor could not be held to be negligent where he or she had exercised the standard of care 'of the ordinary skilled man exercising and professing to have that special skill'. A 'doctor was not negligent if he acted in accordance with a practice accepted as proper by a responsible body of medical opinion'.

However, in *Bolitho*,[2] the then House of Lords held that *Bolam* would be followed only where that body of medical opinion had reached 'a defensible conclusion', that is, where such a conclusion could be rationalized and justified. If the groundswell of medical opinion was outdated and clearly erroneous, the judges would not accept the opinion, even if it came from a respectable medical body.

In the case of an accredited specialist in occupational medicine, the standard of care expected would be higher than for a general practitioner (GP), who works part-time in occupational medicine. Occupational health (OH) professionals are deemed to exercise a standard of care that any reasonably competent OH professional would exercise even if different OH professionals might have come to very different conclusions. This principle would apply to all specialist OH professionals including nurses, ergonomists, and so on.

Duty to inform and warn of risks to health and safety

Employers are obliged to inform their workers, including prospective employees, of inherent risks of the job so that they can accept or decline employment having made an informed choice. Informed choice means the decision is voluntary and that the individual has the capacity in respect of the following:

- Possession of a set of values and goals.
- Ability to understand information and communicate decisions.
- Ability to reason and deliberate.

Any warning does not relieve the employer of the duty to take all reasonable care to guard against reasonably foreseeable risks of injury. The more junior and inexperienced the employee is, the greater the duty there is on the employer to explain the risks of the role and instruct and train the new employee. The principle is that the duty to inform and warn of risks does not extend to every danger and is limited to serious dangers that a person of ordinary common sense would not appreciate.

The defendant employer may raise the defence of *volenti non fit injuria*, in a claim for negligence, that is, that the individual knew about the risk, understood the exact nature of that risk, and *accepted* that risk. However, it has rarely proved to be a successful defence because the risk has to be clearly understood and accepted freely by the claimant and without duress. If the only choice is dismissal or accepting a particular risk at the workplace, the courts will be very slow to accept the defence of *volenti*.

In summary, the employer's duties include obligations to:

- take positive and practical steps to ensure the safety of their employees in the light of the knowledge that they have, or ought to have
- follow current recognized practice, unless in the light of common sense or new knowledge this is clearly unsound
- keep reasonably abreast of developing knowledge and not be too slow in applying it
- take greater than average precautions where the employer has greater than average knowledge of the risk
- weigh up the risk (the likelihood of the injury and the possible consequences) against the effectiveness and the cost and inconvenience of the precautions to be taken to meet the risk.

In *Sutherland* v. *Hatton; Barber* v. *Somerset County Council*,[3] the Court of Appeal gave judgement and guidance on coping with stress at work which they held was a part of the daily strategy of life management:

1. The importance of employers conducting risk assessments and these being used as a pro-active tool, because in civil cases employers owe a duty of care to their employees and should take reasonably practicable steps to maintain a safe workplace.

2. Stress assessments need to include workload and factors such as bullying, harassment, and other discrimination issues. (See the Health and Safety Executive (HSE) website in 'Useful websites'.)

3. There are no special control mechanisms applying to illness or injury due to stress arising from the work an employee is ordinarily required to do.

4. No particular occupation should be regarded as intrinsically dangerous to mental health. The correct approach is to identify the foreseeability of an individual to an adverse stress reaction, balanced against their willingness to do the job.

5. Employers are in the main entitled to take at face value what employees say about their ability to cope with their work and their general mental well-being, unless there are good reasons to think to the contrary. For example, changes in personality and working excessive hours to undertake routine tasks are indications that all is not well with a worker.

6. If an employee advises their employer that they are well and work is not a problem, the employer will not need to conduct 'searching enquiries of the employee or … permission to make further enquiries of his medical advisers'.

7. It is 'useful' for an employer to offer confidential advice, counselling, or treatment services. Even if the employee is at risk, there will be no breach of duty to allow a willing employee to continue in the job.

The Court of Appeal held:

> Many steps might be suggested: giving the employee a sabbatical; transferring him to other work; redistributing the work; giving him some extra help for a while; arranging treatment or counselling; providing buddying or mentoring schemes to encourage confidence; and much more.

> But in all of these suggestions it will be necessary to consider how reasonable it is to expect the employer to do this, either in general or in particular: the size and scope of its operation will be relevant to this, as will its resources, whether in the public or private sector, and the other demands placed upon it. Among those other demands are the interests of other employees in the workplace. It may not be reasonable to expect the employer to rearrange the work for the sake of one employee in a way that prejudices the others.

> As we have already said, an employer who tries to balance all these interests by offering confidential help to employees who fear that they may be suffering harmful levels of stress is unlikely to be found in breach of duty: except where he has been placing totally unreasonable demands upon an individual in circumstances where the risk of harm was clear.

Occupational stress must be considered in relation to external factors with liability accruing for an employer only for 'that proportion of the harm suffered which is attributable to [the employer's] wrongdoing, unless the harm is truly indivisible.'

In an important 'stress' case, *Intel Corporation (UK) Limited* v. *Daw*,[4] the Court of Appeal held that the employer was liable for the personal injury suffered by Mrs Daw as a result of work-related stress. The court held that it is not a rule of law that an employee, who does not resign when stresses at work are becoming excessive, necessarily loses their right of action against their employer.

Some employers believe that offering counselling services could discharge their duty of care in all cases. The Court of Appeal held that whether counselling would discharge the duty of care would depend on the circumstances of each case. In Mrs Daw's case, 'a short term counselling service could not have done anything to ameliorate that risk or help Mrs Daw cope with her stressors. It could not reduce her workload. The most it could have done is advise her to see her doctor. It does not seem to me that on the facts of this case the service provided was a sufficient discharge of the defendant's duty'.

The HSE has produced guidance on stress management including a template for a stress risk assessment, a stress policy, and stress management standards indicator tool (see 'Useful websites').

Balancing the risk

In essence, a cost/benefit analysis must be done. In deciding what is 'reasonably practicable' in eliminating risk and determining what is reasonably foreseeable in terms of injury, the courts have determined a test that balances the quantum of risk against the time, trouble, and expense that the employer must go to, to avert that risk. The greater the risk to health or safety, the greater the time, trouble, and expense the law expects of the employer.

Ignorance is no defence in law. Furthermore, if one member of the employer's staff knows about a risk or a health or safety problem, then (whether this is shared with the employer or not) the employer is deemed to know about it. This is called *constructive knowledge* (see Chapter 3).

The state of the art

The courts will look at the state of knowledge at the time of the alleged act of negligence in judging whether the employer ought to have acted or not. Employers are not expected to be prophets or polymaths, but they are expected to have knowledge of pertinent health and safety matters. They are not permitted to ignore advice and information given to them by their OH professionals merely because other employers do not know about or concern themselves with these issues.

Greater duty of care: 'eggshell skull' principle

The employer owes a higher duty of care to any particularly vulnerable employee with a known, pre-existing medical condition. Those with an 'eggshell skull physique' are more vulnerable to serious injury than others of robust physical health. Those with a fragile personality may suffer greater psychological damage than those with a robust personality. This is defined as the 'eggshell skull' principle, of which *Paris* v. *Stepney Borough Council*[5] is a classic example. Here, the council employed a labourer with only one eye. They failed to ensure that he was wearing eye goggles. Consequently, he injured his other eye at work and was blinded. The courts held that his employers owed him a higher duty of care as he was an individual with an extra risk of serious injury.

It is therefore important for employers to take informed advice from qualified OH professionals on fitness and placement decisions and the need for special arrangements or precautions. Failure to consider whether pre-placement health checks are required and, if so, to arrange for them to be done by properly qualified and trained OH staff, may lead to a successful claim for negligence against the employer. This is all the more important today when disability discrimination claims may be brought and expert evidence required.

Duty owed in mental illness

In several cases, the courts have extended the principle of the employer's common law duty to psychiatric injury. In a case that went to the House of Lords,[5] the negligent party was held liable for the onset of chronic fatigue syndrome precipitated by a car accident.

Although not the first case to establish an employer's duty of care to look after the mental well-being of employees, *Walker* v. *Northumberland County Council*[6] was the first successful claim for damages for not safeguarding the mental health of the employee once he had suffered his first nervous breakdown. The High Court held that it was reasonably foreseeable that in returning to his former post without adequate help and resources, Mr Walker would again become mentally ill—especially in the light of the medical experts' opinions that the nature and the volume of his work was the major contributory factor for his first nervous breakdown. In the *Barber* case in the Court of Appeal,[7] 17 useful propositions were laid down about an employer's duty of care in safeguarding its employees' mental health:

1. There are no unique considerations applying to cases of psychiatric (or physical) illness or injury arising from the stress of doing the work the employee is required to do. The ordinary principles of employer's liability apply.

2. The threshold question is whether this kind of harm to this particular employee was *reasonably foreseeable*. This has two components:
   - an injury to health (as distinct from occupational stress), which
   - is attributable to stress at work (as distinct from other factors).

3. *Foreseeability* depends upon what the employer knows (or ought reasonably to know) about the individual employee. Because of the nature of mental disorder, it is harder to foresee than physical injury, but may be easier to foresee in a known individual than in the population at large. An employer is usually entitled to assume that the employee can withstand the normal pressures of the job unless they know of some particular problem or vulnerability (staff who feel under stress at work should tell their employer and provide a chance for intervention).

4. The test is the same whatever the employment: no occupations should be regarded as intrinsically dangerous to mental health.

5. Factors likely to be relevant in answering the threshold question:
   - Is the workload much more than is normal for the particular job?
   - Is the work particularly intellectually or emotionally demanding for this employee?
   - Are the demands being made of this employee unreasonable when compared with the demands made of others in the same or comparable jobs?
   - Are there signs that others doing this job are suffering harmful levels of stress?
   - Is there an abnormal level of sickness or absenteeism in the same job or the same department?

6. Signs from the employee of impending harm to health:
   - Do they have a particular problem or vulnerability?
   - Have they already suffered from illness attributable to stress at work?
   - Have there recently been uncharacteristically frequent or prolonged absences?
   - Is there reason to think that these are attributable to stress at work, for example, because of complaints or warnings from the individual or others?

7. The employer is generally entitled to take what they are told by their employee at face value, unless the employer has good reason to think to the contrary. It is not generally necessary to make searching enquiries of the employee or seek permission to make further enquiries of their medical advisers.

8. To trigger a duty to take steps, the indications of impending harm to health arising from stress at work must be plain enough for any reasonable employer to realize they should do something about it.

9. The employer is only in breach of their duty of care if they fail to take the steps that are reasonable in the circumstances, bearing in mind the magnitude of the risk of harm occurring, the gravity of the harm that may occur, the costs and practicability of preventing it, and the justifications for running the risk.

10. The size and scope of the employer's operation, its resources, and the demands it faces are relevant in deciding what is reasonable; these include the interests of other employees and the need to treat them fairly, for example, in any redistribution of duties.

11. An employer can only reasonably be expected to take steps that are likely to do some good; the court is likely to need expert evidence on this.

12. An employer who offers a confidential advice service, with referral to appropriate counselling or treatment services, is unlikely to be found in breach of duty.

13. If the only reasonable and effective step would have been to dismiss or demote the employee, the employer will not be in breach of duty in allowing a willing employee to continue in the job.

14. In all cases, therefore, it is necessary to identify the steps that the employer both could and should have taken before finding there has been a breach in duty of care.

15. The claimant must show that that breach of duty has caused or materially contributed to the harm suffered. It is not enough to show that occupational stress has caused the harm.

16. Where the harm suffered has more than one cause, the employer should only pay for that proportion of the harm suffered that is attributable to their wrongdoing, unless the harm is truly indivisible.

17. The assessment of damages will take account of any pre-existing disorder or vulnerability and of the chance that the claimant would have succumbed to a stress-related disorder in any event.

The overall test is that of the conduct of the reasonable and prudent employer taking positive thought for their workers' safety in light of what they ought to know.

Employees' duties

At common law, employees have implied duties, including the duty to work with reasonable care and competence and to serve their employer loyally and faithfully. They are also under a duty to be reasonably competent, to cooperate with their employer, and to obey reasonable lawful instructions. So, for example, an unreasonable refusal to submit to a medical examination by a doctor of the employer's choice and to consent to the disclosure of a medical report could constitute a breach of the duty to cooperate or to obey a reasonable instruction.

Statute law

Health and Safety at Work etc. Act 1974

The Health and Safety at Work etc. Act 1974 (HASAWA) is superimposed on earlier Acts and the duties imposed by some of these (e.g. the Mines and Quarries Act 1954, the Factories Act 1961, and the Offices, Shops and Railway Premises Act 1963) must still be met, although most of their enforcement provisions have been replaced in the new legislation. The HASAWA imposes criminal liability, and the company, individual managers, and employees can be prosecuted for breaches of their statutory duties. Penalties for health and safety offences including failure to comply with an improvement or prohibition notice or for breaches of Sections 2–6 of the HASAWA for offences committed on and after 12 March 2015 include a maximum penalty in a magistrates' court of an unlimited fine, or imprisonment for a term not exceeding 6 months, or both. In the Crown Court, the maximum penalty is an unlimited fine or imprisonment not exceeding 2 years or both.

There is also the statutory crime of corporate manslaughter brought in by the Corporate Manslaughter and Corporate Homicide Act 2007. This renders an organization (not an individual) guilty of the offence of manslaughter if the way in which its activities are managed or organized:

'(a) causes a person's death, and

(b) amounts to a gross breach of a relevant duty of care owed by the organisation to the deceased.'

However, existing health and safety offences and gross negligence manslaughter at common law will continue to apply to individuals.

There have been only a handful of successful prosecutions for corporate manslaughter under the 2007 Act. In one case, the company, OLL Limited, was owned by one man, Peter Kite. He was jailed for 3 years and his company fined £60,000 following the 1993 Lyme Bay canoeing tragedy in which four teenagers died. In another prosecution for corporate manslaughter, the company, Cotswold Geotechnical, was fined £385,000.

There is provision in Section 47 of the HASAWA to permit employees injured at work to sue for their injuries in the civil courts under the Act, but this section has not been implemented to date. Employees who are injured at work as a result of a breach of any other statutory duties can sue in the civil courts, as the other statutory enactments impose both civil and criminal liability. The HASAWA covers everyone at work, including independent contractors and their employees, the self-employed, and visitors, but excludes domestic servants in private households.

There have been many more regulations concerning health and safety since the HASAWA including the Control of Substances Hazardous to Health (COSHH) Regulations 2002, the Management of Health and Safety Regulations 1999 (requiring specific risk assessments to be undertaken), the Maternity and Parental Leave, etc. Regulations 1999 (requiring risks assessments for pregnant women where there may be a specific risk to the health and safety of the pregnant woman or her unborn baby), and the Working Time Regulations 1999 (requiring mandatory rest and work breaks, annual holidays, and limiting the maximum working hours in any week, etc.).

Employers' statutory duties

The HASAWA imposes general duties on employers (Section 2) to ensure, so far as is reasonably practicable, the health, safety, and welfare at work of their employees. See Box 2.1.

Although there is no specific mention of a duty to conduct pre-placement health assessments, part of a safe system of work could be interpreted as ensuring that the staff who have been recruited are fit to perform their duties where there is any question of medical fitness impinging on the work requirements. This can only be done after a job offer has been made and Section 60 of the Equality Act 2010 makes unlawful the asking of any health questions prior to a job offer save for health and safety reasons or where reasonable adjustments may need to be made (see Chapter 3).

Employees' statutory duties

Employees have duties under Sections 7 and 8 of the HASAWA to 'take reasonable care' of their own health and safety, and the safety of others; to cooperate on any matter of health and safety; and to do nothing that could endanger their health and safety or that of others. This duty could be taken to include the disclosure of a relevant medical condition once a job offer has been made. For example, an employee who failed to disclose that they had epilepsy, before starting work in a job where this could pose a hazard, might be in breach of their duty under Section 7 of the HASAWA. Failing to disclose material health information when requested to do so may also constitute grounds for lawful dismissal (see 'Unfair dismissal').

Box 2.1 General duties on employers under the HASAWA

Employers must ensure that:

- there is a safe system of work
- there is a safe place of work
- staff are given information, instruction, and training on matters of health and safety, and are adequately supervised
- there is a safe system for the handling, storage, and transport of substances and materials
- there is a safe working environment

The institutions

The HSE is an executive non-departmental public body now sponsored by the Department of Works and Pensions. It is responsible for the encouragement, regulation, and enforcement of workplace health, safety, and welfare, and for research into occupational risks in Great Britain. As part of its work, the HSE investigates industrial accidents, small and large, including major incidents.

Employment protection legislation (unfair dismissal)

Employees have statutory protection from being unfairly dismissed; the relevant provisions can be found in Section 98 of the Employment Rights Act 1996. However, for "ordinary" unfair dismissal claims, an employee must have at least 2 years' continuous service with the same or associated employer before they are entitled to bring a claim. If the reason for the dismissal is alleged to be a discriminatory or inadmissible reason (e.g. being a member or taking part in trade union activities), then no service qualification is required. Employees who develop illnesses or injuries or who continue to be absent through sickness or injury have certain unfair dismissal rights.

A potential fair reason for dismissal is capability. Section 98(2)(a) of the Employment Rights Act 1996 defines 'capability' in relation to an employee, meaning his or her capability assessed by reference to skill, aptitude, health, or any other physical or mental quality.

Claims for unfair dismissal, discrimination, redundancy payments, certain breach of contract cases, and unlawful deductions from wages claims are heard by employment tribunals (ETs). Straightforward unfair dismissal cases are now only heard by a single employment judge. An employment judge will only sit with a panel of two lay members (one appointed by employers' organizations such as the Confederation of British Industry and one appointed by the Trades Union Congress or other trades union bodies) in discrimination cases.[8] Appeals on points of law or a perverse decision lie with the Employment Appeal Tribunal (EAT), then with the Court of Appeal and the Supreme Court on points of law only and where leave has been given. Cases are only granted leave by petition to appeal to the Supreme Court on matters of public importance. In cases involving questions of European Community law, cases used to be referred directly from ETs to the CJEU. Many of these referrals concerned questions arising from the UK's antidiscrimination legislation, which had been alleged to have failed properly to implement the EU directives. Following Brexit, the UK will no longer refer cases to the CJEU but the UK Courts may still take notice of EU decisions and the case law we have now derived from EU law and CJEU decisions will remain as precedents in the UK until or unless they are overturned with the UK Courts distinguishing the facts in a later case and coming to a different decision.

Grounds for dismissal

Section 98 of the Employment Rights Act 1996 sets out five potentially fair grounds for dismissal. They are conduct, capability, redundancy, illegality, and 'some other substantial reason'. In addition to proving a fair reason for dismissal, there is a requirement for the ET to be satisfied that the employer followed a fair procedure, that it was reasonable in all the circumstances according to equity and the substantial merits of the case. As long as the decision to dismiss fell within the band of reasonable responses that any reasonable employer could have adopted, the dismissal will be fair.

The tests that an employer must satisfy are those found in the leading case of *British Homes Stores* v. *Burchell*,[9] namely:

1. the employer must genuinely and honestly believe in their stated reason for dismissal

2. the employer must have in mind reasonable grounds upon which to sustain that belief

3. the employer, at the final stage at which they formed that belief on those grounds, must have carried out as much investigation into the matter as was reasonable in all the circumstances of the case

ETs are guided by the recommendations of the 'ACAS Code of Practice on Disciplinary and Grievance Procedures' (2015) and to a lesser extent the 'Guidance on the Code of Practice' issued in 2009. Breach of the ACAS code is not in itself unlawful but ETs are required to take its recommendations into account.

Right of representation

Employees are given the statutory right (Section 10 of the Employment Relations Act 1999) to be accompanied by a fellow worker or trade union representative to any grievance meeting or disciplinary meeting that could lead to a formal warning or other disciplinary action. This could include either a directly employed or self-employed contracting OH professional as the definition of a worker could cover an independent OH professional but would not cover an OH professional working for an OH service contracted to provide a service to an employer.

In the public sector, it has been argued that if a professional, such as a doctor or teacher, could be struck off their professional register and as a result be prevented from practice and be dismissed from their employment, then Article 6 of the Human Rights Act 1998 (the right to a fair trial) demands a right to be represented by a lawyer or someone of their own choosing. This may also be the case in relation to the rights of the employee to have the implied term of trust and confidence honoured and respected by their employer.

This was successfully tested in the Court of Appeal in the case of *Kulkarni* v. *Milton Keynes NHS Trust*,[10] by a teacher, in the Supreme Court in *R (on the application of G)* v. *The Governors of X School*,[11] and most recently by a professor of clinical trials at Birmingham University, *Stevens* v. *University of Birmingham*[12] and *Mattu* v. *The University Hospitals of Coventry and Warwickshire NHS Trust*.[13]

In *Kulkarni's* case, Dr Kulkarni was subject to the NHS disciplinary procedure which permitted him to the following express rights of representation:

> At any stage of this process (the investigation) – or subsequent disciplinary action – the practitioner may be accompanied in any interview or hearing by a companion. In addition to statutory rights under The Employment Act 1999, the companion may be another employee of the NHS

body, an official or lay representative of the British Medical Association, British Dental Association or defence organisation; or a friend, partner or spouse. The companion may be legally qualified but he or she will not be acting in a legal capacity.

When he sought representation from the Medical Protection Society (MPS) he was denied the right (the MPS representative had a law degree but was not a qualified solicitor or barrister). K brought a case for interim relief and declaration that he was entitled to the right to be represented by a legally qualified person under his contract and Article 6 of the Human Rights Act 2010 (the right to a fair trial).

The Court of Appeal agreed with him: 'where an NHS doctor faces such serious charges that he/she would be effectively barred from employment in the NHS, the right of legal representation should be given.' It was held that an employer who receives such a request would be well advised to give it fair consideration and when doing so to bear in mind the possibility that a denial of full rights of representation might be held to be a breach of Article 6. It was recommended that the Secretary of State give further thought to question of legal representation in the light of this decision. So far no such guidance has been given by the Department of Health.

In the case of the teacher, in *R (on the application of G)* v. *The Governors of X School*,[11] it was held that there was no requirement for the school's disciplinary proceedings to comply with Article 6; but that there may be circumstances in which legal representation could be a right under Article 6 where the outcome of the dismissal would have a 'substantial influence or effect' on the regulatory proceedings (e.g. a process capable of barring an individual from a profession).

It was noted, however, that where a decision in one set of proceedings determines the outcome in subsequent proceedings that determine a person's civil rights, then the right to a fair hearing, and, by implication, legal representation, may be engaged at that first stage. This may lead to findings in the future that legal representation at disciplinary hearings in such circumstances must be permitted.

In the case of *Stevens* v. *University of Birmingham*,[12] the appellant was a clinical professor, facing very serious allegations about his clinical trials. He was reported to the General Medical Council (GMC), suspended from the university and faced disciplinary action that could lead to his summary dismissal. He requested that his MPS representative attend his disciplinary hearing and represent him at that hearing (the representative had a law degree but was not a solicitor or barrister). The university refused the request because the representative was neither a work colleague nor a trade union official. Professor Stevens claimed that this was a breach of the implied term of trust and confidence. The High Court upheld his claim finding that the refusal to grant him his request for representation was a breach of the implied term of trust and confidence.

They held:

> The companion is not there to act as an advocate. This much is clear from the clearly defined role of the "representative" at the stage of the disciplinary hearing. He or she is there to see fair play (e.g.

in terms of ensuring that the notes of the interview and any statement taken from the employee for potential use in future disciplinary proceedings are accurate and comprehensive) and to help the employee to give a full and sufficiently clear account of everything of relevance so as to enable the investigator to be properly informed, and to understand the employee's response to the allegations.

The court held that in refusing the request to be accompanied by the representative, the relationship of trust between the university and their employee was seriously damaged, and that refusing attendance of the representative was unfair.

'Capability': ill health cases

In order for an employer to justify the fairness of a dismissal on the grounds of ill health (Section 98(4) of the Employment Rights Act 1996), they must obtain an up-to-date medical report from the clinician in charge of the employee's treatment.[14]

Tribunals also have to be satisfied that the employer acted reasonably in all the circumstances of the case, treating that reason as sufficient for dismissal, taking into account the size and administrative resources of the undertaking. In other words, large employers with human resources experts and extensive resources are expected to adopt all the good practices of a model employer, in contrast to a small employer who may be forgiven a failure to follow as thorough a dismissal procedure. The tribunals have given guidance as to what constitutes reasonable conduct on the part of the employer in this regard (see later in this section).

The mere fact that the individual is not prevented from performing all the duties that they are required to perform under their contract, does not affect a decision to dismiss for ill health, as long as the individual is unfit to perform some of the duties and there are no reasonable adjustments including other roles that the disabled individual could do or other duties they could perform. The requirements of the Equality Act 2010 and duty to make reasonable adjustments are now issues for employers to consider concerning long-term health conditions and the decision whether to dismiss (see Chapter 3).

Lying about previous health conditions

Lying has been accepted as being a potentially fair reason for dismissal under the Employment Rights Act 1996 (Section 98(1)(b)), being regarded as 'some other substantial reason for dismissal'. The tribunals have distinguished between lying on a pre-placement health questionnaire and failing to volunteer the information. There is a subtle but important distinction. In some cases, it has been held that there is no duty on employees to 'offer' voluntarily medical information about themselves.

However, it is important to note that Section 60 of the Equality Act 2010 now prevents employers from asking about health conditions at the interview stage. Questions about health conditions should only be asked after interview and an offer of employment (see later in this section). Nevertheless, if a direct question is not answered honestly and to the best of the individual's belief, then not only would a dismissal be potentially fair and non-discriminatory (if justified), but also the employer may be able to reclaim any sick pay. However, the question asked has to be clear, unambiguous, relevant, and job related, otherwise the employer will lose an unfair dismissal claim and possibly a discrimination claim, and will not succeed in reclaiming the sick pay paid.

In *Cheltenham Borough Council* v. *Laird* [15] the council learned a very expensive lesson, which was, to ask the right questions. They asked Mrs Laird, their prospective new chief executive, whether she had 'any ongoing medical condition which would affect [her] employment?' She replied 'no' and did not mention any history of mental health problems. The form contained the following declaration: 'I declare that all the statements on the above answers are true and given to the fullest of my ability and acknowledge that if I have wilfully withheld any material fact(s), I am, if engaged, liable to the termination of my contract of service'.

She subsequently had significant time off for stress and was paid sick pay for a year before the council discovered that she had a history of depression and stress-related illnesses. The council sued her for misrepresentation to reclaim all her sick pay—and lost. The High Court held that as a lay person and not a medical person, Mrs Laird had given an honest answer. At the time of completing the questionnaire she had no ongoing medical condition. The occupational physician admitted that the questionnaire was 'very poorly drafted' and 'quite inadequate'.

According to the Judge:

> The question would reasonably be understood as relating to an ongoing condition that impaired her physical or mental abilities either generally or in January 2002. She was not depressed in January 2002 and had recovered from her previous illness. Similarly, her answer … was not false or misleading because although she had a vulnerability to depression, the vulnerability was ongoing but not the depression … From a lay person's perspective, I consider that the question would reasonably be understood as being directed at a condition that was continually suffered or at least regularly suffered and that her vulnerability was not such a condition.

The judge suggested that a sweeping up question should have been asked, for example, 'Is there anything else in your history or circumstances which might affect our decision to offer you employment?'

Medical evidence and medical reports

In assessing fitness for work, most employers rely on self-certificates for the first 7 days of absence and a Statement of Fitness ('fit note') from the employee's GP thereafter. The current guidance states that after 7 days off sick the employer can ask the employee for a fit note from their doctor or can accept a 'return to work plan' through the Fit for Work scheme instead of a fit note (see 'Useful websites').

Where there is evidence contradicting sickness, the ETs have held that the employer is entitled to look behind the medical certificate, as happened in the case of *Hutchinson* v. *Enfield Rolling Mills Ltd*.[16] Mr Hutchinson was signed off for a week with sciatica but was seen marching in a trade union demonstration in Brighton. His employers took the view that this 'was not consistent with a person who was reputedly suffering from sciatica.

In other words, if you were fit enough to travel to Brighton to take part in a demonstration, you were fit enough to report for work'. The EAT agreed with the employer.

However, contrast Hutchinson's case with that of *Scottish Courage Ltd* v. *Guthrie*[17] where a warning shot was fired across the bows of employers deciding whether or not to pay sick pay in the face of an unchallenged medical certificate. Mr Guthrie's GP had given him a MED 3 (the forerunner of the fit note), but the employer's medical advisers said that he was fit to return to work. Neither medical adviser had suggested that Mr Guthrie's sickness was other than genuine. The employer's sickness absence policy provided that: 'Employees who are absent from work as a result of genuine illness and who fulfil all the requirements of the scheme rules will be eligible for [sick pay]' and 'Payment for sickness absence is conditional upon all appropriate procedures being followed and on management being satisfied that the sickness absence is genuine'. Mr Guthrie had followed the relevant procedures and in the past the company had always paid sick pay where employees produced medical certificates from their GPs. The company also agreed that Mr Guthrie did not have a poor sickness record. Mr Guthrie claimed that an unlawful deduction had been made from his wages. The EAT said that the ET was entitled to test whether the employer reached its decision in good faith. The decision to withhold sick pay was perverse, in that no reasonable employer could have reached it on the evidence gathered. Mr Guthrie was certified sick by his GP and, although the company's doctors differed as to when he could return to work, they had agreed that his illness was genuine. This case emphasizes the need for careful drafting of sick pay policies.

The medical dictionary defines malingering as 'the act of intentionally feigning or exaggerating physical or psychological symptoms for personal gain'. It is not considered to be a mental illness and is thus not classified in the tenth revision of the International Classification of Diseases or the *Diagnostic and Statistical Manual of Mental Disorders*, fifth edition. Malingering often is associated with an antisocial personality disorder and a histrionic personality style.

In *Jeffries* v. *The Home Office* (unreported), the High Court described a malingerer as someone 'who deliberately and consciously adopts the sick role, if necessary deceiving his medical advisers to persuade them that his complaints are true'.

Employers are entitled to 'look behind' fit notes and investigate what the employee is doing while on sick leave, if they are suspected of malingering (e.g. *Hutchinson* v. *Enfield Rolling Mills Ltd* (described earlier)). The employer had evidence that their employee was doing things away from the business that suggested he was fit for work. H was refused sick pay, resigned, and claimed unfair constructive dismissal and lost his claim.

Status of statements of fitness ('fit notes')

If employers choose to rely upon statements of fitness ('fit notes'), then they are entitled to do so, although they are provided for 'Statutory Sick Pay (SSP) purposes only' and have no legal status in their advice to patients or employers. The Department for Work and

Pensions has published very useful advice to GPs, employers, and OH professionals regarding the issuing of fit notes (see 'Useful websites').

Not all duties are suspended when an employee is off sick

The definition of 'incapacity' for Statutory Sick Pay purposes is inability to carry out *any* duties that it is reasonable to expect the employee to do under their contract. The definition requires consideration of the full range of the duties that it would be reasonable to expect the worker to conduct. Where, for example, an employee has their ankle in plaster 6 weeks after an operation, at a time when their consultant advises they can weight bear and walk with crutches, that employee could carry out sedentary tasks, perhaps with adjustments to their working hours to facilitate travel. If the GP continues to sign the employee off sick, careful discussions need to take place between the OH professional and GP in order to resolve any concerns that the GP may have about their patient returning to work with their ankle in plaster. In *Marshall* v. *Alexander Sloan Ltd*,[18] the claimant had called in sick. Her employer asked her to remove the valuable stock from the back of her car, which was left on the road. She refused to do so arguing that her contract was suspended. Not so, said the EAT. It held that someone off sick is only relieved of those duties that the sickness prevents them from doing.

Need for an up-to-date medical report

ETs have made it clear that employers should not rely on fit notes alone, albeit fit notes are more helpful than the former MED 3. In ill health cases, a full up-to-date medical report should be sought before any decision to dismiss is taken. The employer is required to inform the doctor and the employee of the purpose for which the medical report is sought.[19] Typically, the employer will state that the report is needed to plan the work of the department, administer the sick pay scheme, and consider reasonable adjustments and alternative duties. Doctors should always ensure that every employee who attends for an assessment clearly understands its purpose and the intended use of the report and have given their informed consent. In case of doubt, the doctor should explain the situation to the patient prior to any examination and if necessary, write to the originator of the request seeking clarification.

Employers should always advise the doctor as to the purpose of their enquiry, the basic job functions of the individual, and length of absence to date. The employer should obtain prior, written informed consent to do this from the employee. Typically the report will be limited to non-clinical details and a functional assessment. If a medical report is sought from the employee's GP or specialist, then the employer is required under the Access to Medical Reports Act 1988 (see 'Access to Medical Reports Act 1988') to inform the employee of their rights under that Act (which include the right to see the report before it is sent to the employer and the right to withhold it from the employer). If a non-medically qualified person receives a medical report, they may not be able to understand it or the report may be ambiguous or 'woolly'. If so, it should be returned to the doctor with a request for clarification and amplification.

Data Protection Act 1998

Under Article 9(1) of the General Data Protection Regulation 2018 (GDPR), health data are designated as 'special category data' for which 'explicit consent' is required before an employer can process them. 'Processing' means obtaining, inputting, storing, using, disclosing, amending, deleting, erasing, and so on. This data is:

Racial or ethnic origin.

Political opinions.

Religious or philosophical beliefs.

Trade union membership.

Genetic data.

Biometric data for the purpose of uniquely identifying a natural person.

Data concerning health or a natural person's sex life and/or sexual orientation.

Part 4 of the Code of Practice published by the Information Commissioner (see 'Useful websites') provides essential information on how employers must treat health data and the rights of data subjects to give or withhold their consent for data processing. If consent is obtained, employers (as opposed to occupational physicians or other treating doctors) may ask the specialist or GP a range of questions. If an OH professional seeks the medical report, then the employer is entitled to the answers to the model questions listed by the British Medical Association (Box 2.2), although there must be no disclosure of clinical or confidential information.

Under Article 15 of the GDPR, data subjects (i.e. job applicants, employees, ex-employees, and other third parties) have a right of access to such personal data (called a data subject access request—DSAR) whether in electronic or paper form, subject to the restrictions and limitations placed on their rights in the Court of Appeal's judgment in *Durant* v. *Financial Services Authority (FSA)*.[20]

Box 2.2 Model letter to consultant or GP enquiring about an employee's return to work

1. When is the likely date of return to work?
2. Will there be any residual disability on return to work?
3. If so, will it be permanent or temporary?
4. Will the employee be able to render regular and efficient service?
5. If the answer is 'Yes' to question 2, what duties would you recommend that your patient does not do and for how long?
6. Will your patient require continued treatment or medication on return to work?

In Durant's case, the court concluded that 'personal data' does not necessarily mean every document that has the data subject's name on it or in it. The over-riding test is whether the information is significantly biographical and whether the data subject is the focus. The Information Commissioner's Office has issued guidance on what constitutes personal data (see 'Useful websites').

Access to Medical Reports Act 1988

Under the Access to Medical Reports Act 1988, employees are entitled to see any medical report that relates to them, prepared by a medical practitioner responsible for their clinical care. Once an occupational physician (or a member of the OH staff) has treated an employee, the Act will apply to all subsequent medical reports (in Section 2 'care' is defined as including examination, investigation, or diagnosis for the purposes of, or in connection with, any form of medical treatment); but it is less clear whether this may apply to other reports, such as a statement on fitness to work or job placement.

An ET, in a disability discrimination claim, can order an individual to give their consent to the disclosure of their clinical records and reports including correspondence between the OH professional, the consultant, and managers of the company. If the employee refuses their consent to disclosure of medical records or reports, the employment judge will almost invariably strike out the claim, in the interests of fairness to the defendant employer.[21]

Conflicting medical advice

In some cases, employers receive conflicting medical opinions—the employee's doctor stating the individual is unfit for work and the OH professional advising to the contrary. In this dilemma, tribunals have generally accepted that a reasonable employer would rely upon the view of its occupational physician[22] unless:

- the occupational physician has not personally examined the individual
- the occupational physician's report is 'woolly' and indeterminate
- the continued employment of the individual would pose a serious threat to health or safety of the individual or others
- the individual is under a specialist and the occupational physician has not obtained a report from that specialist
- the employee asks the employer to allow him or her to present another specialist opinion.

In the *Heathrow Express Operating Co Ltd*[23] case, the EAT held that:

> provided the employer has taken into account all the evidence reasonably available to it, including if medical issues are raised, sufficiently well-qualified expert medical evidence, then the fact that other evidence is available by the time of the hearing cannot render the treatment unjustified.

Tribunals have accepted that unreasonable refusal by an individual to return to work following the advice of the OH professional constitutes misconduct on their part. The reason for dismissal is 'conduct'—refusing to obey a lawful and reasonable instruction. ETs have not been tolerant of employers who take decisions about the continued employment of an employee in haste, before the medical report is received.[24]

Consultation with the employee

The tribunals have ruled that in ill health dismissal, the employer should normally contact the employee by telephone or, ideally, by visiting them at home. The purpose is to discuss with the employee their incapacity, any possible return date, the continuation or otherwise of company benefits and state benefits, the employment of a temporary or permanent replacement, and the future employment or termination of employment. Consultation like this replaces the warnings that employees are entitled to receive in poor performance or misconduct cases. This was stated in a number of leading cases.[25] Only in exceptional circumstances would an employer succeed in establishing that they had acted reasonably if they failed to consult the employee prior to any decision. This may include advice from the occupational physician on whether the employee qualifies for ill health retirement.[26]

Seeking suitable alternative employment and making reasonable adjustments

The tribunals expect an employer to consider all alternatives other than dismissal and in disability discrimination claims to have considered all reasonable adjustments. This includes looking for alternative employment within the organization or with any associated employers. The 'reasonable adjustments' duty also includes considering whether any modification to the original job is possible. Failure by the employer to seek alternative employment will normally render any dismissal for ill health unfair—see the first House of Lords' decision on a disability discrimination issue, in *Archibald* v. *Fife Council*.[27]

Permanent health insurance benefits or long-term disability benefit

Medical advisers who advise employers offering permanent health insurance (PHI) or long-term disability (LTD) schemes ought to be aware that failure to consider offering such benefits in a particular case could be challenged in the common law courts as a breach of the employment contract.

The House of Lords ruled in *Scally* v. *Southern Health and Social Services Board*[28] that there was a positive duty on employers rather than their medical advisers to inform their staff of those benefits for which the employee must make an application. However, this implied duty on the employer does *not* extend to explaining to a sick employee the financial implications of resigning and taking an LTD scheme.[29] If an employer offers a PHI or LTD scheme, it will be deemed to be a breach of contract to dismiss the employee before allowing them to become eligible for the scheme, as it is regarded as a contractual entitlement that cannot be frustrated by terminating the contract—*Aspden* v. *Webbs Poultry & Meat Group*.[30] If the employee commits gross misconduct, the employer has the right to dismiss them even if this deprives them of their right to PHI—*Briscoe* v. *Lubrizol Ltd*.[31]

Consideration of eligibility for an LTD or PHI scheme, as an alternative to dismissal, may also be viewed by the tribunals as an important factor that could render the dismissal unfair. OH professionals should be familiar with the available benefits so that they can give appropriate advice. If such a scheme exists, the OH professional ought to ask the employer whether the employee has been considered for it.

Early retirement on medical grounds

Some employees may be deemed permanently incapacitated for employment and dismissed and given an early retirement pension. The courts have indicated that the employer must act in good faith in such cases.[32] Medical practitioners must read the exact wording of any pension scheme in this regard, particularly if a medical examination is to be performed to assess eligibility. It would be wise for them to require a copy of the sick pay scheme, PHI scheme, and pension fund rules as they apply to early retirement pensions.

Management's role in sickness decisions

The tribunals have emphasized that the option to dismiss an employee who is off sick and unable to work is a management decision, not a medical one.[33] OH professionals should not be pressured into making such decisions for managers; the OH professional's role is to provide and interpret medical information so that employers are well placed to make proper decisions about the employee's position.

Duty of care in writing OH pre-placement reports

In *Kapfunde* v. *Abbey National Plc*,[34] the Court of Appeal clarified to whom the occupational physician owes a duty of care when writing a report on the fitness for work of a job applicant. In this case, the court made it clear that the person commissioning the report (i.e. the potential employer) was the only person to whom the occupational physician owed a legal duty of care. However, the doctor still owes the patient the normal professional duty of care in clinical matters and must meet the standard expected by the GMC regarding 'Good Medical Practice' (see 'Useful websites'). This includes ensuring that any assessment is conducted to the highest professional standards and that any significant abnormalities detected are notified to the patient and their GP with the subject's informed consent.

Duty to be honest

In a case brought before the ECJ, *X* v. *Commission of the European Communities*,[35] it was ruled that prospective job candidates have the right to be informed of the exact nature of the tests to be carried out and can refuse to participate. In this case, Mr X complained that he had been screened for human immunodeficiency virus antibodies without his consent. The ECJ held that the manner in which the appellant had been medically assessed and declared unfit constituted an infringement of his right to respect for his private life as guaranteed by Article 8 of the European Convention on Human Rights. This right requires that a person's refusal to undergo a test be respected in its entirety; equally, however, the employer cannot be obliged to take the risk of recruitment.

Confidentiality

Ethical questions including the duty of confidentiality are covered in Chapter 4.

Apart from the Article 8(1) right to respect for private life, doctors and nurses are under strict ethical codes of conduct and can be struck off their professional registers for serious breaches. The GMC periodically reviews and publishes guidance concerning confidentiality and the duties of a doctor, including occupational physicians. Guidance that came into force in April 2017 requires that employees must be offered a copy of their report before it is supplied to the employer (see 'Useful websites'). The Faculty of Occupational Medicine has also published guidance on 'Good Occupational Medical Practice' updated in 2017, based on the GMC's Guidance on 'Good Medical Practice' (see 'Useful websites').

The Faculty of Occupational Medicine recognizes that:

> specific additional guidance for occupational physicians arises because their practice differs significantly from that of doctors in most other specialties. The occupational physician usually has responsibilities to employers as well as to workers. Moreover, occupational physicians often work in privately organised occupational health services, and undertake a range of clinical and managerial activities that differ markedly from those of other doctors.

Employers are not entitled to require their staff to undergo health assessments without obtaining their informed written consent on each occasion. This means ensuring that the employee understands the nature of and reasons for assessments. On each occasion, employers must also obtain the employee's written, informed consent to disclosure of the results, or a more detailed report to a named individual in the company. In the absence of written consent, no health assessment or disclosure should take place.

Expert evidence

OH professionals may be asked at some time to give expert evidence, in ETs in ill health dismissals, or disability discrimination cases, or in the High Court in personal injury claims. Expert witnesses give evidence of opinion as opposed to evidence of fact. Expert witnesses are governed by detailed rules and a Practice Direction in the Civil Procedure Rules (Part 1).

Pregnancy, discrimination, and the law

Any form of discrimination on the grounds of a woman's pregnancy is unlawful, constituting direct discrimination (Sections 13, 18, and 19 of the Equality Act 2010). All aspects of pregnancy, pregnancy-related illness, and maternity are covered, including the notification of intention to take maternity leave, the taking of maternity leave, and intention to return to work following maternity leave.

Furthermore, pregnant women and breastfeeding mothers are given statutory protection at work as employers are under a duty to carry out risk assessments and to have adequate control measures where possible. Failing adequate control measures, the woman has a right to be transferred to another safer job, or, if this is not possible, a right to be suspended on normal pay (Section 64 of the Employment Rights Act 1996).[36]

Fathers have the right to take up to 2 weeks' paternity leave and receive statutory paternity pay. Certain statutory conditions must be met before a father is entitled to paid paternity leave. Shared parental leave introduced in April 2015 is designed to give parents more flexibility in sharing child care in the first year following birth or adoption. Parents are able to share maternity leave deciding to be off work at the same time and/or take it in turns to have periods of leave to look after the child. Adoptive parents have rights to the same maternity, parental, and paternity leave as birth parents.

Working Time Directive and Working Time Regulations 1988

The Working Time Directive, which was adopted under the qualified majority voting system, requires member states to legislate for a maximum of 48 working hours in any 7-day period averaged over 17 weeks, with rest breaks and restrictions on the number of hours of work that can be performed at night.

The Working Time Regulations 1998 (SI 1998/1833) provided workers with an entitlement to:

♦ a rest break where the working day exceeds 6 hours

♦ at least 1 whole hour off in each 24 hours

♦ at least 24 hours off in every week.

Other provisions include at least 4 weeks of paid annual leave; restrictions on night work (including an average limit of 8 hours in 24); organization of work patterns to take account of health and safety requirements, and the adaptation of work to the worker; and an average working limit of 48 hours over each 7-day period, calculated over a reference period of 17 weeks (Regulation 4(3) of the Working Time Regulations 1998).

A further statutory instrument, amending the first Working Time Regulations, became law in December 1999—The Working Time Regulations 1999. These regulations simplified the meaning of the unmeasured hours and those workers who work unmeasured hours are now exempt from the 48-hour week; it also amended the requirement for employers to keep records of the hours worked by workers who had opted out of the 48-hour maximum working week.

The directive is littered with derogations that exempt certain types of work. There are some general exceptions that exclude workers in air, sea, rail, and road, inland waterways and lake transport, sea fishing and other work at sea, as well as doctors in training. The major provisions for which there are no derogations are the 4 weeks of paid annual leave and the 48-hour working week.

Other exceptions may arise through national legislation or collective agreements for those whose working time is self-determined or flexible (e.g. senior managers or workers with autonomous decision-taking powers, family workers, and workers officiating at religious ceremonies). In addition, workers may agree voluntarily to work longer hours than those laid down in the directive. In other cases, the workers must be permitted compensatory rest breaks if they work for more than 48 hours in a week (e.g. those whose job involves a great deal of travelling, security and surveillance workers, those whose jobs involve a foreseeable surge in activity such as tourism and agriculture, and emergency rescue workers). In *Landeshauptstadt Kiel* v. *Jaege*,[37] the ECJ ruled that being on call, even if not actually working, constituted working time under the directive. The ECJ held that:

> A period of duty spent by a hospital doctor on call, where the doctor's presence in the hospital is required, must be regarded as constituting in its entirety working time for the purposes of the Working Time Directive, even though the person concerned is permitted to rest at their place of work during periods when their services are not required ... An employee available at the place determined by the employer cannot be regarded as being at rest during the periods of his on-call duty when he is not actually carrying on any professional activity.

In accordance with an important ECJ decision, holidays accrue during sick leave and the employee can opt to take this accrued leave when they return to work even if they have entered a new holiday year.[38]

Other health and safety directives

The 'Six Pack' regulations made it mandatory for employers to carry out risk assessments if there are 'significant and substantial' risks to health or safety and to appoint 'competent' people to assist them (see 'Useful websites'). Employers must maintain, update, and document these risk assessments. Other regulations require regular health surveillance (e.g. COSHH, Regulation 11).

The Health and Safety (Display Screen Equipment) Regulations 1992 ('DSE' Regulations), and Code of Practice and Guidance Notes sought to regulate the use of display screen equipment (DSE). The regulations lay down ergonomic rules relating to the work station, and require employers to provide free eyesight tests and spectacles if required for DSE use. Employers are required to undertake regular risk assessments of the workstation and the work. In addition, the Code of Practice and Guidance Notes recommend rest breaks for habitual users.

Key points

- There are three major legal sources relevant to employment in the UK—the common law, statute law, and European directives. This chapter outlines some of the ways in which the law may affect the employment of people with health issues.
- Following Brexit, domestic health and safety legislation enacting EU directives will remain in force until or unless they are amended or repealed.
- Statutory employment protection in the form of unfair dismissal and disability discrimination legislation have transformed the rights and protection for employees who are injured or become ill at work and cannot work in the short or long term.

◆ OH professionals should have an understanding of the law and the standard of care they are expected to exercise. They should also understand from case law the interplay between disability and ill health.

◆ The chapter includes guidance for OH professionals on their role in long-term or chronic and acute ill health cases and in giving advice on early retirement on the grounds of ill health. It also includes other health/OH issues such as pregnancy and maternity, stress cases, data protection and informed consent, and disclosure of medical records and reports.

Useful websites

Health and Safety Executive. Health and safety regulation	http://www.hse.gov.uk/pubns/hsc13.pdf
Health and Safety Executive. Guidance on management of stress	http://www.hse.gov.uk/stress/
UK Government. Guidance on sick pay and the fit note	https://www.gov.uk/employers-sick-pay/notice-and-fit-notes
Equality and Human Rights Commission (EHRC). Guidance on pre-placement health questions and the Equality Act	https://www.equalityhumanrights.com/en/publication-download/pre-employment-health-questions-guidance-job-applications-section-60-equality
Information commissioner. Guidance on personal data and the Data Protection Act	https://ico.org.uk/media/for-organisations/documents/1554/determining-what-is-personal-data.pdf
General Medical Council. 'Good medical practice' (2014)	https://www.gmc-uk.org/ethical-guidance/ethical-guidance-for-doctors/good-medical-practice
General Medical Council. 'Confidentiality: good practice in handling patient information' (2017)	https://www.gmc-uk.org/ethical-guidance/ethical-guidance-for-doctors/good-medical-practice http://www.gmc-uk.org/guidance/ethical_guidance/confidentiality.asp
Faculty of Occupational Medicine. Good occupational medicine practice	http://www.fom.ac.uk/wp-content/uploads/p_gomp2010.pdf
ACAS. Guidance on employment practice	http://www.acas.org.uk/index.aspx?articleid=1461

Acknowledgement

This chapter contains Parliamentary information and public sector information licensed under the Open Government Licence v3.0.

References

1. *Bolam* v. *Friern Hospital Management Committee* [1957] 1 WLR 582.
2. *Bolitho* v. *City and Hackney Health Authority* [1996] 4 All ER 771.
3. *Sutherland* v. *Hatton; Barber* v. *Somerset County Council* [2002] 2 All ER 1.
4. *Intel Corporation (UK) Limited* v. *Daw* [2007] IRLR 355.
5. *Paris* v. *Stepney Borough Council* [1951] AC 367 House of Lords.
6. *Walker* v. *Northumberland County Council* [1995] IRLR 35.
7. *Barber* v. *Somerset County Council* [2004] UKHL 13.
8. **The Employment Tribunals Act 1996 (Tribunal Composition) Order** 2012.
9. *British Home Stores* v. *Burchell* [1978] IRLR 379.
10. *Kulkarni* v. *Milton Keynes NHS Trust CA* [2009] EWCA Civ 789.
11. *R (on the application of G)* v. *The Governors of X School* [2011] UKSC 30 SC.
12. *Stevens* v. *University of Birmingham* [2015] EWHC 2300 (QB).
13. *Mattu* v. *The University Hospitals of Coventry and Warwickshire NHS Trust* [2012] EWCA Civ 641.
14. *Lindsey District Council* v. *Daubney* [1977] IRLR 181 and *Spencer* v. *Paragon Wallpapers Ltd* [1976] IRLR 373.
15. *Cheltenham Borough Council* v. *Laird* [2009] EWHC 1253 HC.
16. *Hutchinson* v. *Enfield Rolling Mills Ltd* [1981] IRLR 318.
17. *Scottish Courage Ltd* v. *Guthrie.* UKEAT/0788/03/MAA.
18. *Marshall* v. *Alexander Sloan Ltd* [1980] ICR 394.
19. *Whitbread & Co plc* v. *Mills* [1988] IRLR 501.
20. *Durant* v. *Financial Services Authority (FSA)* [2003] EWCA Civ 1746.
21. *Chambers-Mills* v. *Allied Bakeries* [2009] EWCA Civ 1414 and *Elliott* v. *Stobart Group Ltd* [2015] EWCA Civ 449.
22. **Health Work**. Advice for employers – where there appears to be a conflict between GP advice and occupational health advice. 2014. Available at: https://www.healthworkltd.com/News/AdviceForEmployersWhereThereAppearsToBeAConflictBetweenGPAdviceAndOccupationalHealthAdvice.
23. *Heathrow Express Operating Co Ltd* v. *Jenkins* [2007] UKEAT/0497/06.
24. *Wright* v. *Eclipse Blinds Ltd* [1992] IRLR 133 (CA).
25. *Lynock* v. *Cereal Packaging Ltd* [1988] IRLR 510.
26. *First West Yorkshire Limited t/a First Leeds* v. *Haigh.* UKEAT/0246/07.
27. *Archibald* v. *Fife Council* [2004] IRLR 651.
28. *Scally* v. *Southern Health and Social Services Board* [1992] 1 AC 294.
29. *Crossley* v. *Faithful and Gould Holdings Ltd* [2004] IRLR 377.
30. *Aspden* v. *Webbs Poultry & Meat Group* [1996] IRLR 521.
31. *Briscoe* v. *Lubrizol Ltd* [2002] IRLR 607 Court of Appeal.
32. *Mihlenstedt* v. *Barclays Bank International Ltd and Barclays Bank plc* [1989] IRLR 522.
33. *The Board of Governors, The National Heart and Chest Hospitals* v. *Nambiar* [1981] IRLR 196.
34. *Kapfunde* v. *Abbey National plc* [1998] IRLR 583.
35. *X* v. *Commission of the European Communities* [1995] IRLR 320.
36. *Hardman* v. *Mallon t/a Orchard Lodge Nursing Home* [2002] IRLR 516.
37. *Landeshauptstadt Kiel* v. *Jaege* [2003] IRLR 804.
38. *Perada* v. *Madrid Molividad SA* [2009] IRLR 959.

Chapter 3

The Equality Act 2010

Mark Landon and Tony Williams

Introduction

Occupational health (OH) professionals have an important part to play in various areas of equality law, and a critical role with regard to disability. This chapter considers the key legal and practical issues when OH professionals are asked to advise on matters such as the likelihood that a person is disabled; adjustments that are likely to assist someone with a disability to secure work, stay in work, or return to work after a period of absence; and the issues that arise when an OH professional is asked to assess the impact of an employee's health on his/her performance and that of others.

The evolution of equality law

The law governing equality can be found in both anti-discrimination legislation and precedent case law, through which appellate courts and tribunals interpret and clarify the legislation. The importance of precedent case law depends upon the seniority of the deciding court: thus in the context of employment, decisions of the Supreme Court are binding upon the Court of Appeal, whose decisions are binding on the Employment Appeal Tribunal (EAT), which in turn establishes precedent case law for Employment Tribunals (ETs). (Decisions of the European Court of Justice should be followed by all of the aforementioned courts during the UK's membership of the European Union. It is currently difficult to predict exactly what will happen when the UK ceases to become a member state in the near future.)

Anti-discrimination legislation was first introduced in the mid 1970s and initially only outlawed discrimination on the grounds of sex and race. However, the scope of the legislation was subsequently extended: between 1996 and 2006, legislation was introduced which outlawed, among other matters, discrimination on the grounds of disability, religion, sexual orientation, and age. In 2010, pre-existing discrimination legislation was consolidated within one Act. As a consequence, most of the existing discrimination legislation was repealed and replaced by the Equality Act 2010 (EqA), which applies in England, Wales, and (with a few minor exceptions) Scotland. (Equality is a devolved matter for the Northern Ireland administration to address separately. For example, the Disability Discrimination Act 1995 (DDA) currently still applies in Northern Ireland.)

In support of the EqA, the Equality and Human Rights Commission produced a statutory Code of Practice which covers discrimination in employment and which applies to England, Scotland, and Wales ('the Code of Practice').[1] The Code of Practice explains how the EqA should operate in the workplace and, while it doesn't impose legal obligations, the Code of Practice can be used in evidence in legal proceedings and courts, and tribunals must take any relevant guidance from the Code into account (paragraph 1.13, Code of Practice).

Scope of the Equality Act

The protected characteristics

The EqA sets out nine 'protected characteristics', these being the grounds upon which it is unlawful to discriminate against a person (Box 3.1)

The EqA covers discrimination in various contexts, including employment, the provision of goods and services, and education. However, this chapter explains its impact within employment and, while reference is made where relevant to other protected characteristics, the focus is on disability discrimination as this is likely to be of the greatest relevance for those involved with the issue of fitness for work.

Who is protected?

The EqA's provisions covering discrimination in the workplace protect a wide range of individuals, including employees, contract workers, partners, and office holders. However, this chapter focuses on the protection provided for disabled job applicants, current employees, and ex-employees, taking into account the Code of Practice. Given that some of the case law still refers to the DDA which pre-dated the EqA, references to the DDA

Box 3.1 Equality Act protected characteristics

- Age.
- Disability.
- Gender reassignment.
- Marriage and civil partnership.
- Pregnancy and maternity.
- Race.
- Religion or (religious or philosophical) belief.
- Sex.
- Sexual orientation.

('Caste' may be added to the above list although case law already suggests that the definition of 'race' should be broad enough to encompass caste-based discrimination.)

remain: the implications of the relevant judgments should be regarded as applying equally to the disability discrimination provisions of the EqA unless otherwise stated.

Role of the occupational health professional

Although most employers now appreciate the social, moral, and commercial benefits of fulfilling their obligations under equality law, managers often find it difficult to achieve the right approach—particularly as regards disabled people. As the Court of Appeal commented in *Clark* v. *TGC t/a Novacold* [1999][2]:

> Anyone who thinks that there is an easy way of achieving a sensible, workable and fair balance between the different interests of disabled persons, of employers and of able-bodied workers, in harmony with the wider public interests in an economically efficient workforce, in access to employment, in equal treatment of workers and in standards of fairness at work, has probably not given much serious thought to the problem.

OH professionals have an important part to play in various areas of equality law and a critical role with regard to disability, in advising on the likelihood that a person is disabled and, more importantly, on the adjustments that are likely to assist someone with a disability to secure work, stay in work, or return to work after a period of absence.

OH professionals need to take special care when advising about equality issues. For example, they may have to advise on disability-related cases that may lead to claims for discrimination in an ET or for personal injury in the High Court. Employers will often seek their OH adviser's opinion and may require them to give evidence in court. The Faculty of Occupational Medicine's guidance stresses that such advice must be evidence based.

An OH professional's particular expertise lies in assessing the effects of work on health and the impact of the employee's health on their performance and that of others. For example, in sickness absence cases, a key role is to evaluate the functional capacity and limitation of the employee and to advise on adjustments that will help the employee return to work. Where necessary, this advice may require additional information from other medical specialists. It will also help if the OH professional is prepared to learn about disability law so as to understand the issues that may arise.

However, the role of the OH professional does have important limitations in the eyes of an ET. ETs not uncommonly concur with the OH professional's opinion (in contrast to the evidence of a general practitioner (GP)), according to a review of tribunal judgments.[3] However, and as explained later, the question of disability can only be determined finally by the court or tribunal. While prudent managers will seek relevant expert input from OH professionals when managing staff with disabilities and other relevant protected characteristics, the law makes clear that it is the manager who is ultimately responsible for deciding what is reasonable within the workplace, the extent to which an employee's needs can be accommodated, the point at which they should be dismissed by reason of incapability, and so on—albeit that managers are supposed to make well-informed decisions with suitable expert input. OH professionals need to recognize that the manager often has minimal understanding of the law and will turn to the OH professional for expert advice on both interpretation and implementation. OH professionals must ensure they recognize both their expertise and their limitations when doing so.

Joined-up medical advice

In many cases involving an employee with an underlying medical condition (whether or not it amounts to a disability), there may be the opportunity for relevant expert medical input from three practitioners: the OH professional (who is likely to have the best understanding of the particular workplace and job requirements), the GP (who is likely to have the best personal knowledge of the employee involved), and a specialist (e.g. consultant surgeon, cardiologist, or psychiatrist), who will have the best understanding of the specific treatment regimen. Management of the employee is likely to be most successful if the OH professional has the employee's consent to contact the GP and specialist and thereafter provide management with 'joined-up' expert medical guidance. For example, the current treatment may have significant side effects that impact the individual's ability to work effectively. Adjusting the treatment could minimize these side effects while still effectively treating the condition.

GP or specialist evidence?

Many employees with underlying medical conditions or disabilities are not under consultant care. A question then arises from the viewpoint of tribunals as to the standing of generalist advice, as compared with specialist advice.

The evidence from a GP who has been treating the patient does carry weight. In *J* v. *DLA Piper LLP* [2010],[4] the EAT held that a GP was fully qualified to express an opinion on whether a patient was suffering from depression, and on any associated questions arising under the DDA: depression was a condition very often encountered in general practice. However, the EAT qualified this statement by adding that the evidence of a GP would have less weight than that of a specialist and in difficult cases the opinion of a specialist may be valuable. However, that does not mean that a GP's evidence can be ignored if the evidence of a specialist is not available or is inconclusive.

Equally, in *Paul* v. *National Probation Service* [2003],[5] the EAT criticized the OH adviser for only seeking an opinion from the GP and not from the specialist psychiatrist treating Mr Paul. The EAT held that in such cases employers are duty bound to seek 'competent and suitably qualified medical opinion'. (This last situation was complicated by the fact that the GP was not treating Mr Paul's illness.)

Where a 'difficult' medical condition is alleged, employers and OH professionals may elect to seek an additional specialist opinion. This can help in supporting assessment of the diagnosis, prognosis, and causation, as well as assisting the assessment of resulting disability.

Sometimes an OH professional may disagree with the employee's GP over assessment of fitness to work. See 'Medical evidence and medical reports' in Chapter 2 and *Scottish Courage Ltd* v. *Guthrie* [2004],[6] where the employee was denied sick pay on the basis of an OH professional's assessment that the employee was fit for work.

Medical evidence may not only be conflicting but may instead be unclear. The OH professional may be in a position to assist the court in distinguishing between evidence based on fact and evidence based on opinion. For example, a GP might diagnose post-traumatic stress disorder based on reported symptoms from their patient. However, post-traumatic stress disorder as defined in the tenth revision of the International Classification of Diseases, and *Diagnostic and Statistical Manual of Mental Disorders*, fifth edition, has strict criteria that must be met before an expert psychiatrist can diagnose this condition, and the OH professional may assist the tribunal by commenting on this.

The role of the OH professional in specific situations is considered further in this chapter.

Ethical considerations

The OH professional plays a different role from that of other specialists or GPs. This arises because, typically, the OH professional has a formal contractual relationship with the employer, an obligation to remain independent, and an important duty to maintain the employee's confidentiality: this last duty overrides that of disclosure to an employer. Issues of confidentiality and informed consent are dealt with in the Faculty of Occupational Medicine's guidance on ethics for occupational physicians,[7] publications from the General Medical Council, and British Medical Association (including *Medical Ethics Today*, 2012[8]) which states that 'The fact that a doctor is a salaried employee gives no other employee in the company any right of access to medical records or to the details of the examination findings'. See also Chapter 4.

With appropriate informed consent, however, the OH professional can enter into constructive dialogue with managers over reasonable adjustments and support for the employee and other issues such as fitness constraints.

The meaning of 'disability'

In order to be protected against disability discrimination under the EqA, a person must either currently have a disability or must have previously had a disability as defined in the Act. However, both disabled and non-disabled people are protected under the EqA against victimization, and the Act also protects non-disabled people against direct discrimination or harassment by association and by perception, as explained later.

While seeking expert advice about a person's disabled status will help employers to understand when specific legal duties arise under equality legislation, a responsible employer should have due regard to the needs of any staff with an illness or injury, irrespective of whether they are 'disabled' as defined by the EqA. Good medical and employment practice dictates that, even where an employee's medical condition might not qualify as a statutory disability, they should be treated in a similar manner to someone who is disabled, for example, in terms of reasonable adjustments to encourage early return to work or facilitate better performance while at work: such support makes both moral and commercial sense.

The statutory definition

According to section 6(1) of the EqA (as supplemented by Schedule 1 to the Act), a person has a disability if he or she:

- has a physical or mental impairment, which has a
- substantial and
- long-term
- adverse effect on the person's ability to carry out normal day-to-day activities.

Subject to limited exceptions, as explained below, each of the four elements must be satisfied in order for a person to be 'disabled'.

The government has published 'Guidance on matters to be taken into account in determining questions relating to the definition of disability' (the 'Disability Guidance'),[9] which is helpful (and will be relied upon by courts) in understanding how the issue of disability is assessed. A court or tribunal will expect an OH professional to be familiar with the Disability Guidance if being asked to advise as to a person's disabled status.

The EqA also provides protection against discrimination in respect of a *past* disability, even if that person is no longer disabled (section 6(4) and Schedule 1, paragraph 9). For example, it would be discriminatory to unjustifiably reject a job applicant because they had previously experienced a period of mental illness or had cancer that is now in remission.

Physical or mental impairments

Neither mental nor physical impairments are defined in the EqA. Instead, these terms should be given their ordinary and natural meaning. A disability can arise from a wide range of impairments such as:

- sensory impairments, such as those affecting eyesight or hearing
- impairments with fluctuating or recurring effects, such as rheumatoid arthritis and epilepsy
- progressive impairments, such as motor neurone disease and forms of dementia
- organ-specific impairments, including respiratory conditions such as asthma, and cardiovascular diseases
- developmental impairments, such as autistic spectrum disorders and dyslexia
- learning difficulties
- mental health conditions and mental illnesses, such as depression, schizophrenia, and eating disorders
- impairments resulting from injury to the body or brain.

The Disability Guidance states that there is no need for a claimant to establish a medically diagnosed cause for their impairment. It is the effect of an impairment that must be considered and not its cause (paragraph A7). Furthermore, it may not always be possible, and nor is it necessary, to categorize a condition as either a physical or a mental impairment.

The underlying cause of the impairment may be hard to establish and there may be adverse effects that are both physical and mental in nature. Furthermore, effects of a mainly physical nature may stem from an underlying mental impairment, and vice versa. For example physical symptoms such as muscular weakness and cramps were held in *College of Ripon & St John* v. *Hobbs* [2001][10] to be a physical impairment even though a doctor could find no 'organic' cause for them. The Court of Session in Scotland subsequently endorsed this approach in *Millar* v. *HM Commissioners for Revenue and Customs* [2008],[11] where it held that a person may have a physical impairment without knowing what caused it and without having any 'illness'.

The Code of Practice explains that the term 'mental impairment' is intended to cover 'a wide range of impairments relating to mental functioning, including what are often known as learning disabilities' (paragraph 6 of Appendix 1).

People with certain impairments are deemed to be disabled for the purposes of the EqA without having to show that their impairment satisfies the remaining three elements of the statutory definition, namely those who:

- have been diagnosed with cancer, human immunodeficiency virus (HIV) infection, or multiple sclerosis (MS) (EqA Schedule 1, paragraph 6). (These three exceptions were originally introduced in 2005 due to anecdotal evidence that some unscrupulous employers were dismissing staff who had been diagnosed with one of these conditions but who had yet to exhibit any symptoms in the belief that such people would not yet have protection under disability legislation)

- those who are certified as blind, severely sight impaired, sight impaired, or partially sighted by a consultant ophthalmologist (Reg. 7 of The Equality Act 2010 (Disability) Regulations 2010, S.I. no. 2128)

- those with severe disfigurements, with the exception of unremoved tattoos and piercings (paragraph 3, Schedule 1, EqA 2010 and Regulation 5, The Equality Act 2010 (Disability) Regulations 2010).

By contrast, Regulations 3–5 of The Equality Act 2010 (Disability) Regulations 2010 stipulate that certain conditions are deemed *not* to be qualifying impairments for the purposes of the definition of disability, namely:

- addiction to, or dependency on, alcohol, nicotine, or any other substance (other than in consequence of the substance being medically prescribed or administered)

- seasonal allergic rhinitis (e.g. hay fever), except where it aggravates the effect of another condition

- a tendency to set fires

- a tendency to steal

- a tendency to physically or sexually abuse other persons

- exhibitionism

- voyeurism

- disfigurements which consist of a tattoo (which has not been removed), non-medical body piercing, or something attached through such piercing.

These exclusions were included within the original DDA 1995 and reflected a policy view that certain conditions are not 'deserving' of special protection. However, it should be noted that impairments caused by any of these excluded conditions might themselves amount to protected disabilities. In *Power* v. *Panasonic* [2002],[12] the EAT held that depression caused by alcohol abuse was not prevented from being a disability merely because alcohol addiction is expressly excluded from being an impairment. This approach is reflected in the Disability Guidance, which explains that liver disease as a result of alcohol dependency will count as an impairment (paragraph A7).

Substantial

Substantial means 'more than minor or trivial' (section 212(1) EqA). This is a relatively low standard, as confirmed by the EAT in *Vicary* v. *BT* [1999][13] and in *Leonard* v. *South Derbyshire Chamber of Commerce* [2001],[14] in which the EAT gave the following guidance:

- The focus should be on what an employee cannot do or can only do with difficulty, rather than on what they can do easily. The decision-maker should look at the whole picture, but should not attempt to balance what an employee can do against what they cannot do.
- The fact that an employee is able to mitigate the effects of an impairment, for example, by carrying things in small quantities, does not prevent there being a disability.

Examples of what might be regarded as having a 'substantial adverse effect' are listed in the Appendix to the Disability Guidance and include:

- difficulty in getting dressed, for example, because of physical restrictions or a lack of understanding of the concept
- difficulty carrying out activities associated with toileting, or caused by frequent minor incontinence
- difficulty going out of doors unaccompanied, for example, because the person has a phobia, a physical restriction, or a learning disability
- difficulty using transport, for example, because of physical restrictions, pain or fatigue, a frequent need for a lavatory, or as a result of a mental impairment or learning disability
- difficulty operating a computer, for example, because of physical restrictions in using a keyboard, a visual impairment, or a learning disability.

An impairment can have a substantial adverse effect even if the relevant effect is not caused by the impairment directly: in *Kirton* v. *Tetrosyl Ltd* [2003],[15] Mr Kirton experienced incontinence following surgery for bladder cancer. His incontinence was considered to be a part of his disability from cancer as there was a causal link between the two. In the same way, it is important to consider whether symptoms or impairments such as hair loss following chemotherapy might be causally related to the cancer.

Remedial measures

Schedule 1, paragraph 5 of the EqA provides that, in determining whether the effect of an impairment is substantial, any remedial measures (e.g. a hearing aid, medication, or counselling) which are used to treat or correct the impairment should be ignored. The only exception to this is where eyesight is corrected via spectacles or contact lenses. However, where the effect of the treatment is to create a permanent, rather than a temporary, improvement (e.g. corrective surgery), then this permanent improvement should be taken into account.

Recurring effects

If an impairment ceases to have a substantial adverse effect on a person's ability to carry out day-to-day activities, it is nevertheless to be treated as having that effect if that effect is likely to recur (paragraph 2(2), Schedule 1, EqA). The test is whether the particular effect (not, strictly speaking, the impairment) is likely to recur. This might be shown by medical evidence of the prognosis or by statistical evidence. A distinction must, however, be drawn between an impairment which 'recurs' over time and one which is 'repeated' over time:

- A rugby player may fracture an ankle aged 19, fully recover, and fracture an ankle again 10 years later. This is a new condition, not a recurrence of an underlying condition; he does not now have a 'disability' by virtue of an underlying condition lasting 10 years.
- By contrast, a woman with osteoporosis who fractures her wrist aged 50 and who then fractures the same wrist again aged 60 years would have an underlying condition linking the two recurrent events and so would be considered to be disabled.

Progressive conditions

Schedule 1, paragraph 8 of the EqA provides that where an individual has a progressive condition which is likely to have a substantial adverse effect on the individual's normal day-to-day activities at some future stage, then that condition is to be treated as having such a substantial adverse effect now, even if it has yet to do so.

Cumulative effect of impairments

The Disability Guidance states that the effect of an impairment on more than one activity, taken together, could result in an overall substantial adverse effect. Further, the cumulative effect of more than one impairment should be taken into account. For example:

- A person who has poor salivary gland function has to drink a lot with meals. They also have urinary urgency. Together, they result in having to visit the lavatory every half hour and this affects their ability to attend long meetings or travel long distances.
- A person has mild learning disability which makes his assimilation of information slightly slower than normal and he also has a mild speech impairment that slightly affects his ability to form certain words. Neither impairment singly has a substantial adverse effect, but their combined effects have a substantial adverse effect on his ability to converse.

Modification of behaviour: avoidance strategies

The Disability Guidance suggests that if a person can reasonably be expected to modify their behaviour to reduce the effects of an impairment on their normal day-to-day activities then they might not be considered disabled (paragraph B7). The Disability Guidance clarifies, however, that account should also be taken of 'where a person avoids doing things which, for example, cause pain, fatigue or substantial social embarrassment, or avoids doing things because of a loss of energy and motivation'. It states that it would not be reasonable to conclude that a person who employed such an avoidance strategy was not a disabled person (paragraph B9).

Long term

An impairment will have a long-term effect only if:

♦ it has lasted at least 12 months

♦ the period for which it lasts is likely* to be 12 months; or

♦ it is likely* to last for the rest of the life of the person affected (paragraph 2(1), Schedule 1 EqA).

(* In *SCA Packaging* v. *Boyle* [2009],[16] the House of Lords interpreted 'likely' as meaning 'could well happen'.)

Where a substantial adverse effect is deemed to exist because it is likely to recur, the tribunal will take into account the whole period (whether the substantial adverse effect is deemed or actual) in assessing whether it is long term.

Provided that they are related, two consecutive impairments can be aggregated for the purposes of determining the duration of an impairment. For example, a man experienced an anxiety disorder. This had a substantial adverse effect on his ability to make social contacts and to visit particular places. The disorder lasted for 8 months and then developed into depression, which had the effect that he was no longer able to leave his home or go to work. The depression continued for 5 months. As the total period over which the adverse effects lasted was in excess of 12 months, the long-term element of the definition of disability was met.

Normal day-to-day activities

'Normal day-to-day activities' are things that people do on a regular or daily basis, such as shopping, reading, writing, using the telephone, walking and travelling by various forms of transport, and taking part in social activities. 'Normal' should be given its ordinary, everyday meaning and also has to be decided with reference to the sex of the claimant. In *Epke* v. *Metropolitan Police Commissioner* [2001],[17] the EAT stated that just because certain activities were normally done by women (e.g. using hair rollers and applying makeup) they were not disqualified from being normal day-to-day activities.

Section D of the Disability Guidance explains as follows:

> The term 'normal day-to-day activities' is not intended to include activities which are normal only for a particular person, or a small group of people. In deciding whether an activity is a normal

day-to-day activity, account should be taken of how far it is carried out by people on a daily or frequent basis. In this context, 'normal' should be given its ordinary, everyday meaning.

In some instances, work-related activities are so highly specialized that they would not be regarded as normal day-to-day activities, e.g. a watch repairer carrying out delicate work with highly specialized tools, or the pianist who plays to a high standard and performs in public. However, many types of specialist work-related or other activities may still involve normal day-to-day activities, for example:

- In *Paterson v. Commissioner of Police of the Metropolis* [2007],[18] the EAT explained that 'normal day-to-day activities' must be interpreted as including irregular but predictable activities which occur in professional life—in this case taking high-pressure examinations for the purpose of gaining promotion.
- In *Chief Constable of Dumfries and Galloway Constabulary v. Adams* [2009],[19] the EAT held that 'normal day-to-day activities' didn't cover the special skills required specifically of a policeman, but where the activity was a common one across a range of industries then it would be covered. In this case, the EAT held that walking, stair climbing, and driving were normal day-to-day activities even when carried out on a night shift between 2 a.m. and 4 a.m. (given the number of people who carry out night work).

Who should advise an employer about an employee's disabled status?

OH professionals can find themselves in an apparently conflicting situation: in law, only an ET can definitively determine whether an employee satisfies the legal definition of having a disability under the EqA, albeit usually with suitable guidance from a medical expert: cases such as *Vicary v. British Telecommunications PLC* [1999][13] and *Abadeh v. British Telecommunications PLC* [2001][20] have made it clear that the role of the OH professional is to comment upon diagnosis and prognosis, and the effect of medication, but that it is for the tribunal to determine whether an effect is substantial and impacts on day-to-day activities.

However, the EAT subsequently explained in the case of *The Hospice of St Mary of Furness v. Howard* [2007][21] that *Vicary* does not prevent an expert giving evidence as to what may or may not be the consequences of a condition and how serious those consequences may be, or that a particular physical or mental condition could not cause the symptom or functional limitation of which the claimant is complaining. Despite the limitations set out in *Vicary* and *Abadeh*, a tribunal is likely to be assisted by hearing from an independent expert as to their understanding of the limits of a claimant's normal functioning, provided it does not unquestioningly accept whatever the expert says but comes to its own decision on the facts.

Where disability depends solely on diagnosis, such as for HIV, MS, cancer, and being registered blind or partially sighted, it must necessarily be the doctor who effectively decides that the person is disabled.

In addition, ETs will expect an employer to seek guidance from an OH professional or other suitable medical expert about an employee's potential disabled status if there is sufficient reason to do so, for example, because the employee claims to have an underlying medical condition or else a GP's report or sick note refers to one; furthermore, a tribunal will expect an OH professional to provide such an opinion, albeit that it may be caveated by a reminder to the employer that only the tribunal's determination ultimately counts in law.

When seeking a medical opinion about an employee's disabled status, an employer will be expected to provide the medical adviser with any relevant background information about the employee at work (with the employee's prior permission) so that the adviser can make a well-informed decision.

In addition, in the case of *Gallop* v. *Newport City Council* [2013],[22] the Court of Appeal provided important guidance on the responsibilities of employers when seeking and following such OH guidance:

- An employer should not unthinkingly follow an OH professional's opinion that an employee was not disabled where no explanation was given for this opinion. The OH professional should have focused on the four elements of the test for establishing a disability; as it did not do so, the OH report was 'worthless' when Newport CC came to form its own judgement of whether Mr Gallop was disabled.

- Responsible employers have to make their own judgement as to whether an employee is disabled. An employer will usually want assistance from an OH professional or other medical advisers:

  - If such medical guidance advises that the employee is disabled, then the employer will ordinarily respect that judgement unless there is a good reason to disagree.
  - However, where the guidance advises that the employee is not disabled, then the employer must remember that it is the employer, and not the medical advisers, who is responsible for making the final factual judgement. An employer cannot simply 'rubber stamp' a medical adviser's opinion that an employee is not disabled.

- When seeking advice from external clinicians, an employer should not ask general questions about whether an employee is disabled within the meaning of the discrimination legislation. Instead, the employer should ask specific practical questions, directed to the particular circumstances of the employee's potential disability. The answers to these questions will help the employer to judge whether the criteria for disability are satisfied.

Proving disability in tribunal claims

In many tribunal cases there is unlikely to be any doubt about whether a person is (or was) disabled. However, if this is disputed then the burden of proving disability rests with the claimant (as confirmed by the Court of Appeal in *Kapadia* v. *London Borough of Lambeth* [2000][23]). According to the Court of Appeal's decision in *McDougall* v. *Richmond Adult Community College* [2008],[24] whether a claimant is disabled should be assessed on the information known at the relevant time (i.e. the time of the alleged discrimination) and not when the tribunal hearing takes place.

The meaning of 'discrimination'

Types of discrimination

In order for an OH professional to provide advice with regard to the management of people with disabilities in the workplace, it is important to have an understanding of the specific rights provided to such people under the EqA. There are, in fact, six forms of outlawed disability discrimination—albeit that, in practice, one (the duty to make reasonable adjustments) is likely to be more relevant than the others.

The EqA makes it unlawful for an employer to discriminate against a person in respect of any protected characteristic in any of the following ways:

- Direct discrimination (section 13).
- Indirect discrimination (section 19).
- Harassment (section 26).
- Victimization (section 27).

In addition, there are two other forms of outlawed discrimination which are specific to disabled people, namely:

- Discrimination arising from disability (section 15).
- A failure to make a reasonable adjustment (section 21).

Each of these terms is explained below in the context of disability.

Direct disability discrimination: section 13 of the EqA

An employer directly discriminates against a disabled person (e.g. a disabled job applicant or an existing employee) if, because of their disability, the employer treats the disabled person less favourably than it treats or would treat others.

Direct discrimination is the crudest form of discrimination. It is automatically unlawful and (apart from age discrimination) can never be justified. Direct age-related discrimination is lawful if it can be justified, for example, banning people under 17 from driving on health and safety grounds.

For direct disability discrimination to occur, the less favourable treatment must be 'because of' the relevant protected characteristic such as disability. A tribunal will consider the employer's reason for the treatment, which may either be entirely deliberate or at least in part due to his/her subconscious bias. The reason must, however, be the disability itself and not merely something related to the disability (which might instead fall within one of the other forms of outlawed discrimination, as explained below). Furthermore, since the disability itself must be the conscious or subconscious reason for the treatment, there must be some evidence that the employer knew about the disability.

In practice, direct disability discrimination often arises where an employer makes a stereotypical assumption about a disabled job applicant or employee without actually investigating whether their disability will have the anticipated impact (Box 3.2).

THE MEANING OF 'DISCRIMINATION'

Box 3.2 Direct discrimination

John Smith applies for a job with ABC Ltd as a data processor. The job advert explains that the successful candidate must be able to type at a speed of at least 100 words per minute. At the interview, John volunteers the information that he has some arthritis in his hands, but that his condition is well controlled. Rather than assess John's ability to undertake the role, ABC Ltd simply assumes that he will be too slow in inputting data and so doesn't offer John the job.

This would be direct disability discrimination: the failure to offer John the job is less favourable treatment directly related to his condition (arthritis), rather than to any detrimental effect which his arthritis might have and which the company has not even tried to assess.

It is not possible for the employer to balance or eliminate less favourable treatment by offsetting it against more favourable treatment (e.g. extra pay to make up for the loss of job status).

Section 13(3) of the EqA (and paragraph 3.35 of the Code of Practice) makes it clear that it is not direct discrimination to treat a disabled person more favourably than a non-disabled person (e.g. by making reasonable adjustments for the disabled person, as described below).

Section 24 of the EqA (and paragraph 3.10 of the Code of Practice) explains that, for the purposes of establishing direct disability discrimination, it makes no difference that the discriminator is also disabled—it's still discrimination.

Direct discrimination by association and by perception
In two scenarios a non-disabled person may be able to claim direct disability discrimination:

◆ *Discrimination by association* occurs when a non-disabled job applicant or employee is treated less favourably by an employer because of that employee's association with someone who is disabled, rather than because the applicant or employee is themselves disabled. Paragraphs 3.19 and 3.20 of the Code of Practice explain that direct disability discrimination by association can occur in various ways, for example:

   • Where a lone father who cares for a disabled son has to take time off work whenever his son is sick or has medical appointments, and where the employer appears to resent the fact that the worker needs to care for his son and eventually dismisses him, such a dismissal may amount to direct disability discrimination against the worker by association with his son.

◆ It is also direct discrimination by perception if an employer treats an applicant or employee less favourably because the employer mistakenly perceives that they are disabled, for example:

- An employer selects an employee for redundancy on the incorrect belief that they have a progressive illness and is therefore likely to incur significant future sickness absence; this will amount to direct disability discrimination by perception.

Discrimination arising from disability: section 15 of the EqA

Direct discrimination tends to be rare: not many employers set out to treat someone less favourably simply because they are disabled. Far more common is 'discrimination arising from disability', where the unfavourable treatment results from a consequence of the person's disability and cannot be justified (Box 3.3):

'(1) A person (A) discriminates against a disabled person (B) if—

(a) A treats B unfavourably because of something arising in consequence of B's disability, and

(b) A cannot show that the treatment is a proportionate means of achieving a legitimate aim.

[i.e. A cannot justify the unfavourable treatment.]

(2) Subsection (1) does not apply if A shows that A did not know, and could not reasonably have been expected to know, that B had the disability.'

In the case of discrimination arising from disability, there is no requirement for the disabled person to establish that their treatment is less favourable than that experienced by a non-disabled comparator. Instead, the focus is on whether the treatment amounts to a detriment, and, if so, whether it can be justified. This is potentially significant when it comes to the treatment of long-term disability-related sickness absence:

- In considering whether a disabled worker dismissed for disability-related sickness absence amounts to discrimination arising from disability, it is irrelevant whether or not

---

Box 3.3 Discrimination arising from a disability

John Smith applies for a job with ABC Ltd as a data processor. The job advert explains that the successful candidate must be able to type at a speed of at least 100 words per minute. At the interview, John volunteers the information that he has some arthritis in his hands, but that his condition is well controlled. The interviewer explains that this won't be a problem as long as John passes a speed typing test that all candidates are required to undertake. John and the other candidates take the test. John can only type at an average of 80 words per minute and, along with the two other candidates who fail to achieve the minimum typing speed, is not offered a job.

In this case the unfavourable treatment arises from a consequence of John's disability (his slower typing) rather than the disability itself: as such, this would not be direct discrimination but, if the company could not objectively justify the required typing speed (e.g. because, although slower, John was more accurate than the faster candidates and so was more effective overall), then this would amount to discrimination arising from John's disability.

other workers would have been dismissed for having the same or similar length of absence. It is not necessary to compare the treatment of the disabled worker with that of their colleagues or any hypothetical comparator. The decision to dismiss them will be discrimination arising from disability if the employer cannot objectively justify it (paragraph 5.6 of the Code of Practice).

Paragraphs 5.8 and 5.9 of the Code of Practice explain that there must be a connection between whatever led to the unfavourable treatment and the disability: the consequences of a disability include anything which is the result, effect or outcome of a disabled person's disability. There have been a series of recent cases which have examined this causal link:

In *Hall* v. *Chief Constable of West Yorkshire Police* [2015], the EAT confirmed that to establish a claim for discrimination arising from disability there need only be a 'loose' causal link between the disability and any unfavourable treatment. The statutory test requires a connection between whatever led to the unfavourable treatment and the disability: there is a relatively low hurdle for claimants to satisfy section 15 claims. It will be sufficient to show that the unfavourable treatment has been caused by an outcome or consequence of the claimant's disability; the employer's motivation is irrelevant. Employers have an opportunity to redress the balance and defend a claim by showing that either the unfavourable treatment was justified or else that they did not know or could not reasonably have known that the employee was disabled.

The need for only a loose causal link was subsequently reiterated by EAT in *Risby* v. *LB Waltham Forest* [2016]).

In *City of York Council* v. *Grosset* [2018], the Court of Appeal held that discrimination arising from disability had occurred where the employer dismissed a disabled employee without even knowing that an act of misconduct arose from their disability.

- In this case, Mr Grosset, who was a teacher at a school operated by the City of York Council, suffered from cystic fibrosis, which the Council was aware of and conceded amounted to a disability. As a consequence of his condition, Mr Grosset was required to spend up to 3 hours a day in a punishing regime of physical exercise to clear his lungs. Following a change of head teacher, Mr Grosset's workload increased and, as a result of his condition, he struggled to cope with the additional demands placed on him. He suffered stress, which in turn exacerbated his cystic fibrosis. During this period, Mr Grosset took two lessons of 15- and 16-year-olds over the course of which he showed them an 18-rated film. When the head teacher later discovered this, Mr Grosset was suspended and eventually dismissed for gross misconduct. The dismissing panel did not accept that showing the film had been a momentary error of judgement, caused by the level of stress Mr Grosset was under.

- An employment tribunal held that Mr Grosset had not been unfairly dismissed but did find that he had suffered discrimination arising from disability: the tribunal found that his dismissal was unfavourable treatment and that the 'something' that led to it was showing the film. The key question was whether or not that 'something' arose in consequence of his disability. The tribunal held that it did: although the medical evidence available to the Council at the time of dismissal did not suggest a link between Mr Grosset's misconduct and his disability, medical evidence available by the time of the tribunal hearing demonstrated otherwise. The tribunal went on to find that the dismissal was not justified (i.e. a proportionate means of achieving a legitimate aim): the employer had failed to make a number of adjustments that would have helped alleviate Mr Grosset's stress; had it properly addressed the issue of his workload, the situation would not have arisen.

◆ The council appealed unsuccessfully to both the EAT and, subsequently, the Court of Appeal. Both courts rejected the Council's submission that it was not liable unless Mr Grosset could show that it had appreciated that his behaviour was a consequence of his disability. The Court of Appeal explained that there were two distinct causative issues for a tribunal to consider:

- Whether the employer treated the employee unfavourably because of an identified 'something'; and
- Whether that 'something' arose in consequence of the employee's disability.

The first issue involved examining the employer's state of mind, to establish whether the unfavourable treatment occurred because of the employer's attitude to the relevant 'something'. The Council had dismissed Mr Grosset because he showed the film. That was the relevant 'something'.

The second issue was objective: whether there was a causal link between the disability and the 'something'? The tribunal had found that there was a causal link: Mr Grosset had shown the film due to the exceptionally high stress he was suffering, which arose from the effect of his disability under increased work demands. The court held that there was nothing that suggests that there is a need for the employer to be aware of the link between the disability and the 'something' that results in the unfavourable treatment. The court further reasoned that if this were not the case, the defence in section 15(2) (that the employer did not know, or could not reasonably be expected to know, that the employee was disabled) would be redundant. Knowledge is only relevant to the defence under section 15(2) where the employer did not know, and could not reasonably be expected to know, that the employee was disabled. There is no further provision for those cases where the employer did not know that the disability produced a certain consequence. (Going forward, employers who are considering disciplining a disabled employee would be well advised to always consider obtaining medical evidence on whether the employee's actions could in any way be a consequence of their disability.)

Paragraphs 5.11 and 5.12 of the Code of Practice explain the concept of objectively justifying discrimination arising from disability: objective justification will require the employer to be able to show that the treatment is a 'proportionate means of achieving a legitimate aim'. It is for the employer to justify the treatment; it must produce evidence to support the assertion that the treatment is justified and not rely on mere generalizations.

Liability for discrimination arising from disability under section 15 of the EqA cannot occur unless the employer knew (or should have known) about the claimant's disability.

Parliament felt that it would be unfair to judge an employer liable for a type of disability discrimination if the employee in question kept their disability secret (as might be their prerogative). However:

♦ It is not enough for the employer to show that it did not know that the disabled person had the disability; the employer must also show that it could not reasonably have been expected to know about it and an employer must do all that can reasonably be expected to find out if a worker has a disability.

♦ If an employer's agent or employee (such as an OH professional) knows, in that capacity, of a worker's or applicant's disability, the employer will not usually be able to claim that they do not know of the disability and that they cannot therefore have subjected a disabled person to discrimination arising from disability. Therefore, where information about disabled people may come through different channels, employers need to ensure that there is a means—suitably confidential and subject to the disabled person's consent—for bringing that information together to make it easier for the employer to fulfil their duties under the EqA.

Indirect disability discrimination: section 19 of the EqA

Indirect discrimination is concerned with acts, decisions, or policies which are not intended to treat anyone less favourably, but which in practice have the effect of disadvantaging a group of people who share a particular protected characteristic. Where such an act, decision, or policy disadvantages an individual within that group then it will amount to indirect discrimination unless it can be objectively justified.

Indirect discrimination has a fairly complex definition as follows:

(1) A person (A) discriminates against another (B) if A applies to B a provision, criterion or practice which is discriminatory in relation to a relevant protected characteristic of B's.

(2) For the purposes of subsection (1), a provision, criterion or practice is discriminatory in relation to a relevant protected characteristic of B's if—

   (a) A applies, or would apply, it to persons with whom B does not share the characteristic,

   (b) it puts, or would put, persons with whom B shares the characteristic at a particular disadvantage when compared with persons with whom B does not share it,

   (c) it puts, or would put, B at that disadvantage, and

   (d) A cannot show it to be a proportionate means of achieving a legitimate aim (i.e. justify it).

In essence, therefore, indirect discrimination consists of three elements:

♦ The employer's actions have a disproportionately detrimental impact on a group who share a particular disability.

♦ The claimant suffers a detriment as a member of that group.

◆ The employer cannot objectively justify its actions.

Paragraph 4.5 of the Code of Practice explains that 'provision, criterion or practice' should be construed widely so as to include, for example, any formal or informal policies, rules, practices, arrangements, criteria, conditions, prerequisites, qualifications, provisions, or 'one-off' or discretionary decisions.

The EqA defines objective justification as a 'proportionate means of achieving a legitimate aim', the test of which should be approached in two stages:

◆ Is the aim of the provision etc. legal and non-discriminatory, and one that represents a real, objective consideration (e.g. properly evidenced health and safety considerations)?

◆ If the aim is legitimate, is the means of achieving it proportionate—that is, appropriate and necessary in all the circumstances? This involves a balancing exercise, weighing up the discriminatory impact of the provision etc. on the individual as against the employer's reasons for applying it.

In reality, few claimants are likely to rely upon a claim for indirect disability discrimination alone if, as is likely, the application of a disadvantageous provision etc. will also trigger the protection against discrimination arising from disability as well as the duty to make reasonable adjustments (Box 3.4).

Unlike discrimination arising from disability or the duty to make reasonable adjustments, there is nothing to suggest that an employer needs to know about an employee's disability to indirectly discriminate against them.

Failure to comply with the duty to make reasonable adjustments

The duty on employers to make reasonable adjustments is arguably the cornerstone of disability protection and is likely to be of the greatest practical relevance to OH professionals. As such, this duty is explained in detail later.

Box 3.4 Indirect discrimination

John Smith works for ABC Ltd as a data processor. In order to improve performance management, the employer introduces some key performance indicators, which include a new requirement that all data processors must be able to type at least 100 words per minute. John is one of a group of employees who, because of various hand or wrist impairments, have trouble achieving the minimum typing speed. As a result, all of these employees are fearful of being placed on a formal performance management procedure and about their job security. John decides to bring a claim for indirect disability discrimination, arguing that the company cannot justify applying a blanket requirement for 100 words per minute without also considering the accuracy of an employee's work: John can show that he achieves a high level of accuracy which avoids the need to re-enter data, and that overall he is in fact more efficient that many colleagues who can type faster than him.

Harassment: section 26 of the EqA

Three types of harassment are outlawed, including harassment related to a 'relevant protected characteristic', which is defined as follows:

◆ Person (A) harasses another person (B) if A engages in unwanted conduct related to disability and that conduct has the purpose or effect of:

- violating B's dignity, or
- creating an intimidating, hostile, degrading, humiliating or offensive environment for B.

In deciding whether conduct has the effect referred to above, each of the following must be taken into account:

◆ B's perception.

◆ The other circumstances of the case.

◆ Whether it is reasonable for the conduct to have that effect.

In most cases, B will be a disabled person and the unwanted conduct will relate to their own disability. However, and as with direct discrimination, non-disabled people are protected under the EqA against harassment by association and by perception. For example, a person who is harassed because of their spouse's disability would have a claim.

Victimization: section 27 of the EqA

Victimization occurs where a person (A) subjects another person (B) to a detriment because B has done, intends to do, or is suspected of doing or intending to do, any of the following protected acts:

◆ Bringing proceedings under the EqA.

◆ Giving evidence or information in connection with proceedings under the EqA, regardless of who brought those proceedings.

◆ Doing any other thing for the purposes of or in connection with the EqA.

◆ Alleging that the discriminator or any other person has contravened the EqA.

There is, however, no protection if a person makes allegations or gives evidence that they know to be false. However, a person who complains mistakenly but in good faith is protected.

By way of example, victimization would occur where an existing employee has brought a discrimination claim against an employer for failing to stop harassment by colleagues and, subsequently, management fails to promote the employee because he's seen as a 'trouble-maker'.

The duty to make reasonable adjustments: sections 20 and 21 of the EqA

The duty to make reasonable adjustments is a cornerstone of the EqA.

In practice, the majority of employment-related disability issues concern the duty to make reasonable adjustments. An employer will be unlikely to succeed in justifying a step that might amount to discrimination arising from disability or indirect discrimination if it has failed to implement a reasonable adjustment that would have avoided or reduced a disadvantage to the disabled person in question. Many adjustments are likely to require input from an OH professional, for example, with regard to accommodating a disabled new recruit, facilitating a phased return to work from illness, and when redeploying a disabled employee who can no longer continue in their substantive role.

The duty to make reasonable adjustments goes beyond simply avoiding treating disabled job applicants and employees unfavourably; instead, it requires employers to take positive steps to ensure that disabled people can access and make progress in employment. The duty to make reasonable adjustments applies to employers of all sizes, although the question of what is reasonable may vary according to the circumstances of the employer.

Section 21(2) of the EqA explains that an employer discriminates against a disabled person if it fails to comply with the duty to make reasonable adjustments imposed by section 20 of the Act, which in turn imposes three requirements on an employer:

- Where a provision, criterion, or practice applied by or on behalf of an employer puts a disabled person (e.g. a job applicant or an existing employee) at a substantial disadvantage in relation to a relevant matter (e.g. deciding to whom to offer employment or promotion) in comparison with persons (e.g. fellow job applicants or employees) who are not disabled, then the employer must take reasonable steps to avoid the disadvantage (section 20(3) and Schedule 8, paragraph 2(2)(a)).

  - For example, ABC Ltd might reduce their minimum typing speed requirement for applicants and employees who have disabilities which impact their typing, and/or might introduce a broader range of criteria to assess efficiency, such as speed combined with accuracy.

- Where a physical feature of premises occupied by an employer puts a disabled person at a substantial disadvantage in relation to a relevant matter in comparison with persons who are not disabled, then the employer must take reasonable steps to avoid the disadvantage (section 20(4) and Schedule 8, paragraph 2(2)(b)).

  - For example, an employer might need to add stick-on hazard strips to make a glass door more visible for a visually-impaired employee.

- Where a disabled person would, but for the provision of an auxiliary aid or service, be put at a substantial disadvantage in relation to a relevant matter in comparison with persons who are not disabled, then the employer must take reasonable steps to provide the auxiliary aid or service (section 20(5) and (11)).

  - For example, ABC Ltd might provide John Smith with an adaptive keyboard when undertaking the speed typing test if this enables him to type faster.

'Provision, criterion or practice'

Paragraph 6.10 of the Code of Practice explains that the phrase 'provision, criterion or practice' or PCP (which is not defined by the EqA) should be construed widely. For example, a PCP can include both a formal policy as well as a one-off management decision (*British Airways plc v. Starmer* [2005]).[26] It is arguable that a PCP will only give rise to a duty to make reasonable adjustments if it is related in some way to the job, rather than simply to the personal needs of the disabled person. This interpretation is reflected in paragraph 6.33 of the Code of Practice which states that: 'There is no requirement to provide or modify equipment for personal purposes unconnected with a worker's job, such as providing a wheelchair if a person needs one in any event but does not have one. The disadvantages in such a case do not flow from the employer's arrangements or premises.'

Substantial disadvantage

'Substantial' is defined by section 212(1) of the EqA as 'more than minor or trivial'. This is a low threshold and so it will often be relatively easy for a tribunal to conclude that a claimant suffered such a disadvantage:

In *Perratt v. The City of Cardiff Council* [2016],[27] the EAT held that the duty to make an adjustment can apply to any provision criterion or practice which 'bites harder' on the disabled employee than others (regardless of whether it applies equally to all employees).

Physical features

Physical features—whether temporary or permanent—will include steps, stairways, kerbs, exterior surfaces and paving, parking areas, building entrances and exits (including emergency escape routes), internal and external doors, gates, toilet and washing facilities, lighting and ventilation, lifts and escalators, floor coverings, signs, furniture, and temporary or moveable items.

'Auxiliary aids'

Paragraph 6.13 of the Code of Practice explains that an auxiliary aid is something which provides support or assistance to a disabled person. It can include provision of a specialist piece of equipment such as an adapted keyboard or text-to-speech software. Auxiliary aids include auxiliary services; for example, provision of a sign language interpreter or a support worker for a disabled worker.

Employer's knowledge

Job applicants

In the case of a job applicant or potential job applicant, an employer only has a duty to make an adjustment if it knows, or could reasonably be expected to know, that a disabled person is, or may be, an applicant for work.

While there are restrictions (as explained later) on when health or disability-related enquiries can be raised with an applicant, questions are permitted to determine whether reasonable adjustments need to be made in relation to an assessment, such as an interview or other process designed to give an indication of a person's suitability for the work concerned.

Existing employees

For existing disabled employees, an employer only has a duty to make an adjustment if they know, or could reasonably be expected to know, that an employee has a disability and is, or is likely to be, placed at a substantial disadvantage. The employer must, however, do all that it reasonably can to find out whether this is the case: this provision won't protect an employer if, objectively, there is some information or behaviour which ought reasonably to alert the employer to the possibility that an employee has some underlying medical condition which might amount to a disability. What is reasonable will depend on the circumstances and this is an objective assessment. When making enquiries about disability, employers should consider issues of dignity and privacy and ensure that personal information is dealt with confidentially.

If an employer's agent or employee (such as an OH professional or a recruitment agent) knows, in that capacity, of an applicant's (or potential applicant's) or employee's disability, then the employer will not usually be able to claim that they do not know of the disability and that they therefore have no obligation to make a reasonable adjustment. Employers therefore need to ensure that where information about disabled people may come through different channels, there is a means—suitably confidential and subject to the disabled person's consent—for bringing that information together to make it easier for the employer to fulfil their duties under the EqA. In *Hartman* v. *South Essex Mental Health Community Care NHS Trust and other cases* [2005],[28] the Court of Appeal held that if an employee discloses confidential information about their health to their employer's OH provider and does not consent to release of this information to the employer, the employer should only be deemed to have knowledge of the information actually provided to it by the OH provider. However, the position may be different if the worker consents to the disclosure of the information.

When is an adjustment 'reasonable'?

An employer will not breach the duty to make adjustments unless it fails to make an adjustment which is 'reasonable'. This is a fact-sensitive question. In *Smith* v. *Churchill's Stairlifts plc* [2005],[29] the Court of Appeal held that the test of reasonableness is objective and is to be determined by the tribunal. There is no objective justification defence available in respect of an employer's failure to make reasonable adjustments: the proposed adjustments are either reasonable or they are not.

The EqA does not specify any particular factors that should be taken into account in determining whether an adjustment is 'reasonable'. Instead, this is explained in paragraphs 6.23–6.29 of the Code of Practice and includes the following:

- Whether the proposed adjustment would be effective in preventing the substantial disadvantage.
- The practicability of making the adjustment.
- The financial and other costs of making the adjustment and the extent of any resulting disruption.

◆ The extent of the employer's financial or other resources: it is more likely to be reasonable for an employer to make more costly adjustments if it has substantial financial resources.

◆ The availability to the employer of financial or other assistance when making an adjustment (such as advice through Access to Work).

◆ The type and size of the employer.

Examples of reasonable adjustments

Paragraphs 6.32–6.35 of the Code of Practice provide many examples of reasonable adjustments, some of which are likely to be of particular relevance to OH professionals when considering matters such as rehabilitation or redeployment, for example:

◆ Allocating some of the disabled person's duties to another person.

◆ Transferring the disabled person to fill an existing vacancy (e.g. an employer should consider whether a suitable alternative post is available for an employee who becomes disabled, or whose disability worsens, where no reasonable adjustment would enable the employee to continue doing their current job).

◆ Altering the disabled person's hours of working or training (e.g. allowing a disabled person to work flexible hours or permitting part-time working or different working).

◆ Assigning the disabled person to a different place of work or training, or arranging home working.

◆ Allowing the disabled person to be absent during work or training hours for rehabilitation, assessment, or treatment.

◆ Giving, or arranging for, training or mentoring.

◆ Acquiring or modifying equipment.

◆ Modifying procedures for testing or assessment.

◆ Allowing a disabled employee to take a period of disability leave (e.g. an employee who has cancer needs to undergo treatment and rehabilitation, and their employer allows a period of disability leave and permits the employee to return to their job at the end of this period).

The concept of transferring the disabled person to fill an existing vacancy has been developed over the years via a number of cases, such that the following principles have emerged:

◆ As long as the candidate is capable of undertaking the vacant role (perhaps with suitable training), it may be reasonable to place them into that role ahead of any other candidate: in *Archibald* v. *Fife Council*,[30] the House of Lords stated that reasonable adjustments include allowing disabled persons to take precedence over fellow applicants for new jobs, even if a disabled employee is not the best candidate, provided that the disabled employee is suitable to do that work.

- While some form of competitive assessment must be reasonable so as to ensure that a disabled candidate meets the core competencies of the job (*Wade* v. *Sheffield Hallam University* [2013]),[31] employers may have to adapt their assessment procedures (e.g. where a disabled candidate would struggle to cope with a current competitive interview for a post, by basing an assessment of their suitability on existing appraisals from previous posts) (*Waddingham* v. *NHS Business Services Authority* [2015]).[32]
- While the Code of Practice refers only to an 'existing vacancy', an employer might in some circumstances be required to redeploy a disabled employee even where no vacancy exists:
  - In *Southampton City College* v. *Randall* [2006],[33] the EAT upheld a tribunal's decision that it would have been reasonable for an employer to create a new job which took into account the employee's disability: in this case, the employer was undertaking a reorganization and accepted that it had 'a blank sheet of paper' so far as job specifications were concerned.
  - Swapping with another employee: in *Chief Constable of South Yorkshire Police* v. *Jelic* [2010],[34] the EAT upheld an ET's decision that:
    - swapping the claimant's role with an existing role that was already filled by another police officer was capable of being a reasonable adjustment. While the tribunal recognized that the current post holder would have to be consulted before being transferred, it found that he could have been ordered to move whether he liked it or not, since the police force was a 'disciplined service'
    - swapping jobs was not equivalent to 'bumping' for redundancy purposes, because the person being transferred was not losing his job but was instead being given another role. It was also not the same as creating a role, as the post already existed.

While it should be borne in mind that the EAT made it very clear that the 'special nature of the police service was an important part of the factual matrix in this case', it does appear that swapping people between jobs to accommodate disabled employees might now constitute a reasonable adjustment in certain circumstances (e.g. if the employer has an express contractual power to move staff between roles). That said, there should be proper consultation with any non-disabled colleague before management decide to transfer them to a suitable alternative role, so as to free up their current role for the disabled employee. If the non-disabled employee puts forward good reasons why they should not be transferred out of their current role (e.g. health or domestic related) then these reasons must be properly considered by management before deciding upon a particular course of action.

Employee involvement and the cooperation of other employees

While there is no onus on a disabled person to suggest adjustments and it is principally for the employer to explore the possibility of making them (*Cosgrove* v. *Caesar and Howie* [2001]),[35] paragraph 6.24 of the Code of Practice points out that it is good practice for the employer to ask the disabled employee about possible adjustments and case law has established that adjustments can only be implemented with an employee's agreement. In practice, employers are most likely to achieve a positive outcome when considering possible adjustments by working in close partnership with the employee, their representative, and the OH professional, subject as always to issues of confidentiality and consent.

Paragraph 6.35 of the Code of Practice explains that in some cases a reasonable adjustment will not work without the cooperation of other employees. Subject to considerations about confidentiality, employers must seek to ensure that such cooperation is given. It is unlikely to be a valid defence to a disability claim under the EqA that staff were obstructive or unhelpful: any employer would at least need to be able to show that it took such behaviour seriously and dealt with it appropriately.

The cost of making reasonable adjustments

Section 20(7) of the EqA makes it clear than an employer/prospective employer is not (subject to an express provision to the contrary) entitled to require a disabled person to contribute to the cost of making any reasonable adjustments. Nonetheless the cost of the possible adjustments, together with the financial and other resources available to the employer, will be relevant to whether the adjustments will be reasonable. However, paragraph 6.25 of the Code of Practice warns:

> Even if an adjustment has a significant cost associated with it, it may still be cost-effective in overall terms – for example, compared with the costs of recruiting and training a new member of staff – and so may still be a reasonable adjustment to have to make.

The employer's duties towards disabled job applicants and employees

Part 5 of the EqA makes it unlawful for an employer to discriminate against a disabled person in relation to the recruitment, employment, or the retention of staff. Management are likely to seek OH professional input at various stages of the employment relationship.

Job applicants

According to section 39(1) of the EqA, it is unlawful for an employer to discriminate against or victimize a disabled person:

- in the arrangements which it makes for deciding to whom it should offer employment
- as to the terms on which it offers that person employment (e.g. pay and other benefits)
- by not offering that disabled person employment.

Discrimination in this context includes a failure to make a reasonable adjustment for a job applicant as well as harassing the applicant. 'Arrangements' are construed broadly.

Employers must therefore take care to avoid discriminating against disabled people throughout the recruitment process, for example:

- When specifying job descriptions, which should accurately describe the job in question and exclude unnecessary or seldom-used requirements.

- When advertising roles: job adverts should accurately reflect the requirements of the job and only include criteria that relate to health, physical fitness, etc. where these can be objectively justified by the job in question.
- When establishing the application process and thereafter undertaking the selection, assessment, and interview process.
- When deciding to whom to offer the job.

The above-listed provisions are particularly relevant where an OH professional is advising on medical standards for employment. Blanket bans on certain conditions will only be acceptable if there is either a statutory prohibition on employment or such a ban can be justified (as opposed to considering each candidate on their merits via a health assessment, for example). There have been a number of successful challenges to policies that seemed reasonable at the time (e.g. medical students with disabilities have increasingly been allowed to train, even though limited from some duties such as surgical procedures and resuscitation).

Prohibition of pre-placement health questions

Evidence exists to suggest there is discrimination against disabled people (particularly those with mental health issues) in recruitment, and people are often put off even applying for jobs because of pre-placement health questions. Section 60 of the EqA is intended to address this problem. Save for very limited reasons, it prohibits an employer from asking any job applicant about their health or any disability until the person has either been:

- offered a job either outright or on conditions, or
- included in a pool of successful candidates to be offered a job when a position becomes available (e.g. if an employer is opening a new workplace or expects to have multiple vacancies for the same role but doesn't want to recruit separately for each one).

This prohibition includes asking such a question as part of the application process or during an interview. Questions relating to previous sickness absence count as questions that relate to health or disability. This prohibition applies whether the employer asks the question of the applicant or of some other person, such as the applicant's former employer by way of a reference request. Further, the Code of Practice clarifies that the prohibition applies where an agent or employee of the employer (such as an OH professional), rather than the employer itself, asks the questions, except again in the very limited circumstances described below.

As paragraph 10.39 of the Code of Practice explains, job offers can be made conditional on satisfactory responses to pre-placement disability or health enquiries or satisfactory health checks, and an employer can ask questions once it has made a job offer or included someone in a group of successful candidates. At that stage, an employer can make sure that a candidate's health or disability would not prevent them from doing the job, having proper regard, of course, as to whether there are reasonable adjustments that would enable them to do the job: employers must not discriminate against job applicants on the back of the results of such enquiries or checks.

Section 60 does, however, permit an employer to ask questions about health or disability in limited circumstances, including for the purpose of:

- finding out if an applicant needs any reasonable adjustments to be made to the recruitment process (e.g. to an assessment test or for an interview)
- finding out if a person, whether they are a disabled person or not, can take part in an assessment as part of the recruitment process, including questions about reasonable adjustments for this purpose
- where the question relates to a person's ability to carry out a function that is intrinsic (i.e. absolutely fundamental) to that job, whether with or without adjustments.

It is important in these circumstances to ensure that mechanisms are in place to complete the enquiries about disability and health in a timely manner and to ensure as far as possible that the job candidate does not start work until these enquiries are complete. Where the person has already started the role, employment may still be terminated lawfully provided that the offer letter clearly identifies this as a possible outcome following receipt of the medical assessment. Good medical practice mandates that all pre-placement health assessments relating to high-risk and safety-critical posts should be completed before work is started.

While some doubt remains, it's safe to assume that section 60 also applies to internal promotions as well as external recruiting.

Existing employees

According to section 39(2) of the EqA, it is unlawful for an employer to discriminate against or victimize a disabled employee:

- as to the employee's terms of employment (e.g. pay, working hours, occupational pensions, sickness or maternity and paternity leave and pay)
- in the way that the employer affords the disabled employee access to, or by not affording access to, opportunities for promotion, a transfer, training or for receiving any other benefit, facility or service
- by dismissing the disabled employee (which includes 'constructive dismissal'*); or
- by subjecting the employee to any other detriment.

Discrimination in this context includes a failure to make a reasonable adjustment for an employee as well as harassing him/her.

(*Constructive dismissal refers to the situation in which, because of the employer's alleged conduct, the employee resigns on the basis that there's been an irreparable breakdown in relations.)

Employers must therefore take care to avoid discriminating against disabled employees throughout their employment with regard to the following:

- *Terms and conditions of service, and benefits*: it might be a reasonable adjustment to allow an employee to work flexibly (paragraphs 17.11 and 17.12 of the Code of Practice) and employers must not discriminate in respect of the provision of contractual and other benefits.

◆ *Induction, training, promotion, transfer, and career development*: paragraphs 17.67–17.76 of the Code of Practice explain the significance of avoiding discrimination in this regard (e.g. by selecting staff for training and promotion on a non-discriminatory basis and by implementing adjustments to enable disabled staff to undergo training). An employer should also think about whether other staff need to be trained to enable them to work safely and effectively with a disabled colleague (provided the disabled person has given permission for other staff to know about their situation).

◆ *Appraisals*: paragraphs 17.80 and 17.81 of the Code of Practice explain that employers should be aware of the duty to make reasonable adjustments when discussing past performance (e.g. would performance have been more effective had a reasonable adjustment been introduced earlier?) and that appraisals provide an opportunity for workers to disclose a disability to their employer, and to discuss any adjustments that would be reasonable for the employer to make in future.

◆ *Disciplining staff*: paragraph 17.93 of the Code of Practice explains that employers should ensure that when conducting disciplinary and grievance procedures they do not discriminate against a worker because of a protected characteristic. For example, did an employee with a learning impairment fully understand the relevant rule that was breached? Does the discipline or grievance procedure need to be adjusted to enable the employee to fully participate in the process?

◆ *Performance management*: where an employer is addressing an employee's poor performance, good practice and employment law requires that management reviews the factors which may be contributing to the underperformance, explains the standards required of the employee, warns about the consequences of failing to improve, puts in place any relevant measures to assist the employee in achieving the required improvement, and allows a reasonable timeframe for that improvement. Where the underperformance is contributed to in whole or in part by one of more protected characteristics such as age (e.g. where an employee's physical abilities are deteriorating as they get older) and/or an underlying medical condition which may amount to a disability, then the employer will need to guard against discriminating when managing the poor performance. As part of this, management should consider seeking expert medical and other advice (e.g. with regard to health and safety) about the extent of the employee's capabilities and what supportive adjustments might be made.

◆ *Redundancy exercises*: when undertaking a redundancy exercise, an employer must ensure that neither the selection procedure nor criteria discriminate against any employee.

  • For example, a manufacturer is making some employees redundant. One of the selection criteria is flexibility, in the sense that the manufacturer wants to retain people who can operate every machine on the production line. A disabled person cannot operate one of the machines because of the nature of their impairment. The employer decides that it is a reasonable adjustment to the criterion to adjust the employee's mark so as to ignore the absence of that machine, so they score the same as a worker who has operated that machine to a satisfactory standard.

- An employer also needs to ensure that any disabled person being considered for redundancy or who wishes to apply for voluntary redundancy does not face a disadvantage when receiving communications about the redundancy.

- *Managing sickness absence*: one aspect of employee management which is most likely to involve the input of an OH professional is with regard to sickness absence, be this a pattern of frequent/short absences or a long-term sickness absence, and where there might be an underlying medical condition which may amount to a disability and/or involve some other protected characteristic such as age or maternity.

Although many people with qualifying disabilities take little or no sickness absence, others do, with attendant costs to employers in sick pay and loss of productivity. Employment law, including the EqA, requires that management adopts a fair procedure when addressing sickness absence, that managers make well-informed decisions with input from relevant experts such as OH professionals, and that any action taken is justified; otherwise, employees with disability-related absences are likely to bring claims for discrimination arising from disability, indirect discrimination, and a failure to make reasonable adjustments.

Paragraphs 17.16–17.24 of the Code of Practice explain the following:

- It is important to ensure that sickness absence policies and procedures are non-discriminatory in design, and are applied to workers who are sick or absent for whatever reason without discrimination of any kind. This is particularly important when a policy has discretionary elements such as decisions about stopping sick pay or commencing attendance management procedures.

- When taking attendance management action against a worker, employers should ensure that they do not discriminate because of a protected characteristic. In particular, it will often be appropriate to manage maternity or disability-related absences differently from other types of absence. Recording the reasons for absences should assist that process.

- Employers are not automatically obliged to disregard all disability-related sickness absences, but they must disregard some or all of the absences by way of an adjustment if this is reasonable. If an employer takes action against a disabled worker for disability-related sickness absence, this may amount to discrimination arising from disability, indirect discrimination and/or a failure to make a reasonable adjustment if the decision cannot be justified.

On the other hand, employees need to appreciate that poor attendance can lead to a fair dismissal on grounds of capability.

- The EAT in *Royal Liverpool Children's NHS Trust* v. *Dunsby* [2005][36] confirmed that:

  - 'The provisions of the DDA 1995 [as succeeded by the EqA] do not impose an absolute obligation on an employer to refrain from dismissing an employee who is absent wholly or in part on grounds of ill health due to disability.

- It is rare for a sickness absence procedure to require disability-related absences to be disregarded. An employer may take into account disability related absences in operating a sickness absence procedure.'

The management of disability-related sickness absence continues to create challenges for managers and to result in case law: in *Griffiths* v. *The Secretary of State for Work and Pensions* [2015],[37] the Court of Appeal:

- Held that an absence management policy, under which all employees, both disabled and non-disabled, were treated equally, was capable of placing a disabled employee at a substantial disadvantage and that therefore the duty to make reasonable adjustments was engaged. The Court of Appeal held that the relevant PCP was the requirement to maintain a certain level of attendance at work in order not to be subject to the risk of disciplinary sanctions: this was a requirement that would substantially disadvantage disabled employees whose disability increases the likelihood of absence from work.

- The court emphasized that the duty to make reasonable adjustments goes beyond equal treatment and requires employers to take positive steps. Thus an employer should have regard to the duty to make reasonable adjustments when issuing disciplinary warnings for sickness absence. This didn't mean that such warnings should not be issued, but rather that an employer should consider whether it would be reasonable not to issue them or to vary them in some way (e.g. by adopting a more lenient trigger point).

- Stated that whether or not an adjustment is reasonable is a question for determination by the tribunal, and the court's only role was to determine whether the conclusion reached by the tribunal, that the adjustments were not reasonable, could be sustained on the evidence.

With regard to sickness absence management, OH professionals are likely to be involved in advising as to:

- whether absences are caused by an underlying medical condition and whether this amounts to a disability. This includes the expected level of absence for this particular circumstance such as recovery from a surgical procedure in the absence of complications, or whether the stated symptoms are expected in relation to treatment side effects
- what workplace adjustments and/or lifestyle choices might be made to help an employee reduce their sickness absence
- what workplace adjustments might be made to facilitate an earlier return to work from (potentially) longer-term sickness absence (e.g. as part of a phased rehabilitation plan)
- what workplace adjustments might be implemented to avoid the need to dismiss an employee by reason of their sickness absence, including the possibility of retraining and/or redeployment to a suitable alternative role.

The key issue for most employers is to determine what is reasonable in the circumstances of the case. An OH professional may be asked to determine this, but should exercise due caution as the ultimate decision rests with the employer:

- In *The Board of Governors, The National Heart and Chest Hospitals* v. *Nambiar* [1981] IRLR 196,[38] the EAT stated that any decision as to whether or not to dismiss was a management decision not a medical one. 'Seeking a report from a medical consultant did not carry with it the implication that the (employer) would be bound by any opinion that the consultant expressed.'

Advice from the OH professional should be limited to views on which absences have been related to the disability, what would be expected in the circumstances, what future absence might be expected, and what reasonable adjustments could be made if any. A person with well-controlled diabetes would not be expected to have frequent sick leave from minor respiratory infections, but may need time off for treatment of recurrent leg ulcers arising from peripheral vascular disease. Any advice must be based on evidence and the facts known to the OH professional.

An OH professional might also be required to provide advice about absences that are linked to other protected characteristics. For example, is an absence maternity related such that it should be excluded from any calculation of sickness absence for disciplinary purposes?

After the termination of employment: section 108 of the EqA

Where a disabled person's employment has come to an end, it will still be unlawful for their former employer to discriminate against the disabled person or to harass them, provided that the discrimination or harassment arises out of the employment relationship which has come to an end and is closely connected to it, and would, if it had occurred during the employment relationship, have been unlawful. As such, it is possible that an OH professional may be asked to provide guidance to management about an ex-employee.

Liability, enforcement, and remedies

Liability of employers and principals

In order to ensure that employers and principals take their obligations under the EqA seriously, the law holds that:

- employers will be vicariously liable for the discriminatory acts of their employees if those acts are committed in the course of employment and the employer failed to take reasonable steps to prevent such action*; and
- principals will be liable for the discriminatory actions of their agents which are carried out when acting under the principal's authority.

(*In order to successfully rely upon this so-called 'reasonable steps' defence, an employer will typically need to demonstrate that it operated an equal opportunities policy, educated staff about their obligations towards disabled colleagues, sought and acted upon relevant expert advice when necessary, and investigated complaints and disciplined those who unreasonably failed to adhere to the employer's equal opportunities approach, etc.)

In addition, the employee or agent concerned can be personally liable for discriminating against, or harassing, another employee.

Enforcement

Disabled job applicants, employees, and former employees who believe that they have suffered discrimination may present a complaint to an ET. A person must bring a claim within 3 months of the alleged discriminatory conduct (the time limit can be extended at the tribunal's discretion in certain circumstances).

If an ET finds in favour of the claimant in a case then it can make:

◆ a declaration regarding the rights of the complainant and/or the respondent

◆ order compensation* to be paid for the financial loss which the claimant has suffered (e.g. loss of earnings), and damages for injury to feelings

◆ an appropriate recommendation that the employer take action to remove or reduce the adverse effect in question within a given period.*

(* There is no maximum limit on the amount of the compensation that a tribunal may award. Compensation can include injury to feelings and compensation for personal injury, and can be substantial (e.g. where the act of discrimination has resulted in the loss of a job, or the loss of future earnings prospects). A tribunal will typically order sufficient compensation so as to put the claimant in the same position, as far as possible, that they would have been in if the unlawful act had not taken place.)

Key points

◆ Occupational health professionals have a critical role in advising on the likelihood that a person is disabled and, more importantly, on the adjustments that are likely to assist someone with a disability to secure work, stay in work, or return to work after a period of absence; a thorough understanding of the EqA is therefore essential.

◆ Disability is determined by the effect the condition has on the individual and not by the diagnosis except in MS, cancer, HIV, and blindness.

◆ The duty on employers to make reasonable adjustments is arguably the cornerstone of disability protection and is likely to be of the greatest practical relevance to OH professionals. When managing staff with disabilities, it is the manager who is ultimately responsible for deciding what is reasonable within the workplace.

◆ When seeking a medical opinion, it is essential that an employer provides the medical adviser with all relevant background information about the employee at work (with the employee's prior permission) so that the adviser can make a well-informed decision.

◆ In difficult cases where employment may be terminated or there is a possibility of an ET, management of the employee is most likely to be successful if the OH professional has the employee's consent to contact the GP and specialist and provide management with 'joined-up' expert medical guidance.

Useful websites

The Equality Act 2010 (Specific Duties and Public Authorities) Regulations 2017	https://www.legislation.gov.uk/ukdsi/2017/9780111153277
Equality and Human Rights Commission. 'Employment: statutory code of practice'	https://www.equalityhumanrights.com/en/publication-download/employment-statutory-code-practice
Government Equalities Office. 'Equality Act 2010: how it might affect you'	https://www.gov.uk/government/publications/equality-act-guidance

Acknowledgements

This chapter contains public sector information licensed under the Open Government Licence v3.0, http://www.nationalarchives.gov.uk/doc/open-government-licence/version/3/.

This chapter also contains extracts from the Equality and Human Rights Commission's Equality Act 2010 Statutory Code of Practice on Employment ('Code of Practice') who have kindly given permission for references to the Code of Practice to be included in this chapter. Please note that:

- the references to the Code of Practice are adapted from the original source (see 'Useful websites')
- the copyright in the Code of Practice and all other intellectual property rights in that material are owned by, or licensed to, the Commission for Equality and Human Rights, known as the Equality and Human Rights Commission ('the EHRC').

References

1. **Equality and Human Rights Commission**. *Equality Act 2010 Statutory Code of Practice: Employment*. London: The Stationery Office; 2011.
2. *Mummery LJ. Clark v. TGC t/a Novacold* [1999] EWCA Civ. 1091.
3. **Williams AN.** Are tribunals given appropriate and sufficient evidence for disability claims? *Occup Med* 2008;**58**:35–40.
4. *J v. DLA Piper LLP* [2010] UKEAT/0263/09.
5. *Paul v. National Probation Service* [2003] EAT/0290/03.
6. *Scottish Courage Ltd v. Guthrie* [2004] UKEAT/0788/03/MAA.
7. **Faculty of Occupational Medicine**. *Ethics Guidance for Occupational Health Practice*. London: Faculty of Occupational Medicine; 2012.
8. **British Medical Association**. *Medical Ethics Today*. London: British Medical Association; 2012. Available at: https://www.bma.org.uk/advice/employment/ethics/medical-ethics-today.
9. **Office for Disability Issues**. *Equality Act 2010 Guidance: Guidance on Matters to be Taken into Account in Determining Questions Relating to the Definition of Disability*. London: Department for Work and Pensions; 2010.

10. *College of Ripon & St John* v. *Hobbs* [2001] No. EAT/585/00.
11. *Millar* v. *HM Commissioners for Revenue and Customs* [2006] Court of Session IRLR 112.
12. *Power* v. *Panasonic* [2002] EAT/747/01.
13. *Vicary* v. *British Telecommunications plc* [1999] EAT/1297/98.
14. *Leonard* v. *South Derbyshire Chamber of Commerce* [2001] IRLR 19.
15. *Kirton* v. *Tetrosyl Ltd* [2003] EWCA Civ 619 A1/2002/2039.
16. *SCA Packaging* v. *Boyle* [2009] UKHL 37.
17. *Epke* v. *Metropolitan Police Commissioner* [2001] EAT/1044/00.
18. *Paterson* v. *Commissioner of Police of the Metropolis* [2007] UKEAT/0635/06.
19. *Chief Constable of Dumfries and Galloway Constabulary* v. *Adams* [2009] UKEATS/0046/08/BI.
20. *Abadeh* v. *British Telecommunications plc* [2001] EAT/1124/99.
21. *The Hospice of St Mary of Furness* v. *Howard* [2007] UKEAT/0646/06/MAA.
22. *Gallop* v. *Newport City Council* [2013] EWCA Civ. 1583.
23. *Kapadia* v. *London Borough of Lambeth* [2000] CA A1/1999/0869.
24. *McDougall* v. *Richmond Adult Community College* [2008] ICR 431.
25. *Hall* v. *Chief Constable of West Yorkshire Police* [2015] UKEAT/0057/15/LA.
26. *British Airways plc* v. *Starmer* [2005] EAT/0306/05/SM.
27. *Perratt* v. *The City of Cardiff Council* [2016] UKEAT/0079/16/RN.
28. *Hartman* v. *South Essex Mental Health Community Care NHS Trust and other cases* [2005] EWCA Civ 06.
29. *Smith* v. *Churchill's Stairlifts plc* [2005] EWCA Civ 1220.
30. *Archibald* v. *Fife Council* [2004] UKHL 32.
31. *Wade* v. *Sheffield Hallam University* [2013] UKEAT/0194/12/LA.
32. *Waddingham* v. *NHS Business Services Authority* [2015] ET/1804896/2013 and ET/1805624/2013.
33. *Southampton City College* v. *Randall* [2005] UKEAT/0372/05/DM.
34. *Chief Constable of South Yorkshire Police* v. *Jelic* [2010] UKEAT/0491/09/CEA.
35. *Cosgrove* v. *Caesar and Howie* [2001] No. EAT/1432/00.
36. *Royal Liverpool Children's NHS Trust* v. *Dunsby* [2005]. IRLR 351.
37. *Griffiths* v. *The Secretary of State for Work and Pensions* [2015] EWCA Civ 1265.
38. *The Board of Governors, The National Heart and Chest Hospitals* v. *Nambiar* [1981] ICR 441.

Chapter 4

Ethics in occupational health

Steve Boorman and Diana Kloss

Introduction

Ethics, or moral philosophy, is an attempt to define principles that govern how people should behave in society. Ethics may be described as the principles underlying the distinction between right and wrong and how we make that distinction. Healthcare is practised within communities and must reflect the cultural and ethical values of society as a whole. Professional codes of ethics are not unique to healthcare, but from as early as the fifth century BC, ethical behaviour has been acknowledged as a cornerstone of good medical practice. The relationship between a health professional and a patient is one where power lies predominantly with the health professional and the various biomedical ethical codes seek, among other things, to redress that balance (Box 4.1).[1]

In some situations, the principles can be opposing and each health professional must decide on the right course of action in those circumstances and be accountable for their decision. There are many sources of advice to help deal with such dilemmas including the General Medical Council (GMC), British Medical Association (BMA), Faculty of Occupational Medicine (FOM)[2] and the World Medical Association (see 'Useful websites').

Ethics in occupational health

The issues in occupational health (OH) may differ from those in other branches of healthcare but the same principles apply. A therapeutic relationship is uncommon in OH and blanket use of the term 'patient' in describing ethical duties may therefore be unhelpful. Internationally, the term 'worker' is used much more widely in ethical guidance and this is the terminology that will be used throughout this chapter, whether or not a therapeutic relationship exists.

Ethical guidance in OH has tended to be produced at national level, by and for individual professional groups within the discipline.[2,3] This has its benefits but does not reflect well the multidisciplinary nature of most OH teams or the increasing globalization of the workforce. The International Commission on Occupational Health (ICOH) has produced a code of ethics[4] that applies to all OH professionals and which is particularly helpful for those with international responsibilities.

> ### Box 4.1 Underpinning biomedical ethics are four main principles or shared moral beliefs first articulated by Beauchamp and Childress in the 1970s
>
> ◆ Respect for autonomy of the individual.
>
> ◆ Non-maleficence (do no harm).
>
> ◆ Beneficence (do good).
>
> ◆ Justice (fairness and equality).
>
> Source: data from Beauchamp TL, Childress JF. (2013) *Principles of biomedical ethics*, 7th edn. New York, US: Oxford University Press. Copyright © 2013 OUP.

Ethical guidance reflects consensus views on appropriate action but it is also important to understand that there is not always a right or a wrong answer and that contrary actions may be ethically justifiable according to circumstance. This can potentially be confusing, particularly for less experienced healthcare professionals, hence the importance of being able to access sources of advice to inform and support when necessary.

There is sometimes confusion between acting ethically and acting lawfully. They are not the same. Laws sometimes allow health professionals to opt out on ethical or moral grounds (e.g. termination of pregnancy). Where that is not the case, professionals should reflect carefully, consult with appropriate colleagues, and follow their conscience in full knowledge of any potential consequences for themselves of breaking the law. Simple legal compliance does not guarantee ethical behaviour and acting ethically may be unlawful. The hallmark of a professional is taking responsibility for one's own actions and acting with probity—that may be difficult but the application of sound ethical analysis can ease the process.

Governance

The concept of good clinical governance focuses on activities being undertaken in a way that promotes engagement, transparency, openness, due process, accountability, and clear communication. Good governance should also provide a sound audit trail in the event of adverse consequences that require examination or investigation. It therefore applies to all aspects of OH practice, not only clinical activity but also the organizational aspects of health and the commercial elements of providing a service. Many organizations have developed their own corporate values and ethical codes which OH staff will be expected to follow and they should satisfy themselves that there is no conflict with their professional ethics. However, OH professionals have a further duty over and above their business colleagues to promote the health and well-being of workers.

Professional standards

OH professionals have a personal responsibility to continuously improve their own standard of practice and to promote the transfer of knowledge to others. Practice should be based upon the best evidence available and OH professionals should contribute to the knowledge base by disseminating findings from their own practice. They should develop protocols based on current evidence and undertake clinical audit to facilitate continuous improvement. Audit should be kept separate from any performance management system so that there is clarity of purpose for both activities. Lifelong learning for oneself and staff for whom one has leadership or managerial responsibility should be encouraged and issues such as budgetary constraints or service delivery requirements should be managed so as not to compromise essential education, training, or revalidation. OH professionals should contribute to the information, instruction, and training of workers in relation to occupational hazards and more generally to both clinical and non-clinical members of the team. Those providing or procuring services should give consideration to how they can help ensure the maintenance of professional expertise for the future. The FOM has published guidance[5] which was originally specifically for occupational physicians, but which now has wider applicability.

Commercial occupational health

Much OH provision is delivered on a commercial basis and the pressures inherent in this type of professional market can lead to ethical difficulties. OH professionals must abide by sound principles of business and biomedical ethics in their dealings with their client organizations and each other in order to safeguard their own reputations and that of the discipline as a whole. Potential areas of difficulty include advertising, competence, competitive tendering, transfer of services, resourcing, and contractual terms.

OH providers may wish to advertise their services but many OH professionals are subject to constraints imposed by their professional bodies[6] limiting them to the provision of factual information about professional qualifications and services. OH professionals should only accept or perform work which they are competent to undertake and recognize areas where specific expert knowledge is required. The terminology used to describe OH staff should be consistent with the definitions applied by relevant professional bodies.[7–9] Services themselves should work to appropriate standards and be subject to quality accreditation, such as SEQOHS (Safe Effective Quality Occupational Health Service) as administered by the FOM (see 'Useful websites'). Competitive tendering exercises should be conducted with integrity, which implies not only honesty but also fair dealing and truthfulness. Competitors should not be denigrated in any way and great care should be taken not to damage their professional reputations. It is important to recognize circumstances in which a conflict of interest may arise, for example, when contacts with a procurer of services via alternative routes may give knowledge not available to other bidders.

Clients change providers and the abiding principle in transferring OH services should be to safeguard the health, safety, and welfare of the workers. Early consideration should be given to issues such as the transfer of equipment, hazard information, and OH records with the interests of the affected workers, rather than commercial considerations, having primacy. Resources should be suitable and sufficient to meet the agreed needs of the client and, in particular, appropriate access to accredited specialist expertise must be ensured. It is important for OH staff to be aware of contractual service specifications since they could include provisions that are lawful but unethical, such as inappropriate access to clinical records. Where doubt exists, it is prudent to seek advice from representative bodies or medical defence organizations.

Protecting health and promoting well-being

The scope of OH has broadened over time from simply addressing health issues of the workforce to considering the impact of work, its inputs, and its outputs on society as a whole. In parallel, the focus has shifted to include well-being, which incorporates the positive dimension of health in which citizens can realize their potential, work fruitfully, and contribute to society.[10] While the focus on the health of the individual worker remains undiminished, the levers to effect improvements are increasingly recognized as being work organization and health behaviours in the workplace. Advancements in screening technologies and methods may enable prognostic understanding of future risk, due to genetic or other identified risk factors. It is important that such information is used to benefit the individual and not to their disadvantage, for example, in relation to the provision of pensions or insurance cover. Individuals should be given the opportunity to understand the consequences of screening and given the choice of whether or not to consent to such.

It is the ethical duty of OH professionals to do no harm and this is consistent with the risk management hierarchy applied by businesses and the health and safety community. However, OH professionals also have a duty to do good which does not necessarily translate into traditional management practice. In consequence, OH professionals may find themselves acting as advocates for management action for which there is no legal requirement and commenting on areas of company activity (e.g. organizational design) which have not traditionally been viewed as health related.

Organizational health

The culture of an organization and the way that it conducts its activities can have a profound effect upon the health of the workforce. Management style is an important determinant of mental health and competencies[11] have been developed to help organizations train managers better. Workload, control, and change can also affect health and the perception of justice in the way the organization behaves is increasingly seen as being critical.[12] Some OH professionals still focus only on the narrower issues of hazardous exposures and individual capability, thereby potentially neglecting their wider duty to protect health and promote the well-being of people of working age. Only a few will be in a position to influence behaviour directly at an organizational or wider societal level, but all should flag the issues on an opportunistic basis and link them, where valid, to individual cases on which they are advising.

Health promotion

The increasing prevalence of non-communicable diseases, including mental health problems, is a global issue[13] and lifestyle is critical. Promoting behavioural change in the work environment is particularly effective in public health terms and delivers benefits not only to the individual worker and society but also to the employing organization.[14] OH professionals are well placed to promote health and well-being and respect for the autonomy of the individual should be paramount. The evidence should be presented in a balanced way that helps workers make their own decisions. Participation should be voluntary and OH professionals should oppose compulsion, even if well meaning. A clear distinction should be drawn between fitness programmes designed to improve operational capability (e.g. service personnel, firefighters), which may well rightly be compulsory, and those with more general aspirations to improve health status, which should not.

Pre-placement assessment

The rationale for having any pre-placement health assessment process should be established before it is implemented and the system should be reviewed periodically to ensure that it remains fit for purpose. Criteria to justify such a scheme might include statutory requirements, significant safety risks to the individual, the safety of others, or a material risk to the business by virtue of a critical position held or the associated financial exposure. A number of organizations, including the BMA,[15] recommend engagement at the pre-placement stage with a light-touch process asking selected candidates if they have a health problem or disability for which they might need assistance. OH professionals should reflect on whether activity in this area is driven by benefit to their clients and workers rather than to themselves.

The content of pre-placement assessment should reflect the nature of the work to be undertaken. There is rarely any justification for standardized general assessments of health, whether by physical examination or by completion of a health questionnaire. Invading the privacy of individuals by requiring them to disclose sensitive personal information which is not relevant to the assessment process is unethical and may infringe their human rights. In the European Union, including the UK, it also contravenes the principles enshrined in data protection legislation[16] which require that information sought is adequate, relevant, and not excessive in relation to the purpose and that it is only used for the declared purpose. Some jobs have health standards and OH professionals setting these should ensure that they are based on capability and function, rather than a specific diagnostic category, and that they are underpinned by robust evidence. Where health standards exist, they should be transparent and made available to applicants at an early stage in the recruitment process so that they do not have unrealistic expectations of a job offer.

Hazard control

Where an individual is at risk because of a particular vulnerability to a hazard at work, there is a balance to be struck. The clinician may have to weigh the autonomy of the worker to decide the acceptability of a risk to their own health or safety against the clinician's duty to do no harm. A paternalistic approach, whereby the clinician makes the decision for the worker, is not acceptable. OH professionals should help the worker make an informed decision about the level of risk that they find acceptable and then decide how to act. Every effort should be made to achieve a consensual decision but if the clinician feels that the risk of harm to the individual is too high, regardless of the worker's willingness to accept it, they should follow their conscience and refuse to provide health clearance for the activity. Where the risk of harm includes others, the ethical analysis is different because the balance is shifted from autonomy towards non-maleficence. The duty to the worker conflicts with the duty to protect others and the public interest may justify putting the interests of third parties before those of the worker.

Immunization

Immunization against occupational biohazards is another aspect of hazard control. The ethical issues are influenced by whether the programme is primarily for the protection of the individual worker or for the protection of others. An ethical complication of immunization, unlike most health assessments, is that the procedure itself may cause harm to the individual worker and it may not always confer the desired protection. Immunization is also invasive and failure to obtain consent is therefore not just unethical but, potentially, a battery. OH professionals should ensure that policies are clear about how workers who fail to develop the anticipated immunity following vaccination will be managed, and that individuals have been apprised of this information before entering the programme. Similarly, the approach to dealing with workers who decline immunization should be determined and promulgated in advance of implementing a programme. Some immunizations, notably against influenza, are offered partly for the protection of workers and those they come into contact with, but also to mitigate the operational disruption of sickness absence. OH staff should understand the reasons behind such programmes and must not misrepresent the benefits to workers. It is unethical for OH professionals to be party to the coercion of workers to undergo immunization based on operational or business needs, but it is acceptable to try to persuade workers of the public interest in maximizing the fitness of healthcare workers in caring for patients.

While it is sometimes tempting to rely on immunization or vaccination to reduce risk, it is salient to remind organizations that the principle of hierarchy of control promotes avoidance of exposure (containment and avoidance of risk of infection) before the use of protective measures.

Health screening

Well-person health screening may be offered by employers for a variety of reasons but, once accepted, is an activity for the sole benefit of the individual worker. It must be differentiated from statutory health surveillance which is an activity undertaken as part of a hazard control programme or to ensure continuing fitness to work where there are specific health criteria. Health screening programmes should be evidence based and should satisfy established criteria such as those published by the UK National Screening

Committee.[17] Screening is a voluntary activity and while OH professionals may encourage and promote participation, they must avoid being complicit in compulsion. Arrangements must be in place for the follow-up of abnormal results including referral with consent to the worker's own medical professionals. If aggregated results of workforce screening are used, data must be anonymized and presented so that linkage to identifiable individuals is prevented.

Health surveillance

While health screening is voluntary, health surveillance is not and may be a condition of employment in a given role and mandated by law. Adverse outcomes of health surveillance results may have high consequences, and potentially restrict employment options. Decisions must be based on sound evidence which should be confirmed if there is material doubt. Professional judgement must be objective and must not be swayed unduly by emotion, and compassion should be shown in communicating adverse results to the worker. Matters requiring medical intervention should be referred on appropriately and agreement should be sought from the worker to communicate the employment advice (but not the health issues) to the employer. If the worker refuses consent for the outcome to be communicated, the OH professional must consider whether a public interest disclosure is indicated or whether it will suffice to advise the employer that health surveillance could not be completed because of withdrawal of consent.

Providing an issue identified by health surveillance would not create additional risks to other workers or the public, there may be circumstances in which a worker may choose to decide to continue at work, despite an increased personal health risk. This is also providing they fully understand the consequences to their own health and are able to make an informed decision. Unless specific legislation prevents this, or the potential for harm to others is clear, it may be ethical to support the worker in continuing. In such circumstances, careful documentation of the information provided and the individual's decision is important to protect the OH professional.

Drug and alcohol testing

Drug and alcohol testing programmes should only be introduced after careful consideration of their full implications. Clarity of purpose is essential and acceptance is more likely if introduced for safety critical tasks than if put in place to enhance corporate image. The consumption of alcohol is lawful in most countries and the pharmacokinetics are relatively predictable. The illegal nature of many other recreational drugs, the potential for confusion with prescribed medication, the lack of easily demonstrable dose–effect relationships, and the persistence of some substances in the body create practical problems as well as potential civil liberties and human rights issues. No programme should be introduced without a detailed policy that sets out the reasons for testing, the procedures to be followed, and the role of OH staff. This issue is the subject of detailed guidance produced by the BMA.[18] Many organizations employ specialist contractors to conduct testing programmes which reduces the potential conflict of interest for OH staff and removes confusion among workers about the role of the service. Expert interpretation of results of such testing is important as the consequences of error may be great.

Genetic testing and monitoring

Neither genetic testing nor monitoring is yet well developed, but knowledge is increasing rapidly and tests are becoming more widely available. In the US, employers are prohibited from using genetic testing in the workplace for most purposes. In the UK, the Human Genetics Commission and the Information Commissioner have advised that employers should not demand that an individual takes a genetic test as a condition of employment and it should not be used in an effort to obtain information that is predictive of a worker's future general health.[19,20] Employers can ask for information that is relevant to health and safety or other legal duties, but the provision of the information should be voluntary.

Health and work

OH professionals are often engaged to provide an impartial opinion on a worker's functional capacity and adjustments to overcome obstacles to effective working. Opinions may also be the gate to financial benefits for the worker from pension schemes, insurers, and so on. There are therefore multiple stakeholders to satisfy and professionals must resist inappropriate pressures to sway their objective and evidence-based judgement. Balancing these multiple responsibilities according to ethical principles is consistent with the injunction to 'make the care of your patient your first concern'.[21] That does not mean taking the side of the worker regardless of the circumstances but rather ensuring that clinical issues are given primacy. OH professionals should ensure that decisions are based on good evidence and that the rationale for their opinion is clear.

Supporting the sick worker

OH professionals may engage with sick workers while they are still working, but often OH input is only sought once they have commenced a spell of sickness absence. Such referrals may be part of an absence management process and OH professionals should ensure that their prime focus remains the individual worker and not absence levels. Workers must be treated with courtesy and respect, recognizing that an OH assessment may well be a new experience which can feel threatening or intimidating. Clinical concerns should be explored and followed up without undermining the worker's confidence in the treatment they are receiving from their own professionals. Informed consent is required to ensure protection of the worker's rights to confidentiality, unless the information provided is solely related to factual confirmation of non-attendance or withdrawal of consent to a report.[21]

Recommending adjustments

OH professionals should use their training and experience to define adjustments that will help workers' rehabilitation. Recommendations must be practicable for the worker and the employer. The OH professional who recommends totally unrealistic measures is behaving neither responsibly nor ethically. Permanent adjustments and alternative duties may be more difficult to accommodate in the workplace than temporary measures. OH professionals should give careful consideration before issuing advice that may impact a worker's future employability. Many workers have a naïve view of the power of OH professionals and think that guidance they give must be followed by employers when the decision as to what is reasonable is that of the manager. Recommendations that offer a desirable benefit to the worker at the expense of costing them their job do not represent sound ethical judgement.

Health-related pension benefits

OH input is often sought in relation to enhanced benefits payable for medical retirement and in some cases for injury awards. The foremost responsibility in these cases is to the pension scheme. Difficulties may arise when, subsequent to an assessment process, a worker seeks to withdraw consent to provide a report that they consider adverse to their expectations. OH professionals should ensure they understand and carefully follow authorized procedures to avoid becoming compromised, but should stand by their professional opinion even if it is challenged, though errors of fact and opinions based on those errors should be corrected.

Information

Confidentiality and the associated issues of disclosure and consent constitute the main area of ethical challenge within OH. Data must be collected, stored, and processed ethically as well as to comply with legal requirements and professional standards. OH professionals must ensure that workers' personal information is kept confidential and that any disclosure is both appropriate and normally only made with consent. The principle of confidentiality is an important ethical obligation for all health professionals and is also a legal duty under the common law, data protection legislation, and the Human Rights Act 1998. However, the duty of confidentiality is not an absolute one and it may be broken if required by the law or on the grounds of public interest. In 2017, the GMC published revised and updated guidance for doctors.[22]

Collection of information

OH professionals generally obtain personal information about workers either by conducting a clinical assessment or by communicating with third parties. Clinical assessments may be carried out face-to-face or undertaken remotely using electronic communication. Whatever the medium, the ethical requirements are that the OH professional must aim to ensure that the worker understands from the outset the purpose, nature, and process of the consultation and, as far as possible, the potential outcomes. OH professionals have a similar duty when obtaining reports from third parties to explain why, what, and how information is to be sought and then how it is to be used. In both cases, the consent of the worker is mandatory. The primary purpose of a clinical record is to facilitate the OH care of the worker and it should therefore be contemporaneous, accurate, balanced, readily retrievable, and accessible to others who may need to use it in future. FOM guidance[2] highlights the important distinction between a clinical record, which the OH professional is responsible for maintaining and protecting, and a record of statutory health surveillance, which is the responsibility of the employer to maintain to comply with legislation, such as the Control of Substances Hazardous to Health Regulations 2002.

Storage

Clinical records must be kept secure to minimize the risk of unintended disclosure and whether data is recorded on paper or electronically. Filing cabinets must be lockable with a secure key system and databases must be password protected. Access rights must be defined with suitable training on ethical issues for system administrators. Responsibility for administrative and IT systems may be delegated but accountability for the security of the clinical information rests with the OH professional. If it is necessary to transfer records between sites, a secure system should be established with particular care paid to mobile equipment such as laptops and memory sticks. A file tracking system should be in place along with a process for informing subjects if their information is lost. Modern data security requires knowledge and maintenance of systems to avoid the loss of data or data corruption by malicious computer programmes. Data protection laws were extended and strengthened from May 2018 when the General Data Protection Regulation came into force.[16]

Retention and transfer of records

It is good practice not to keep information for longer than is necessary and in the UK this is enshrined as one of the data protection principles. Some retention periods are set by law but in general, it is left to data controllers to define what is reasonable and to justify their decision if questioned. In-house OH professionals are rarely data controllers in this context, but independent OH provider organizations usually assume this role. The range of retention periods for OH records is wide and can vary from 1 year to 50 years after the worker leaves that employment; 6 years is a common timeframe. Statutory retention periods may apply to some records of statutory health surveillance and these records should be kept separate from clinical OH records. They must be preserved even if a new OH provider is appointed. Records which have become redundant must be destroyed appropriately so that, as far as possible, unauthorized disclosure cannot occur. Shredding is the normal practice for paper records and specialist IT advice should be sought about the destruction of electronic files since simple deletion or overwriting is not sufficient. If OH records are transferred between providers, the responsible OH professional in the outgoing service has a duty to ensure that transfer is to an appropriate person for the new provider. For clinical information this should only be into the custody of the healthcare professional responsible for the new service.

Seeking individual worker consent to transfer records is usually impractical but the workforce should be advised of the change and be given the opportunity to opt out of any transfer.

Disclosure

Disclosure relates to personal information which the OH professional has acquired either directly from the worker or from a third party with the worker's consent. If an OH professional is asked by an employer or pension scheme to give a view on data which are already in their possession, that simply represents an interpretation of data, not a disclosure, and further consent is unnecessary.

Disclosures should normally only be made with the consent of the worker concerned. Disclosure can be made without consent if required by law but it is only ethical (as opposed to lawful) if the OH professional believes the law to be just. Disclosure without consent can also be made where circumstances dictate that it is in the public interest but the onus is on the OH professional to demonstrate that it is justified. Before making a disclosure without consent, the OH professional should make all reasonable efforts to obtain consent from the worker and should only act against their wishes after due consideration, which would normally include taking suitable advice.

In writing reports for employment purposes, OH professionals should avoid disclosing unnecessary clinical detail. In general, the information required for employment purposes relates to functional capacity and workplace adjustments rather than specific medical information. There is, however, often a need to put the report into context with non-specific information about the nature of a health problem and complete avoidance of all medical issues can render a report so bland as to be meaningless.

Workers may ask for disclosure of their OH records and full disclosure should be made as speedily as practicable provided there is no perceived risk of harm to the worker's physical or mental health and references to a third party who has not consented to disclosure are redacted. It should be noted that the risk of criticism or malpractice litigation against OH staff or colleagues is not a justification for non-disclosure. In 2015, after the publication of the report of the Francis Inquiry into the Mid-Staffordshire Hospital,[23] the GMC and Nursing and Midwifery Council (NMC) declared that their members have an ethical duty of candour to reveal mistakes and failures of care to patients and to cooperate with investigations into alleged malpractice.[24] People acting on behalf of a worker or an employer (e.g. solicitors, trade unions) may seek the disclosure of information but the consent of the individual should be sought. The BMA and the Law Society have produced a standard form of consent, designed for use in England and Wales, for the disclosure of health records.[25]

Consent

Consent is a process whereby an individual agrees to a proposed action after having been provided with full information about it and understanding the consequences—it may be implied or express. Implied consent should only be relied upon in circumstances where it is obvious, routine, and generally accepted. In most OH practice, express consent, preferably in writing, is required. Consent is a continuous process which is only valid for the stipulated purpose and which can be withdrawn at any time. Some OH professionals provide treatment, including immunization, and comprehensive guidance on consent has been produced by bodies such as the GMC.[26]

The overriding principle which OH staff should apply in producing reports on workers is one of 'no surprises'. The reason for a referral and the content of the assessment should be explained at the beginning of a consultation in a way that the worker understands and express consent to proceed should be obtained. The content of the report should be explained during the consultation and it is good practice for the OH professional to offer to show the worker a copy before sending it to the recipient. This latter element has been included in GMC guidance on disclosing information for insurance, employment, and similar purposes since 2009.[27] It is becoming common practice to copy all reports to workers as a routine in the interests of openness and transparency. Updated GMC guidance[28] states that if consent is informed and given at the beginning of the commissioning of a report, provided that the patient has not specifically requested further review, a report may be released without additional consent, but it should not contain any unexpected detail and the advice to offer the patient a written copy of the report before it is sent to management and at that stage allow withdrawal of consent is repeated.

Problems can be minimized by having clarity throughout the process, demonstrating integrity in behaviour, and firmly resisting attempts to alter opinion. If a worker withdraws consent for the release of a report having had the opportunity to read it then the OH professional must accept that and advise the commissioning body of what has happened. The only exceptions are where the worker is a hazard to others and public interest justifies disclosure without consent, or where there is a legal duty to disclose as, for example, under the Public Health Act 1984 or the Terrorism Act 2000. The employer, or other body, may then act based on the information available to them and this may not be in the best interests of the worker. Where consent to release a report is withdrawn, a copy should be retained within the OH record, clearly marked that consent has been withdrawn and that it has not been and will not be released.

Social media

The use of social media is expanding rapidly at home and at work with the boundaries between the two sometimes blurred. Workers and OH professionals may use networking sites to communicate with friends, colleagues, and customers as well as to seek information and to answer specific queries. OH professionals should not be deterred from using this technology appropriately but should be aware of the potential dangers of mixing personal and professional activities. Workers for whom one has a professional responsibility should not normally be accepted as 'friends' on social sites and privacy settings should be set conservatively. If professional discussion forums are used, care should be taken in relation to the release of information regarding individual cases and details that would allow the identity of a worker or employer to be determined must not be given.

Covert surveillance

Increasing use is being made, particularly in benefit and personal injury cases, of covert recording. OH professionals should not be party to commissioning such evidence, since (by definition) it is obtained without consent. They should also be wary of commenting on it as a substitute for a properly constituted assessment. If an OH professional does comment on surveillance material relating to a worker of whom they have no previous professional knowledge, then there can be no disclosure and consent is not required. Consent would, however, be required if the OH professional is asked to comment on material concerning a worker whom they had previously assessed or obtained confidential reports upon, unless the request is simply to confirm the identity of the individual.

Working with others

Many OH professionals work in multidisciplinary teams which may be purely clinical or may include colleagues with a non-clinical background. The qualities and values that should be displayed towards colleagues are set out in *Good Occupational Medicine Practice*.[5]

Clinical and non-clinical teams

Sharing information within a clinical team for the benefit of a worker's health is invariably good practice but the 'need to know' principle should be applied and it should be made clear to those accessing a service that this is the unit's way of working and its value. Sharing clinical information within a wider non-clinical team, without specific informed consent, is not ethically acceptable. Where information obtained in a clinical setting is shared for use by non-clinical colleagues for the benefit of workers it must be anonymized and presented as group data. Care should be taken to ensure that sample sizes are large enough and that other identifiers do not compromise confidentiality.

Other health professionals

It is likely to be beneficial to a worker for their primary care physician to be aware of work-related facts which may have a bearing on their health. OH professionals should therefore obtain consent to share information in this way when appropriate but consent must not be assumed. Requests for information from a worker's own health professionals should be specific, relate only to the matter in hand, and explain the context of the enquiry. Blanket requests for a complete set of records can rarely be justified in OH practice. Written consent for the provision of a report must be obtained from the worker in advance under the Access to Medical Reports Act 1988[29] and the worker must be given the opportunity to see the report before it is sent.

Others in the workplace

Workers sometimes ask to have a friend or trade union representative accompany them to an OH consultation. Most OH professionals would normally agree but it is prudent to clarify the role of the representative, which is to provide support to their colleague rather than to act as a spokesperson.

Legal departments in organizations have no greater right of access to OH records than any other representative of the employer and worker consent or a court order is required before disclosure. Non-clinical managers of services should not normally require access to clinical records. If there are concerns about the ability to maintain appropriate privacy in a department, managers may be asked to sign a confidentiality agreement. Similarly, auditors of an OH service (as opposed to those undertaking clinical audit) should not be given access to clinical records without the consent of subjects. The information required for a service audit should be obtained from other sources even if this is administratively less convenient for the auditor.

Others outside the workplace

Normal ethical principles should be applied to dealings with government officials and information obtained in confidence should normally only be disclosed with suitable consent. The number of agencies with powers to seize documents has increased significantly in recent years and legal advice should be sought if disclosure is sought. Any court order to release records must be complied with. OH professionals may become aware of information relating to adverse health effects arising from an organization's operations. In such circumstances, a public interest disclosure may be considered and it would be prudent to take appropriate advice. It would be rare to make such a disclosure without having discussed matters fully with the organization concerned. Disclosure of this type may attract legal protection but may still result in adverse consequences for the 'whistle-blower', though where workers or the public are being placed at significant risk there may be an ethical duty to disclose to the proper authorities, such as the Health and Safety Executive. The GMC advises that doctors have an ethical duty to protect patients which may involve disclosing information about colleagues' poor practice. OH professionals may be approached by the media to comment on issues. Information given should be limited to scientifically determined facts and evidence-based opinions. On no account should the health of individuals be discussed.

Occupational health research

Research is central to the development of evidence-based practice in OH. The need to undertake research may be a training requirement or arise as part of professional practice, for example, investigating a cluster of disease or emerging occupational risk factors. Most funded research in OH is carried out through academic centres that should have established procedures and access to expertise in ethics but all OH professionals should have an understanding of the main issues that might arise.

A common area of difficulty for OH professionals is deciding whether the activity they wish to undertake constitutes research or not. Problems may arise in differentiating research from clinical audit and service evaluation since there can be considerable overlap. The main issue for most OH professionals is determining if there is the need for an *independent* ethical review of the work, generally by a research ethics committee. This will arise if there is a specific statutory requirement (e.g. under the UK Human Tissue Act) or if the governance arrangements of the controlling organization require independent ethical review. The majority of universities and the UK NHS require independent ethical review for research but not for audit and service evaluation. It is therefore essential to consider ethical issues from the outset in relation to all programmes. This is a precursor to deciding whether reference to a research ethics committee is warranted and independent review is not a substitute for reflective analysis.

The decision on whether it is ethical to embark on a particular study involves weighing the risk of potential harm to the research participant against the possible benefits to society. There are several international codes and guidelines, principally the Declaration of Helsinki and its subsequent amendments. Emanuel and colleagues have defined seven requirements that provide a systematic and coherent framework for determining whether clinical research is ethical[30] and these can form a useful template for potential researchers.

Those recruited to a research study must give free and informed consent. Issues can arise in a workplace setting in relation to whether participation is truly 'voluntary'. Coercion must not be used and attention should be paid to whether workers might feel that participation would affect their employment position. Similarly, misrepresentation of the societal importance of the research or the possible impact on workers' personal health status is unethical.

If it is proposed that routine OH records or personal exposure data might be used to generate anonymized information for research purposes, the OH professional must ensure that employees are informed prospectively. Effective communication is important not just at the point of recruitment into a study but throughout the research. In particular, there should be a plan for communication of results as part of the study protocol. Where the research topic is sensitive and of interest to the public, there may be pressure from the media to disclose information when the full implications are not clear. In such cases, it is particularly important to handle the timing of communication to workers in relation to the media release. In general, individual results from studies are not disclosed. However, the individual worker should have the right of access to their own results and procedures should be put in place to communicate those appropriately. If in the pursuit of research a worker is found to have a clinical issue requiring further intervention, it is important that the researcher is able to inform and explain the implications of the condition and with appropriate informed consent able to communicate the relevant information to the worker's nominated health carer, but where the survey is anonymous, this will not be possible. The research protocol should advise that in the event of any concerns the worker should seek assistance from their general practitioner.

Key points

◆ Principles of law and ethics are not always the same and simple legal guidance does not always guarantee ethical behaviour.

◆ Guidance on ethics for occupational health professionals has been published by regulatory bodies including the FOM, GMC, and NMC, and also internationally by the ICOH.

◆ Pre-placement assessments and assessments of fitness for work should reflect the nature of the work to be undertaken and not be standardized general assessments of health or be based on stereotypical assumptions.

◆ Confidential information should not be disclosed to third parties without informed consent, but if a worker poses a potential risk to third parties the OH professional is entitled, indeed may have an ethical duty, to report to the appropriate authority.

◆ Clinical OH records must be kept securely and only retained as long as is necessary, usually while the worker remains in employment and a few years thereafter, except for research and statistical purposes. Records of statutory health surveillance should be kept for longer, in the case of some regulations for 40 years.

Useful websites

General Medical Council. 'List of ethical guidance' http://www.gmc-uk.org/guidance/ethical_guidance.asp

British Medical Association. 'Medical ethics' https://www.bma.org.uk/advice/employment/ethics/medical-ethics-today

World Medical Association. 'International Code of Medical Ethics', 2006. https://www.wma.net/policy/

Safe Effective Quality Occupational Health Services
Standards for occupational health services https://www.seqohs.org

References

1. **Beauchamp TL, Childress JF.** *Principles of Biomedical Ethics*, 7th edn. New York: Oxford University Press; 2013.
2. **Faculty of Occupational Medicine of the Royal College of Physicians.** *Ethics Guidance for Occupational Health Practice*. London: Faculty of Occupational Medicine of the Royal College of Physicians; 2018.
3. **Nursing and Midwifery Council.** The code: standards of conduct, performance and ethics for nurses and midwives. 2015. Available at: http://www.nmc-uk.org/Publications/Standards/The-code/Introduction/.
4. **International Commission on Occupational Health.** International code of ethics for occupational health professionals. 2012. Available at: http://www.icohweb.org/site_new/multimedia/core_documents/pdf/code_ethics_eng.pdf.

5. **Faculty of Occupational Medicine.** Good occupational medicine practice. 2017. Available at: http://www.fom.ac.uk/gomp/gomp-2017.

6. **General Medical Council.** Good medical practice: probity. 2013. Available at: https://www.gmc-uk.org/guidance/good_medical_practice/probity_information_about_services.asp.

7. **Faculty of Occupational Medicine.** Qualifications and training in occupational medicine. Available at: http://www.facoccmed.ac.uk/about/qualstra.jsp.

8. **Nursing and Midwifery Council.** Specialist community public health nursing. Available at: http://www.nmc-uk.org/nurses-and-midwives/specialist-community-public-health-nursing/.

9. **British Psychological Society.** Becoming an occupational psychologist. Available at: http://www.bps.org.uk/careers-education-training/how-become-psychologist/types-psychologists/becoming-occupational-psychol.

10. **World Health Organization.** Mental health: a state of wellbeing, 2014. Available at: http://www.who.int/features/factfiles/mental_health/en/index.html.

11. **Health and Safety Executive.** Line manager competency tool, 2009. Available at: http://www.hse.gov.uk/stress/mcit.htm.

12. **Kieselbach T, Triomphe TE, Armgarth E, et al.** Health in restructuring: innovative approaches and policy recommendations (HIRES). DG Employment, Social Affairs and Equal Opportunities, European Commission; 2009. Available at: http://citeseerx.ist.psu.edu/viewdoc/download?doi=10.1.1.626.9093&rep=rep1&type=pdf.

13. **World Health Organization.** Global status report on non-communicable diseases. 2014. Available at: http://www.who.int/nmh/publications/ncd-status-report-2014/en/.

14. **World Economic Forum.** Workplace Wellness Alliance. Available at: https://www.weforum.org/reports/workplace-wellness-alliance-making-right-investment-employee-health-and-power-metrics.

15. **British Medical Association.** The occupational physician. 2017. Available at: https://www.bma.org.uk/advice/employment/occupational-health/the-occupational-physician.

16. **Data Protection Act.** 2018; General Data Protection Regulation 2016, in force 25 May 2018. Available at: https://ico.org.uk/for-organisations/guide-to-data-protection/.

17. **UK National Screening Committee.** Programme appraisal criteria. 2015. Available at: http://www.screening.nhs.uk/criteria.

18. **British Medical Association.** *Alcohol, Drugs and the Workplace: The Role of Medical Professionals*, 2nd edn. London: British Medical Association; 2016.

19. **Human Genetics Commission.** Genetics and employment. Available at: http://webarchive.nationalarchives.gov.uk/20120504105138/http://www.hgc.gov.uk/Client.

20. **Information Commissioner.** Data Protection: Employment Practices Code, Part 4, 2011. Available at: https://ico.org.uk/media/for-organisations/documents/1064/the_employment_practices_code.pdf.

21. **General Medical Council.** Good medical practice: duties of a doctor. Available at: http://www.gmc-uk.org/guidance/good_medical_practice/duties_of_a_doctor.asp.

22. **General Medical Council.** Confidentiality: good practice in handling patient information. 2017. Available at: http://www.gmc-uk.org/guidance/ethical_guidance/confidentiality.asp.

23. **Francis R (Chair).** *Report of the Mid-Staffordshire NHS Trust Public Inquiry.* HC 947. London: TSO; 2013.

24. **General Medical Council and Nursing and Midwifery Council.** Openness and honesty when things go wrong: the professional duty of candour. 2015. Available at: https://www.gmc-uk.org/-/media/documents/openness-and-honesty-when-things-go-wrong--the-professional-duty-of-cand_____pdf-61540594.pdf.

25. **BMA and the Law Society.** Consent form for the release of health records. 2011. Available at: https://www.bma.org.uk/advice/employment/ethics/confidentiality-and-health-records/access-to-health-records.

26. **General Medical Council**. Consent guidance: part 2: making decisions about investigations and treatment. 2008. Available at: http://www.gmc-uk.org/guidance/ethical_guidance/consent_guidance_part2_making_decisions_about_investigations_and_treatment.asp.

27. **General Medical Council**. *Confidentiality: Disclosing Information for Insurance, Employment and Similar Purposes*. London: General Medical Council; 2017.

28. **Faculty of Occupational Medicine**. GMC guidance on confidentiality and occupational physicians. FAQ. 2010. Available at: http://www.fom.ac.uk/wp-content/uploads/m_gmcconf_qa.pdf.

29. **Access to Medical Reports Act. 1988, c.28**. Available at: http://www.legislation.gov.uk/ukpga/1988/28/contents.

30. **Emanuel EJ, Wendler D, Grady C.** What makes clinical research ethical? *JAMA* 2000;**283**:2701–11.

Chapter 5

Health promotion in the workplace

Steve Boorman

Introduction

While there are a number of subtly different definitions for health promotion, at its simplest, health promotion aims to give people the awareness, capability, and skills to control and thereby improve their own health. Health is a complex concept and has become inextricably linked with the equally complex concept of well-being. Both concepts have a continuum between positive (good health and well-being) and negative (ill health or poor well-being) and both are subjective in terms of having an individual focus and potential for variation.

This chapter considers the definition of health promotion and its potential in public and occupational health (OH) practice. Workplace health promotion provides an opportunity to deliver health messages and reach groups such as 'blue-collar men' who may be less accessible to health information delivered through other routes. Practical examples are used to illustrate health promotion techniques. Communication techniques are discussed, with exemplars of successful campaigns. Examples are given of the range of evaluation measurements used to demonstrate impact. It is also fair to highlight debate regarding the strength of evidence related to the impact of workplace health promotion. In the UK, the evidence base is less well developed than overseas publications.

Defining health promotion

The World Health Organization (WHO) defined health in 1946 as a 'state of complete, physical, mental and social well-being and not merely the absence of disease or infirmity'.[1] This was developed further in 1986, with the Ottawa Charter for Health Promotion, in which WHO proposed that, rather than being a static state, health should be regarded as 'a resource for everyday life, not the objective of living. Health is a positive concept emphasizing social and personal resources, as well as physical capacities'.[2]

Successive conferences and statements from WHO global assemblies since Adelaide in 1988 to Bangkok in 2005[3] have refined and built upon the Ottawa Charter—emphasizing health as a basic human right and establishing health promotion as a process of enabling people to increase control over their health and its determinants. Subsequent WHO conferences have continued to call for government and societal support to support health improvement, as typified by the 2013 WHO conference statement agreed in Helsinki.[4]

This is inextricably linked with public health improvement and recognizes that reducing health inequalities and improving public health is vital to economic success and sustainability. Political, economic, and cultural influences play significant roles in creating a supportive environment to help people make positive health choices which will underpin successful healthy public policy.

Being aware that there have been many attempts to clearly define 'well-being', it is perhaps simpler to consider well-being as subjective contentment with similar physical, mental, and social components.

Whatever the definitions used, it is clear that both concepts are more than just about the presence or absence of disease or injury, and authors have repeatedly reinforced the importance of the 'health triangle'—physical, mental, and social well-being components, interacting to influence health and well-being status. Influences on health are summarized in Box 5.1.

It follows therefore that some determinants of health may be difficult to modify or change, although in the case of genetic or sex-determined components, awareness may enable choices to modify or reduce the risk of expression or impact. For example, if an individual knows they have a genetic predisposition to cardiovascular disease, they can choose to modify other risk factors that may act to promote the disease.

Other health determinants may be modified by personal decisions or behavioural changes, such as increasing exercise to reduce the risk of disease related to being overweight. These factors, often described as 'lifestyle risk factors', are popularly targeted in traditional workplace health promotion campaigns. The simple underlying principle is that increased awareness of risk behaviour can enable and encourage an individual to modify that behaviour. However, evidence of sustained, significant health-improving behaviour change is too often not documented in many health promotion programmes.

Environmental risk factors may be modified by personal intervention (individual awareness and control), or may be beyond individual control with varying opportunities for direct influence. For instance, working conditions may be changed by negotiation and political decisions will depend on systems of administration, both of which offer opportunities to change, but macro environmental factors, such as temperature, rainfall, or availability of local resources, may be less easy to alter.

Box 5.1 Influences on health

- Predetermined: sex, genetic predisposition to disease.
- Environment: social status and income, education employment conditions.
- Behaviours and lifestyle: smoking, alcohol use, drug consumption, exercise.
- Access to healthcare or support: economic, political, and cultural considerations.

Health promotion and public health

Health promotion is often interpreted as simply offering advice to individuals, but increasingly broader opportunities to influence public health have seen the concept extended to encompass societal, environmental, and organizational interventions. This is exemplified by the concept of 'health-promoting workplaces'.

The detailed Marmot review, *Fair Society, Healthy Lives: A Strategic Review of Health Inequalities in England Post-2010*, explored the underlying basis of health inequalities across the UK.[5] The review highlighted that productivity losses due to health inequalities cost the UK £31–33 billion a year with a further £20–32 billion of cost to the economy from lost taxes and increased welfare payments and direct cost to the NHS of £5.5 billion. The Marmot review also concluded that without measures to address risk factors for ill health, this situation may worsen—increasing obesity, for example, was associated with £2 billion of illness costs in 2010, but this could rise to £5 billion by 2025. Marmot identified six policy areas where improvement was needed to reduce health inequalities (see Box 5.2).

Giving every child the best start in life was the highest priority recommendation, focusing on reducing inequalities in early development, better maternity and childcare services, and building resilience in young children.

Marmot clearly identified components of work that contribute to reducing ill health, effectively defining 'good work'. Additional work by Waddell and Burton, *Is Work Good for Your Health & Well-being?*, provided evidence for the ill health created by 'worklessness' and concluded that good work was beneficial to health.[6] Marmot's work identified the components of good work, concluding that ten features ranging from job security, individual control, and workload through to issues around work/life balance are important (see Chapter 9, Box 9.3 'Characteristics of good work').

Two key areas, relevant to this chapter, included the workplace as a health and well-being promoting environment, and the opportunity for work to reintegrate those with sickness or disability. It is possible therefore to think of health promotion as addressing needs at different levels—individual, organizational, and societal.

Box 5.2 Six policy areas to reduce health inequality according to Marmot

- Giving every child the best start in life.
- Enabling people of all ages to maximize capabilities and control their lives.
- Creating fair employment and good work.
- Ensuring a healthy standard of living.
- Creating and developing healthy and sustainable places and communities.
- Improving ill health prevention.

At a societal level, governments are responsible for establishing conditions to create environments in which the populations they serve can lead healthy lives. Social justice is a key part of this, and the case has been made that healthy public policies in the short term will drive the conditions to improve health, creating increased productivity and economic success. Technology, changes in population demographics, globalization, and political, economic, and ecological change all represent significant challenges to which public health policy will need to adapt.

Throughout the emergence of the modern health promotion agenda a number of key themes have remained:

- The creation of supportive environments, where people can live and work with reduced exposure to hazardous agents.
- The need to improve food and nutrition and access to safe water, reducing hunger and malnutrition and enabling healthy food choices.
- The reduction of dependence on harmful substances such as alcohol, tobacco, and other drugs hazardous to health.
- The improved capacity of communities to support enhanced personal skills to improve health.
- The development of health services orientated to support health-promoting communities.

In the UK, this agenda is driven on behalf of government by Public Health England, created in 2013 from over 100 agencies with influence on public health matters.

Health promotion in the workplace

Work is a major component within this agenda. Not only does work create the economic success needed to fund improvements, it creates social cohesion and forms the place where many in a community spend a significant proportion of their waking time, providing the opportunity for effective health promotion awareness.

Many workplaces still consist of workforces with a high proportion of one sex; for instance, men predominate in heavier manufacturing, labouring, and the armed forces whereas women predominate in some service industries such as the NHS. In addition to gender diversity, some types of work may also involve workers in lower social classes, for instance, construction. Work of this nature may also have geographical and ethnic variation.

Research confirms that different groups in society access health information in different ways and to a variable extent. Throughout global societies, women are consistently more receptive and interested in health messages. Public health policy has sought to exploit this, targeting women's networks to carry health messages to communities and using women as health-promoting 'champions'. The concept of champions is also used in the 'Health Trainer' model in which lay workers can be trained to recognize and support workplace health issues and help signpost colleagues to sources of advice. In the NHS, the

NHS England Healthy Workforce Programme is encouraging staff to take responsibility for their own health, to lead as 'ambassadors for health' and promote healthy behaviours for their own benefit and for their patients. Staff are also encouraged to 'make every contact count'—using every contact with patients or relatives to actively promote health-improving behaviours.

In the UK, there is a clear differential in the use and access to health services—women either in themselves or in their role as the main carer for dependents are more likely to attend clinics, pharmacies, or other health services. Literature targeted at a female audience contains more health content than that targeted at men. There is a wealth of evidence that suggests that men's health behaviours are different, with a tendency to minimize symptoms and present later for health advice. This differential results in a number of common health conditions having generally higher morbidity and mortality among men, while being no more frequent in incidence.

A good example of this is the condition of malignant melanoma.[7] Data collated by the European Men's Health Forum clearly show that more women than men get the disease, perhaps due to the desirability of having tanned skin, yet more men die from the disease—not because the disease has a different virulence in this sex, but rather because their health behaviours result in late presentation with more advanced disease.

At a societal level, the health promotion agenda relies on political decisions to influence the allocation of resources to create the environment to support positive change. To some extent this is also true of the approach needed to health promotion at an organizational level. Developing health-promoting workplaces has featured in successive government public health policies recognizing that quality employment is important in maintaining a healthy population. This recognition is not new! Historically, a number of forward-thinking employers have recognized this and also understood that a healthy workforce is good for business—with better overall productivity.

Workplace health promotion case studies

Royal Mail appointed a workplace doctor in 1855, with objectives which included 'improving and maintaining the health of the Royal Mail workforce'. Another well-known example lies in the Cadbury business; after nearly 70 years of trading in the nineteenth century, George Cadbury, the son of John Cadbury who started the business in 1824, recognized that the developing rail network enabled his business to develop away from the poor conditions workers experienced in many parts of London. As he built the business in south Birmingham, he recognized an opportunity 'to alleviate the evils of modern more cramped living conditions' and purchased 120 acres of land around their factory to create a village to house their workers—Bournville. Aside from the improved living conditions for workers afforded by the 313 cottages built across the estate, the Cadbury Quaker beliefs also banned alcohol. This example of a health-promoting workplace is a good one as it clearly recognizes the social dimension of good health as well as seeking to raise awareness of lifestyle risk factors that may adversely impact physical or mental health.

The example is also a good one as the move created conditions that enabled a transformation in the business's productivity and quality, enabling it to successfully compete in an increasingly competitive international marketplace.

While Royal Mail's approach was initially a traditional 'medical model', with a company doctor examining and advising sick employees, this business also recognized the impact that social distress had on its workforce and importantly the potential for this to reduce business success. In the mid-twentieth century, Royal Mail created a welfare service, training workplace 'welfare officers' to support workers. This support deliberately extended beyond the walls of the workplace, helping staff to find cost-effective housing, supporting those with debt or relationship problems, providing advice in crisis, and helping with bereavement or legal problems. In some organizations, trade unions provided similar functions; in others, philanthropic employers recognized that looking after their workers enabled them to retain a committed and loyal workforce.

Aside from the health benefits, caring for workers' health is associated with psychological benefits—reinforcing the 'psychological contract'. This concept recognizes that as well as any formal contractual relationship between employer and employee, workers' commitment to an employer or a business has psychological elements. In circumstances where employees feel they share common perceptions and beliefs with their employer, enhanced loyalty is generated and this may be associated with enhanced productivity, quality, and reduced losses associated with grievance or absence. This is increasingly referred to as 'engagement'.

MacLeod and Clarke formally examined this association in their 2008 review, 'Engaging for Success: Enhancing Performance through Employee Engagement'.[8] The review provided multiple business case studies to support its findings and the authors concluded that 'the correlation between engagement, well-being and performance is repeated too often for it to be a coincidence'. The review encouraged employers to consider the value of developing better bonds with workers and reinforced evidence that employers who support the health of their workers have higher engagement and better business performance. The recommendations of this review were accepted in full by the UK government.

The association between worker well-being and productivity and performance was also illustrated by the 2009 Department of Health-commissioned review of the health and well-being of the NHS workforce.[9] The review was part of the government's response to the Black report, *Working for a Healthier Tomorrow*, which highlighted the economic losses associated with ill health among the working age population.[10] With over 1.3 million workers, the NHS is one of Europe's largest employers and research was undertaken exploring the association between NHS workers' health and organizational performance. The review highlighted that those NHS trusts which had better staff health and well-being also had improved financial performance including lower sickness absence costs, reduced turnover, and less need for investment in agency staff cover. Importantly, they also had improved patient outcomes including satisfaction and less illness from hospital-acquired infection and better performance against regulatory targets for quality of service and use of resources. The review drew on research from Aston University which has also shown that patient outcomes are better in NHS organizations that have better staff feedback relating to their own health. Since this report, NHS leadership has supported measures to improve workforce well-being including, from 2016, a financial incentive (CQUIN), rewarding NHS organizations that introduce measures to improve staff health.

National campaigns

Business in the Community, a third-sector organization, has studied this association in many national and international major businesses.[11]

Its well-being campaign, supported by business case studies from employers, promotes the role of well-being and engagement in driving sustainable business performance.

The Workwell model has been developed with the support and involvement of leading businesses and has five dimensions supporting workplace well-being and engagement (see Box 5.3).

Supported by guidelines on public reporting using the model as a company reporting template across these areas, the model affirms an integrated strategic approach to health promotion at an organizational as well as an individual level. The Workwell model cites research from the Work Foundation suggesting good job design that increased investment in employee engagement would significantly improve UK business productivity.

Business in the Community has also worked in association with Public Health England,[12,13] producing in 2016/2017 toolkits to help employers tackle musculoskeletal and mental health issues, including the issue of employee suicide. This has resulted in resources focused on both prevention and postvention of suicide (dealing with the aftermath). A large and well-known employer who had been impacted by the suicide of a young employee supported the public launch of the resources, with the involvement of a wide range of representatives from businesses and public health.

These themes are echoed in a number of national initiatives. Under the auspices of public health improvement, the 'Responsibility Deal' seeks to engage businesses, government, and specialist stakeholders by signing up to health improvement-related pledges.[14] Its targets include producers, retailers, employers, and communities and its aims include

---

Box 5.3 Supporting workplace well-being and engagement according to the Workwell model

- Better work.
- Better relationships.
- Better specialist support.
- Better physical and psychological health.
- Working well.

to encourage healthy eating, responsible alcohol use, increased exercise, and healthy workplaces. Organizations participating in the workplace health strand are encouraged to make pledges to actively support their workforces to lead healthier lives. This includes pledges to measure and report employee health, target smoking cessation, provide healthier workplace nutritional programmes, provide good quality advice on common health issues, and use good quality (accredited) OH services. Public Health England has incorporated its multiple health improvement campaigns under the 'One You' brand (see 'Useful websites').

A number of schemes actively promote and reward workplace health promotion. The Investors in People scheme now incorporates health management and health promotion within its measurement framework of good management practice. In England, the Workplace Wellness Charter seeks to encourage organizations to measure and recognize good support for workplace health.[15] There are equivalent health workplace awards schemes in Scotland and Wales. The Scottish Health at Work Scheme encourages organizations to support individual employees, to seek measures to improve the working environment, and to intervene to improve organizational structures and working practices.[16] Participation in schemes such as these help employers to access simple toolkits with good quality health awareness advice and by their nature these schemes seek to involve workers in getting actively involved in health-improving activities.

Communication techniques

Health promotion seeks to firstly raise awareness among its target audiences, be they individuals, employers, politicians, or leadership role models. This is an exercise in good communication and the most effective communication is planned in the knowledge of how best to attract the attention of the recipient. Unless health promotional materials are targeted to their audience they risk being ignored or discarded. For instance, male-dominated blue-collar workforces may respond better to material that includes humour and simple cartoons, while other groups may find this style less attractive.

As well as raising awareness, the factual content of health promotion messages needs to convince of the need to modify behaviours, supporting change. Factors influencing behaviour may be complex—stark messages such as 'smoking may kill' are not always persuasive and individual risk perception may vary based on past experiences, cultural beliefs, or other influences, such as the attitude of peers.

Effective planning has a key role to play in increasing the impact and efficacy of health promotion messages. Simple considerations may make a big difference to the priority and retention of information materials. For example, a health promotion event delivered to manual workers during working time as a 'toolbox talk' will be better attended than an event at the end of a working shift, or on the same evening as a key sports event.

The approach to delivery may also clearly influence uptake—visually attractive material with an obvious presence in a prominent part of the workplace is more likely to attract attention than a low-key presence in a remote location. However, for some health promotion or health surveillance programmes the latter may be preferable— for example, in a large, male-dominated manual workforce, a mobile cervical screening programme achieved significantly better uptake from female workers when the screening vehicle was parked 'discreetly' (allowing access without male workers overlooking).

Creativity is needed to attract attention. This may involve a 'tagline'—a catchy phrase or branding that encourages recognition. The Health and Safety Executive campaign 'Good health equals good business' is a good example.[17] 'The mindful employer' is another simple phrase carrying a clear message informing of a campaign's aims.[18] The language and style of campaigns also needs consideration—jargon or slang can in some cases improve accessibility, but if its use confuses the message the converse may be true. Associating a health message with a product or service, particularly one linked to the workplace concerned, may strengthen the message. In Royal Mail, the simple branding of health promotion under the banner 'Feeling First Class' has lasted for over a decade, resonating clearly with the core activities of the business.

The Men's Health Forum is a charitable organization promoting men's health in the UK.[19] It worked with the Royal Mail to raise awareness of a forthcoming health promotion week. Millions of stamps were cancelled with the words 'Delivering male health'—a pun on the function of the mail service provider while deliberately raising awareness of the series of events.

Knowing the target audience can also influence the best mode of communication to use for effective health promotion. Some groups respond best to face-to-face communication, while other groups may favour provision of online electronic information that can be accessed with privacy, particularly where a health topic may be seen as embarrassing or 'sensitive'.

Gimmicks, giveaways, and gadgets can also be used to promote retention of material and messages. These include items directly contributing to the issue being promoted, for example, a pedometer being used to promote exercise. The Global Corporate Challenge is a good example of an international initiative that has gained widespread support to encourage physical activity.[20] Alternatively, the health message may be attached to a commonly used item that is likely to be retained, such as notepads, pens, or memory sticks.

There is much commonality here between the skills of the advertising/marketing professions, and those designing health promotion campaigns. In both cases, the aim is to generate sufficient attention and interest from the recipient that a key message is understood and then retained, with the aim of influencing future behaviour.

As with other disciplines, health promotion must embrace the benefits of technology, which allows a wider range of audiences to be reached. Digital information can be amended and updated more easily and with lower cost, may be replicated and widely dispersed, and can be designed to be interactive. Interactivity has benefit in allowing health promotion messages to be further tailored or targeted to individual need (e.g. generating specific nutrition or lifestyle information), and can also engage other techniques to improve retention and interest. Computer technology-based programmes can, for example, generate an element of competition or challenge to encourage participation. By introducing fun to repetitive tasks such as exercise they can help to reduce attrition associated with lost interest. Increasingly, such programmes may also include follow-up or prompts—emails or other contact to remind participants of tasks and encourage compliance. Coupled with wearable technology, giving users real-time feedback on biometric data, there has been rapid growth in app-based health-promoting programmes ranging from sleep improvement to mental health improvement.[21,22]

The advent of social media, and increasingly sophisticated portable technology such as 'smartphones' and tablets, further increases the flexibility of communications media to deliver health promotion messages. While some working populations (lower-income groups, for example) may traditionally have been excluded from access to such modes of communication, increasingly the ubiquitous nature of games, access to music, and video media, mean that such technology now reaches substantial proportions of the population and cannot be ignored as a mode of health promotion delivery.

Although it may be more difficult to measure the positive impact this has on families of workers, many businesses interested in workplace health promotion will extend programmes to include families. This may originate from knowledge that health issues in dependants may impact the productivity of the worker. This can be from the perspective of sickness absence, leave requested to support an ill family member, or from the direct impact on worker health from worrying about issues arising. The family unit may also be a more receptive target for health promotion messages. Delivering health promotion materials to the home may enable other family members or contacts to use their awareness to influence the worker's behaviour more effectively.

UK national workforce health promotion examples

A large UK organization successfully ran smoking cessation programmes involving the individual worker's spouse. Providing smoking cessation materials to the home enabled the spouse and other family members to help motivate change. This approach has been echoed in effective television advertising campaigns—children in the household being used to promote a positive message regarding smoking cessation.

Targeting is now generally considered essential rather than just a good idea. This can be based on a number of criteria such as occupation, age, geographical location, culture, and gender. Male-specific targeting of health information and services is a relatively new concept. The Men's Health Forum has pioneered UK approaches, working to articulate the business case for targeting male health promotion in the workplace (see Box 5.4).

Box 5.4 Men's Health Forum: National Men's Health Week policy paper

Health improvement initiatives delivered in the workplace are of particular importance for men because:

- Men are less likely than women to make use of almost all other forms of primary health provision. For example, men see their general practitioner an average of only three times annually compared to five times for women; men are less likely than women to have regular dental check-ups (just over half of men compared with two-thirds of women); and are less likely to seek health advice at a pharmacy. Men are also acknowledged to be less likely to participate in public health improvement programmes of all kinds.

- Men spend far more of their lives in the workplace. Overall there are more men than women in paid employment (17 million men compared with 15 million women)[49] and men are twice as likely to work full-time. However, changes to pension eligibility has seen a rise in female employment rates in 2016, 79.3% of men aged 16–64 were in work (little change from previous year), while 70% of women in this age group worked, the highest female employment rate since 1971. Men also work much more overtime (30% of men work more than 45 hours per week compared with 10% of women) and because of the traditional differential in the retirement age, men still tend to work to a greater age.

- Men develop many serious illnesses earlier than women—10–15 years earlier in the case of heart disease, for example (there are nearly five times as many male deaths as female deaths from coronary heart disease in the 50–54 age group); 16% of men compared to 6% of women die while still of working age.

- There is an increasing and convincing body of evidence that health improvement initiatives in the workplace are not only effective at engaging men but are also welcomed and valued by men. In this sense, workplace interventions have gained an endorsement from men that may have been lacking in previous population-level initiatives.

Source: data from Men's Health Forum, www.menshealthforum.org.uk. Copyright © 2012 Men's Health Forum.

There are sound social and economic reasons for an effective programme of health promotion in the workplace.[23]

Recent work would suggest that the delivery of services, including health promotion, is in fact 'hard to reach' for many men and is a contributory factor for the significant differences in morbidity and mortality between the sexes. Although men are more than one and a half times as likely to develop bowel cancer, they remain less likely to participate in the NHS Bowel Cancer Screening Programme (57% female uptake compared with 51% male uptake).[24] A European Commission report into the health of men in Europe had similar conclusions.[25] Many of the key issues concerning gender differences in access to health services are set out in a 2008 Department of Health-commissioned report, *The Gender and Access to Health Services Study*.[26]

Strategic reviews

The importance of actions tailored to meet the needs of different groups within the workforce, including men, has been recognized more widely. Dame Carol Black's review of the health of the working age population, *Working for a Healthier Tomorrow*, observed that successful health programmes are those that are specifically designed to meet employee needs—'there is no *one size fits all*'.[8]

The Black report also acknowledged the potential importance of gender-sensitive approaches in enhancing the effectiveness of workplace health improvement initiatives, a point also made in a report from the World Economic Forum, *Working Towards Wellness: Practical Steps for CEOs*.[27,28] This report highlighted the successful health improvement initiatives undertaken by a UK-based telecommunications company in support of its global workforce and acknowledged both that 'different strategies and messaging are required for men and women' and that 'men are a much more resistant audience and require special attention'.

The workplace is considered to be an ideal setting for health promotion initiatives; approximately one-third of waking hours are spent at work and it provides regular access to a relatively stable population, many of whom are men. Importantly, workplace health promotion is associated with a reduction in health risks, and with improvements in economic and productivity factors including reduced medical costs, compensation benefits, employee absenteeism, and increased job satisfaction. The value of workplace health promotion was identified in the Health Promotion Strategy and 'Developing a Health Promoting Workplace' provides a framework and guidelines for the development of workplace health promotion policies.[29]

A prostate health awareness programme run for postal workers in the West Midlands not only produced a significant increase in awareness levels, it also gathered a range of qualitative data that demonstrated men's willingness to engage with this sort of initiative. An academic analysis of the project concluded that 'it has shown that the workplace can provide an ideal setting in which to deliver health promotion to men'.[30] Another good example of a similar successful workplace campaign to raise awareness on this issue is exemplified by JCB, who promoted prostate screening widely across its workforce.

A study of men and indigestion, conducted by Bournemouth University found that, overall, nearly 70% of the men sampled felt that health issues should be discussed at work and concluded that 'going to where men are' with health campaigns and services would be useful in terms of improving their health and offering screening.[31]

Trade union involvement

The 'Work Fit' project is another example of a 'male-friendly' approach to health improvement. A UK-based telecommunications company (BT) worked with a specialist provider to help the company target public health issues linked to obesity, an ageing workforce, sedentary lifestyles, and the associated health implications.

The overall aim of Work Fit was to contribute to the development of a healthy workplace culture within BT by encouraging staff to make sustainable improvements to their lifestyle. Key objectives included encouraging and enabling BT staff to maintain a healthy weight, to seek advice from their general practitioner if needed, and to develop a model for health improvement interventions, usable within BT and other workplace settings.

Liaison with the two main trade unions, Connect and the Communication Workers Union, was identified as crucial to the project's ability to succeed and they were both involved from the outset. Focus groups were also undertaken to involve employees in the development process, to test proposed resources, and to gain feedback on how best to market health improvement messages to the workforce.

Work Fit was designed as a lifestyle-management programme focusing on nutrition and physical activity. It was delivered entirely through the BT company intranet and open to all 90,000 male and female employees as individuals or as part of a team. The 16-week programme incorporated weekly challenges, email prompts, and online help from independent health advisors. Information supplied allowed participants to monitor their own progress online and gave the project team the ability to review progress and trends against critical success factors. On registration, participants were sent a tool kit including a pedometer, tape measure, and a health advice booklet designed to look like a Haynes' car manual.[32]

It was also recognized that to be effective, all employees needed to be aware of the programme and any fears concerning confidentiality should be allayed. Over 20 half-day road-shows were organized, in conjunction with the Communication Workers Union and with active support from Connect, as a form of community outreach and incorporated an information stall providing background information, general advice, and health 'MOTs' to employees. Internal and external marketing channels were also used to get the message across, including the in-house newspaper, workplace posters, and the national press.

Work Fit was extremely successful. Its target of 5000 participants was achieved within 24 hours of going live. Over 16,000 participants were eventually registered, 75% of whom were male, accurately reflecting the ratio of male/female workers at BT; 4377 of these lost a combined weight of over 10,000 kg, representing an average of 2.3 kg per person. Most significant is that up to two-thirds of participants reported sustained changes to their lifestyle as a direct result of the Work Fit programme.

Other workplace-based diet and physical activity initiatives aimed at men have also achieved positive results. The 'Keeping It Up' campaign in Dorset aimed at middle-aged men resulted in almost three-quarters of participants reducing their body mass index, 58% increased their physical fitness (as measured by a step test), and almost half reduced their percentage of body fat.[33] The Bradford Health of Men project has also successfully engaged with men at workplaces.[34]

Making the business case

Business benefits of health promotion can be hard to calculate but a study by PricewaterhouseCoopers commissioned by the Health Work Wellbeing Executive in 2008 suggested that improving employee health is good for business.[35] The study identified a number of benefits of staff wellness programmes including reduced levels of sickness absence, lower staff turnover, and greater employee satisfaction. Where these benefits were costed against staff performance, they demonstrated a measurable return against the financial investment. The study concluded that 'workplace wellness makes commercial sense' and suggested that the workplace offers considerable untapped potential as a setting for the improvement of population health.

These are not just theoretical assertions. The potential of action to improve health at work is clearly shown by work to reduce absenteeism undertaken by Royal Mail. Royal Mail employs 180,000 people. A report by the London School of Economics found that the company achieved significant reductions in absence—from 7% to 5%—between January 2004 and May 2007, equivalent to an extra 3600 employees in work.[36] Raising the health awareness of staff formed an important element of Royal Mail's approach. The London School of Economics calculated that if the 13 sectors in the economy with the highest absence rates followed Royal Mail's example, the resultant reduction in absenteeism would be worth £1.45 billion to the UK economy.

The arguments for cost benefits associated with health promotion have been better developed in the US, where the financial differences in healthcare organization place greater emphasis on the potential benefits of prevention. US literature contains many references to cost/benefit analysis of health promotion programmes. Burton et al. document the increased likelihood of lost working days and productivity losses linked to identified health risks.[37] Loeppke et al. have published data showing the benefits of health promotion in modifying health risks,[38] and further work from Burton et al. cites the productivity improvements gained by modifying health risks.[39] Edington's research cites an annual saving of $143 per annum per person (from 2001) for each health risk reduced.[40]

An OH scheme pilot commissioned by the Health and Safety Executive and carried out in Leicestershire between 2004 and 2006 demonstrated that it is possible to achieve a high take-up of voluntary health checks in another industry with workers that may be hard to access with healthcare messages.[41] More than 1700 construction workers had health checks during the programme. One-third of those checked suffered from general health issues such as high blood pressure and respiratory illness. Problems arising from OH risks, such as vibration or excess sound levels, were also common. Overall, one-third of those checked needed to be referred to their own general practitioners. Significantly, the pilot found that the main barrier to delivering OH to construction workers was at the managerial level, and not a lack of interest from workers.

Another project with construction workers—addressing skin cancer prevention—also achieved positive results. All the workers considered the workplace an appropriate setting in which to address health issues with men, 68% of the men attending awareness-raising workshops said they were now more aware of the dangers of sun exposure, and 69% said they would now protect themselves in sunlight.[42]

The Institute of Occupational Safety and Health has also run regular campaigns highlighting the risks of occupational-related cancer—their sun awareness campaign 'No Time to Lose' being a good example from 2017.[43]

A 2003 study found that delivering self-testing kits for chlamydia screening via workplaces is potentially an effective way of increasing take-up among men.[44] Of those people submitting urine samples for analysis in the study, 78% were male, compared with only 13% of those screening for chlamydia in the National Chlamydia Screening Programme at the time. The proportion of men being screened in the National Chlamydia Screening Programme has increased significantly since this work due to better targeting. The programme's men's strategy, *Men Too*, published in 2007, identifies workplaces as one of several accessible venues for men.[45]

A study commissioned by the Food Standards Agency found that a workplace intervention can produce positive change in awareness of the impact of salt on health and can contribute to positive changes in workers' health behaviours.[46] For example, there were significant increases between baseline and follow-up in the proportion of workers who believed salt intake to be associated with heart disease (51% to 62%), heart attack (46% to 61%), and stroke (32% to 43%). There were also significant increases in the proportion of workers who were able to correctly identify the advised maximum daily intake of salt between baseline and follow-up (29% to 64%). The evaluation showed that men are likely to value different methods of delivery from women and concluded that gender sensitivity is therefore important in both the design and implementation of a workplace intervention.

A health initiative run by Lambeth Primary Care Trust (PCT) at two ARRIVA bus garages also produced positive results.[47] The interventions used in this project included nurse-led 'MOT' health checks, advice, support, signposting to relevant services, on-site interventions such as stop smoking support, and a weight-loss competition. The MOT consisted of a cardiovascular check (body mass index, blood glucose, blood pressure, smoking status, nutrition, alcohol, and physical activity), counselling, advice, support, service referral, and a 3-month post-contact follow-up. The checks also provided an opportunity for sexual and mental health issues to be addressed through health education and signposting. The PCT confirmed that engaging with men in the workplace about their health was effective: 162 men had MOT checks at both garages, 20–30% of whom were referred for lifestyle support because of their cardiovascular risk.

In 2017, the Society of Occupational Medicine published a summary of the value proposition for OH.[48] In its articulation of the business case for good OH, health promotion was included as a key component.

Key points

- The workplace is an effective forum for health-promoting activities and the examples highlight that careful planning and targeting may increase the likelihood of success.
- Many employers expect such programmes to have a high cost, or be difficult to organize, but the increasing resources available from third-sector and public health programmes may be accessed by partnership approaches to deliver high-quality programmes, with minimal cost.
- Comprehensive OH should encompass prevention and health promotion, within the continuum ranging from proactive health support to more reactive intervention to address injury or illness.
- This chapter provides multiple examples of successful workplace-based health promotion initiatives.
- While debate continues regarding the evidence base for outcomes, workplace health promotion is seen as valuable by many employees and employers.

Useful websites

Public Health England. 'One You'	https://www.nhs.uk/oneyou
Men's Health Forum	https://www.menshealthforum.org.uk/
Business in the Community	https://www.bitc.org.uk/
Workplace Wellbeing Charter.	http://www.wellbeingcharter.org.uk/

Acknowledgements

The author would like to thank David Wilkins from The Men's Health Forum and Dr Ian Banks from the European Men's Health Forum for support and research contributing to this chapter.

References

1. **Preamble to the Constitution of The World Health Organization as adopted by the International Health Conference,** New York, 19 June–22 July 1946; signed on 22 July 1946 by the representatives of 61 States (Official Records of the World Health Organization, no. 2, p. 100) and entered into force on 7 April 1948.
2. **World Health Organization.** *Ottawa Charter for Health Promotion.* First International Conference for Health Promotion, Ottawa; 1986.
3. **World Health Organization.** *Milestones in Health Promotion: Statements from Global Conferences.* Geneva: World Health Organization; 2009.
4. **World Health Organization.** The 8th Global Conference on Health Promotion, Helsinki, Finland, 10–14 June 2013: The Helsinki statement on Health in All Policies. Available at: http://www.who.int/healthpromotion/conferences/8gchp/statement_2013/en/index1.html.

5. **Marmot M** (Chair). *Fair Society, Healthy Lives. A Strategic Review of Health Inequalities in England post-2010* (The Marmot Review). London: The Marmot Review; 2010. Available at: http://www.instituteofhealthequity.org/projects/fair-society-healthy-lives-the-marmot-review/fair-society-healthy-lives-full-report.

6. **Waddell G, Burton AK.** *Is Work Good for Your Health & Well-Being?* London: TSO; 2006.

7. **Cancer.Net. Melanoma.** Available at: http://www.cancer.net/cancer-types/melanoma/statistics.

8. **MacLeod D, Clarke N.** *Engaging for Success: Enhancing Performance through Employee Engagement. A Report to Government.* London: Department for Business, Innovation & Skills; 2009.

9. **Boorman S** (Lead reviewer). *NHS Health & Well-Being: Final Report.* London: Department of Health; 2009.

10. **Black C.** *Working for a Healthier Tomorrow.* London: Department of Work and Pensions; 2008.

11. **Business in the Community.** *Public Reporting Guidelines: Employee Wellness and Engagement.* London: BiTC; 2011.

12. **Business in the Community.** Musculoskeletal health toolkit for employers. Available at: https://wellbeing.bitc.org.uk/all-resources/toolkits/musculoskeletal-health-toolkit-employers.

13. **Business in the Community.** Suicide prevention toolkit. Available at: https://wellbeing.bitc.org.uk/all-resources/toolkits/suicide-prevention-toolkit.

14. **Department of Health.** Public health responsibility deal. 2011. Available at: http://responsibilitydeal.dh.gov.uk/.

15. **Liverpool NHS Primary Care Trust.** *The Workplace Wellbeing Charter.* Liverpool: Liverpool NHS Primary Care Trust; 2011.

16. **Healthy Working Lives, Scotland.** Homepage. Available at: http://www.healthyworkinglives.com.

17. **Entec UK Ltd.** *Evaluation of the Good Health is Good Business Campaign.* Entec UK Contract Research report for HSE No. 272/2000. London: Entec UK; 2000.

18. **Mindful Employer®.** *Line Managers' Resource: A Practical Guide for Supporting Staff with a Mental Health Condition.* Exeter: Devon Partnership NHS Trust; 2011.

19. **Men's Health Forum.** Homepage. http://www.menshealthforum.org.uk

20. **Batman DC.** Hippocrates: 'Walking is man's best medicine'. *Occup Med* 2012;**62**:320–2.

21. **Sleepio.com.** Sleepio™. Available at: https://www.sleepio.com/.

22. **Headspace.com.** Headspace®. Available at: www.headspace.com/.

23. **Men's Health Forum.** *Improving Male Health by Taking Action in the Workplace: A Policy Briefing Paper.* Men's Health Week Policy Paper. London: Men's Health Forum; 2008.

24. **Wilkins D.** *Slow on the uptake? Encouraging Male Participation in the NHS Bowel Cancer Screening Programme.* London: Men's Health Forum; 2011.

25. **White A.** *The State of Men's Health in Europe: Extended Report.* Brussels: European Commission; 2011.

26. **Men's Health Forum/Bristol University report for Department of Health.** *The Gender and Access to Health Services Study: final report.* London: Department of Health; 2008.

27. **World Economic Forum.** *Annual Report 2007/2008.* Geneva: World Economic Forum; 2008.

28. **Litchfield P.** *Working Towards Wellness: Practical Steps for CEOs.* Geneva: World Economic Forum; 2003.

29. **Chu C, Driscoll T, Dwyer S.** The health-promoting workplace: an integrative perspective. *Aust N Z J Public Health* 1997;**21**(4 Spec No):377–85.

30. **Dolan A, Staples V, Summer S, et al.** 'You ain't going to say ... I've got a problem down there': workplace-based prostate health promotion with men. *Health Educ Res* 2005;**20**:730–8.

31. **Hemingway A, Taylor G, Young N.** *Quit Bellyaching: The Men and Indigestion Pilot Study.* London: Men's Health Forum; 2004.

32. **Men's Health Forum**. Man manuals. Available at: http://www.menshealthforum.org.uk/mini-manuals/19009-mens-health-forum-mini-manuals.

33. **Wilkins D.** Promoting weight loss in men aged 40–45: the 'keeping it up' campaign. In: Davidson N, Lloyd T (eds), *Promoting Men's Health*, pp. 131–8. London: Bailliere Tindall; 2001.

34. **White AK, Cash K, Conrad P, Branney, P.** *The Bradford & Airedale Health of Men Initiative: A Study of its Effectiveness in Engaging with Men.* Leeds: Leeds Metropolitan University; 2008.

35. **Price Waterhouse Coopers LLP for Department of Work and Pensions.** *Building the Case for Wellness.* London: Price Waterhouse Coopers LLP; 2008.

36. **Marsden D, Manconi S.** *The Value of Rude Health: A Report for the Royal Mail Group.* London: London School of Economics; 2008.

37. **Burton W, Chen CY, Conti DJ, et al.** The association of health risks with on-the-job productivity. *J Occup Environ Med* 2005;**47**:769–77.

38. **Loeppke R, Edington D, Beg S.** Impact of the prevention plan on employee health risk reduction. *Popul Health Manag* 2010;**13**;275–84.

39. **Burton W, Chen CY, Conti DJ, et al.** The association of health risk change and presenteeism change. *J Occup Environ Med* 2006;**48**:252–63.

40. **Edington R.** Emerging research: a view from one research center. *Am J Health Prom* 2001;**15**:341–9.

41. **Institute of Employment Studies.** *Constructing Better Health: Final Evaluation Report.* London: Health and Safety Executive; 2007.

42. **Twardzicki M, Roche T.** Addressing skin cancer prevention with outdoor workers. In: Davidson N, Lloyd T (eds), *Promoting Men's Health: A Guide for Practitioners*, pp. 123–30. London: Bailliere Tindall; 2001.

43. **Institute for Occupational Safety and Health.** 'No Time to Lose' campaign. Available at: https://www.iosh.co.uk/News/Safety-and-health-professionals-sun-safety.aspx.

44. **Men's Health Forum.** *The Men and Chlamydia Project 2002–2004.* London: Men's Health Forum; 2005.

45. **National Chlamydia Screening Programme.** *Men Too: Strategy to Support Equitable Access to Chlamydia Screening for Men Within the National Chlamydia Screening Programme.* London: Health Protection Agency; 2007.

46. **Men's Health Forum.** *With a Pinch of Salt: Men and Salt—A Workplace Intervention.* London: Food Standards Agency; 2008.

47. **Local Government Association.** All Aboard for Better Health. Available at: https://www.local.gov.uk/our-support/our-improvement-offer/care-and-health-improvement/integration-and-better-care-fund/new.

48. **Society of Occupational Medicine.** Occupational health: the value proposition. 2017. Available at: https://www.som.org.uk/sites/som.org.uk/files/Occupational %20health %20-%20the %20value %20proposition_0.pdf.

Chapter 6

Health screening in occupational health

David Koh and Tar-Ching Aw

Introduction

Screening refers to a test or a series of tests to which an individual submits to determine whether enough evidence of a disease exists to warrant further diagnostic examination by a physician. Health screening has been defined by the US Commission on Chronic Illness as 'the presumptive identification of unrecognized disease or defect by the application of tests, examinations or other procedures which can be applied rapidly'. The commission describes screening tests as tests that 'sort out apparently well persons who probably have a disease from those who probably do not' although cautioning that 'A screening test is not intended to be diagnostic. Persons with positive or suspicious findings must be referred to their physicians for diagnosis and necessary treatment'.

In occupational health (OH) practice, health screening programmes focus on working populations rather than the general population. Several distinct types of health screening, with different specific aims, can be identified:

- Detecting pre-existing, unrecognized ill health that may pose a risk to the individual or to third parties in the workplace (co-workers, members of the public).
- Health surveillance: detecting effects resulting from workplace exposure to hazards. Some health surveillance is statutory.
- Using the workplace as an opportunity for health promotion, to provide general health screening for health effects that may not be directly related to specific occupational exposures, but which may be used to influence positive health behaviours in a workforce.

It is important that the correct type of screening test is used, and that the characteristics and interpretation of test results for both the individual and the population are understood.

Screening in occupational health practice

In OH settings, screening examinations are performed at different times and for various purposes.

Pre-placement examination

In some countries, pre-employment examinations are prohibited under disability discrimination laws and health assessments should not be carried out unless or until a job offer has been made. For example, in the UK, the Equality Act 2010 stipulates that, with few exceptions, employers should now not ask about the health of prospective employees before a job offer.

However, pre-placement examinations are often required of persons embarking on a new job. The distinction between the terms is that pre-employment examination is usually performed before an individual is offered a job, and confirmation in the post is contingent upon passing the 'medical examination'. In pre-placement examination, the clinical assessment is conducted after a person is offered a job based on qualifications, experience, recommendations, and other considerations, rather than health considerations.

The purpose of a pre-placement examination is to determine whether there may be health reasons why an individual should not be placed in a particular workplace, and/or make any necessary workplace adjustments. The reason that is often stated for excluding an individual from a specific job is that the safety of the individual or third parties may be compromised because of the health status of the prospective employee (e.g. an infectious hepatitis B carrier proposing to perform surgical procedures). For a proper evaluation of fitness, the examining health professional should be aware of the requirements of the job and the working environment, in addition to assessing the health status of the person.

Another reason for the pre-placement examination is to establish baseline health information for subsequent health surveillance. It could also be used to assess health status for medical insurance purposes, and to defend or support a subsequent compensation claim for occupational illness. It is uncertain how much use is made of such baseline information, or whether the records are readily retrievable should there be a need to refer to baseline findings from pre-placement assessments.

Many occupations do not require high standards of physical fitness. The probability of discovering disease that might significantly impair job performance in apparently healthy job applicants, especially among young adults, is low. Thus, the rejection rate for fitness to work based on medical grounds is generally low. In a national audit of pre-employment assessments for healthcare workers, the rejection rate for applicants was less than 1%.[1]

The components of any pre-placement assessment should be justified on the basis of necessity and risk, and based on sound evidence that the specific questions asked or examinations performed are warranted for the proposed job.

If warranted, instead of subjecting every job applicant to the same general pre-placement screening, the examination should be tailored to the specific demands of the job. A self-administered health declaration or questionnaire that is processed by an OH professional may be adequate for most clerical or administrative jobs. However, it has been advocated (albeit, with controversy) that more comprehensive screening be conducted for selected 'high-flier' candidates, where substantial investment in training and resources is required. A recent evidence-based review on pre-placement examinations indicated that there was conflicting evidence on whether these procedures prevent injury or ill health, or reduce sickness absence. It reaffirmed the view that, if indicated, pre-placement examinations should be job specific.[2]

Health screening prior to job transfers

Health screening is often performed for employees prior to job transfers or job reassignment, especially in large multinational organizations. In cases of posting overseas for a prolonged period, the employee may be accompanied by their family, and therefore the examination can also be offered to accompanying family members (often for health insurance purposes or where the employer has responsibility for healthcare costs of the individual and the family) (see Chapter 17).

Health surveillance

The periodic clinical and physiological assessment of workers for exposure to workplace hazards[3] or for monitoring general health status forms an integral part of OH practice. For the prevention of work-related illness, emphasis should be on the former.

Biological monitoring and biological effect monitoring

Biological monitoring and biological effect monitoring are procedures used as part of screening in OH practice.[4] Biological monitoring screens for exposure, and biological effects monitoring attempts to detect early effects. As in other forms of screening, the principle is to detect adverse exposure or early alterations in biochemical parameters following workplace exposures, and then to take appropriate preventive measures to prevent the onset of overt health effects or clinical disease.

Biological monitoring involves the analysis of biological samples (urine, blood, or breath) for the presence of the chemical to which the individual worker is exposed, or for a metabolite. Examples amenable to monitoring are lead and mercury, and organic solvents such as trichloroethylene and xylene. Metabolites of organic solvents that can be detected in urine samples are trichloroacetic acid for trichloroethylene and 1,1,1,-trichloroethane, and mandelic acid for styrene. Some metabolites are non-specific and can result from several different exposures, both occupational and non-occupational (e.g. hippuric acid in the urine can occur from benzoate in foods or from occupational exposure to toluene). Other metabolites are more specific (e.g. methyl-hippuric acid in urine following exposure to xylene).

Biological effect monitoring attempts to detect changes in one or more biochemical parameters as an early effect of occupational exposure. Examples are the detection of elevated free erythrocyte protoporphyrin level in blood among those exposed to inorganic lead, and depression of serum cholinesterase in workers exposed to organophosphates. Tests such as the detection of DNA adducts in biological samples for exposure to carcinogens[5] and markers of oxidative stress in workers exposed to pesticides[6] are available, but are not indicated for routine biological effect monitoring.

Specific screening tests

In many countries, there are national regulations that stipulate pre-placement and periodic medical examination for specific occupational groups, or persons exposed to specific hazards at work (e.g. workers exposed to inorganic lead). A variety of laboratory and clinical investigations may be used for screening of individuals exposed to specific hazards. Examples include the following:

• *Exposure to noise*: audiometric screening is required under noise regulations in many countries. (See Chapter 31.) Noise surveys to determine and reduce sources of excessive noise should have precedence over audiometry as a means for effective prevention.

• *Exposure to hand-transmitted vibration*: UK legislation and guidance on screening for hand–arm vibration syndrome requires an initial screening questionnaire for all workers before they start work involving exposure to vibration, and an annual screening questionnaire for surveillance of exposed workers. Different tiers of screening are required for those reporting symptoms. (See Chapter 18.)

• *Lung function tests*: spirometry, serial peak flow readings, and other tests of lung function are considered in workers exposed to the risk of obstructive or restrictive lung disease. Some of these tests are also used for diagnostic purposes (e.g. serial peak flow rates for occupational asthma), or for following up the efficacy of treatment or prevention. (See Chapter 27.)

• *Vision screening*: in the UK, workers who regularly use computers and other display screen equipment in the course of their work are entitled to vision testing. (See Chapter 30.)

• *Tests of liver or renal function*: attempts have been made to explore the use of bile acid clearance to indicate acute and chronic liver damage from chemicals but this marker remains experimental. Serum transaminases and transferases are elevated in liver disease but they are not specific enough for use as a screening tool. Similarly, there is no good indication for the use of indices of renal function, such as blood urea and electrolytes, for occupational health screening. (See Chapters 33 and 36.)

• *Other specific screening procedures*: such as periodic chest X-rays for exposure to fibrogenic dusts, urinary screening for microscopic haematuria and detection of malignant cells in those exposed to bladder carcinogens, and examination of the skin in workers exposed to mineral oils are covered in greater detail elsewhere.[7]

Executive health screening

A Cochrane review of general health checks among adults for reducing morbidity and mortality from disease concluded that such checks did not reduce morbidity or morbidity, and are unlikely to be beneficial.[8]

However, personnel in managerial and senior posts in an organization are sometimes subjected to 'executive health screening'. The screening may involve determination of biochemical profiles, exercise electrocardiograms (ECGs), scans, and endoscopies. These periodic, multiphasic medical examinations may be advocated by some patients and their physicians with the rationale that early detection of disease in highly paid executives has economic benefit to the company; but there is only anecdotal evidence to support this.[9,10]

As executive medicals are usually offered on a voluntary basis, the tendency would be for the highly motivated and health conscious to participate in the examination. In contrast to these 'worried well', those who are less concerned with their personal health (and who may have a greater need for counselling and lifestyle interventions), seldom participate in screening. Hence, any illness that may be present in this latter group remains undetected. This paradoxical phenomenon has been called the 'inverse care law'.[11] In time, executive health screening may well have a benefit with regard to the individual or to the organization as a return on investment,[12] but for the moment they are viewed as a 'perk' for selected groups within an organization.

Genetic screening

Several markers have been developed that attempt to detect those at higher risk of disease following specific exposure. Examples are alpha-1-antitrypsin deficiency as an indicator of increased risk of emphysema in those exposed to cadmium, and human leucocyte antigen (HLA) gene markers, specifically HLA-DPB1, as a factor associated with the development of chronic beryllium disease.[13] There is no indication that these methods are sufficiently well developed to warrant their routine use in OH practice. There are also ethical constraints over the use of such tests.

In regard to other screening for susceptibility, the determination of atopic status for workers who may be exposed to asthmagens, for example, is of limited use for screening in OH. Since atopy in the general population is common, this would result in exclusion of a significant proportion of job applicants.

Screening for drugs and alcohol

In OH practice, this is best considered in the context of a clear organizational policy on the consequences of a positive result, on whether testing is voluntary or mandatory, and whether it should apply to all levels of staff regardless of seniority (see also Chapter 14).

Theoretical and practical issues in screening

Characteristics of a screening test

Wilson and Jungner suggested several criteria which screening should meet. These relate to the condition to be screened, and the test to be used for screening (Table 6.1). The principles are applicable to screening for occupational as well as non-occupational diseases. With the advent of new screening tools, these criteria have been reviewed.[14] However, they remain applicable, especially for OH where there are limited advances in procedures for effective screening.

Table 6.1 Characteristics of diseases and tests that are appropriate for screening

Disease	Screening test

Clinically important:
    Significant morbidity/mortality
    Prevalent
	Acceptable
	Safe
	Sensitive

Has recognizable latent stage	Specific Easily done
Amenable to treatment	Relatively cheap

Sensitivity, specificity, and predictive value of a screening test

The *sensitivity* of a test is its ability to detect those with the condition being tested. A test with 100% sensitivity will produce a positive test result for everyone affected by the condition. Thus, it will not produce any false-negative results.

The *specificity* of a test is its ability to detect those who do not have the condition for which testing is being done. A test with 100% specificity will produce a negative result for everyone not affected by the condition. Thus, it will not produce any false-positive results.

No test is 100% sensitive and 100% specific. The likelihood of anyone with a positive test result actually having the disease, the *positive predictive value* (PPV) of the test, depends on the prevalence of the disease in the population being tested. While sensitivity and specificity are often described as constant characteristics of any screening test, the PPV of a test will vary with the population in which the test is being applied. If the disease prevalence is low in the population tested, there will be a greater likelihood of false-positive results, so that a given positive test has a low PPV.

The *negative predictive value* (NPV) of a test is the probability that a person is disease free in the presence of a negative screening test result. This value will also be affected by the disease prevalence in the population that is tested. For a rare disease, the NPV is expected to be high, as virtually all who are screened will be disease free. Besides the disease prevalence, the sensitivity and specificity of the test will also affect the predictive values.

In summary (see Table 6.2):

◆ *Sensitivity* = $a/(a + c) \times 100\%$

is the probability of a positive test in people with the disease.

Table 6.2 Sensitivity, specificity, and predictive value of a screening test

Test result	Disease or condition	
	Present (+)	**Absent (−)**
Positive (+)	a	b
Negative (−)	c	d

a = true positive, b = false positive, c = false negative, d = true negative.

- *Specificity = d/(b + d) × 100%*

  is the probability of a negative test in people without the disease.

- *PPV = a/(a + b) × 100%*

  is the probability of having the disease when the test is positive.

- *NPV = d/(c + d) × 100%*

  is the probability of not having the disease when the test is negative.

The relationship between disease prevalence, sensitivity, specificity, and predictive value is shown in the worked example in Table 6.3, where:

- PPV increases with increasing disease prevalence

- PPV increases with increasing sensitivity of the screening test

- PPV decreases for a rare disease, but increases for a common disease with increasing specificity of the screening test.

A similar example can also be worked out for NPV.

Likelihood ratios

Likelihood ratios (LRs) of tests indicate how many times more likely patients with a disease are to have that particular result, compared to those without the disease. It is the ratio of the probabilities of specific test results among the diseased to those who are disease free.

A test with a LR above 1 indicates that it is associated with presence of the disease. Conversely, a test with a LR below 1 is associated with absence of the disease. As a rule of thumb, a test with a LR of 10 or more provides good evidence to indicate the presence of disease, while a test with a LR of less than 0.1 gives a good indication to rule out the disease.

Receiver operating characteristic curves

There are often practical difficulties in the definition of a positive or negative screening result. If the screening test result is a variable measured on a continuous scale, the cut-off point for a positive result can be varied to produce a test with either high sensitivity and low specificity, or high specificity and low sensitivity. An important question is, 'How does one determine an appropriate cut-off point for the screening test?'

One method is to express these values of the test in a visual form as a receiver operating characteristic (ROC) curve. In a ROC curve, the vertical axis of such a plot is the sensitivity of the test, while the horizontal axis is (1 − specificity). The individual points represent the sensitivity and specificity obtained using different cut-off values, and the optimal cut-off value for the screening test is the point that is furthest from the 45° diagonal.

As an example: an occupational physician needs to determine an effective cut-off point for the blood level of chemical X to screen workers with significant exposure and a high likelihood of developing toxic effects. They conduct a study and measure the blood concentration in workers who either have or do not exhibit clinically significant toxicity to chemical X. From these data (Table 6.4), a ROC curve can be plotted (Figure 6.1).

Table 6.3 How disease prevalence, sensitivity, and specificity of a screening test affect its positive predictive value. Consider screening tests for two diseases in a population of 1000 people: let a = true positive, b = false positive, and PPV = a/(a + b)

	True + ve (a)	False + ve (b)	PPV [a/(a + b)]
Rare disease (20 cases in 1000)			
Sensitivity low (20%)	4		
Specificity low (20%)		196	2.0%
Specificity 50%		490	0.8%
Specificity high (80%)		784	0.5%
Sensitivity high (80%)	16		
Specificity low (20%)		196	7.5%
Specificity 50%		490	3.2%
Specificity high (80%)		784	2.0%
Sensitivity 50% and specificity 50%	10	490	2.0%
Specificity low (20%)		196	
Sensitivity low (20%)	4		2.0%
Sensitivity 50%	10		4.9%
Sensitivity high (80%)	16		7.5%
Specificity high (80%)		784	
Sensitivity low (20%)	4		0.5%
Sensitivity 50%	10		1.3%
Sensitivity high (80%)	16		2.0%
Common disease (400 cases in 1000)			
Sensitivity low (20%)	80		
Specificity low (20%)		480	14.3%
Specificity 50%		300	21.1%
Specificity high (80%)		120	40.0%
Sensitivity high (80%)	320		
Specificity low (20%)		480	40.0%
Specificity 50%		300	51.6%
Specificity high (80%)		120	72.7%
Sensitivity 50% and specificity 50%	200	300	40.0%
Specificity low (20%)		480	
Sensitivity low (20%)	80		14.3%
Sensitivity 50%	200		29.4%
Sensitivity high (80%)	320		40.0%
Specificity high (80%)		120	
Sensitivity low (20%)	80		40.0%
Sensitivity 50%	200		62.5%
Sensitivity high (80%)	320		72.7%

Table 6.4 Blood concentration of chemical X, presence of clinically significant toxicity, and sensitivity and false-positive rate of a screening test at different cut-off points

Blood concentration of chemical X	Sensitivity	1 – specificity (false positive)
21.5	0.941	0.550
24.0	0.882	0.500
27.5	0.882	0.300
32.5	0.765	0.200
37.5	0.765	0.150
41.0	0.647	0.150
43.5	0.588	0.150
46.5	0.412	0.100
49.0	0.412	0.050
52.5	0.294	0.050
55.5	0.235	0.050
57.0	0.176	0.050
59.0	0.059	0.050
61.0	0.000	0.000

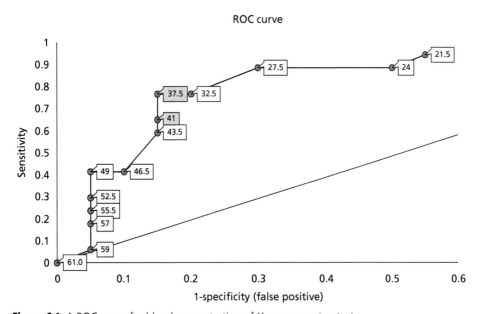

Figure 6.1 A ROC curve for blood concentration of X as a screening test.

Based on the table and the curve:

- If a blood concentration of 41 is adopted as a cut-off point, the test would have a sensitivity of 65%, and a 15% false-positive rate.
- If a blood concentration of 37.5 is adopted as a cut-off point, the sensitivity is increased to 76%, while the false-positive rate remains at 15%

This method to determine the most appropriate cut-off point is not applicable for a test with a dichotomous outcome. The method also assumes an equal weight (or value, or importance) for sensitivity and specificity. An equal weight given to sensitivity and specificity may not necessarily be desirable, depending on the nature and natural history of the disease, and also the consequences of false-positive and false-negative results.

Practical and ethical aspects of screening

Scope of the screening examination

Screening procedures could include symptom review, clinical assessment, medical examination, and special investigations. The physical examination is unlikely to reveal significant abnormalities in an apparently healthy person. A wide range of ancillary tests and laboratory investigations are available to screen for health disorders such as vascular, neoplastic, metabolic, haematological, ophthalmological, otological, and mental disorders (and substance abuse), and infectious diseases (see 'Useful websites'). Two useful website addresses for guidance are from the US Preventive Services Task Force[15] and the Canadian Task Force on Preventive Health Care.[16]

Frequency of examination

The frequency of screening and whether the tests are performed on specific occasions will depend on the conditions to be detected, the resources available, and on presenting opportunities. For situations where screening can be effective, the recommended frequency of examination varies with age and the natural history of the disease. Commonly, frequency of examination varies from annually to once every 3–5 years.

In occupational asthma, if sensitization to an inhaled agent in the workplace occurs, it is more likely in the early stages of employment and exposure. Hence, the UK Health and Safety Executive advice on lung function testing for workers exposed to asthmagens puts emphasis on greater frequency of screening during initial employment. For diseases with a long latent period between first exposure and subsequent health effects, there are no clinical reasons for advocating screening in the earlier years following initial exposure.

Advantages and disadvantages of health screening

Health screening may detect sentinel cases of disease in populations exposed to hazardous materials. The detection of these cases will signal the need for preventive measures. The principle behind instituting health screening is therefore appealing: detect disease early, and take preventive action. In practice, there are good examples where this is effective, for example, screening for cardiovascular risk factors followed by measures to reduce risk. There are also examples where the benefits of screening are limited. Periodic chest X-rays for exposure to fibrogenic dusts such as silica particles or asbestos fibres may enable earlier detection of pulmonary fibrosis, but there may be little that can be done to halt the progression of the disease.

Early detection of disease may produce an apparent gain in the duration of life between detection and death, although the mean age at death of those screened is not altered. All that screening does in these cases is to alert the screened individuals to the occurrence of disease, without necessarily affecting disease outcome. Earlier diagnosis as a result of screening can cause an improvement in survival time (interval from diagnosis to death), but this can be due to lead time and length time bias, instead of actual prolongation of life.[17] In any case, early detection is part of secondary prevention. Prevention of occupational disease through reduction of exposure (primary prevention) is preferable.

Adverse effects of screening can arise with the indiscriminate use of screening tests. A false-positive test result causes unnecessary anxiety and worry in the subject. A false-positive test often leads to further investigations, with their associated risk of morbidity and further expense. False-negative results can provide false reassurance and cause complacency. They may be viewed as an 'all clear' until the next round of screening and can even lead to the person ignoring future early warning symptoms.

For example, the exercise ECG (stress ECG), when used for screening coronary artery disease (CAD) in an apparently healthy general population, has a PPV of less than 30%.[18] Hence, seven of ten persons who are stress ECG positive are subjected to unnecessary and potentially harmful further investigations. Even in cases of suspected CAD, the PPV for stress ECG is only 51%.[19] In addition to causing anxiety, a false-positive stress ECG may also have negative consequences for occupational and insurance eligibility, or other leisure opportunities. While the introduction of coronary computed tomographic angiography has enabled the non-invasive evaluation of CAD, it could still have a false-positive rate of up to 35%.[20] Among symptomatic patients without known CAD, positive and negative predictive values have been reported as 85% and 92%, respectively.[21]

There is an evolving range of opinions on screening of asymptomatic workers in occupational groups. Various organizations and expert groups have recommended the stress ECG for job categories including airline pilots, firemen, police officers, bus and truck drivers, and railroad engineers. For athletes, there is a suggestion that stress ECG could be considered for younger (aged <45 years), asymptomatic individuals if they have multiple cardiovascular risk factors.[22] The American College of Cardiology and the American Heart Association[23] indicate that exercise testing in healthy asymptomatic persons is not recommended, but may be considered in occupations where public safety may be affected. For example, stress ECG testing may be indicated for applicants for a large goods or public service vehicles driving licence, if there is possible underlying cardiovascular disease.

The US Preventive Services Task Force also recommend against routine screening with stress ECG testing for asymptomatic adults.[24] A review of the published evidence on ECG screening of asymptomatic adults concluded that ECG abnormalities are associated with a risk of cardiovascular events, but 'the clinical implications of these findings are unclear'.[25] However, for people in certain occupations involving public safety, considerations other than benefit to the individual may influence the decision to perform screening.

Ethical considerations

There is a key difference between clinical consultation and health screening. In the clinical consultation, the patient approaches the doctor for advice or treatment for a health complaint and has to give consent to certain diagnostic procedures and therapy having been advised of some limitations or even possible adverse effects. In health screening, however, the doctor reviews an apparently healthy person for the possible presence of asymptomatic disease. In so doing, there must be a good understanding of the efficacy and safety of the screening tests, and patients should similarly be informed of the possible consequences of false-positive and false-negative results following screening.

A test procedure that is ethically justifiable on diagnostic grounds may not necessarily be applicable when used for screening asymptomatic people. Holland points out that there is a lack of evidence that some health screening procedures are beneficial.[26] The disadvantages of introducing anxiety and expense from health screening have been discussed earlier in this chapter. From a preventive perspective, the energy and expense of general health screening could perhaps be better diverted to promote measures to encourage proper diet, weight control, regular exercise, smoking cessation, moderation in alcohol consumption, and stress management, or control of workplace hazards. Modifications in lifestyle behaviour require motivation and effort on the part of the individual, whereas health screening is essentially a passive process, where an individual is seemingly reassured that all is well after a negative examination. This is perhaps the reason why general health screening has popular appeal.

Evaluation of screening programmes

A common error in evaluating the potential of a screening test is to adopt the sensitivity and specificity of the test when it is first evaluated in people with the disease. As the population considered for screening by OH practitioners consists mainly of asymptomatic persons who may or may not have disease, the application of findings of the screening test in a diseased population to the general population is not appropriate and could lead to erroneous conclusions about the usefulness of the test.

In evaluating screening programmes, the potential for bias should be considered. Different categories of possible bias are summarized in Table 6.5. Screening programmes should also be reviewed and audited periodically to ensure that the basis and procedures for such screening remain valid.

Table 6.5 Possible biases in the evaluation of screening programmes

Selection bias	Occurs when those who participate in screening programmes are volunteers. Such volunteers are generally more health conscious than those who do not participate in screening programmes
	As such, even without screening, these persons who volunteer for the screening test are more likely to have better health outcomes from their disease as compared with the general population or those who do not participate in the screening
Lead-time bias	The evaluation of the usefulness of screening examinations may sometimes be influenced by the apparent long survival of a patient (e.g. a patient with cancer) who is diagnosed early by screening
	This long survival in fact may only be a manifestation of *lead-time bias*, where screening brings forward the time of diagnosis and thus lengthens the disease knowledge time without actually prolonging life
Length bias	There is a tendency for screening to detect the less serious conditions. More rapidly advancing illnesses, by their nature, will only be present in the population for a relatively short time, and so miss being detected
	As more slowly progressing illnesses than aggressive conditions are found on screening, this also gives the erroneous impression that detecting these conditions early has improved survival

Key points

◆ Health screening is a useful tool in OH practice, but theoretical and practical issues should be considered before beginning such screening for any group of workers.

◆ Several distinct types of health screening, with different specific aims, can be identified. Screening for fitness to work can be done prior to job placement or transfers, whereas health surveillance is performed for workers to detect effects resulting from workplace exposure to hazards.

◆ General health screening may be used to promote health and influence positive health behaviours in a workforce.

◆ Legal requirements for screening will vary from country to country and will influence what is provided.

◆ Proper communication with the workforce, employer, and OH and safety professionals is essential for implementing successful health screening programmes.

References

1. **Whitaker S, Aw TC.** Audit of pre-employment assessments by occupational health departments in the National Health Service. *Occup Med* 1995;**45**:75–80.

2. **Mahmud N, Schonstein E, Schaafsma F, et al.** Cochrane review—pre-employment examinations for preventing injury and disease. *Cochrane Database Syst Rev* 2010;**8**:CD008881.

3. **Koh DSQ, Aw TC.** Surveillance in occupational health. *Occup Environ Med* 2003;**60**:705–10.

4. **Aw TC.** Biological monitoring. In: Gardiner KG, Harrington JM (eds), *Occupational Hygiene*, pp. 160–9. Oxford: Blackwell Publishing Ltd; 2005.

5. **Al Zabadi H, Ferrari L, Laurent A-M, et al.** Biomonitoring of complex occupational exposure to carcinogens: the case of sewage workers in Paris. *BMC Cancer* 2008;**8**:67.

6. **Astiz M, Arnal N, de Alaniz MJ, et al.** New markers for screening for pesticide exposure—oxidative stress biomarkers? *Env Toxicol Pharmacol* 2011;**32**:249–58.

7. **Aw TC.** Health surveillance. In: Sadhra SS, Rampal KG (eds), *Occupational Health: Risk Assessment and Management*, pp. 288–314. Oxford: Blackwell Science; 1999.

8. **Krogsbøll LT, Jørgensen KJ, Grønhøj Larsen C, Gøtzsche PC.** General health checks in adults for reducing morbidity and mortality from disease. *Cochrane Database Syst Rev* 2012;**10**:CD009009.

9. **O'Malley PG, Greenland P.** The annual physical: are physicians and patients telling us something? *Arch Intern Med* 2005;**165**:1333–4.

10. **Oboler SK, Prochazka AV, Gonzalez R, et al.** Public expectations and attitudes to annual physical examinations and testing. *Ann Intern Med* 2002; **136**:652–9.

11. **Hart JT.** The inverse care law. *Lancet* 1971;**1**:405–12.

12. **Komaroff AL.** Executive physicals: what's the ROI? *Harv Bus Rev* 2009;**87**:28.

13. **McCanlies EC, Ensey JS, Lefant JS Jr, et al.** The association between HLA-DPB1Glu69 and chronic beryllium disease and beryllium sensitization. *Am J Ind Med* 2004;**46**:95–103.

14. **Andermann A, Blancquaert I, Beauchamp S, et al.** Revisiting Wilson and Jungner in the genomic age: a review of screening criteria over the past 40 years. *Bull World Health Organ* 2008;**86**:s317–9.

15. **US Preventive Services Task Force.** The guide to clinical preventive services. Available at: https://www.uspreventiveservicestaskforce.org/BrowseRec/Index.

16. **Canadian Task Force on Preventive Health Care.** CTFPHC Guidelines. Available at: http://www.canadiantaskforce.ca/.

17. **George PJM.** Delays in the management of lung cancer. *Thorax* 1997;**52**:107–8.

18. **Petch MC.** Misleading exercise electrocardiograms. *Br Med J* 1987;**295**:620–1.

19. **Maffei E, Palumbo A, Martini C, et al.** Stress-ECG vs. CT coronary angiography for the diagnosis of coronary artery disease: a 'real-world' experience. *Radiol Med* 2010;**11**:354–67.

20. **Mowatt G, Cook JA, Hillis GS, et al.** 64-Slice computed tomography angiography in the diagnosis and assessment of coronary artery disease: systematic review and meta-analysis. *Heart* 2008;**94**:1386–93.

21. **Arbab-Zadeh A.** Stress testing and non-invasive coronary angiography in patients with suspected coronary artery disease: time for a new paradigm. *Heart Int* 2012;**7**:e2.

22. **Freeman J, Froelicher V, Ashley E.** The ageing athlete: screening prior to vigorous exertion in asymptomatic adults without known cardiovascular disease. *Br J Sports Med* 2009;**43**:696–701.

23. **American College of Cardiology/American Heart Association Task Force on Practice Guidelines.** ACC/AHA guidelines for exercise testing: executive summary. *Circulation* 1997;**96**:345–54.

24. **Agency for Healthcare Research and Quality.** The Guide to Clinical Preventive Services 2014 Recommendations of the U.S. Preventive Services Task Force. Available at: https://www.ahrq.gov/professionals/clinicians-providers/guidelines-recommendations/guide/index.html.

25. **Chou R, Arora B, Dana T, et al.** Screening asymptomatic adults with resting or exercise electrocardiography: a review of the evidence for the U.S. Preventive Services Task Force. *Ann Intern Med* 2011;**155**:375–85.

26. **Holland WW.** Screening: reasons to be cautious. *BMJ* 1993;**306**:1221–2.

Chapter 7

The older worker

Steven Nimmo

Introduction

According to Benjamin Franklin, there are only two certainties in life: death and taxes. One of the key messages of this chapter is that people are surviving until older ages, and will need to work longer and contribute more in tax to support themselves and others in retirement. One of the biggest challenges for occupational health (OH) professionals is helping to facilitate this.

Throughout the developed world, birth rates are falling and people are living longer, so populations are getting older. This is causing a substantial change in population demographics and an increase in the ratio of people traditionally regarded as 'retirement age' to those regarded as 'working age'. People are also living longer in retirement, further increasing the cost to society of supporting them. To maintain funding for pensions and other social benefits, the pattern of working life and the social and political structures that underpin it have to change to match the changing needs of society. In particular, people in the developed world must expect to work for longer, a change that has implications both for employees and employers. OH professionals have an important role to play so that older workers can be 'healthy, happy, and here' in the workplace for longer.

The demographic background

It is estimated that by 2050 the number of people aged over 60 in Europe will have doubled to 40% of the population. Populations in developing countries show a broad-based, rapidly tapering structure characterized by a high birth rate and a high infant mortality rate (Figure 7.1). However, the pattern in the developed world is characterized by falling birth rates and longer life expectancy.

European countries are also undergoing demographic change due to the large numbers of children born post World War II between the late 1940s and the mid 1960s (the 'baby boomers'). These individuals have produced fewer children than their parents and so as they age, there will be a relative decline in the proportion of people of working age supporting them economically (Figure 7.2). The 'age dependency ratio', that is, the number of people of retirement age compared to the number of people of working age, is likely to almost double from about 1:3 to about 2:3. This is the basis of the so-called pensions crisis. The mass immigration of younger workers since 2000 will not meet this challenge

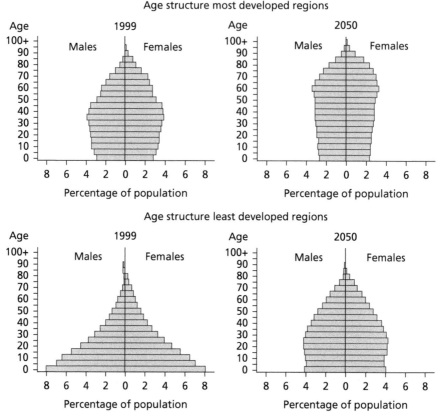

Figure 7.1 The changing age structure of developed and developing countries.

Reproduced with permission from Professor David Wegman, from the keynote speech, Society of Occupational Medicine, Annual Scientific Meeting, 2003. Source: data from United Nations, Department of Economic and Social Affairs, Population Division (2015). *World Population Ageing, 1999*. New York, US: United Nations. Copyright © 1999 United Nations.

entirely, especially for the UK, where the population density is already high. The Brexit vote to leave the European Union (EU) is likely to reduce free movement of workers. Young workers grow old, so the problem is postponed, not solved. There is therefore a need for workers to increase their lifetime contribution to the funding of pensions and other benefits. This means working longer, although not necessarily full-time or without work adjustments. It also means increasing opportunities for people who are under-represented in the current workforce, such as women and people with disabilities.

According to the Office for National Statistics in 2016, the UK population is projected to:

♦ increase by 3.6 million (5.5%), from an estimated 65.6 million in mid 2016 to 69.2 million in mid 2026:

  • England will grow more quickly than the other UK nations: 5.9% between mid 2016 and mid 2026, compared with 4.2% for Northern Ireland, 3.2% for Scotland, and 3.1% for Wales

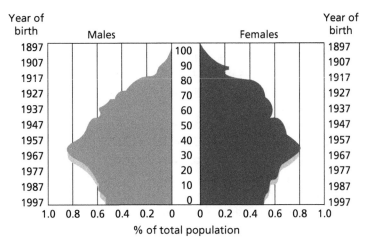

Figure 7.2 How Europe is ageing (based on 11 European member states).
Source: data from Eurostat, http://europa.eu.int/comm/eurostat/. Copyright © 2012 European Union.

- almost half (46%) of UK population growth will result from more births than deaths, with 54% resulting from net international migration
- pass 70 million by mid 2029 and be 72.9 million in mid 2041.

The rate of immigration is likely to change following the UK referendum vote to leave the EU in 2016 (Brexit), and the UK is likely to curtail free movement of EU citizens across its borders. The UK migration strategy may not be entirely clear before completion of Brexit negotiations in 2019. However, labour market gaps and government spending on public services to support the increasing population will create a need for more nurses, teachers, doctors, and other skilled workers.

Importing young people from abroad may offer a partial solution but this may produce a net drain on resources if they do not have the skills to enable them to contribute to the economy. Migrants are currently important for a number of UK industry sectors including agricultural labour and hospitality where it has been difficult to recruit indigenous workers. However, once migrants are settled, they tend to 'go native' and adopt the habits and lifestyle of the host country. They will also inevitably grow older. More new immigrants are then needed to plug the gaps and support them and the cycle is repeated.

For several decades, societal attitudes, consumer pressures, and legislation have all been driving business organizations towards becoming 'lean, mean, and young'. The skills and experience of older workers have been largely sidelined by the movement of information away from personal experience, knowledge, and books, and into information technology systems. This has been driven by computerization, the global standardization of processes across industry, and by the need to reduce manufacturing process variability, all driven by consumer pressures for higher quality and reliability of goods, and services at reduced cost.

As the population ages, expectations and norms will need to change as will social institutions. In an increasingly competitive world, all age groups will need to provide for themselves and for one another, and for their own periods of low productivity and low earnings (e.g. pregnancy, sickness, and retirement). Concepts of 'rights' and 'entitlements' will have to evolve, as the UK's earning capacity in the world changes relative to the developing economies, primarily in China, and the Far East. However, the global picture is complex and China also has an ageing population. Economic competitiveness of the West with new emerging economies which have significantly younger age profiles, will require the UK workforce to 'work smarter', as 'working harder' may not be practicable as the working population ages.

It is clear that the current situation with a reducing number of younger people in work supporting a growing number of older people in retirement is not sustainable in the long term.

There are many barriers to older workers remaining in work including physical and psychosocial factors.[1] There is evidence that there is significant ageism and intergenerational exclusion of older workers in the workplace.[2] However, multicomponent interventions including adequate healthcare provision, coordination of services, and work adjustments have been shown to improve retention of older workers.

The United Kingdom

Historically, the state pension age in the UK has been 65 for men and 60 for women. The average life expectancy for men did not reach 65 until the 1950s so prior to this most men did not live long enough to reach retirement age. Following the Turner report in 2006, state pension age will steadily rise to 68 for both men and women over the next four decades.[3] Under current plans, people born between 1970 and 1978 will be unable to claim the state pension until the age of 68. The age at which women can claim the state pension will rise from 60 to 65 by November 2018. Between October 2018 and October 2020, both men and women's state pension age will rise to 66 and between 2026 and 2028, it will rise to 67.

Recognizing the impact of the ageing workforce, the British Medical Association occupational medicine committee published a report summarizing the issues in 2016.[4] The Faculty of Occupational Medicine has also highlighted the issues in the UK in a position paper on age and employment.[5] See Box 7.1.

This is probably an unduly pessimistic interpretation. In the UK, Employment and Support Allowance (disability benefit) is more generous than Job Seekers Allowance (unemployment benefit) and it is well documented that in places where traditional industries, such as steel making and coal mining, have closed down, redundant workers often seek sickness certification rather than claim less lucrative unemployment benefits.

Box 7.1 Age and employment

'The majority of non-working men [in the UK] aged between 50 and 65 are economic-ally inactive (i.e. retired, sick or caring for others and unavailable for work) rather than unemployed (one in ten of this non-working age group). The number of people over 50 and on incapacity benefit has trebled in the last 20 years. Of those not seeking work, approximately half are on sickness or disability benefit (over 1 million people) and nearly half a million, mainly women, are full time carers. Individuals in this age group are more likely to experience low self-esteem, ill health and poverty. Thirty-seven per cent of 55–64 year olds say they have a limiting long-standing illness. Depression, so-cial exclusion, and marital problems are also more common in this age group. Most of those not working have been out of employment for long periods, many having pre-viously been in long standing jobs. Involvement in other activities (such as charitable work) is also declining in this age group.'

Source: data from Faculty of Occupational Medicine. (2004) *Position Paper on Age and Employment, 2004.* London, UK: Faculty of Occupational Medicine. Copyright © 2004 Faculty of Occupational Medicine.

General age-associated changes

Ageing

Ageing in the biological sense refers to loss of adaptability over time. As we age, we be-come less able to respond to challenges from our external and internal environments. Homoeostatic responses become less sensitive, less effective, and less well sustained. For most people, loss of adaptability may not be obvious until very late in life, as we live in physically non-challenging environments that rarely bring individuals to the limit of their functional capacity. However, as they grow older, most people go about their work and daily life with diminishing functional reserves.

The exact cause of cellular ageing is unclear but telomere shortening and DNA damage appear to underlie the process. The loss of adaptability that characterizes ageing is due to the accumulation of unrepaired and partially repaired damage to body systems.

In humans, the first age-related changes become apparent at about the age of 12 years when cell mortality rates start to increase, and is then a continuous, lifelong process. It is not a process that starts around the age of retirement. Indeed, determinants of disease and disability in later life can often be identified in childhood and even *in utero*.

Differences between younger and older people

Comparing younger people with older people[6] can be deceptive because differences be-tween these groups also arise through processes other than ageing (Table 7.1).

Table 7.1 Differences between young and old

Non-ageing	True ageing
Selective survival	*Primary*:
Cohort effects	Intrinsic
Differential challenge	Extrinsic
	Secondary:
	Individual adaptation
	Specific adaptation

Some differences occur, not because older people have changed as a result of ageing, but because they have always been different from the younger people to whom they are being compared.

Selective survival is the result of people with better genetics, better social environment, or healthier lifestyles, surviving longer.

Cohort effects are the differences between generations of people born at different times and therefore exposed to different influences and experiences, particularly early in life. Cohort differences can be considerable. A major part of what may appear in cross-sectional studies to be age-associated change in some types of psychological functioning is due to cultural, especially educational, differences between generations.[7] Although most prominent in psychological function (which may reflect education and experience in childhood) cohort effects also contribute to age-associated variation in physical variables such as height, serum lipids, and obesity. Cohort comparisons reflect differences between generations in their lifestyle and behaviour as well as in changes in physical environment.

Differential challenge. Adaptability may also be affected by offering different challenges at different ages. Challenges for older people may be more severe than those for younger people, and the differences in outcome may then be attributed to the effects of ageing.

It may be difficult to distinguish the effects of pathology from the effects of 'true' ageing, and in scientific terms the distinction is meaningless. True ageing refers to the ways in which individuals change over time. Some of the processes involved may be labelled as diseases and some as senescence.

Primary ageing is loss of adaptability due to the effects of processes in the tissues of the body. These processes are the product of interactions between *extrinsic* (environmental and lifestyle) and *intrinsic* (largely genetic) factors. Physical exercise, for example, affects a wide range of body systems. Healthy eating is important in ageing through dietary deficiencies and intake of unhealthy foods. Other dietary factors are also probably involved in ageing, for example, due to free radicals (highly reactive oxygen molecules) that may damage cellular components including DNA.

Secondary ageing refers to adaptations due to natural selection that counter the effects of ageing. At the individual level, secondary ageing is most obvious in terms of psychological and behavioural function. Mildly obsessional behaviour (e.g. inflexible routines and list writing) to compensate for short-term memory loss is a common and successful adaptation. Older workers may develop apparently idiosyncratic ways of carrying out familiar tasks, for example, to accommodate a painful joint.

Social factors are also important. One of the most significant correlates of healthy ageing is higher educational attainment. This may be due to the health benefits of relative affluence and being in occupations that are less physically challenging. Educational level is also important for the ability to be aware of medical advances and to understand implications for prevention and treatment. Social class effects on health and disability are highly complex. There are also subtle psychosocial and work-related determinants of health in middle age and later life. People in lower-status jobs may have less job control and less job reward, and this may lead to 'stress' with chronic arousal, associated with changes in endocrine and immune function. These may have adverse effects on susceptibility to illness and disability, including risk of cardiovascular disease.[8]

The effects of ageing also depend on baseline function. Women on average start with less muscle than men and are more likely to become less mobile and less strong in later life. The same applies to bone density, and to the higher rates of fractures in older women, although women also experience a higher rate of bone loss than men with ageing. Two important determinants of how quickly declining brain function, for example, as a result of Alzheimer-type dementia, becomes apparent, are the intelligence and educational level of the individual. The better the pre-morbid brain function, the longer it can compensate for progressive damage.

Because people start from different baselines, inherit different genes, and live different lives, they age at different rates and in different ways. There may therefore be significant differences between apparent biological and chronological age in different cohorts. Although we all deteriorate with age, some people in their 80s will function better than some people in their 30s. It is therefore inaccurate and unscientific to make judgements about individuals' capabilities purely on the basis of their chronological age.

Increasing frailty is a well-recognized feature of ageing and frailty 'symptoms' are relatively common in workers aged 50–65.[9] The frailty 'phenotype' is a good predictor of adverse health events and work problems including accidents, sickness absence and worklessness. Struggling with work demands and slow walking speed are also associated with frailty. Frailty, and 'pre-frailty', are therefore a potential target for workplace interventions.

Is the pattern of ageing changing?

Data from the US and the UK indicate that over the last few decades people have been living longer on average and that the prevalence of disability in later life has been falling. People are therefore living longer and are healthier for longer in retirement.[10] This may be partly due to the adoption of healthier lifestyles and better nutrition, and partly due to better medical care, and the less challenging environments in which most people live and work. But there are other factors that have caused a decline in morbidity, especially cardiovascular disease. In particular, reductions in cigarette smoking and control of urban and industrial air pollution have reduced the prevalence of cardiovascular and pulmonary disease in the last three decades. Less reassuringly, British data suggest that social class differences in mortality and morbidity have been widening. The reasons for this are complex, and include changes in the composition of the various social classes, but also include failure of some of the population to benefit as much as others from social and medical advances.

There are signs that the epidemic of cardiovascular disease has peaked, although the incidence may still be rising in some population groups, notably immigrants from the Indian subcontinent. Rates of cardiovascular disease in Scotland also remain relatively high. If the improvements in the patterns of disability in older people are sustained, this would improve the prospects of people working longer, and living long enough to enjoy an active period of retirement.

Age-associated changes in function

Physical activity

Sarcopenia is the loss of muscle mass with age and there is a 30% decline in both sexes from the third to the eighth decades. There is physiological muscle atrophy with predominantly a reduction in type II fibres and loss of cross-sectional fibre area, reducing the force of contraction. Because women start life with lower muscle mass than men they are more likely to suffer from limitation in muscle strength in later life.[11] In addition to muscular strength and endurance, joint flexibility also declines with age. Changes in the structure of collagen fibres also reduce joint elasticity. There is some evidence that this can be ameliorated by 'warm-up' exercises.

Endurance—the ability to maintain high levels of physical activity over prolonged periods—is limited by muscular power and exercise tolerance, and also by pulmonary and cardiac function. All of these tend to decline with age and limits on exercise capacity are usually muscular or cardiac in origin.

Older workers in physically strenuous jobs may be working closer to their physical limits than younger workers, especially when the work is externally paced, and they may become more easily fatigued. Older workers may cope with heavy physical exertion as long as the work is interspersed with recovery periods of sufficient frequency and duration. But they may find the demands of continuous, fast-paced lighter work more difficult to sustain.[12] There is evidence that a mismatch between physical job demands and physical capabilities increases the risk of injury in older workers. Older people in jobs with high work demands with a higher need for recovery are relatively more likely to be planning to retire earlier.

Part of the age-associated loss of muscular function is due to lower levels of exercise in older age groups. Training can recover some of the loss of function by increasing muscle bulk, as well as improving muscle function and endurance.

Hearing

Some age-associated loss of sensitivity to higher frequencies (presbycusis) is virtually universal. However, some hearing loss may be due to chronic noise exposure.[13] People who have worked in noisy industries for many years with inadequate hearing protection or those with noise exposure in the armed forces frequently have occupationally induced hearing loss from their mid-50s onwards. High frequencies are less important in the comprehension of speech but before the process becomes sufficiently severe to produce overt hearing loss, it can result in slower 'decoding' of speech. This in turn can produce de facto functional cognitive impairment due to slowing of processing and the missing of some information.[14] In the workplace, this effect may be compounded by high ambient background noise levels.

Sufferers lose the ability to accurately distinguish soft consonants, notably 'b', 'd', 't', 'p', and 's' sounds. They may mishear words and have difficulty in following one voice in conversation. The natural reaction when talking to someone with hearing loss is to speak louder. However, the cochlea may show a disproportionate response to the increase in volume known as 'recruitment', and loud sounds can become more distorted. In some working environments, loss of accurate understanding of verbal instructions will have implications for safety and efficiency. Some individuals can compensate for hearing loss by lip-reading, and colleagues can help by making use of gestures and facial expressions. In some hazardous working environments, use of visual signals and other safe systems of work can improve safety. A wide range of adaptive technologies now exist to support the hearing impaired worker (see Chapter 31).

Up to a third of older people suffer from tinnitus, of which the commonest cause is occupational noise-induced hearing loss. Most people manage to accommodate to tinnitus but for others it can become very intrusive and distressing. There are some effective treatments including psychological therapies and tinnitus masks.

Vision

There are age-associated changes in visual perception, due to both peripheral and central factors. With increasing age, the lens becomes less elastic and the intrinsic muscles weaker, so that accommodation for near vision becomes limited. Hence the increasing need for reading glasses with increasing age. The lens and vitreous of the eye become less transparent and may acquire a yellowish tinge that can interfere with colour perception. This may have consequences for workers who require normal colour vision. Due to the loss of transparency, and also because of changes in the retina, the older eye requires higher light intensities and greater contrast in print for accurate reading. Cataracts become more common, reducing visual acuity and also scattering incoming light, causing dazzle. This may be particularly significant for night driving at work.

Also relevant to driving safety is a tendency for the functional visual field to contract, so that stimuli in the peripheral vision may not be noticed, even though formal testing of the visual fields shows no defect.[15] This is thought to be one factor in the increase with age in road traffic collisions at road intersections and it may represent some form of central sensory inattention.

Macular degeneration is more common in the older worker and is the commonest cause of severe irreversible vision loss in the over 60s. There are now treatments available that can reduce loss of vision and slow progression of the disease. Modifications to computer keyboards and display screen equipment, and scanning cameras to assist in reading may be helpful (see Chapter 30).

Touch and proprioception

Dexterity and sensation may deteriorate with age, especially if chronic exposure to trauma leads to thickening of the skin and subcutaneous tissues of the hands. The risk of falls increases in both sexes after the age of 65. The risk is higher at all ages in women, who also show a bimodal risk with an earlier transitory peak around the age of 50.[16] Although the risk of falls is related to muscle strength and joint stiffness, there also seems to be a general age-associated impairment of global proprioception.

Joint proprioception, as tested by standard clinical examination (joint position sense or the Romberg test, for example), is unlikely to be objectively impaired in the absence of specifically diagnosable conditions, such as vitamin B12 deficiency. Global proprioception, in the sense of accurate awareness of the body's position, orientation, and movement in space, is the product of continuous integration of input from the eyes, semicircular canals, and a range of peripheral proprioceptors, especially in cervical joints, the feet, and the Achilles tendons. As a consequence of degeneration in cervical joints and peripheral nerves, the information from these various sources may be attenuated or delayed in the central nervous system.

Cognitive function

The prevalence of dementia worldwide is around 46 million, with the number expected to reach 75 million by 2030 and 130 million by 2050. The prevalence of dementia in the UK is around 850,000, with numbers set to rise to over 1 million by 2025 and 2 million by 2050. Dementia is relatively uncommon under the age of 70, although there are some types with earlier onset, for example, Lewy Body dementia.

Mild cognitive impairment affects 5–20% of the over 65s. It affects memory, cognition, language, attention, and visual depth perception. By definition, it does not have a substantial effect on activities of daily living; however, it may be considered to be a 'pre-dementia' state. About 10–15% of individuals with mild cognitive impairment progress to dementia per year. There is little research on the effect of mild cognitive impairment on work; however, it may have some effect in occupations requiring a high degree of cognitive function.

There are differences in cognitive function between older and younger people that may need to be considered in matching older workers to occupational tasks. Some of the apparent cognitive differences may be due to cohort effects rather than ageing. Cohort effects should be taken into account when designing training programmes for older workers with lower levels of educational attainment.

The various factors that make up human intelligence fall between the 'crystalline' and the 'fluid'. Crystalline intelligence solves problems by applying learned strategies or known paradigms. Fluid intelligence solves problems by innovation and analysis from first principles. As people grow older, they tend to rely more on crystalline than fluid processes. As long as the paradigm is appropriate, crystalline intelligence can be an effective problem-solving strategy. However, it may fail in dealing with novel situations that require original thinking.

The dominant problem in mental ageing is impaired memory. It is an oversimplification to think of memory as consisting of an immediate working memory linked to a long-term memory. Some information passes from working memory to long-term memory and can be retrieved later. Both types may show deterioration with age although difficulties with short-term memory tend to be more obvious. In age-related memory decline, and in the early stages of Alzheimer-type dementia, a dominant feature is an apparent problem with the link between short-term and long-term memory, so that new material is not written into long-term storage or cannot be retrieved from storage. This difficulty is commonly mislabelled as a defect in short-term memory, even though the ability to remember telephone numbers long enough to dial them may still be normal.

Employers of older workers should encourage the use of memory-supporting strategies: list-writing, notice boards, and electronic prompters, for example. Indeed, the value of checklists for workers of all ages is formally recognized for safety critical workers such as airline pilots and surgeons.

Ageing is also associated with a slowing of mental processing and a reduction in channel capacity—the capacity to process several different streams of data simultaneously—that is, multitasking. Decisions may take longer and mistakes may be made in complex multitasking situations. These processes are thought to contribute to the rise in accident rates among older car drivers, for example.

Specific age-associated system changes and pathology

Cardiovascular function

There are age-associated changes in the structure and function of the cardiovascular system. The prevalence of cardiovascular diseases increases with age and cardiovascular diseases remain a leading cause of death, disability, and premature retirement.

The heart

With ageing, cardiac muscle becomes stiffer, so that diastolic filling may be impaired.[17] Contraction time is lengthened and ventricular relaxation is delayed, also contributing to diastolic dysfunction. There is a reduction in mechanical and contractile efficiency. Stroke volume falls, resulting in reduced cardiac output. In response to exercise, cardiac output rises less through increasing heart rate and more by increasing stroke volume, compared to a younger heart. VO_2 max (a measure of oxygen carrying capacity) remains well preserved up to the age of 55 in men and then begins to decline. Cardiac reserve falls with age, even in the absence of ischaemic heart disease (IHD) or ventricular dysfunction.

IHD is common after middle age, especially in men. Risk factors include hypertension, smoking, dyslipidaemia, diabetes, obesity, and lack of exercise. Risk of IHD can be reduced by modification of risk factors at any age and there is no justification for excluding older people from prevention or treatment. For reasons that remain unclear, angina may be a less prominent symptom in older people. In later life, limited cardiac output due to IHD or other causes may present as muscular fatigue on exertion rather than as chest pain or dyspnoea.

Effective treatments for acute coronary syndrome and myocardial infarction including angioplasty and coronary artery stents have reduced long-term morbidity and levels of disability. People are more likely to return to work and are more likely to retain good cardiac function.

Blood pressure

Systolic blood pressure tends to rise with age. High blood pressure is associated with an increased risk of vascular disease, especially stroke and IHD. There are changes in vascular matrix composition and increased elastolytic and collagenolytic activity. This leads to thickening and stiffening of the arterial wall and increased vascular tone and afterload. This in turn can lead to left ventricular hypertrophy as the left ventricle has to work harder to pump blood into the stiffer arterial system.

Epidemiological evidence suggests that the rise of blood pressure with age is largely due to extrinsic factors including obesity. As a risk factor for vascular disease, hypertension interacts with other risk factors such as cigarette smoking, and the combination of smoking, hypertension, and diabetes is particularly problematic. The benefits of treatment are at least as great for older people as for younger people. For older people, first-line drug treatment includes calcium channel blockers and diuretics. Other options include angiotensin-converting enzyme inhibitors and alpha blockers. The difference in treatment algorithms for younger and older people probably reflects the difference in aetiological factors.

Cerebrovascular disease

Epidemiological data suggest that cerebrovascular disease has been reducing in incidence for several decades in Western countries. However, other conditions may mimic stroke including hypoglycaemia in type 1 diabetics. An epileptic seizure may be mistaken for a stroke or transient ischaemic attack (TIA). A cerebral tumour presenting as a stroke-like syndrome will usually come to light in the course of subsequent assessment, as will emboli from atrial fibrillation or valvular heart disease.

Cerebrovascular disease is also a cause of dementia either through the step-wise accumulation of small strokes, or by the less well understood 'small vessel disease' thought to underlie the periventricular white matter damage (leucoaraiosis) seen on magnetic resonance imaging of the brain. TIAs are often recurrent and may imply a high risk of stroke requiring anticoagulation as preventive treatment. They are characterized by focal neurological deficit lasting less than 24 hours. Other conditions may mimic TIA, including vasovagal syncope, cardiac arrhythmia, and transient global amnesia.

Peripheral vascular disease shares risk factors with other forms of vascular disease but smoking and diabetes are especially important. The typical presentation is intermittent claudication, that is, pain in the calves induced by walking and resolving rapidly with rest. Treatment may include angioplasty, stenting or arterial bypass surgery.

Respiratory system

There is impaired gas exchange in the lung and a decrease in vital capacity. A decline in the elasticity of the bony thorax and loss of muscle mass affects muscles of respiration. The alveolar surface area for gas exchange decreases. There is also loss of elastic support of the airways leading to increased collapsibility. Closing capacity increases to encroach on tidal volume, which can lead to a ventilation/perfusion mismatch. Central nervous system responsiveness to hypoxia and hypercapnoea also reduces. These factors all combine leading to declining lung function with increasing age.

The kidney

The mass of the kidney peaks in the fourth decade and then reduces by 25% by the ninth decade. This is primarily cortical with relative sparing of the medullary tissue. There is reduced surface area for filtration and a reduction in renal blood flow of 10% per decade after the age of 30. A reduction in the number of glomeruli and an increase in glomerular and vascular sclerosis is accompanied by increasing tubular atrophy and fibrosis. This leads to a reduction in glomerular filtration rate. The kidney also becomes more susceptible to acute ischaemia. Renal excretion of drugs is impaired which can be a significant problem in older people.

Nervous system

Brain mass, predominantly grey matter, reduces by 30% by the age of 80. There is a reduction in motor, sensory, and autonomic fibres in the peripheral nervous system with a significant reduction in afferent and efferent nerve conduction velocities. A reduction in neurotransmitters including serotonin may affect mood and memory. Speed of processing may be affected by depletion of neurotransmitter binding sites and reduction in dopamine transport. Sympathetic tone increases, increasing vascular resistance. There is reduced sensitivity of aortic arch and carotid sinus baroreceptors to changes in arterial pressure which may lead to postural hypotension. Haemodynamic homeostasis is impaired by a combination of autonomic and baroreflex dysfunction leading to hypotension with dehydration or diuretic use. Changes in the autonomic nervous system partially mediate impaired thermoregulation, increasing the risk of adverse reactions to hot or cold environments.

Immune system

Older people are more prone to infection, and recovery may be delayed. Macrophage, B-cell, and T-cell function all reduce with age. There is impaired production of other important mediators such as cytokines, interleukin 1, and nitric oxide, and an increased risk of reactivation of dormant viral infections and tuberculosis. Autoimmune conditions also become more common.

Gastrointestinal system

There are a number physiological changes associated with ageing. Swallowing is a multi-stage process involving voluntary contraction of skeletal muscles in the pharynx, then involuntary relaxation of sphincter muscles between the pharynx and oesophagus, and finally smooth muscle peristalsis in the oesophagus. With ageing, these processes can become desynchronized and discoordinated, leading to impaired swallowing.

There is decreased gastric secretion of hydrochloric acid and pepsin leading to changes in gastric pH. There is some evidence of reduction in absorption of some substances including vitamin B12, an increase in transit time, and an increase in the incidence of constipation.

Cancer

Virtually all cancers increase in incidence with age. Fear of cancer may be an unspoken element in any medical consultation with an older person. Lung, colon, prostate, and breast are currently the commonest sites of cancers in the UK.

Work-related cancer remains a concern and older workers may have had longer periods of exposure to occupational carcinogens. Some cancers, for example, asbestos-related mesothelioma, have very long latencies but may present in older workers prior to retirement age. A small increase in the risk of breast cancer in older women doing shift work including nights for more than 20 years has been reported[18] but there is conflicting evidence regarding this risk (see Chapter 29).

Skeletal changes

Osteoarthritis is a common problem from later middle age. One possible aetiological factor is cumulative overuse at work. The hip, knee, shoulder, and hand are particularly susceptible. Non-occupational factors (e.g. obesity, trauma, and pre-existing developmental abnormalities) also contribute to lower limb osteoarthritis. Hip and knee replacements are increasingly common in younger patients and are a significant cause of sickness absence from middle age. However, the great majority of patients do return to work, with early return associated with male sex and younger age.[19]

Apart from pain arising directly from degenerating joints, cervical and lumbar disc prolapse can produce acute painful entrapment neuropathies. The most serious consequence of cervical spondylosis is cervical myelopathy, affecting the long tracts of the spinal cord. One of the subtler effects of cervical spondylosis is the loss of proprioceptive feedback from cervical joint receptors that contributes to control of body stability and movement. This may increase the risk of falls.

Low back pain is a leading cause of disability and lost productivity, and osteoarthritis is one of the causes of this in older workers. The risk of metastatic disease increases with age. In older workers with severe, unremitting, non-mechanical back pain, the cancers that commonly metastasize to bone including bowel, breast, prostate, and thyroid should be considered. Osteoarthritis of the spine is more common in older workers, particularly in the cervical and lumbar regions than in the less mobile thoracic spine. However, in occupations that involve bending and twisting of the upper body, pain radiating from thoracic spondylosis does occur and can mimic cardiac pain. Other diseases of thoracic vertebrae, including tuberculosis, metastases, and osteoporotic collapse, can cause similar symptoms.

Osteoporosis is largely but not exclusively a disease of older women. Both sexes lose bone mass throughout adult life, but women start with less and have accelerated bone loss following the menopause. The older female worker may therefore be more likely to suffer a wrist fracture in a fall on an outstretched hand, or to experience the effects of spinal osteoporosis such as compression fracture. Thoracic and lumbar vertebrae are most at risk, the most commonly affected vertebrae being those near the thoracolumbar junction. Spinal osteoporosis may follow a painless and insidious course with increasing kyphosis and loss of height. At the other extreme, acutely painful vertebral collapse may occur in a fall or follow apparently minor trauma. Although most pathological spinal fractures in middle-aged women are due to osteoporosis, metastatic disease, especially from the breast, should be in the list of differential diagnoses.

Older workers in physically demanding jobs may be at increased risk of pathological fracture. For example, older workers in residential psychiatric units where physical intervention in patients with challenging behaviour may be required and healthcare workers dealing with acutely confused patients in emergency departments and medical assessment units. Each case must be risk assessed on its individual merits based on the degree of osteoporosis and the risk of physical attack requiring restraint. The requirements of equality legislation in terms of age, gender, and disability must be taken into account when making decisions on fitness for work.

Genitourinary problems

Older men and women may experience various genitourinary problems. Urgency, frequency, and incontinence—or the fear of incontinence—can interfere with work as well as with sleep and social activities.[20] Benign prostatic hypertrophy is common in older men. Affected individuals may be embarrassed about discussing their symptoms even with their general practitioner (GP), and urinary problems are typically worsened by anxiety. Older workers may need more frequent rest periods especially from externally paced work, and easy access to appropriate toilet facilities. Surveys have indicated that people with incontinence have often not received expert advice on managing their symptoms.

Depression

It is unclear whether the older brain is more susceptible or less susceptible to depression. However, late middle age is a time when particularly distressing life events and experiences are liable to happen. Bereavement, relationship breakdown, children leaving home, and financial worries are all common. Although there have been some changes in societal attitudes to mental illness, older people are less willing than younger adults to accept the idea of being mentally ill and may somatize their symptoms of depression. Chronic illness, persistent pain, or tinnitus may become the focus of depressive thoughts and feelings. There are also important cultural differences in the physical and behavioural manifestations of depression in a multicultural and multi-ethnic society.

Suicide risk increases with age. While para-suicide is relatively common in younger women, middle-aged and older men living alone have a higher incidence of successful suicide. The presence of chronic symptomatic illness and higher social class are also recognized risk factors, as is accessibility to means of self-harm, such as prescribed medication. Mechanism of suicide is often linked to occupation, for example, access to drugs and toxins.

Iatrogenic factors

There is a high prevalence of iatrogenic illness in older people, often due to polypharmacy. The taking of a careful drug history is particularly important for older people. Many problems arise from failing to take into account interactions between multiple prescription drugs or the co-use of over-the-counter or alternative medicines, especially by people from ethnic minorities. Pharmacokinetic issues with drugs excreted mainly through the kidney can cause problems in the presence of renal impairment. Pharmacodynamic factors, such as age-associated increased sensitivity to the effects of sedatives, may also be an issue.

The *British National Formulary* is a source of information on drugs (see 'Useful websites'). In older people, adverse effects from antihypertensives are common, and include postural hypotension and erectile dysfunction. Diuretics may cause urinary frequency and incontinence. Impairment of exercise tolerance by beta blockers may be significant for older workers in physically demanding occupations, especially in externally paced work.

Alcohol: in general, the problems associated with alcohol and the means of dealing with them are the same for workers of all ages and are dealt with in Chapter 14.

Health maintenance and service issues

Nutrition, diet, and exercise

Few of today's older workers received any advice about diet and nutrition in their early lives. However, research suggests that older workers may be more likely to have a greater understanding of nutrition than younger workers. Evidence from the US suggests that the most successful educational interventions are aimed at families, neighbourhoods, and communities, especially when supported by legislation, the media, and marketing.

In the ageing population, those with greatest health needs include members of minority groups and recent immigrants. These groups are often overlooked when designing and implementing health promotion programmes.[21,22]

During the 1960s and 1970s, government health education encouraged the UK population to reduce salt, sugar, and fat in their diets. Quality protein, salads, and fruit were then more expensive than foods containing high concentrations of saturated fats. Ready meals and other processed foods containing large quantities of salt, sugar, and saturated fats became popular with the spread of microwave ovens. The changes in eating and lifestyle habits of different socioeconomic groups resulted in wealthier groups eating a healthier diet. The consequences of this are seen in today's poorer older workers, in higher rates of heart, lung, and liver disease, diabetes, and in reduced life expectancy. Only vegetarians and vegans have bucked the trend of a widening gap between the life expectancy of rich and poor.

In the past 30 years, year-round salads, fruit, and frozen food have become accessible to almost all of the population. However, habits acquired in the 1960s and 1970s have been hard to change, with those in the poorer socioeconomic groups changing least. Poorer people are more likely to be overweight because less healthy, calorie-dense foods tend to be cheaper. Smoking has been more persistent in lower socioeconomic groups, increasing the life expectancy gap still further.

There is some evidence that workers over the age of 50 have more positive health behaviours, stronger beliefs about the value of healthy behaviour, and better self-assessed health. In addition, they are more likely to participate in workplace health promotion activities. This may to some extent be related to healthy worker and survivor effects. Physical activity should continue in older workers, even though stamina and strength may decrease. Regular exercise sufficient to raise the heart rate at least five times a week is key. There is evidence that those with a body mass index (BMI) of 30 or more die earlier and that all age groups benefit from regular exercise. The myth of 'fat but fit' has been debunked and even metabolically normal obese individuals have a 28% increase in the risk of IHD. BMI should ideally be kept under 25, even though there is a natural tendency for body fat to move centrally, with age. Accumulation of intra-abdominal fat is especially prominent in men and central obesity is strongly associated with the metabolic syndrome.

Health checks

There is a lack of evidence that regular health checks improve health or work outcomes even for older workers. However, health promotion activities focusing on reducing smoking and improving diet and exercise may be beneficial for workers of all ages and health checks can provide an opportunity to impart health promotion information.

Sickness certification

Under guidance from the Department of Work and Pensions, hospital doctors are responsible for providing sickness certification for both in-patients and out-patients under their care. However, in practice, the task is often delegated to the GP who may have no specialist knowledge of the effect on work of the health condition. 'Fit notes' are intended to provide information to support return to work. Healthy alliances with better coordination between primary and secondary care (as described in the government documents *Health of the Nation*[23] and *Our Healthier Nation*[24] may improve fitness for work advice for older workers who are more likely to be suffering from chronic conditions.

Workability and employability

Degenerative diseases and the chronic illnesses of older age often have adverse effects on work capacity, leading to impaired attendance and performance at work. In the past, older workers were often placed on unofficial 'light duties' with heavy manual handling tasks allocated to younger workers. However, as the proportion of older workers increases, this is becoming less feasible. The concept of 'workability', rather than 'disability', as advocated in the Faculty of Occupational Medicine's 'Position Paper on Age and Employment',[5] requires a change of mindset away from the concept of medical restrictions and a more person-focused approach to fit the task to the person and not vice versa. Indeed, this is already a legal requirement under the UK Management of Health and Safety at Work Regulations 1992.

Job analysis, skills assessment, job coaching, retraining, and job matching are all components of an effective management system. There are now a number of job content and employee capability assessment tools available. These build up a worker capability profile which can then be matched with a list of job requirements allowing better matching of the job to the person. This is a dynamic process requiring regular reassessment of workers as they age or recover from incapacity. The benefits include transparency, flexibility of labour, and retaining older workers in suitable jobs.

Ageing and recovery from illness or injury

Ageing and age-associated loss of adaptability not only increase the risk of disease and injury, but increase the risk of complications, prolonged healing, and recovery time. Patterns of sickness absence vary with age. Younger workers tend to take more frequent but shorter periods of absence, with social and domestic factors being more prominent, whereas older workers take fewer but longer periods of absence, mainly related to significant illness. Overall, older workers do not take more sickness absence than younger workers and are often more careful to conserve sick leave as a 'buffer' for serious illness.[25]

Enhanced rehabilitation programmes are particularly important for older workers. While rest may be necessary initially, inactivity is detrimental to older people and can lead to a permanent reduction in level of function. Active rehabilitation and physiotherapy are often vital in returning older people to the workforce. Psychological as well as physical needs may also need to be addressed. Older workers may suffer from loss of confidence following an accident or illness. Combined with a phased return to work, active and repeated encouragement and reassurance will help to rebuild confidence and restore function.

Older people often recover more slowly than younger people. However, there may be wide variations in recovery time, depending on previous health, availability of health services, motivation, job status and job satisfaction, support of colleagues, managers' attitudes, and the availability of a phased return to work monitored by OH professionals. The myth that workers should be 100% recovered or 100% pain free before returning to work should be actively discouraged, particularly for older workers. Competent functional assessment in the work environment is key to early and successful reintegration into work, especially for acute musculoskeletal conditions.

Delayed return to work increases costs for employers and leads to loss of income and sometimes loss of job for employees. It also leads to physical deconditioning and loss of work hardening which can be difficult to reacquire for older people. Early access to functional assessment, active rehabilitation, and treatment services, will minimize absence. Proactive intervention and case management (e.g. early access to physiotherapy and individually tailored exercise programmes) may also prevent significant injury in those at risk and those displaying early symptoms. It may also prevent progression to chronicity and permanent loss of function. Older workers usually welcome early access to assessment and treatment, enabling them to stay in work and avoid sickness absence. See Box 7.2.

This is the most cost-effective and efficient way of returning older people safely to work and results in a reduction in long-term sickness absence. Dialogue between the GP and the OH professional may help in the decision regarding return to work or ill health retirement.

There may be a positive cost/benefit ratio in proactively expediting early outpatient investigation and specialist treatment ahead of normal NHS waiting times. Some larger employers will fund private medical treatment particularly for employees who are critical to the running of the business.

Retraining and redeployment

There are many myths about the shortcomings of older workers. However, they are often more reliable and make fewer mistakes than younger workers. Some UK employers actively recruit older workers because of this. Lower staff turnover in older workers has financial benefits in reduced recruitment costs and better returns from training. However, content and delivery of older workers' training may need to be structured differently from that for younger workers. Trainers need to understand and utilize the different strengths and weaknesses, and different learning styles of both groups and tailor their programmes

---

Box 7.2 Elements of an integrated approach to return to work

- Early outpatient investigation and specialist assessment of the illness.
- Supportive treatment and work conditioning plan.
- Graded and phased return to work on fewer and shorter shifts.

accordingly. For example, older workers may respond better to didactic teaching styles than small group-based learning.[26]

Multiple career changes and retraining are now the norm as people often work to age 70 and even beyond. New technologies will require training in specific skills and adaptation to change, and there is a risk that if older workers don't retrain and adapt then they will become effectively obsolete. Training costs will inevitably rise in the future.

Many semi-retired workers seek part-time employment to supplement their pensions. Part-time and flexible work in the UK service industry sector now provides many jobs. These often have low rates of pay although this may be ameliorated by the minimum wage and the more recent living wage. Working on controversial zero hours contracts is becoming more common. Personal safety for older people with direct contact with the public may be a concern. When handling cash is involved, the older worker may be physically more vulnerable to injury or threats than the younger worker. However, the trend in the UK has been a steady fall in violent crime for the last few decades so this may not be a significant issue.

Ethical issues

Expectations will need to change for employers and employees. With an increased retirement age there will need to be sufficient employment opportunities for older people. There will also be a need for more varied and flexible working as the retirement age rises.

There may also be ethical consequences for OH professionals. The economic necessity for manpower reduction, downsizing, and voluntary redundancy may result in conscious and unconscious discrimination against older workers.[27] Age discrimination is often based on inaccurate and outdated assumptions and stereotypes about older workers. See Box 7.3.

In one study, it was reported that 80% of employees between the ages of 34 and 67 years said that they had been victims of age discrimination. However, at least one major UK national retail store chain has opted for positive age discrimination, actively recruiting older workers for their greater experience of dealing with customers' needs. UK legislation has now removed the traditional default retirement age except in some roles covered by statute, thereby outlawing age discrimination. However, whether employers will seek ways around the legislation remains to be seen.

Some managers still subscribe to the myth that all workers with cancer will die or will never return to productive work. Younger managers often have little or no personal experience of serious illness. Many older workers expect and want to stay in work, in spite of serious illness.[28,29] However, there is often a mismatch between the expectations of managers and those of older workers.

The issue of ill health retirement is covered in detail in Chapter 12. There are many differing definitions and criteria for 'ill health' or 'medical' retirement in different occupations with different pension schemes. Criteria for eligibility may become 'flexible' if organizational accommodations are believed to be too difficult or expensive to achieve.

Box 7.3 The benefits of older workers

Older workers often have accumulated experience or learned strategies that may be valuable in contributing to business success. The published literature does not support the popular misconception that work performance declines with age. Older workers are noted to perform generally more consistently and to deliver higher quality, matching the performance of younger colleagues. In practice, despite an age-related decline in physical strength, stamina, memory, and information processing, this rarely impairs work performance. Older workers may use knowledge, skills, experience, anticipation, motivation, and other strategies to maintain their performance. Older workers also bring the benefits of often being more conscientious, loyal, reliable, and hardworking and having well-developed inter-personal skills. On balance, older workers do not have more absence from the workplace than workers of other ages. Older workers are also less prone to accidents. Lower staff turnover in the older age groups has financial benefits in reduced recruitment costs, and also in terms of better returns from training initiatives.

Source: data from Faculty of Occupational Medicine. (2004) *Position Paper on Age and Employment, 2004*. London, UK: Faculty of Occupational Medicine. Copyright © 2004 Faculty of Occupational Medicine.

Older workers working with adjustments may also be more vulnerable to dismissal on the grounds of incapability.

The OH professional must maintain an objective and consistent position, and be robust in the face of management pressure to remove an individual from the workforce if they are simply perceived as being unlikely to return to pre-illness levels of productive work. There may be a need to request medical reports from the treating specialist or GP to get a full picture of the patient's health and long-term prognosis. Although a recommendation for ill health retirement may be the outcome, this should normally be the last resort. It may also be useful to hold a 'case conference' involving line management, human resources, OH, and the employee and their representative.

As people expect to work longer, attitudes to career trajectories will need to change. Whether employers whose core business requires heavy or repetitive externally paced work should be required by law to make lighter work available is open to debate. There is a requirement under the Equality Act 2010 to make reasonable adjustments. Case law defines 'reasonable' as largely a cost/benefit analysis based on the size and nature of the business. The adjustments should not be economically unviable, and the expectations of a large multinational company are very different to the expectations of small and medium-sized enterprises. The reality is that every employee and employer is different, and this must be judged on a case-by-case basis.

Pre-retirement courses run by many large employers should include a session on staying healthy in retirement delivered by a healthcare worker. These courses provide a valuable opportunity to guide prospective retirees in lifestyle choices and to encourage them to remain active and healthy in retirement or in part-time work.

Organizational issues

Management and social aspects

Some UK managers may perceive that older workers are more expensive than younger workers. While capabilities and patterns of sickness absence are different, this is not necessarily true. There is a degree of ambivalence in the attitude of trade unions to older workers remaining economically active for longer. Society will need to address these issues, and one option is for positive discrimination in favour of the older worker. However, this is bound to be controversial, and if older workers are receiving preferential treatment at the expense of younger workers, then there will be a difficult conflict of interests for employers, employees, and trade unions.

Increasingly, as people remain healthier for longer, retirement is seen as a time for new interests and the pursuit of new goals. Part-time working, job-sharing, and other semi-retirement options can all help the older worker to achieve a work–life balance that suits their capabilities and personal circumstances. This enables workers to retain the social contact and support networks of the working environment without the pressure and commitment of full-time work. However, in some industries this flexibility may be difficult to achieve as employers find job-sharing expensive and time-consuming, especially if illness or family responsibilities disrupt the agreed work pattern and employees require additional support.

Shift work

Many workers find working rotating shifts, particularly those including nights, more difficult as they age, and may seek a medical reason to withdraw from night working.[30] People aged over 40 starting shift work for the first time—for example, late entrants to nursing—experience difficulty adapting to different sleeping and eating times. Those who have worked shifts for decades may start to notice fatigue at night, difficulty sleeping in the day, and feel lethargic and less well. Older workers' performance at night may be worse than that of younger workers. There is evidence that the time to exhaustion is reduced by a significant amount (20%) for older shift workers during the recovery period from night shift working.[31] In addition, there is evidence that a faster forward-rotating shift pattern is more suitable for older workers than a slower backward-rotating pattern which is consistent with recovering from jet lag.

Sleep disorders are more common in older workers.[32] The older worker may be at risk of losing their job if regular day shift work cannot be provided. In addition, older workers who travel regularly back and forth across several time zones by air, either as aircrew or passengers, take longer to recover their circadian rhythms with increasing age. However, some older individuals who have wider natural circadian rhythm swings and the apparent ability to reset their body clocks more quickly appear to cope better so this is not universal. If performance is adversely affected, redeployment within the employing organization may prove difficult (e.g. for pilots or senior doctors). Employers should be sympathetic to making adjustments to accommodate such requests where possible. It was traditional for hospital doctors to come off the night time on-call rota in their late 50s. However, as the medical workforce ages and a higher proportion of doctors are over 55, this has become increasingly unworkable and may lead to considerable conflict.

There are some health conditions that may be exacerbated by night working including epilepsy, type 1 diabetes mellitus, depression, and gastrointestinal disorders. Some of these may be more common in older workers. Also use of prescription medicines for which the timing is critical is more common in older workers, for example, insulin or the use of tricyclic anti-depressants for pain.

Hours of work

The EU Working Time Directive (implemented in UK law by the Working Time Regulations 1998) requires workers to opt out if they wish to work more than 48 hours per week averaged over a 17-week reference period. In addition, other requirements include a minimum rest period of 11 consecutive hours a day and that night working must not exceed 8 hours a night on average.

A culture of long working hours is more prevalent in the UK than in other European countries. Lucrative additional hours of work (e.g. 12-hour shifts, weekend overtime, and additional shifts) are often welcomed by younger workers. Older workers may be less enthusiastic, especially those in poor health. The incentives for the self-employed to work longer hours and to take less time off for illness remain. The Turner Report[3] urged the UK government to consider incentives to keep older workers in work for longer. These incentives will need to be flexible regarding part-time working and accompanied by changes in taxation and employment legislation to ensure that they achieve the desired result. In addition, the older self-employed and teleworkers will need to be included in these arrangements.

Ergonomics: input into the design of processes

Mass production and service industry job design requires early ergonomic involvement, including effective monitoring of process developments and changes. Feedback of information learned from current processes and incorporating ergonomic improvements into new manufacturing and service delivery processes is in the interests of all workers, regardless of age. Failure to do so can lead to costly work reorganization and/or legal claims from workers suffering from musculoskeletal injuries. The older worker who develops these conditions is likely to take longer to recover than the younger worker, and is more likely to progress to a chronic state, requiring permanent adjustments or redeployment.[33]

Ergonomic improvements should ideally be innovative, individual, and inexpensive. Adaptation of workplaces may be needed to accommodate physically restricted older workers. Ideally, job rotation should be 2–4-hourly, rather than daily or weekly, to accommodate temporarily or permanently restricted workers. The introduction of robots or other mechanical equipment and improved workplace and component design are examples of improvements that would preferentially protect older workers and improve their overall flexibility in the workforce.

Additional training may be needed for ergonomists to enable them to understand the abilities and limitations of older people regarding muscular strength, static loads, the risk of injury, and the effect of shift patterns and rest periods in relation to fatigue. Expert ergonomic input into processes and risk assessments should ensure that they are relevant and appropriate for workers of all ages.

Older workers and younger managers

This is the first generation in which the majority of managers and supervisors, commonly in their 30s and 40s, are managing groups of people who may be from their parents' (or even their grandparents') generation. The cultural 'generation gap' between a 25-year-old manager and a 65-year-old employee born before computers, the Internet, and smartphones, is likely to be quite considerable. Often, the younger manager has no concept of living with chronic ill health or chronic pain and the effect they have on performance and on enjoyment of work.

Research has shown that younger managers often rate older job applicants as less economically beneficial to the organization than younger applicants. The older worker is sometimes seen by the younger manager as being slow, work-shy, uncooperative, and resistant to change. The younger manager, in turn, is sometimes seen as overbearing, inconsistent, and arrogant. Inflexible handling of misunderstandings by the younger manager can lead to resentment, mistrust, and ultimately demotivation. Older workers may fear for their job security, especially if already coping with discomfort and disability associated with chronic illness. This can lead to emotional distress and, not uncommonly, to sickness absence. Aggressive management style, blame culture, and other organizational 'blue' and 'black' flags may exacerbate these problems (see Chapter 10). Individual productivity may suffer. In an ageing population, these situations are likely to occur more frequently. All parties can benefit from improved training in communication, conflict resolution, and in improved knowledge and understanding of the strengths, capabilities, and reasonable expectations of different age groups. The OH professional will often require patience and great sensitivity in managing these situations.

Care commitments

A survey of UK employers showed that 86% believe that care issues for older relatives of employees will be a key concern in the future. A 2017 study showed that average lifespan in the UK increased between 1991 and 2011.[34] But over the same period, there was also an increase in the 'high dependency' state of 1.3 years on average for women and 0.9 years for men. On average, older men spend 2.4 years and older women 3.0 years with substantial care needs. The study concluded that further population ageing will require an extra 71,215 care home places by 2025.

Table 7.2 Active age management strategies

Strategy	Descriptors
Job flexibility	Adjusting schedules or hours Adapting employee roles or job responsibilities as abilities change Phased retirement
Comprehensive benefits package	Flexible benefits Wellness programmes Retirement, financial, and personal counselling and support to help find child care and elder care
Professional growth and development	Emphasis on a lifelong career with the company, with continuing development opportunities Retirees as mentors as part of the 'knowledge transfer' process for newer employees; can continue to work part-time while drawing a pension Preparing current employees for future roles
Other workplace accommodations	Job safe practices for keeping employees healthy and injury free A process for responding to worker requests for work and workplace adjustments Use of specialized equipment to reduce physical occupational demands

Source: data from British Medical Association (BMA). (2016) *Ageing and the workplace*. Copyright © 2016 BMA.

Adult social care in the UK is currently a cause for concern as demand outstrips supply. One of the consequences of this is 'bed blocking', where patients fit for discharge are unable to leave hospital because of a lack of social care beds. Older people living in the community may struggle to get domiciliary social care. With workers' elderly relatives living into their 90s and becoming highly dependent, career expectations, earnings, and savings, will all need to change. As will legislation, taxation, pensions, and provision of social care (Table 7.2).

Key points

◆ In the developing world, populations are ageing and people are living longer in retirement, often with substantial care needs. People need to work for longer to cover the cost of looking after the retired and elderly population.

◆ As people age, there are changes in function that may impact work ability.

◆ Older people are valuable members of the workforce with useful knowledge and skills whose attendance and performance usually equal that of younger workers.

◆ Adjusting working hours and duties and considering flexible retirement options may help to retain people in work for longer.

◆ Wellness programmes and personal and financial counselling may benefit older workers.

Useful websites

Office for National Statistics. Life expectancy	http://visual.ons.gov.uk/how-has-life-expectancy-changed-over-time/
UK Government. State pensions	https://www.gov.uk/browse/working/state-pension
World Health Organization. 'Ageing and Life Course'	http://www.who.int/ageing/en/
OECD. Ageing and employment policies	http://www.oecd.org/els/emp/ageingandemploymentpolicies.htm
British Medical Association. 'Healthy ageing'	https://www.bma.org.uk/collective-voice/policy-and-research/public-and-population-health/healthy-ageing
British National Formulary	http://www.bnf.org.uk

References

1. **Carr E, Hagger-Johnson G, Head J, et al.** Working conditions as predictors of retirement intentions and exit from paid employment: a 10-year follow-up of the English Longitudinal Study of Ageing. *Eur J Ageing* 2016;**13**:39–48.
2. **North MS, Fiske ST.** Resource scarcity and prescriptive attitudes generate subtle, intergenerational older-worker exclusion. *J Soc Issues* 2016;**72**:122–45.
3. **Pensions Commission.** *A New Pension Settlement for the Twenty-First Century: The Second Report of the Pensions Commission.* London: Department for Work and Pensions; 2006.
4. **British Medical Association (BMA).** *Ageing and the Workplace: A Report from the BMA Occupational Medicine Committee.* London: BMA; 2016.
5. **Faculty of Occupational Medicine.** *Position Paper on Age and Employment.* London: Faculty of Occupational Medicine; 2004.
6. **Grimley Evans J.** How are the elderly different? In: Kane RL, Grimley Evans J, Macfadyen D (eds), *Improving the Health of Older People: A World View*, pp. 50–68. Oxford: Oxford University Press; 1990.
7. **Schaie KW, Strother CR.** A cross-sequential study of age changes in cognitive behavior. *Psychol Bull* 1968;**70**:671–80.
8. **Grimley Evans J.** Ageing and disease. In: Evered D, Whelan J (eds), *Research and the Ageing Population* pp. 38–57. Chichester: John Wiley and Sons Ltd; 1988.
9. **Palmer KT, D'Angelo S, Harris EC, et al.** Frailty, prefrailty and employment outcomes in Health and Employment After Fifty (HEAF) Study. *Occup Environ Med* 2017;**74**:476–82.
10. **Manton K, Gu X.** Changes in the prevalence of chronic disability in the United States black and non-black population above age 65 from 1982 to 1999. *Proc Nat Acad Sci USA* 2001;**98**:6354–9.
11. **Aittomaki A, Lahelma E, Roos E, et al.** Gender differences in the association of age with physical workload and functioning. *Occup Environ Med* 2005;**62**:95–100.
12. **Snook SH.** The effects of age and physique on continuous-work capacity. *Hum Factors* 1971;**13**:467–9.
13. **Goycoolea MV, Goycoolea HG, Rodriguez LG, et al.** Effect of life in industrialized societies on hearing in natives of Easter Island. *Laryngoscope* 1986;**96**:1391–6.
14. **Pichora-Fuller MK.** Cognitive aging and auditory information processing. *Int J Audiol* 2003;**42**(Suppl. 2):S26–32.

15. **Ball K, Owsley C, Beard B.** Clinical visual perimetry underestimates peripheral field problems in older adults. *Clin Vis Sci* 1990;**5**:113–25.

16. **Winner SJ, Morgan CA, Grimley Evans J.** Perimenopausal risk of falling and incidence of distal forearm fracture. *BMJ* 1989;**298**:1486–8.

17. **Lakatta EG.** Cardiovascular aging without a clinical diagnosis. *Dialogues Cardiovasc Med* 2001;**6**:67–91.

18. **WHO IARC Working Group.** Carcinogenicity of shift – work, painting and firefighting. *Lancet Oncol* 2007;**8**:1065–6.

19. **Sankar A, Davis AM, Palaganas MP, Beaton DE, Badley EM, Gignac MA.** Return to work and workplace activity limitations following total hip or knee replacement. *Osteoarthritis Cartilage* 2013;**21**:1485–93.

20. **Wu EQ, Birnbaum H, Marynchenko M, et al.** Employees with overactive bladder: work loss burden. *J Occup Environ Med* 2005;**47**:439–46.

21. **Bagwell MM, Bush HA.** Improving health promotion for blue-collar workers. *J Nurs Care Qual* 2000;**14**:65–71.

22. **Infeld DL, Whitelaw N.** Policy initiatives to promote healthy aging. *Clin Geriatr Med* 2002; **18**: 627–42

23. **Secretary of State for Health.** *The Health of the Nation. A Strategy for Health in England.* Cm1986. London: HMSO; 1992.

24. **Secretary of State for Health.** *Our Healthier Nation. A Contract for Health.* CM 3852. London: The Stationery Office; 1998.

25. **Cant R, O'Loughlin K, Legge V.** Sick leave—cushion or entitlement? A study of age cohorts' attitudes and practices in two Australian workplaces. *Work* 2001;**17**:39–48.

26. **Bongers PM, de Winter CR, Kompier MAJ, et al.** Psychosocial factors at work and musculoskeletal disease. *Scand J Work Environ Health* 1993;**19**:297–312.

27. **Vahtera J, Kivimäki M, Pennti J.** Effect of organisational downsizing on health of employees. *Lancet* 1997;**350**:1124–8.

28. **Kinne S, Probart C, Gritz ER.** Cancer-risk-related health behaviors and attitudes of older workers. Working Well Research Group. *J Cancer Educ* 1996;**11**:89–95.

29. **Verbeek J, Spelten E, Kammeijer M, et al.** Return to work of cancer survivors: a prospective cohort study into the quality of rehabilitation by occupational physicians. *Occup Environ Med* 2003;**60**:352–7.

30. **Tepas DI, Duchon JC, Gersten AH.** Shiftwork and the older worker. *Exp Aging Res* 1993;**19**:295–320.

31. **Hakola T, Harma M.** Evaluation of a fast forward rotating shift schedule in the steel industry with a special focus on ageing and sleep. *J Hum Ergol (Tokyo)* 2001;**30**:315–9.

32. **Reid K, Dawson D.** Comparing performance on a simulated 12 hour shift rotation in young and older subjects. *Occup Environ Med* 2001;**58**:58–62.

33. **Salvendy G, Pilitsis J.** Psychophysiological aspects of paced and unpaced performance as influenced by age. *Ergonomics* 1971;**14**:703–11.

34. **Kingston A, Wohland P, Wittenberg R, et al.** Is late-life dependency increasing or not? A comparison of the Cognitive Function and Ageing Studies (CFAS). *Lancet* 2017;**390**:1676–84.

Chapter 8

Women's health and other gender issues at work

Blandina Blackburn and Patrick Bose

Introduction

The workforce of the twenty-first century contains more women than at any previous time. Many women work part-time and having children makes it more not less likely that they will stay at work. As demographics change and people stay at work for longer, this will probably apply to women too.

Within their working lives women experience normal physiological changes such as pregnancy and the menopause, as well as specific health problems related to menstrual, cervical, ovarian, or uterine conditions. Some of these have associated psychological consequences, which may require adjustments at work to enable women to continue contributing to commercial productivity and societal responsibilities. The newer treatments for many conditions such as infertility and cancers may also require repeated appointments and considerable time off work.

This chapter also includes a section on gender identity issues, increasingly encountered in the occupational health (OH) clinic. While society learns to view these issues as normal, and we learn to conceptualize these as normal, much stigma and intolerance will be experienced by these workers in employment.

Employment statistics

There were 742,000 men and 448,000 women aged 65 and over in employment in the UK in May to July 2016 compared to 301,000 men and 177,000 women in 1992.[1] In August 2017, 80% of men aged 16–64 were in work, which is the highest recorded rate since 1991, and 71% of women aged 16–64 were in work, the highest female employment rate recorded since comparable records started in 1971.[1] The increase in the employment rate for women was influenced by ongoing changes to the state pension age for women, resulting in fewer women retiring between the ages of 60 and 65.[2] See Figures 8.1 and 8.2.

The occupations most heavily populated by female workers are health, education, social care, and hospitality. Few women work in the manufacturing sector, other than at an administrative level.[2]

Of those workers aged between 50 and 64, 47% are women which is the joint highest level since records began in 1971.[1] Within this population, a total of 1.7 million (5%)

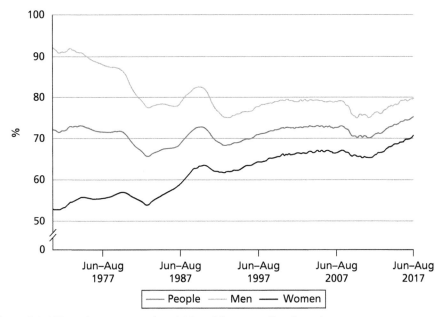

Figure 8.1 UK employment rates (aged 16 to 64), seasonally adjusted.

Reproduced from The Office for National Statistics (ONS) (2017) Labour Force Survey. Copyright © 2017 ONS.

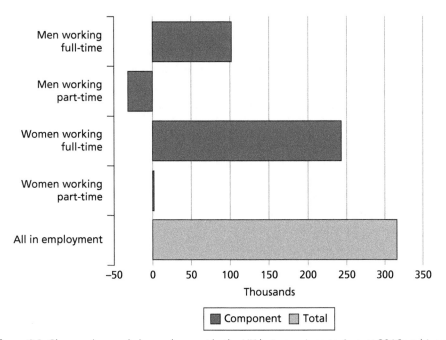

Figure 8.2 Changes in people in employment in the UK between June to August 2016 and June August 2017, seasonally adjusted.

Reproduced from The Office for National Statistics (ONS) (2017) Labour Force Survey. Copyright © 2017 ONS.

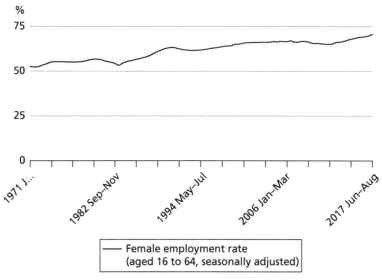

Figure 8.3 Sickness absence rate: by sex, UK, 1993 to 2016.
Reproduced from The Office for National Statistics (ONS) (2017) Labour Force Survey. Copyright © 2017 ONS.

women could be adversely affected by menopausal symptoms. A full understanding of the complex and poorly researched relationship between women's health and performance at work is still to be elucidated (Figure 8.3).

Analysis by the Office for National Statistics (ONS) suggests that mothers with young children are more likely to go back to or begin full-time work now than 20 years ago.[4] The proportion of mothers with children aged between 3 and 4 who are in employment increased by almost 10 percentage points over the past two decades. In England, there were around 133,000 more mothers, whose youngest child is a toddler, in employment in 2017 (65%), compared with 1997 (56%). This was largely driven by an increase in full-time employment (Figure 8.4).[4]

Sickness absence

Although loss of working days due to sickness and injury in the UK has fallen to its lowest recorded level (from 7.2 days per worker in 1993 to 4.3 days in 2016),[3] the causes of work absence due to gynaecological causes are not well researched.

Causes of sickness absence in women (Labour Force Survey) include:[1]

◆ minor illnesses (33%)

◆ musculoskeletal problems (14%)

◆ other (13%).

For women, genitourinary problems (including urine infections and pregnancy-related problems) were the reason for 5% of sickness absences.[3] As women now constitute a large

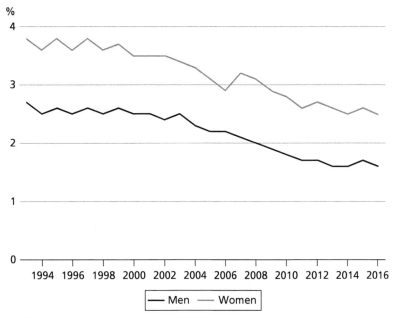

Figure 8.4 Sickness absence rate: by sex, UK, 1993–2016.
Reproduced from The Office for National Statistics (ONS) (2017) *Labour Force Survey*. Copyright © 2017 ONS.

proportion of the workforce, it is important to consider their gender-related health issues and needs at work.

Gynaecological conditions from menarche to menopause

Benign gynaecology

Many benign gynaecological problems that are frequently encountered in the workplace could have an impact on attendance and performance.

◆ *Polycystic ovary syndrome (PCOS)*: PCOS affects 2–26% of women[5] and is diagnosed according to the Rotterdam criteria (i.e. 2 out of 3 of >12 ovarian follicles on ultrasound scan, hyperandrogenism, and anovulation). PCOS predisposes to diabetes, sleep apnoea, depression, endometrial thickening, and, in some phenotypes, cardiovascular disease. Presenting symptoms can include central obesity (carbohydrate intolerance), acne, excess facial hair, and menstrual dysfunction. The mainstay of treatment is control of carbohydrate metabolism (commonly metformin or Inofolic® (400 mcg folic acid + 4 g of myo-inositol)) and menstrual regularization.[5] Women with PCOS should be reassured that although they may take longer to conceive, their lifetime fertility is nevertheless not impaired, and that modest weight loss (5–10%) can restore normal fecundity.[5,6]

◆ *Endometriosis*: this is a benign but complex condition that affects 10% of women of reproductive age.[7] Characterized by the presence of hormonally reactive endometrial tissue around ovaries, pelvis, bladder, and bowel, endometriosis commonly presents with dysmenorrhoea, menorrhagia, general pelvic pain, dyspareunia, and discomfort when going to the toilet. In addition to the cost of hospital treatment, a prospective study showed that losses in productivity were twice those of the direct healthcare costs.[7] In the UK, the estimated cost of endometriosis approaches £14 billion per year, and this points to the need for prompt referral to a specialist centre.

◆ *Menorrhagia/heavy menstrual bleeding*: this is defined as menstrual loss of greater than 80 mL of blood or bleeding sufficient to interfere with emotional, social, and material quality of life. Diagnosis relies on excluding common primary causes of excessive haemorrhage such as submucous fibroids, endometrial polyps, coagulation disorders, platelet disorders, or (rarely) neoplasia. One-stop clinics employing transvaginal ultrasound and outpatient hysteroscopy facilitate early diagnosis. Use of hormonal manipulation (such as the progesterone-releasing intrauterine system (IUS)), endometrial ablation, myomectomy, and uterine artery embolization as an alternative to hysterectomy have resulted in a significant fall in morbidity and mortality post hysterectomy.[8]

Hysterectomy

Hysterectomy is traditionally indicated for heavy periods, long-term pelvic pain (e.g. endometriosis/adenomyosis), prolapse, non-cancerous tumours (fibroids), ovarian cancer, uterine cancer, cervical cancer, or cancer of the fallopian tubes. Depending on the type of hysterectomy being performed, accompanying organs such as the fallopian tubes, ovaries, and cervix are often removed at the same time. Abdominal, vaginal, and laparoscopic (keyhole) approaches are available. Recovery rates range from 2 to 6 weeks depending on indication and surgical approach (Table 8.1).[9]

Long-term complications include early menopause, impaired sexual function, dyspareunia, injury to bladder or ureters, and occasionally psychological effects.[10] The advent

Table 8.1 Risk of serious complications from abdominal hysterectomy

Complication	Risk
Overall	40/1000
Damage to the bladder and/or the ureter	7/1000
Haemorrhage requiring blood transfusion	23/1000
Pelvic abscess/infection	2/1000
Venous thrombosis or pulmonary embolism	4/1000
Damage to the bowel	4/10,000
Risk of death within 6 weeks	32/100,000

of pharmacological therapies, such as the progesterone-releasing IUS, and less invasive surgical alternatives, such as endometrial ablation techniques, have seen a steady fall in rates of hysterectomy for benign conditions.[10]

It is important for women to make their own decision about whether to have a hysterectomy, which can be a difficult and emotional process. Women need to be well informed about the procedure so they can confidently discuss all available options with their gynaecologist.

Depression following hysterectomy is more common if the operation takes place due to cancer or severe illness rather than as an elective operation. Women experiencing these symptoms following a hysterectomy should talk to their general practitioner (GP) or appropriately trained counsellor.

Occupational health management of hysterectomy or other gynaecological operations

The likelihood of fibroids or idiopathic menorrhagia increases with age. The duration of sickness absence for an uncomplicated hysterectomy procedure in a healthy woman should be less than 3–4 weeks. However, associated medical conditions can delay recovery and this must be considered when advising on fitness to work and adjustments. The type of work, especially heavy manual work, must also be taken into account. Evaluation of physical strain on a surgical scar must be considered in the assessment to minimize the risk of scar rupture and subsequent incisional herniation.

The psychological impact of straightforward surgery is usually minimal, but can delay recovery in some cases. See Chapter 11 for return to work times after breast and gynaecological surgery.

Fibroids

Fibroids are non-cancerous growths (myomas or leiomyomas) that develop in or around the uterus. They vary in size and many are asymptomatic, but reported symptoms include heavy periods or painful periods, abdominal pain, lower back pain, urinary frequency, constipation, and pain or discomfort during sex.

Fibroids are linked to the hormone oestrogen and are thought to develop more frequently in women of African-Caribbean origin. They occur more often in overweight women due to increased levels of oestrogen. They tend to shrink when oestrogen levels are low, such as after the menopause, and over time they will often diminish and disappear. Treatment is not indicated for asymptomatic fibroids. Selective progesterone receptor modulators reduce their size and are currently advocated to reduce large fibroids before surgery. Trials are ongoing with regard to long-term use.[11]

Occupational health management of fibroids

Menstrual problems can affect young females in their teenage years, at a time when they may be entering university or employment. The symptoms that impact work or study include persistent pain, especially during menstrual periods, irregularities of menstruation, or side effects of contraception, often exacerbated by the psychological impact of hormonal monthly changes. This can produce an effect on work attendance and productivity. An assessment of personal health, potential side effects of any treatment, and social factors that may affect recurrence or persistence of symptoms should be factored into any advice about adjustments. Associated conditions include PCOS, endometriosis, and sexually transmitted disease.

Physical consequences of heavy bleeding, such as anaemia and associated fatigue, are usually manageable. Short-term adjustments to work patterns may be helpful, but the effectiveness of treatment should be monitored and any OH advice modified with regard to the need for continuation of adjustments or for further support.

Fertility and pregnancy

Recovery from surgical termination of pregnancy

Following surgical intervention to terminate a pregnancy, most women will continue to bleed for around 1–2 weeks.[12] Symptoms of nausea, vomiting, and tiredness usually stop within 3 days but breast tenderness may take 7–10 days to disappear. Ibuprofen or paracetamol may be necessary for the pain. Most women are physically ready to return to work within 48 hours.

Recurrent miscarriage

Defined in the UK as three consecutive pregnancies lost prior to 24 weeks, recurrent miscarriage affects 2% of pregnancies. A high proportion, 50–75%, are unexplained[13] but medical causes include advanced maternal age, antiphospholipid syndrome, parental balanced reciprocal (Robertsonian) translocation, embryonic aneuploidy, uterine anomalies, maternal endocrine disorders, and thrombophilias. Investigation should be performed in specialist centres and treatments should be limited to evidence-based procedures, unless offered within appropriate clinical trials. There can be significant, and often unrecognized, psychological and psychiatric trauma for both mother and partner. Online support is available from the Miscarriage Association (see 'Useful websites'). When women who have experienced miscarriage become pregnant again, anxiety, fear, and overprotection are common as a result of fear of another miscarriage. Reassurance, encouragement, and provision of work flexibility are supportive measures to help women stay at work while maintaining a safe pregnancy.

Pregnancy

Normal pregnancy in a healthy mother-to-be should not give rise to any particular health problems although fatigue is common (especially in the first and third trimester). The potential impact of the gradually increasing size of the pregnancy on the ability to carry out physical work can also hamper work activities. However, employers have a responsibility to carry out a risk assessment.

Legislation to protect the health and safety of new and expectant mothers at work includes the:

◆ Management of Health and Safety at Work Regulations 1999 (MHSWR)

◆ Workplace (Health, Safety and Welfare) Regulations 1992 (the Workplace Regulations)

◆ Equality Act 2010.

Regulation 3 of the MHSWR places a legal duty on all employers to assess the health and safety risks to which their employees are exposed while at work. Once these risks have been assessed, the employer is then required to put in place the appropriate health and safety measures that may be required to control any identified risks. Specific health and safety requirements relating to new and expectant mothers at work are mainly contained in regulations 16–18 of the MHSWR. An initial pregnancy risk assessment should be undertaken by the manager as soon as pregnancy is reported, and appropriate adjustments made, in accordance with regulation 16 of the MHSWR (Box 8.1).

Every employer and OH service should be familiar with the risks to the pregnant worker in their particular occupation. A risk assessment flow chart for employers is available at the Health and Safety Executive (HSE) website (see 'Useful websites'). This provides guidance for employers and employees on health and safety during pregnancy.[14] It also lists risks that employers should assess.

If employees are of childbearing age, and a workplace risk is identified for pregnant women or new mothers, then the risk assessment must include a 'specific' risk assessment of exposure to work risk factors from any processes; working conditions; and physical, biological, and chemical agents that may be encountered. This includes women who have given birth in the last 6 months and for as long as they are breastfeeding, as well as any women who may have had a stillbirth after the 24th week of pregnancy. If the risk assessment identifies such a risk, then advice to the employer should suggest reasonable steps to remove it or prevent exposure to it.[15]

A risk assessment must also consider personal risk factors that may impact pregnancy (e.g. gestational diabetes, gestational high blood pressure, and hyperemesis). Again, as these are temporary adjustments, they are usually feasible for employers to implement, and depending on severity, generally should not result in an absence from work.

Exposure to infection of the pregnant mother within healthcare and educational settings is a risk that should be assessed and reduced, including by vaccination where

---

Box 8.1 Factors to consider in a pregnancy risk assessment

◆ Physically demanding work.

◆ Prolonged standing.

◆ Long hours, shift work, or night work.

◆ Hazards: radiation exposure, chemicals/anaesthetic gases.

appropriate. If the pregnant mother is exposed to high risks such as radiation or the lifting of heavy loads as part of routine duties, then this must be carefully assessed and prevented or reduced as per HSE guidance.

The infographic in Figure 8.5 has been produced by the Physical Activity and Pregnancy Study, commissioned by the UK Chief Medical Officers.[16]

The guiding principle of risk management is to ensure that employer and employee both abide by current legislation in order to maintain the safety of both mother and baby. The employer, on guidance from OH, should robustly assess the feasibility of instituting suggested adjustments within the service they provide, be that to patients or service users, or with regard to commercial deadlines, or indeed any other occupational obligations in order to maintain the health of the pregnant employee and her baby.

Impact of medication

Side effects of treatment during pregnancy, and the monitoring of pregnant workers coming off certain treatment, are additional factors to be considered and advised on by OH professionals, for instance, coming off medication for mental health disorders.

Pregnancy-related time off

Time off work for pregnancy-related medical conditions can be difficult, and should be addressed jointly with the employee, manager and human resources (HR). Maternity leave should be decided according to symptoms, and if all remains well, can be delayed for as long as possible, or until just before delivery. However, if there are continuous pregnancy-related symptomatic illnesses for which adjustments have not worked, then the pregnant employee should be advised to contact HR to discuss the best possible solution for both the employer and the employee regarding the start of maternity leave.

Pregnant employees have four key rights:

◆ Paid time off for antenatal care (which includes antenatal classes if recommended by a healthcare professional).

◆ Maternity leave.

◆ Maternity pay.

◆ Protection against unfair treatment, discrimination, or dismissal as a consequence of being pregnant, or on maternity leave.

Reciprocally, they are required to inform their employers that they are pregnant, the week the baby is expected to be born, and when they would like maternity leave and pay to commence. All pregnant employees are entitled to 52 weeks of maternity leave—26 weeks of ordinary maternity leave and 26 weeks of additional maternity leave.

Maternity leave

Pregnant women can start maternity leave as early as 29 weeks, and must not work for 2 weeks after the birth of their baby. While it might be possible for some women to work up

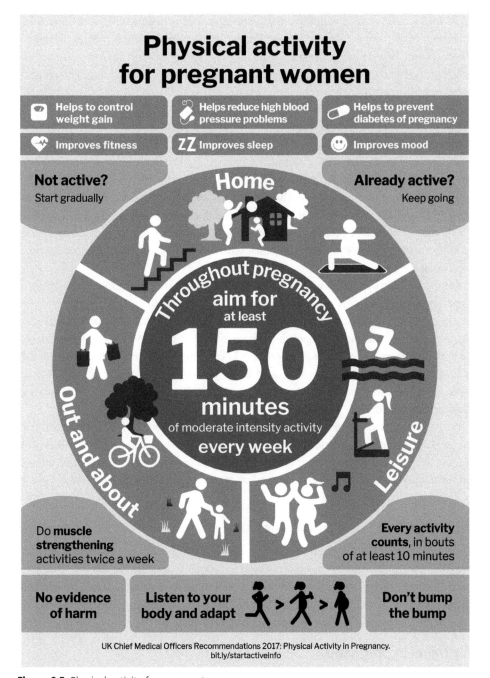

Figure 8.5 Physical activity for pregnant women.

Reproduced from Department of Health and Social Care (2018) Start active, stay active: infographics on physical activity. © Crown copyright, 2018.

to 38 weeks, most women will stop around 36 weeks. 'Term' begins at 37 weeks, with a 1 in 15 chance of delivery within the ensuing 7 days. Approximately 25% of women deliver between 38 and 39 weeks of gestation. By the due date, just over half of all pregnant women will have delivered. Women with a twin pregnancy, or higher-order multiple pregnancy, are especially likely to deliver prematurely, often between 32 and 37 weeks. A woman will be eligible for statutory maternity pay if she meets the required conditions.

Pregnancies with additional factors, such as multiple pregnancies, pregnancy following *in vitro* fertilization (IVF), pregnancies associated with a fetal abnormality, or pregnancies associated with uncertainty due to possible exposure to infection, should be assessed for their potential impact on the duties performed, as well as for the impact on the psychological well-being of the mother-to-be. Reassurance is often helpful, and regular contact with OH until the time of commencement of maternity leave can be helpful. In such cases, contact with OH prior to returning to work is often reassuring to all concerned as adjustments or advice to mitigate against biosocial factors or new health conditions is important.

Mental health in pregnancy is a serious issue that needs to be carefully considered, as the expectant mother may well be reluctant to take or continue treatment, and there is a tendency to non-compliance of treatment in the interest of protecting the fetus. During this time, expectant mothers may be susceptible to exacerbations of existing mental health conditions. In the postnatal period, it is even more important that such individuals are reassessed prior to any return to work, especially if postnatal depression is an issue. They may need guidance, reassurance, or specific temporary work adjustments of reduced hours or duties.

Pregnancy-related illness will need to be carefully considered with regard to the impact on work. The burden of reduced duties for the pregnant worker frequently falls on colleagues and this can lead to feelings of guilt in the person who needs to take time off or is on restricted duties. Guidelines on work adjustments are available from the Royal College of Physicians[17] and the HSE.[14]

Breastfeeding and postnatal health

Employers are legally required to provide suitable rest facilities for workers who are breastfeeding. Employers are also encouraged to provide a healthy, safe, and private environment for nursing mothers to express and store milk, although not a legal requirement. Importantly, new mothers are also entitled to paid time off for postnatal care (i.e. health clinic appointments), as is the case for antenatal care visits.

Air travel in pregnancy

There is no evidence that air travel increases the risk of complications in pregnancy such as preterm labour, rupture of membranes, or abruption. The radiation dose to the fetus from flying is not significant unless frequent long-haul air travel occurs in pregnancy. Body scanners that utilize ionizing radiation for security checks do not pose a risk to mother or fetus. Flights lasting more than 4 hours are associated with a small increase in the relative risk of venous thrombosis, but overall the absolute risk is very small. A specific venous thromboembolic risk assessment should be made in pregnant women who are travelling by air. Graduated elastic compression stockings are recommended for women flying medium- to long-haul flights and low-molecular-weight heparin for those with significant risk factors such as previous thrombosis or morbid obesity. Low-dose aspirin provides insufficient thromboprophylaxis for air travel. Some airlines request a 'fit to fly letter' after 26 weeks of gestation. 'Twin pregnancies' are advised not to fly after 32 weeks and women with singletons are advised not to fly after 36 weeks of gestation.[18]

Infertility

One in seven (14%) of couples will experience difficulty conceiving. Success rates for IVF vary significantly by age, but a quarter of cycles started using a woman's own fresh eggs result in a live birth. For women aged under 35, this figure is one-third. Sixty per cent of IVF is now privately funded with the average cost per cycle being approximately £4000.[19] Couples who have not conceived after 1–2 years of regular unprotected intercourse are advised to seek the help of a specialist. The variety of treatments varies enormously by diagnosis and maternal age, but a couple should expect to need 10–12 appointments, that is, a minimum of 10–12 days off work to attend the necessary appointments.

Initial consultations are performed face-to-face in clinic but increasingly telephone/video consultations are becoming available. Basic investigation includes semen analysis to exclude male factors. The women will then undergo a blood test to assess ovarian reserve (anti-Mullerian hormone) and usually a transvaginal ultrasound to exclude uterine abnormality and a test for tubal patency (e.g. hysterosalpingogram (HSG) or hysterosalpingo-contrast-sonography (HyCoSy)). Following initial testing, a review consultation will be offered to establish the diagnosis and decide on the best variant of treatment. The commonest form of fertility treatment is IVF.

Consent is an important part of Human Fertilisation and Embryology Authority regulation and most units require a specific appointment with an IVF nurse specialist to provide informed consent and teach safe injection techniques etc. Each attempt at IVF is called an IVF cycle. Depending on the protocol, three or four transvaginal ultrasounds over a 2-week period will be required to monitor ovarian response.

Two days after an appropriate response has been observed on scanning, egg collection will be arranged. This process often requires sedation and rarely may require general anaesthetic. Patients are advised to take 2 days to recover from egg collection. Eggs can either be stored (social egg freezing for women wishing to use them at a later date), fertilized, and re-implanted as a fresh cycle, or fertilized and stored as frozen embryos for future use if the 'fresh' cycle is unsuccessful.[19]

Embryo transfer is performed 2–5 days after egg collection, assuming fertilization has occurred *in vitro*. This does not usually require sedation. Sixteen days after egg collection urine can be tested for the pregnancy hormone human chorionic gonadotropin. Many IVF units will monitor pregnancy for 6 weeks with an ultrasound scan to confirm a fetal heartbeat. The success rate is 25–50% per cycle using fresh embryos but advances in storage technology has meant IVF cycles using frozen eggs are now similar. This is particularly significant for single women requiring social egg freezing when they are waiting to meet the right partner.

Occupational health management of infertility treatment

The number of women taking up IVF treatment is increasing. Such efforts tend to be accompanied by anxiety about the success of the process and the financial implications. Employers and employees need to confer as to arrangements that might be suitable to both parties regarding allowances for time taken off to attend IVF clinics, and for the purpose of making adjustments for any temporary side effects of the process or treatments. The distress related to failure of IVF treatment should be carefully considered and, wherever possible, emotional support should be arranged in order to maximize support for continued subsequent work attendance or performance.

IVF also carries a risk of multiple pregnancy. This needs to be considered with respect to shift work, long hours, or exposure to radiation or chemicals such as dry cleaning fluids, or noxious gases that could have an adverse impact on the high-risk pregnancy. The HSE provides clear guidance[14] on assessment of pregnancy risks with regard to substances that may pose a risk in the workplace. Nevertheless, in the case of an individual who is pregnant by virtue of IVF treatment, extra caution should be taken and any foreseeable risks removed or reduced as far as possible, and additional emotional support provided.

Menopause

Natural menopause is defined as the permanent cessation of menstrual periods, determined retrospectively after a woman has experienced 12 months of amenorrhea without any other obvious pathological or physiological cause. It occurs normally at a median age of 51.4 years and is a reflection of complete, or near complete, ovarian follicular depletion, with resulting hypo-oestrogenaemia and high follicle-stimulating hormone concentrations.[20] Menopause before the age of 40 years is considered to be abnormal and is referred to as primary ovarian insufficiency (premature ovarian failure). The menopausal transition, or perimenopause, occurs after the reproductive years, but before the menopause. Menopausal transition begins on average 4 years before the final menstrual period and includes a number of physiological changes that may affect a woman's quality of life. It is characterized by irregular menstrual cycles and marked hormonal fluctuations, often accompanied by hot flushes, sleep disturbance, mood symptoms, and vaginal dryness.[20,21] Up to 80% develop hot flushes (the most common menopausal symptom), but only 20–30% seek medical attention for treatment.[20] In addition, changes in lipids and bone loss begin to occur, both of which have implications for long-term health.

Comprehensive information about the endocrine and clinical manifestations of the menopausal transition comes from a number of longitudinal cohort studies of midlife women, the largest of which, the Study of Women's Health Across the Nation (SWAN), has followed a multi-ethnic, community-based cohort of over 3000 women aged 42–52 years for 15 years.[22]

For most women, the menopause causes no significant problems, but some women, perhaps 20–25%, report considerable difficulties in both their personal and working lives.[23] During their menopausal transition, some women report that fatigue and difficulties with memory and concentration affect work. Those who experience problematic hot flushes report them as a source of embarrassment and distress at work. Although the evidence is as yet inconclusive, some women report that they believe that their symptoms impact negatively on their work performance. Some report that they work particularly hard during this time to overcome perceived performance detriments. Whatever the case, women do report concern over such issues, and that they feel less confident than usual at work. For some, it is clearly a challenging time.

Occupational health support during menopause

Women are sometimes reluctant to disclose their menopausal status and related problems at work. This is particularly the case where they have male managers or managers who are younger than them, regardless of gender. The provision of training programmes about menopause and work for women and for managers could be offered, as well as advice about how to broach a discussion about menopause and work.[24] There is evidence that a cognitive behavioural therapy approach helps women deal with hot flushes and night sweats.[25]

Information about menopause and signposting to further sources of advice can be provided within the workplace. There are many examples of online guidance for the management of menopausal symptoms for particular working conditions as well as generic guidance (see 'Useful websites'). The guidance from the Faculty of Occupational Medicine is a valuable tool for both employees and employers (Figure 8.6).[26]

Employers should have a sympathetic and pragmatic understanding of the impact of the menopause on the female workforce. Engendering a culture whereby employees feel comfortable disclosing health problems, can work flexibly with agreement, and manage any work-related stress that adds to the burden of symptoms would be very helpful. Women themselves have suggested that flexible working helps during periods of poor sleep. In an administrative work environment, adjustments can be made more readily as the work is usually sedentary and can be flexible. With current IT support, work can also be done remotely from the office, (e.g. at home), especially during symptomatic phases.

Menopausal bleeding irregularities should be clinically assessed, and the resultant situation then addressed accordingly within the workplace. This will require provision for clinical appointments for symptomatic issues (e.g. menorrhagia/associated mental health issues). If cognitive function (e.g. mild forgetfulness, concentration, and fatigue) is an issue, then consider OH assessment with advice to ensuring safety or adjustments such as temporary reduction or redefinition of the workload while an equilibrium is still being reached during menopausal physiological changes. Existing mental health conditions can be aggravated, and the individual may benefit from review or reassurance.

In addition, simple environmental measures such as providing easy access to cold drinking water and toilets and reviewing workplace temperature and ventilation could further help in accommodating symptoms during the period of physiological changes.

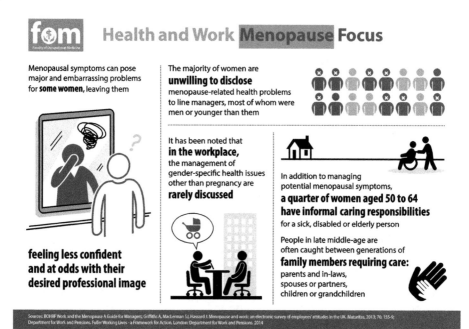

Figure 8.6 'Health and Work: Menopause Focus' infographic from the Faculty of Occupational Medicine.
Reproduced from Department of Health and Social Care (2018) Start active, stay active: infographics on physical activity. © Crown copyright, 2018.

Where women are required to wear uniforms, consider allowing a more flexible approach, for example, with layering, or with changes to the types of fabric used.

A number of qualitative studies[27, 28] have explored women's views about the nature of supportive employer and manager behaviour (Box 8.2).

Box 8.2 Workplace recommendations for the menopause

- Employers and managers should have more knowledge and awareness about the menopause.
- Employers and managers should be better able to talk about the menopause.
- Specific needs during the menopause should be assessed with agreement of appropriate work adjustments.
- Staff should be provided with appropriate training and supportive policies should be developed.
- Working conditions should be assessed to consider the specific needs of menopausal women and ensure that the working environment will not make their symptoms worse.

Cancers of the reproductive system

Endometrial cancer

Endometrial cancer accounts for 3% of female cancers, and is the fourth most common cancer diagnosed in women after breast cancer, lung cancer, and cancer of the colon and rectum (see Cancer Research UK website, listed in 'Useful websites'). In the UK, about 8475 new cases of uterine cancer are diagnosed each year, mainly in postmenopausal women aged 40–74. Other risk factors include nulliparity, obesity, diabetes, and Lynch syndrome (aka hereditary nonpolyposis colorectal cancer). Ninety per cent of endometrial cancers present with postmenopausal bleeding, intermenstrual bleeding, vaginal discharge, anaemia, or thrombocytosis.

Staging with magnetic resonance imaging or computed tomography scans are commonly used to help a multidisciplinary specialist team within a cancer centre determine the most appropriate treatment. Shared decision-making has been an integral part of the NHS since 2010.[29] Surgery is the mainstay of treatment, although radiotherapy and chemotherapy may be required in advanced stages. Five-year survival rates range from 95% at stage I to 15% for stage IV endometrial carcinoma.

Cervical cancer

In the UK, 2800 women are diagnosed with cervical cancer annually. It usually affects women over the age of 20 with the highest rates in women aged between 30 and 34. The NHS cervical screening programme is available to women aged 25–64 in England. GP-registered eligible women receive an invitation every 3 years while women aged 50–64 receive invitations every 5 years. Early screening/detection prevents 75% of cancers.

Human papillomavirus (HPV) causes 99.7% of cervical cancers. HPV is transmitted through sexual contact and can be prevented by a two-dose vaccination (Gardasil®). In most cases, the immune system will clear HPV without the need for treatment but smokers are at higher risk. HPV has over 100 subtypes and hence HPV-positive women should be referred for colposcopy. If high-risk HPV is not detected, women may return to routine screening.[30]

Biopsies taken at colposcopy may confirm the pre-invasive (non-cancerous) condition known as cervical intraepithelial neoplasia (CIN). CIN is graded I–III and is most commonly treated with large loop excision of the transformation zone or loop electrosurgical excision.

Invasive cancers (squamous cell carcinoma and adenocarcinoma, adenosquamous carcinomas, clear-cell carcinoma, and small-cell carcinoma) are staged and graded. Treatment depends on location, size, and metastasis. Treatments include surgery or a combination of chemotherapy and radiotherapy (chemoradiotherapy). The advent of radical trachelectomy (removal of cervical cuff and retention of uterus and vagina rather than hysterectomy) has enabled nulliparous women to have IVF and children following major surgery.

Ovarian cancer

Ovarian cancer affects 7000 women per year and a woman's lifetime risk of developing ovarian cancer is about 1.3%. Symptoms such as bloating, pain, urinary frequency, change in bowel habit, fatigue, and unexplained weight loss are non-specific and presentation of ovarian cancer is often at an advanced stage (75% at stage III or IV). Risk factors include advancing age, family history of *BRCA1* or *BRCA2* gene mutations, and use of hormone replacement therapy. Treatment depends on grade and staging and consists of a combination of surgery or chemotherapy. Palliative debulking surgery may be offered to maintain quality of life in advanced stages. Five-year survival rates vary by stage and subtype, ranging from 90% at stage I to 6% for stage IV (see Cancer Research UK website, in 'Useful websites').

Occupational health management of gynaecological cancers

The implications of breast and gynaecological cancers for fitness for work are covered in Chapter 29. Any diagnosis of cancer has a huge and understandable psychological impact on the affected individual. The majority of women who respond well, return to or remain at work and perform all duties normally. Others who have disabling side effects may require permanent adjustments, being either psychologically unable to recover completely, or else cautious about the kind of duties they undertake, or being limited by lymphoedema, pain, and scarring. These should be assessed independently on a case-by-case basis, and case-specific adjustments suggested to maintain work attendance and performance. A multidisciplinary meeting with HR included can be useful.

Same-sex preference and gender identity issues

LGBTQ

Approximately 10% of people identify as lesbian, gay, bisexual, transgender, or questioning their gender (LGBTQ). Health and well-being issues relating to these groups are numerous and poorly understood by health professionals.

Depression and suicide

Young gay men account for 30% of completed suicides[31] and 40% of LGBTQ youths have either attempted or seriously contemplated suicide. Gay men are six times more likely to attempt suicide than heterosexual men and lesbians are twice as likely to attempt suicide as heterosexual women. Suicide attempts by gay men are more severe than their heterosexual counterparts with risk factors including non-conforming to gender (e.g. men in more feminine gender roles), self-identification as gay or bisexual at a young age, first homosexual experience at an early age, history of sexual or physical abuse, and rejection from important social support.

Substance misuse

Early reports on drug and alcohol use in the LGBTQ community suggested that substance abuse affected about a third of the adult gay population.[32] Comparisons of lesbian and heterosexual women showed no differences in alcohol consumption, although lesbians and bisexual women were more likely to report being recovering alcoholics. Gay men abuse a wider variety of drugs, such as marijuana, 'poppers' (amyl nitrite or butyl nitrite), and amphetamines. Although causality cannot be determined, a history of consistent use of inhalants, amphetamines, and cocaine is strongly associated with HIV seroconversion, independent of injection drug use. Cigarette smoking is also increased and healthcare professionals should actively assess the extent and context of substance misuse in their LGBTQ patients.

Cervical cancer

In a recent US national survey,[32] only 54% of lesbian and bisexual women had undertaken a cervical smear within the past year, and 7.5% had never had cervical screening. This is partially due to the misconception among both lesbians and healthcare professionals that lesbians are not at risk of cervical cancer. In one study, 30% of lesbians and bisexual women had a history of sexually transmitted disease. Physicians should recommend cervical screening according to current guidelines and teach safe sex techniques to prevent the transmission of HPV between sexual partners.

Breast and endometrial cancer

Lesbian and bisexual women are less likely to use oral contraceptives, more likely to be nulliparous, and more likely to smoke cigarettes than heterosexual women, all of which are risk factors for breast and endometrial cancer. Healthcare professionals should recommend breast screening according to guidelines.

Transgender health (gender dysphoria)

In recent years, transgender issues have arisen with increasing frequency within the workplace. These issues should be assessed with sympathy as society gradually learns to normalize their perspective. Transgender persons maintain a strong and persistent cross-gender identification, not merely a desire for any cultural advantages of being the opposite sex. Transgender persons are considered to have gender dysphoria. Those who are transgender (transsexual) face novel challenges compared to lesbians, gays, and bisexuals. They are a minority within a minority group. Therefore they are at greater risk of depression, suicide, substance abuse, and violence, although this has not been formally quantified.

Transsexuals may seek gender reassignment surgery. The process of gender reassignment is long and involves psychiatric, endocrine, and surgical evaluation. In addition to the risk of thromboembolism and liver abnormalities secondary to prolonged oestrogen use, there is also the rare possibility of pituitary prolactinoma. For female-to-male transgender persons, androgen therapy carries an increased risk of heart disease, endometrial hyperplasia, and subsequent endometrial carcinoma.

Gender reassignment surgery may cause sexual dysfunction. Clinicians need to be sensitive to the psychosocial and medical status of transgender patients.[33]

Occupational health assessment around gender reassignment

Sympathetic support while undergoing reassignment assessment is of great importance. The issues to be considered during the treatment phase would be time required to attend appointments, side effects of any treatment both medical as well as surgical, needs to be recognized, and adjustments advised accordingly. A major issue would be the psychological impact before and after the conversion into the opposite gender. Within the workplace, due to stigma, there may be unkind (intentional or non-intentional) comments from colleagues. This requires careful handling of the psychological understanding of the colleagues and managers as well as the employee themselves. If there are any underlying mental health issues, these need to be monitored carefully as they are often exacerbated while coping with the stresses of a gender conversion process. Healthcare professionals should create a safe, non-judgemental environment for patients. In addition, OH professionals should be aware of community support systems within schools and workplaces.

This is often the time and setting for bullying and harassment to prevail and the employee needs support and appropriate signposting for specific help. HR may need to be part of the support by reducing intolerance among colleagues, and addressing bullying behaviour in the workplace.

Tolerance of homosexuality is far better now than in the past, but some can still experience a detrimental attitude at work that could result in mental health problems. Training and reducing stigma in the workplace is an employer responsibility but OH has a part to play in enhancing the well-being of such employees and enabling them to work securely in their workplace.

Key points

- Women constitute a valuable part of the labour workforce and contribute economically to the commercial welfare of the country.

- Provision of good childcare also helps in maintaining the wellness at work of women and of men who have childcare duties. With newer technology, it is easier to make flexible working hours more possible and hence enable parents to work productively within their health limitations.

- As women work longer, their physiological changes such as menopause may need to be addressed in the workplace. The comfort of work places, especially temperature, is important for all employees but can be particularly helpful during perimenopause.

- As medical treatments advance and expectations of women with female gender-related cancers change, OH professionals need an up-to-date understanding of the treatment processes and side effects in order to give specific and helpful advice to the employee and employer.

- Those with same-sex preferences or gender identity issues may seek OH advice. They need reassurance and support in the workplace as much as other employees, and training of employers and colleagues will help reduce stigma.

Useful websites

Royal College of Physicians. Pregnancy: occupational aspects of management	https://www.rcplondon.ac.uk/guidelines-policy/pregnancy-occupational-aspects-management
Faculty of Occupational Medicine. Advice on the menopause	http://www.fom.ac.uk/health-at-work-2/information-for-employers/dealing-with-health-problems-in-the-workplace/advice-on-the-menopause
Royal College of Obstetricians and Gynaecologists	https://www.rcog.org.uk/en/careers-training/resources-support-for-trainees/advice-and-support-for-trainees/working-during-pregnancy-advice-for-trainees/carrying-out-your-normal-duties-during-pregnancy/
Human Fertilisation and Embryology Authority	http://www.hfea.gov.uk
Health and Safety Executive	http://www.hse.gov.uk/mothers/flowchart.htm http://www.hse.gov.uk/mothers
Miscarriage Association	http://www.miscarriageassociation.org.uk
Tommys	https://www.tommys.org
Trades Union Congress (2011). Supporting women through the menopause	http://www.tuc.org.uk/extras/Supporting_Women_Through_the_Menopause.pdf
Royal College of Nursing (2016). The menopause and work: guidance for RCN representatives	https://www.rcn.org.uk/professional-development/publications/pub-005467
National Union of Teachers (2014). Teachers working through the menopause.	https://www.teachers.org.uk/files/menopause-a4-for-web--9968-.pdf
Department of Health and Social Care. Infographics on physical activity	https://www.gov.uk/government/publications/start-active-stay-active-infographics-on-physical-activity
UK government. Statutory maternity pay	https://www.gov.uk/maternity-pay-leave/eligibility
Cancer Research UK	https://www.cancerresearchuk.org

Acknowledgement

The authors are grateful to Amanda Griffiths for her contribution on the menopause.

References

1. **Office for National Statistics.** Labour Force Survey performance and quality monitoring reports. Available at: https://www.ons.gov.uk/employmentandlabourmarket/peopleinwork/employmentandemployeetypes/methodologies/labourforcesurveyperformanceandqualitymonitoringreports.

2. **Office for National Statistics.** UK labour market: June 2017. Available at: https://www.ons.gov.uk/employmentandlabourmarket/peopleinwork/employmentandemployeetypes/bulletins/uklabourmarket/june2017.

3. **Office for National Statistics.** Sickness absence in the UK labour market: 2016. Available at:https://www.ons.gov.uk/employmentandlabourmarket/peopleinwork/labourproductivity/articles/sicknessabsenceinthelabourmarket/2016.

4. **Office for National Statistics.** UK labour market: October 2017. Available at: https://www.ons.gov.uk/employmentandlabourmarket/peopleinwork/employmentandemployeetypes/bulletins/uklabourmarket/october2017.

5. **Kuchenbecker WK, Groen H, van Asselt SJ, et al.** In women with polycystic ovary syndrome and obesity, loss of intra-abdominal fat is associated with resumption of ovulation. *Hum Reprod* 2011;**26**:2505–12.

6. **ESHRE Capri Workshop Group.** Health and fertility in World Health Organization group 2 anovulatory women. *Hum Reprod Update*, 2012;**18**;586–99.

7. **Simoens S, Dunselman G, Dirksen C, et al.** The burden of endometriosis: costs and quality of life of women with endometriosis and treated in referral centres. *Hum Reprod* 2012;**27**:1292–9.

8. **National Institute for Health and Care Excellence (NICE).** *Heavy Menstrual Bleeding: Assessment and Management.* NICE clinical guideline [NG44]. London: NICE; 2016. Available at: https://www.nice.org.uk/guidance/ng88.

9. **NHS.** Recovering from a hysterectomy. 2016. Available at: https://www.nhs.uk/conditions/Hysterectomy/#recovering-from-a-hysterectomy.

10. **Aarts JW, Nieboer TE, Johnson N, et al.** Surgical approach to hysterectomy for benign gynaecological disease. *Cochrane Database Syst Rev* 2015;**8**:CD003677.

11. **Murji A, Whitaker L, Chow TL, Sobel ML.** Selective progesterone receptor modulators (SPRMs) for uterine fibroids *Cochrane Database Syst Rev* 2017;**4**:CD010770.

12. **British Pregnancy Advisory Service.** After an abortion. Available at: https://www.bpas.org/abortion-care/after-an-abortion.

13. **Royal College of Obstetricians and Gynaecologists.** *Recurrent Miscarriage: Investigation and Treatment of Couples.* Greentop Guideline 17. London: Royal College of Obstetricians and Gynaecologists; 2011 (updated 2017).

14. **Health and Safety Executive.** New and expectant mothers at work. 2013. Available at: http://www.hse.gov.uk/pubns/indg373.pdf.

15. **Maternity Action UK.** Work and benefits. Available at: https://www.maternityaction.org.uk.

16. **UK Chief Medical Officers.** Physical Activity and Pregnancy Study. Department of Health and Social Care; 2016. Available at: https://www.gov.uk/government/publications/start-active-stay-active-infographics-on-physical-activity.

17. **Royal College of Physicians.** Pregnancy: Occupational aspects of management. 2013. Available at: https://www.rcplondon.ac.uk/guidelines-policy/pregnancy-occupational-aspects-management.

18. **Royal College of Obstetricians and Gynaecologists.** Air Travel and Pregnancy. RCOG Scientific Impact Paper No. 1. 2013. Available at: https://www.rcog.org.uk/en/guidelines-research-services/guidelines/sip1/.

19. **Human Fertilisation and Embryology Authority**. Fertility treatment 2014–16: Trends and figures. 2018. Available at: https://www.hfea.gov.uk/media/2544/hfea-fertility-treatment-2014-2016-trends-and-figures.pdf.

20. **Casper, R.F.** Clinical manifestations and diagnosis of menopause. *UpToDate* Oct. 2017. Available at: https://www.uptodate.com/contents/clinical-manifestations-and-diagnosis-of-menopause.

21. **Burger HG.** Unpredictable endocrinology of the menopause transition: clinical, diagnostic and management implications. *Menopause Int* 2011;**17**:153–4.

22. **Bromberger JT, Schott LL, Kravitz HM, et al.** Longitudinal change in reproductive hormones and depressive symptoms across the menopausal transition: results from the Study of Women's Health Across the Nation (SWAN). *Arch Gen Psychiatry* 2010;**67**:598–607.

23. **Griffiths A, Hunter M.** Psychosocial factors and the menopause: the impact of the menopause on personal and working life. In: Davies SC (ed), *Annual Report of the Chief Medical Officer 2014 – The Health of the 51%: Women*, pp. 109–20. London: Department of Health; 2015. Available at: https://www.gov.uk/government/publications/chief-medical-officer-annual-report-2014-womens-health.

24. **Hardy C, Griffiths A, Hunter M.** What do working menopausal women want? A qualitative investigation into women's perspectives on employer and line manager support. *Maturitas* 2017;**101**:37–41.

25. **Hardy C, Griffiths A, Norton S, Hunter M.** Self-help cognitive behaviour therapy for working women with problematic hot flushes and night sweats (MENOS@Work): a multicentre randomised controlled trial. *Menopause* 2018;**25**:508–19.

26. **Faculty of Occupational Medicine**. Guidance on menopause and the workplace. 2016. Available at: http://www.fom.ac.uk/health-at-work-2/information-for-employers/dealing-with-health-problems-in-the-workplace/advice-on-the-menopause.

27. **Hardy C, Griffiths A, Hunter MS.** What do working menopausal women want? A qualitative investigation into women's perspectives on employer and line manager support. *Maturitas* 2017;**101**:37–41.

28. **Griffiths A, Ceausu I, Depypere H, et al.** EMAS recommendations for conditions in the workplace for menopausal women. *Maturitas* 2016;**85**:79–81.

29. **Department of Health and Social Care**. *Equity and Excellence: Liberating the NHS*. London: Department of Health and Social Care; 2010.

30. **Public Health England**. NHS Cervical Screening Programme: laboratory quality control and assurance for human papillomavirus testing. 2017. Available at: https://www.gov.uk/government/publications/cervical-screening-laboratory-testing-for-human-papillomavirus/nhs-cervical-screening-programme-laboratory-quality-control-and-assurance-for-human-papillomavirus-testing.

31. **Paul JP, Catania J, Pollack L, et al.** Suicide attempts among gay and bisexual men: lifetime prevalence and antecedents. *Am J Public Health* 2002;**92**:1338–45.

32. **Russell ST, Fish JN.** Annual review of clinical psychology mental health in lesbian, gay, bisexual, and transgender (LGBT) youth. *Annu Rev Clin Psychol* 2016;**12**:465–87.

33. **Lee R.** Lesbian, gay and bisexual patients the issues for general practice. *West J Med* 2000;**172**:403–8.

Chapter 9

Sickness absence

Richard Preece

Introduction

Sickness absence is an important issue for workers, managers, and occupational health (OH) services. Most employees suffer health problems at some time during their career, and face decisions on fitness in relation to their work. All employers will occasionally be concerned about the fitness to work of absent employees and what actions they might take to address this. Advising on sickness absence management and the fitness to work of absentees, individually and collectively, is a major activity for OH professionals.

Epidemiology of sickness absence

An estimated 137 million working days are lost each year in the UK due to sickness absence.[1] International comparisons of sickness absence rates are uncommon but reveal marked variations.[2] Sickness absence rates vary by sex, age, occupation, sector, region, pay grade[3] (see Figure 9.1), and the size of the workplace[4] and a large number of other psychosocial factors relating to employees' attitudes and behaviour.[5]

The principal causes of long-term sickness absence among manual workers (across all sectors in the UK) are musculoskeletal injuries, followed by acute medical conditions, back pain, and stress. Among non-manual workers (across all sectors), the leading causes are acute medical conditions, stress, mental health problems (such as depression and anxiety), minor ailments, and musculoskeletal injuries.[4] Many different factors influence sickness absence. Illness is usually accepted as the reason for an episode of sickness absence, but very little of the variance in absence rates among individual employees is explained by illness. In a large study in Wales, only 4% of the variance in sickness absence rates was explained by illness.[6,7] This observation is important as it emphasizes the importance of addressing the non-biological elements of the biopsychosocial model.

Theoretical models of sickness absence management

Three models of sickness absence are popular: the expected utility model of absenteeism, the stress model, and the organization model.[8]

The *expected utility model* assumes that workers have some choice whether or not they will report sick and that they consider the costs and rewards in making a decision to

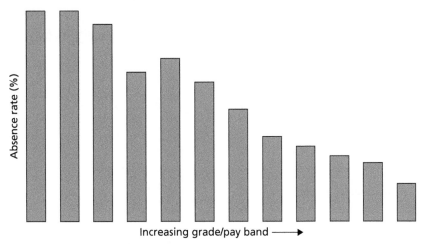

Figure 9.1 Absence rate relationship with grade/pay.
Source: data from National Health Service (2011) *Managing Sickness Absence in the NHS*. Health Briefing February 2011. London, UK: NHS. Copyright © 2011 Audit Commission.

attend or not. Approaches based on this model should aim to set a high threshold for being absent and a low threshold for resuming work when absent.

The occupational *stress model* focuses on the negative effects of the work environment and the coping abilities of workers. Some people are more resilient and have better coping strategies than others. Approaches based on this model focus on reducing stressors, improving social support, and building resilience.

The *organization model* focuses on rewarding work, including job content, fairness, status, and social relationships, to improve satisfaction and motivation. Approaches based on this model focus on promoting well-being.

These three models all have merit. In practice, they are often combined to form an *integrated model* which aims to alter the balance of costs and rewards, reduce stress, and promote resilience and well-being.

Promoting attendance

Engagement

Engagement is 'a workplace approach designed to ensure that employees are committed to their organisation's goals and values, motivated to contribute to organisational success and are able at the same time to enhance their own sense of wellbeing'.[9]

In recent years, measures of staff engagement have been increasingly recognized as important indicators of performance across the private and public sectors. Macleod et al.[9] found that engaged employees have lower sickness absence rates than those who are disengaged with beneficial effects on competitiveness and performance. Staff with high levels of engagement displayed a number of positive behavioural traits. See Box 9.1.

Box 9.1 Positive traits of staff with high engagement

- ◆ Increased commitment.
- ◆ A belief in their organization.
- ◆ A desire to work to make things better.
- ◆ Suggesting improvements.
- ◆ Working well in a team.
- ◆ Helping colleagues.
- ◆ A likelihood to 'go the extra mile'.

Four broad enablers are critical to employee engagement: leadership (strategic narrative), enabling managers, employee voice, and, integrity.[9]

A positive working environment is good for health and well-being with evidence from the largest staff survey in the UK that higher levels of staff engagement are associated with lower levels of sickness absence (Figure 9.2).[10]

Manager attitudes and behaviour

Line managers are important to promoting attendance. See Box 9.2.

The behaviour of line managers is a major influence on whether employees remain in work and resume work successfully following a period of sickness absence.[11] The most

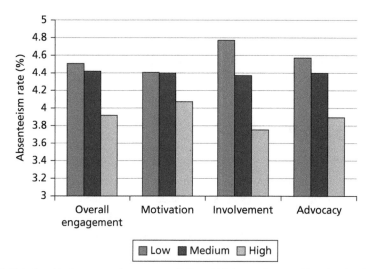

Figure 9.2 Relationship between absence rate (%) and high, medium and low levels of staff engagement (n = 154,726).

Adapted from West, M. et al. *NHS Staff Management and Health Service Quality*. London, UK: Department of Health. © Crown Copyright 2011.

Box 9.2 Line management responsibilities

◆ Setting objectives.

◆ Designing work arrangements.

◆ Supporting employees (whether they face health issues or not).

◆ Making adjustments to work.

important attributes of managers are good people management skills, including effective communication, and sensitivity to, and understanding of, the individual and the context.

Managers who do not believe that sickness absence can be reduced tend to underestimate its impact and are less likely to tackle the problem proactively. This may be a particular issue for managers who have only ever worked in a sector with relatively high sickness absence rates and have not experienced anything different. In these circumstances, managers' attitudes will undermine the effectiveness and bring into doubt the value of interventions. It becomes critical to understand and change managers' beliefs about improving attendance if improvement is to be achieved.[12]

What is good work?

In his review of the most effective evidence-based strategies for reducing health inequalities, Marmot reported that being in 'good' employment is protective of health and getting people into work is therefore of critical importance. Marmot described ten core components of work that protect good health and promote health[13] (Box 9.3).

Although good work is desirable, there is a danger that its importance is both overstated and idealistic, leading everyone to conclude that their own work and the work of those they manage is not good. It is difficult to show the health benefits of work; the evidence for physical health benefits remains limited but there is now strong evidence that employment reduces the risk of depression and improves general mental health.[14] In encouraging and supporting attendance, the focus should emphasize that work is usually good for health and that with some effort it can be even better.

Measuring and monitoring absence

The starting point in managing sickness absence is to measure and report it. The system of measurement should reflect the size and complexity of the organization. In smaller businesses, the impact of absence is often immediate and stark—there is simply nobody else to do the work.

For larger organizations, managers will need to measure and respond to the impact on their teams' activities. The immediate and short-term impact may seem small as work carries on. Senior managers in larger organizations will need to measure and respond to the wider organizational impact on performance and productivity.

Box 9.3 Characteristics of good work

'Good' work (is):

- Free of the core features of precariousness, such as lack of stability and high risk of job loss, lack of safety measures (exposure to toxic substances, elevated risks of accidents), and the absence of minimal standards of employment protection.

- Enables the worker to exert some control through participatory decision-making on matters such as the place and the timing of work and the tasks to be accomplished.

- Places appropriately high demands on the worker, both in terms of quantity and quality, without overtaxing their resources and capabilities and without doing harm to their physical and mental health.

- Provides fair employment in terms of earnings reflecting productivity and in terms of employers' commitment towards guaranteeing job security.

- Offers opportunities for skill training, learning, and promotion prospects within a life course perspective, sustaining health and work ability and stimulating the growth of an individual's capabilities.

- Prevents social isolation, discrimination, and violence.

- Enables workers to share relevant information within the organization, to participate in organizational decision-making and collective bargaining, and to guarantee procedural justice in case of conflicts.

- Aims at reconciling work and extra-work/family demands in ways that reduce the cumulative burden of multiple social roles.

- Attempts to reintegrate sick and disabled people into full employment wherever possible by mobilizing available means.

- Contributes to workers' well-being by meeting the basic psychological needs of experiencing self-efficacy, self-esteem, sense of belonging, and meaningfulness.

Reprinted from Department for International Development (2010) *Fair society, healthy lives: the Marmot Review: strategic review of health inequalities in England post-2010.* London, UK: Department for International Development. © Crown Copyright 2010.

The act of measuring and reporting absence accurately can serve to prompt intervention and to identify trends. Typically, organizations will measure sickness absence rates in terms either of days of absence or percentage of lost working time. However, this seemingly simple measure may not be straightforward, for example, in counting:

- the number of working days (e.g. public holidays and weekends)
- absence for only part of a working day

◆ absences of part-time workers
◆ absences of those working variable length shifts.

$$\text{Sickness absence rate}(\%) = \frac{\text{Total absence (hours or days) in the period}}{\text{Possible total (hours or days) in the period}} \times 100$$

Many organizations prefer instead to emphasize and report the positive measure of attendance rate.

The second typical measure is one that provides an indication of the frequency of periods of sickness absence:

$$\text{Frequency rate} = \frac{\text{No. of spells of absence in the period}}{\text{No. of employees}} \times 100$$

These two measures give some indication of the impact of sickness absence on the organization. However, they offer little insight into the nature of the underlying absence in terms of causes, patterns, and the impact arising from absent subgroups within the workforce.

The cause of absence can be monitored by recording the reasons cited by employees and their doctors on certificates, but data gathered in these ways can be difficult to interpret. The actual reason or reasons for sickness absence may not be the one(s) declared. Moreover, the impact of work and potential for intervention at work may not be clear.

A summary sickness absence rate gives no indication of the underlying pattern of absence. Other measures are needed to demonstrate the contribution from distinct episodes of short and long duration. Long periods of absence usually contribute most to the overall lost time but may not have such a dramatic effect on business continuity as managers have time to make plans in response and maintain output. In contrast, short, frequent episodes may contribute less to overall lost time but may be highly disruptive with a disproportionate impact on productivity.

Inception rates indicate the number of new episodes starting in the measurement period—expressed as a proportion (%) of the average number of staff employed in that period. This may be useful as a measure of longer periods of absence. (Termination rates, the number of episodes ending in the measurement period, are a related alternative and have a potential advantage as the reason for absence may be known.)

$$\text{Inception rate} = \frac{\text{No. of spells of absence which start in the period}}{\text{No. of employess}}$$

Many workers will not be absent at all during a monitoring period and some will be absent on several occasions. The overall rates do not give any indication of absence behaviour. Frequent absences may be an indication of a long-term underlying health problem but more often it is because the worker has a lower threshold for not attending (e.g. due to carer responsibilities or illness behaviour). Measuring the organizational impact of workers taking frequent episodes of sickness absence can prompt management intervention:

$$\text{Frequency episodes rate} = \frac{\text{No. of employees absent on more than} \times \text{occasions in the period}}{\text{No. of employees}} \times 100$$

While some workers will be absent frequently, the majority will not. Many workers rarely take any sickness absence. Some illness is inevitable and it is not possible for all employees to attend all the time. In some cases, attending when ill can have a detrimental impact on productivity (presenteeism) or on colleagues and customers (e.g. due to infectious diseases). Full attendance during a time period does, however, provide some indication of engagement and commitment:

$$\text{Full attendance rate} = \frac{\text{No. of employees who take no sickness absence at all in the period}}{\text{No. of employees}} \times 100$$

Recording sickness absence in 'real time' enables managers to intervene swiftly to provide support and to take action to encourage attendance.

Trigger points

Typically, management protocols will define 'trigger points' at which managers should consider formal action to require improved attendance. Trigger points can provide a consistent approach to attendance management but there is a risk that they institutionalize absenteeism by establishing an acceptable level of absence. In setting trigger points, it is important to emphasize that the objective is full attendance of all employees and to emphasize the importance of management discretion in considering the period(s) of absence within the whole picture for an individual employee.

Trigger points may be based upon any or all of:

◆ the cumulative number of days of absence in a time period

◆ the number of episodes of absence in a time period

◆ the pattern of episodes (e.g. on a public holiday or immediately before or after a holiday/weekend).

Organizations may adopt a trigger point based on a combination of days and episodes. The best known example of this is the Bradford score (also known as factor, formula, and index) which is designed to provide an indication of the disruption caused by persistent periods of short-duration sickness absence. The Bradford score combines measures of both frequency and duration of absence, with a greater emphasis placed on frequency. The formula S^2D or $S \times S \times D$, is used to calculate a score or index for a given period (usually a rolling year), where S is the number of spells of absence, and D is the aggregate number of days absent.

The Bradford score appears to have been derived from Bradford's law (of scatter). Samuel Clements Bradford (1878–1948) was a practising librarian and one of the pioneers of bibliometrics. He found that most of the papers on a certain subject were published in a few journals and some articles were scattered in many borderline journals, and so proposed a mathematical formula to describe the large contribution from a small number.[15]

The utility of the Bradford score is even less certain than its provenance. Its effectiveness has not been demonstrated. There is a danger that use of the Bradford score, or another scoring system, leads to undue focus on employees with long-term health conditions who are prone to short-term exacerbations but whose overall attendance is above average, and employees with significant carer responsibilities.

For example, an employee taking five individual days of sickness absence in a year would have a higher Bradford score ($5 \times 5 \times 5 = 125$) than an employee having two episodes each totalling 4 weeks ($2 \times 2 \times 20 = 80$). The first employee's absence may be significantly below average and the second employee's well above average, but if the organization has set a trigger point of 100 then only the first employee would face formal management action. However, many employers are comfortable with this as they place greater weight on disruptive periodic absences.

Statement of Fitness for Work (fit note)

The Statement of Fitness for Work (known as a 'fit note') was introduced in the UK in 2010. It was designed to allow clinicians to provide their patients with advice on fitness for work and to encourage patients to resume some work as soon as they have recovered sufficiently. However, clinicians do not provide fitness advice on the great majority of fit notes.[16] Mild to moderate severity mental illnesses are the commonest diagnoses recorded on fit notes.[17] Factors associated with issue of a longer-term fit note include male patients, older patient age, and higher social deprivation.

As yet, the benefit of the fit note has not been convincingly demonstrated.[18] This is especially the case for mental illness. However, it has been suggested that provision of fitness for work advice may be improved through training[16] and case-specific guidance.[19]

In 2016, the UK government reported that the fit note was 'not fully achieving what it set out to do' and announced a review of the fit note system, including extension of the certification from doctors to other healthcare professionals.[20]

Policy and procedure

Employers should establish a policy that explains the responsibilities of managers and employees when an employee is absent due to sickness. This should describe the expectations, actions, and terms and conditions of employment. Organizations pay employees to attend work, so attendance is accepted as the norm. While employers recognize that some limited absence is inevitable, their aim is to facilitate a return to work at the earliest opportunity when provided with appropriate support and assistance.[21]

Box 9.4 Effective interventions in sickness absence

- Appropriate health support for absentees should be available from their GP and other relevant clinicians.

- Absentees should provide consent to share some confidential information with specified parties.

- Absentees and employers should be in regular contact to plan and execute any agreed activities.

- The person planning, coordinating, or delivering support should have the relevant experience, expertise, and credibility.

- Account should be taken of the employee's age, illness, and the nature of their work.

- Activities need to be tailored to the individual's condition and perceived (or actual) barriers to returning to work.

- Organizational sickness absence policies and health and safety practices should be implemented.

Prerequisites to interventions

The National Institute for Health and Care Excellence (NICE) described a number of pre-requisites for effective action.[22] See Box 9.4.

NICE suggests that there is evidence that actively helping to implement something (e.g. physiotherapy) can be more effective than encouraging the absentee to do something for themselves (e.g. advising regular physical activity or to make contact with another organization).

Managing short- and medium-term absence

Short-term absences can be highly disruptive. In some organizations these absences may be common. They have the potential to significantly influence attendance culture, potentially legitimizing absence among peers and setting a benchmark that encourages workers to expect even longer periods of absence in the event of more serious illness.

There is no commonly agreed definition of short-term absence but usefully a short-term absence can be considered as up to 7 days as this can be self-certificated. Medium-term absence is therefore 8 days up to 4 weeks. Reasons for short-term self-certificated absences are likely to differ from those that are longer and certificated by the employee's general practitioner (GP).

Two interventions have been popularized for preventing short-term sickness absence—the use of triggers and return-to-work interviews. However, their popularity is founded on reputation rather than persuasive evidence.

Table 9.1 Employers' experience of managing short-term absence

	Proportion of respondents using this approach (%)			Proportion believing it to be among the most effective interventions (%)		
	2003	**2010**	**2016**	**2003**	**2010**	**2016**
Triggers	68	83	79	28	56	52
RTW interviews	77	88	70	60	68	60

RTW, return-to-work.

Source: data from Chartered Institute of Personnel and Development (CIPD). (2016) *Annual absence management surveys*. London, UK: CIPD. Copyright © 2016; and CIPD (2003) *Employee absence 2003: a survey of management policy and practice*. London, UK: CIPD. Copyright © CIPD 2003; and CIPD (2010) *Annual survey report 2010: absence management*. London, UK: CIPD. Copyright © CIPD 2010.

The Chartered Institute of Personnel and Development (CIPD) annual survey has been influential in developing management practice. Respondents to the survey have repeatedly shared their opinions that triggers and return-to-work interviews are effective but this has not been substantiated by empirical research. Practice experience has strengthened a belief in the effectiveness of these two interventions and they are widely used (Table 9.1).[2,4,24] However, the value of return-to-work interviews is not certain and their use has diminished recently.

Irrespective of the evidence on effectiveness there is an expectation that managers both talk to an employee who has been absent on their return (a return-to-work interview) and use some sort of threshold to initiate a discussion about improved attendance (trigger point). The focus of these activities is to identify the support that might enable an employee to attend work more consistently. In some cases, the discussion between the employee and the manager will identify a health need that may result in referral for OH advice. Referrals should not be automatic as unnecessary consultations are not likely to be valued by the employee, the manager, or the OH professional.

The use of return-to-work interviews and triggers is not without difficulty. Return-to-work interviews can be time-consuming, especially if formally recorded. A large amount of management time is invested for each employee who is ultimately dismissed for poor attendance and, even if effective, there should still be doubt about their cost-effectiveness and the effort to conduct them as efficiently as possible. These concerns should be balanced against the importance of taking action and the need to reinforce the responsibility of managers in promoting a healthy workplace and attendance culture.

A trigger point approach to management action can be useful but can also over-simplify attendance management. Setting the threshold too low generates a considerable volume of work of doubtful value for managers, while setting it too high defeats its purpose.

The role of OH services in the management of short-term absence is usually limited. In many cases, there will only be a pattern of unrelated and relatively minor ailments. Where short-term absences arise from an underlying long-term health condition, the OH team will provide advice to both the manager and the patient on actions that might promote well-being and attendance. The advice may include an opinion as to whether, taking account of health factors, the patient is likely to provide regular and effective attendance and performance in the future.

Short- and medium-term absence is common. The lack of evidence of effectiveness for interventions in short-term absence remains an important and costly gap in knowledge that should be addressed by new research.

Predicting future absence

A large number of factors associated with sickness absence have been reported in epidemiological studies. Some are related to working conditions and may be modified by the employer, such as the flexibility and support provided at work. Most of the factors related to the individual employee cannot be modified, including age, gender, location, and type of occupation (skilled vs unskilled). The individual factors that can be modified include the treatment for any underlying conditions and the behaviours associated with health.

An important role for OH professionals in managing sickness absence is to identify whether an employee has any underlying medical conditions and make sure that the appropriate treatment and advice is being provided. However, improving treatment of underlying medical conditions is unlikely to significantly improve attendance most of the time (as differences in health explain very little of the variation in individual sickness absence). Interventions that change individual behaviour, in response to health and well-being issues, may have a more enduring impact on attendance in many situations.

Workplace interventions to prevent sickness absence have not generally been effective.[25,26] However, they might reduce the cumulative duration of sickness absence.[27] As benefits may be small and interventions may not be cost-effective, employers must use their judgement in applying the uncertain evidence in their workplaces.[28]

Employees' beliefs about when they might be justified in taking sickness absence directly influences future absence. Those whose perception of their own health means they believe they would have been justified in taking time off work at least five times in the past year are likely to be absent more often in the future.[29]

Past sickness absence is an important indicator of future absence and the risk of future sickness absence increases with the number of prior episodes.[30] A recent systematic review concluded that sickness absence data from the past 2 years helps to identify employees who are likely to have above-average sickness absence and it is not necessary to go further back than 2 years in an employee's history to predict this.[31] The review found that:

◆ days of sickness absence in the past year predict future days of sickness absence

◆ episodes of sickness absence in the past 2 years predict future episodes of sickness absence.

Tools are being developed to assist in identifying employees at higher risk of sickness absence but further validation is needed before these can be widely adopted.[32]

Changing health behaviours is possible in theory, but difficult in practice. This is a major reason why there is limited evidence of effectiveness for interventions for frequent episodes of absence.[33] However, the potential for success will be greater with approaches that focus on the psychosocial context rather than underlying health.

Long-term absence

NICE has defined long-term sickness absence as absences from work lasting 4 or more weeks. Long-term absence explains a significant proportion of total sickness absence. The proportion varies according to the type of work, the business sector, and the size of the organization (Table 9.2).[21] The proportion of total absence is likely to be closely related to the amount of (paid and unpaid) time a worker's terms and conditions of employment allow before an absentee's contract is terminated. The proportion of absence due to long-term sickness absence is biggest in large and public sector organizations.

In 2009, NICE commissioned an evidence review and published guidance on interventions in the workplace and community to help people return to work after sickness absence and/or incapacity.[22] The evidence review aimed to identify any relevant interventions, policies, strategies, or programmes that help people return to work after sickness absence and/or incapacity.[34,35] Of the thousands of reports considered, more than 50 met

Table 9.2 The proportion of total days of absence due to short-, medium-, and long-term periods for different employees and employers

	1–7 days (%)	8–28 days (%)	>28 days (%)
All employees	64	16	19
Manual employees	62	17	22
Non-manual employees	73	12	15
Industry sector			
Manufacturing and production	71	16	14
Private sector services	72	14	14
Public services	52	18	29
Non-profit organizations	57	20	22
Number of UK employees			
1–49	78	12	9
50–249	70	16	14
250–999	61	16	23
1000–4999	56	20	25
5000+	46	20	34

Source: data from Chartered Institute of Personnel and Development (2011) *Annual survey report 2011: absence management*. London, UK: CIPD. © CIPD 2011.

well-defined criteria for inclusion, quality, appropriateness to the scope, and applicability to specific populations and settings in England. The evidence was considered by a multi-disciplinary committee comprising professional, lay, and academic experts. This review is the most comprehensive to date and provides a robust foundation for managing sickness absence. Since the initial publication, NICE has consulted on the need for revision on two occasions and concluded there has been no significant change in evidence that would warrant a revision of the guidance. NICE suggests a three-step approach: initial enquiries, detailed assessment, and coordinating and delivering interventions and services.[22,35]

Initial enquiries

1. Identify someone who is suitably trained and impartial to undertake initial enquiries with the relevant employees.

2. Make sure that initial enquiries are undertaken in conjunction with the employee, ideally between 2 and 6 weeks of a person starting the period of sickness absence:

   - To determine the reason for the sickness and their prognosis for returning to work (i.e. how likely it is that they will return to work) and if they have any perceived (or actual) barriers to returning to work (including the need for workplace adjustments).

   - To decide on the options for returning to work and jointly agree what, if any, action is required to prepare for this.

3. If action is required, consider identifying:

   - whether or not a detailed assessment is needed to determine what interventions and services are required and to develop a return-to-work plan

   - whether or not a case worker should be appointed to coordinate a detailed assessment, deliver any proposed interventions, or produce a return-to-work plan.

Detailed assessment

1. Arrange for a relevant specialist/s to undertake an assessment (or different components of it) in conjunction with the employee (and in communication with the line manager) which includes referral to an OH professional or another appropriate health specialist.

2. Conduct a combined health and work assessment that evaluates the following:

   - The employee's health, social, and employment situation: this includes anything that is putting them off returning to work, for example, organizational structure and culture (such as work relationships) and how confident they feel about overcoming these problems.

   - The employee's current or previous experience of rehabilitation.

   - The tasks the employee carries out at work and their physical ability to perform them (dealing with issues such as mobility, strength, and fitness).

- Any workplace or work equipment modifications needed in line with the disability provisions of the Equality Act 2010 (including ergonomic modifications).

3. Prepare a return-to-work plan that identifies the type and level of interventions and services needed (including any psychological support from someone trained in psychological assessment techniques) and how frequently they should be offered. The report could also specify whether or not any of the following are required:

    - A gradual return to the original job by increasing the hours and days worked over a period of time.

    - A return to some of the duties of the original job.

    - A move to another job within the organization (on a temporary or permanent basis).

The detailed assessment should be coordinated by a suitably trained case worker (Box 9.5).

Coordinating and delivering interventions and services

NICE further recommends that the delivery of planned health, occupational, or rehabilitation interventions or services and any return-to-work plan developed following initial enquiries or the detailed assessment is coordinated. People who have a 'poor' prognosis

---

Box 9.5 Case worker

A case worker has been defined as a person responsible for managing an assessment and coordinating delivery of interventions and services to help a person return to work (NICE).[22] The purpose of the role is to make sure that support and intervention is co-ordinated so that it is provided in a timely way to help employees to resume their usual or adjusted work as soon as they can. While there is no commonly agreed description of case working, there is some emerging consensus on the importance of:

- monitoring absence data in real time
- coordinating any required assessments
- timetabled actions to eliminate delays between milestones
- initiation of formal interventions
- prompt and tracked actions
- providing periodic reports to stakeholders.

Goal-setting approaches, including problem-solving and motivational interviewing, are increasingly used by case managers. Their principle is to engage the employee in actively identifying and planning to overcome their barriers to return to work, or at least to be an active stakeholder in this process.

for returning to work are likely to benefit most from more 'intensive' interventions and services; those with a 'good' prognosis are likely to benefit from 'light' or less intense interventions and services. Liaison of all parties (e.g. line managers and OH staff) should occur. NICE advises the following:

1. Where necessary, arrange for a referral to relevant specialists or services. This may include referral via an OH professional (or encouragement to self-refer) to a GP, a specialist physician, nurse, or another professional specializing in OH, health and safety, rehabilitation, or ergonomics. It could also include referral to a physiotherapist.

2. Where necessary, employers should appoint a case worker to coordinate referral for any required interventions and services. This includes delivery of the return-to-work plan including modifications to the workplace or work equipment if required. The case worker does not necessarily need a clinical or OH background. However, they should have the skills and training to act as an impartial intermediary and to ensure appropriate referrals are made to specialist services.

3. Ensure employees are consulted and jointly agree all planned health, occupational, or rehabilitation interventions or services, and the return-to-work plan (including workplace or work equipment modifications).

4. Encourage employees to contact their GP or OH service for further advice and support as needed.

5. Consider offering people who have a poor prognosis for returning to work an 'intensive' programme of interventions (e.g. counselling about a return to work, workplace modifications, and vocational rehabilitation including training).

6. Consider offering specific interventions for common psychological and musculoskeletal problems where the evidence supports the success of such intervention.

The annual CIPD[4,21,23,24] survey has indicated that some of the recommendations made by NICE are becoming more commonplace (Table 9.3), especially the availability of work adjustments (changes), rehabilitation, and psychological support (e.g. counselling). However, despite the evidence of benefit, active case management is still relatively uncommon.

The CIPD surveys indicate that almost all interventions are more commonly used in the public sector where sickness absence rates are measured and long-term absence is more common. A notable exception is the provision of private medical insurance which is provided by up to 29% of private sector employers but by only 7% in the public sector.[4]

Timeliness

A consistent theme in guidance on managing attendance is the need for early intervention. Studies have not yet been conducted that provide evidence for the best timing for intervention. However, it is assumed that in many cases there is not likely to be benefit from delaying the provision of effective advice and treatment and in some cases this will be detrimental. The longer someone is not working, the less likely they are to return to

Table 9.3 Options adopted by managers in cases of long-term absence

	% of surveyed organizations using this approach			
	2003	**2010**	**2011**	**2016**
Referral to OH	66	77	74	61
Stress counselling	36	45	43	34
Employee assistance programme	24	46	47	40
Rehabilitation	28	46	40	28
Changes to work	41	63	61	51
Nominated case manager	17	22	26	22
Return-to-work interviews	74	85	86	69

Source: data from Chartered Institute of Personnel and Development (CIPD). (2016) *Annual absence management surveys*. London, UK: CIPD. Copyright © 2016; and CIPD (2011) *Annual survey report 2011: absence management*. London, UK: CIPD. © CIPD 2011; and CIPD (2003) *Employee absence 2003: a survey of management policy and practice*. London, UK: CIPD. © CIPD 2003; and CIPD (2010) *Annual survey report 2010: absence management*. London, UK: CIPD. © CIPD 2010.

work; consequently, most benefit claimants absent for 6 months or more have an 80% chance of being off work for 5 years.[13]

NICE suggested the time to intervene was within the first 2–6 weeks.[22] Others have concluded there is insufficient evidence to recommend intervention within the first 1 or 2 weeks.[36] Recent research has demonstrated the effectiveness of early and intensive telephone-based intervention for sickness absence management.[37,38]

Dame Carol Black, in her report, *Working for a Healthier Tomorrow*, highlighted the importance of early intervention[39] and identified three key principles. See Box 9.6.

Effective early intervention combines action by managers with early support from OH services and the timeliness of intervention is an important component when monitoring the effective case management and quality of service provision in OH.

Box 9.6 Key principles in early intervention in absence management

◆ A biopsychosocial approach that simultaneously considers the medical condition, the psychological impact, and the wider social determinants including work, home, or family situation.

◆ Multidisciplinary teams able to deliver a range of services tailored to the needs of the individual patient.

◆ Case workers who can help the individual navigate the system and facilitate communication.

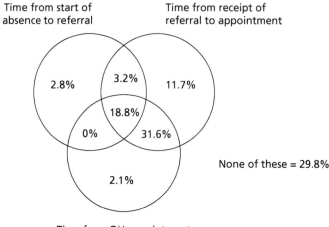

Time from start of absence to referral

Time from receipt of referral to appointment

2.8%

3.2%

11.7%

18.8%

0%

31.6%

None of these = 29.8%

2.1%

Time from OH appointment to issue of report

Figure 9.3 Proportion of English NHS organizations measuring the timeliness of intervention.
Reproduced with permission from Royal College of Physicians (RCP), Faculty of Occupational Medicine. (2011) *Implementing NICE public health guidance for the workplace: a national organisational audit of NHS trusts in England.* London, UK: RCP. Copyright © 2011 Royal College of Physicians.

The timeliness of referrals to OH services has been best described by audit in the NHS where one-quarter of organizations routinely measured the time from start of absence to referral to OH (see Figure 9.3).[40] However even in this setting, where all employees had access to OH, one-third were not assessed until they had been absent for more than 3 months.[41]

Occupational health reports

Effective attendance management relies on collaboration between line managers, human resources managers, OH professionals, and others. The main output from OH is usually a report providing advice to the manager. There is no commonly agreed standard for OH reports although guidance has been published (Box 9.7).[42] There is a clear expectation that the report is issued with the informed consent of the patient and that medical information is omitted unless there is a good reason it must be brought to the attention of the recipient.

Communication with other specialists

The benefit of good advice from experts on health and work must not be underestimated. Studies in the UK and elsewhere have shown the importance of OH professionals influencing colleagues in secondary care to change the work-related illness behaviour of patients (and potentially the sickness certification behaviour of primary care clinicians).[43,44]

Box 9.7 Ingredients of a suitable OH report

a. Must use language that can be easily understood by a non-medical audience and be of practical value to managers and the employee.

b. Should be focused and deal with matters of employment and fitness for work.

c. Should, with the employee's consent, contain relevant and appropriate medical information, including any interventions being planned to allow management to achieve a full understanding of the employee's situation.

d. Should include details of any functional limitations or relevant disabilities that may temporarily or permanently affect the employee's ability to carry out their job.

e. Should include guidance in relation to the timescale for a return to full or restricted duties, expected duration of any limitations, and whether a review is necessary.

f. Should indicate if further information needs to be obtained from the employee's GP or hospital doctor to enable a better understanding of the underlying medical condition.

g. Should advise whether the condition is likely to be covered by the disability provisions of the Equality Act 2010, if adjustments to the job would be appropriate, and if these are likely to be temporary or permanent.

h. Should indicate if it appears that the employee's medical condition is related to their work, including any allegations of internal disputes that may require management assessment.

i. Should provide an opinion on the impact of the employee's health condition on future attendance or performance and whether retirement on health grounds may be appropriate.

j. Should indicate if a meeting between the OH professional and management would be helpful, or if a workplace visit would provide further information that would assist in providing advice.

Source: data from Addley K et al. Occupational health reports: Top 10 tips. *Occupational Health & Wellbeing*. 2009; 61:28. Copyright © Reed Business Information.

It should not be assumed that patients receive good health and work advice from their specialists. A substantial proportion of professional advice is out of line with the research literature.[45] Advice is more likely to be correct when it refers to up-to-date research literature. OH professionals who ask for advice should always ask for the evidence supporting the advice and should provide information to colleagues that might improve their practice. There is a growing body of resources providing evidence-based and consensus-based guidance on when patients can return to work.

Occupational rehabilitation

Occupational rehabilitation is whatever helps someone with a health problem stay at, return to, or remain in work.[46] It is an approach more than an intervention or a service and considers all of a person's needs for getting or keeping work. Early intervention is important because the challenge of returning an employee to work only increases as a period of sickness absence continues. Effective occupational rehabilitation is dependent on coordinating work-focused healthcare with accommodating workplaces.

OH professionals should provide advice on rehabilitation that combines guidance for both the patient and the employer. The rehabilitation plan should describe the capabilities of the patient on resuming work and the adjustments that might need to be accommodated by the employer to enable this. Research by the Health and Safety Executive suggests the rehabilitation plan should describe the complete patient journey—including intermediate milestones—from resuming adjusted work to resuming all the usual work activities (or to resuming all the work activities with any permanent adjustments that might be needed)[47] (Box 9.8). The expectations of employee and employer should be clearly defined.

Rehabilitation, including adjustments to work, is covered in further detail in Chapter 10.

Presenteeism and productivity

Presenteeism is defined in terms of the lost productivity that occurs when employees come to work ill and perform below par because of that illness.[48] The cost of presenteeism may exceed the cost of absenteeism. Reduced productivity due to reduced health at work is important but its impact has not been fully established.[49] There is limited evidence from the UK on the costs of presenteeism.[48]

It has been suggested that rigorous management of sickness absence may increase presenteeism and could, in theory, be counterproductive.[50] However, there is very little evidence to suggest this happens in practice.[51]

The risk of presenteeism should not be used as a justification for neglecting management of attendance. The risk of presenteeism is a justification only for providing the

---

Box 9.8 Key features of a return to work plan

- Details of any temporarily adjusted work arrangements with a timeframe.
- Clearly specified goals which are achievable and can be measured as milestones.
- A timeframe which provides a start and end point, with appropriate steps.
- Defined review points.

Data from Hanson, MA. et al. (2006) *The costs and benefits of active case management and rehabilitation for musculoskeletal disorders* (RR493). London, UK: Health and Safety Executive. Copyright © 2006 Health and Safety Executive.

appropriate support for employees with health needs at work and for trying to change beliefs about capability of those workers. Most employees with health needs if appropriately supported will remain productive and the impact of presenteeism will be minimized.

Most workers face health concerns at certain times during their career. It is important that employers invest in the health of their workforce to enhance performance and productivity. The foremost solution to presenteeism should be to encourage action that enables employees to continue their activities when health problems arise, by making adjustments and providing effective OH support.

Key points

- Health-related absence from work is common.
- Illness only explains a small proportion of the variance in sickness absence—it is important to recognize the contribution of other factors.
- Evidence of the benefit of early intervention to support absent workers absent is increasing.
- Patients may not get evidence-based advice on resuming work from the specialists treating their illness.
- If a return-to-work plan is needed, it should determine the level, type, and frequency of interventions and services needed.

Useful websites

NICE. 'Workplace health: long-term sickness absence and incapacity to work'	https://www.nice.org.uk/guidance/ph19
Health and Safety Executive. 'Managing sickness absence and return to work'	http://www.hse.gov.uk/sicknessabsence/
Advisory, Conciliation and Arbitration Service (Acas). 'Managing staff absence: a step-by-step guide'	http://www.acas.org.uk/index.aspx?articleid=4199
Fit For Work	https://fitforwork.org/about/

References

1. **Office for National Statistics.** *Sickness Absence in the Labour Market: 2016.* London: Office for National Statistics; 2017.
2. **European Foundation for the Improvement of Living and Working Conditions (EFLIWC).** *Absence from Work.* Dublin: EFLIWC; 2010.
3. **Audit Commission.** *Managing Sickness Absence in the NHS, Health Briefing.* London: Audit Commission; 2011.

4. **Chartered Institute of Personnel and Development**. *Annual Survey Report 2016: Absence Management*. London: CIPD; 2016.

5. **Miraglia M, Johns G.** Going to work ill: a meta-analysis of the correlates of presenteeism and a dual-path model. *J Occup Health Psychol* 2016;**21**:261–83.

6. **Wynne-Jones G, Buck R, Varnava A, Phillips C, Main CJ.** Impacts on work absence and performance: what really matters? *Occup Med* 2009;**59**:556–62.

7. **Preece R.** (Lack of) Impacts on work absence and performance. *Occup Med* 2010;**60**:81.

8. **Steensma H.** Sickness absence, office types, and advances in absenteeism research. *Scand J Work Environ Health* 2011;**37**:359–62.

9. **MacLeod D, Clarke N.** *Engaging for Success: Enhancing Performance through Employee Engagement*. London: Department for Business, Innovation and Skills; 2008.

10. **West MA, Dawson JF.** *Employee Engagement and NHS Performance*. London: The King's Fund; 2012. Available at: https://www.gov.uk/government/uploads/system/uploads/attachment_data/file/215455/dh_129656.pdf.

11. **Yarker J, Munir F, Donaldson-Feilder E, Hicks B.** *Managing Rehabilitation: A Competency Framework for Managers to Support Return to Work*. London: BOHRF, 2010.

12. **Walker V, Bamford D.** An empirical investigation into health sector absenteeism. *Health Serv Manage Res* 2011;**24**:142–50.

13. **Marmot M** (Chair). *Fair Society, Healthy Lives. A Strategic Review of Health Inequalities in England post-2010* (The Marmot Review). London: The Marmot Review; 2010. Available at: http://www.instituteofhealthequity.org/projects/fair-society-healthy-lives-the-marmot-review/fair-society-healthy-lives-full-report.

14. **van der Noordt M, IJzelenberg H, Droomers M, Proper KI.** Health effects of employment: a systematic review of prospective studies. *Occup Environ Med* 2014;**71**:730–6.

15. **Bradford SC.** Sources of information on specific subjects. *Engineering* 1934;**137**:85–6.

16. **Coole C, Drummond A, Watson P, Nouri F, Potgieter I.** *Getting the Best from the Fit Note: Investigating the Use of the Statement of Fitness for Work*. Leicestershire: IOSH; 2015.

17. **Gabbay M, Shiels C, Hillage J.** Factors associated with the length of fit note-certified sickness episodes in the UK. *Occup Environ Med* 2015;**72**:467–75.

18. **Dorrington S, Roberts E, Hatch S, Madan I, Hotopf, M.** Fit note use in UK clinical practice 2010–2016: a systematic review of quantitative research. *Eur Psychiatry* 2017;**41**:S618.

19. **Nordhagen HP, Harvey SB, Rosvold EO, Bruusgaard R, Blonk A, Mykletun.** Case-specific colleague guidance for general practitioners' management of sickness absence. *Occup Med* 2017;**67**:644–7.

20. **Department of Work and Pensions and Department of Health.** *Improving Lives: The Work, Health and Disability Green Paper*. London: HMSO; 2016.

21. **Chartered Institute of Personnel and Development (CIPD).** *Absence Measurement and Management: Fact Sheet*. London: CIPD; 2011.

22. **National Institute for Health and Clinical Excellence (NICE).** *Workplace Health: Management of Long-Term Sickness and Incapacity for Work*. Public health guideline [PH19]. London: NICE; 2009.

23. **Chartered Institute of Personnel and Development (CIPD).** *Employee Absence 2003: A Survey of Management Policy and Practice*. London: CIPD; 2003.

24. **Chartered Institute of Personnel and Development (CIPD).** *Annual Survey Report 2010: Absence Management*. London: CIPD; 2010.

25. **Odeen M, Magnussen LH, Maeland S, Larun L, Eriksen HR, Tveito TH.** Systematic review of active workplace interventions to reduce sickness absence. *Occup Med* 2013;**63**:7–16.

26. **Amlani NM, Munir F.** Does physical activity have an impact on sickness absence? A review. *Sports Med* 2014;**44**:887–907.

27. **van Vilsteren M, van Oostrom SH, de Vet HC, Franche RL, Boot CR, Anema JR.** Workplace interventions to prevent work disability in workers on sick leave. *Cochrane Database Syst Rev* 2015;**10**:CD006955.

28. **Palmer KT, Harris EC, Linaker C, et al.** Effectiveness of community- and workplace-based interventions to manage musculoskeletal-related sickness absence and job loss: a systematic review. *Rheumatology* 2012;**51**:230–42.

29. **Bergström G, Bodin L, Hagberg J, Aronsson G, Josephson M.** Sickness presenteeism today, sickness absenteeism tomorrow? A prospective study on sickness presenteeism and future sickness absenteeism. *J Occup Environ Med* 2009;**51**:629–38.

30. **Shiels C, Gabbay M, Hillage J.** Recurrence of sickness absence episodes certified by general practitioners in the UK. *Eur J Gen Pract* 2016; **22**: 83–90

31 **Roelen CA, Koopmans PC, Schreuder JA, Anema JR, van der Beek AJ.** The history of registered sickness absence predicts future sickness absence. *Occup Med* 2011;**61**:96–101.

32. **Roelen CA, van Rhenen W, Groothoff JW, van der Klink JJ, Bültmann U, Heymans MW.** The development and validation of two prediction models to identify employees at risk of high sickness absence. *Eur J Public Health* 2013;**23**:128–33.

33. **Rick J, Carroll C, Hillage J, Pilgrim H, Jagger N.** *Review of the Effectiveness and Cost Effectiveness of Interventions, Strategies, Programmes and Policies to Reduce the Number of Employees Who Take Long Term Sickness Absence on a Recurring Basis.* Brighton: Institute for Employment Studies; 2008.

34. **Hillage J, Rick J, Pilgrim H, Jagger N, Carroll C, Booth A.** *Review of the Effectiveness and Cost Effectiveness of Interventions, Strategies, Programmes and Policies to Reduce the Number of Employees Who Move from Short-Term to Long-Term Sickness Absence and to Help Employees on Long-Term Sickness Absence Return to Work.* Brighton: Institute for Employment Studies; 2008.

35. **Gabbay M, Taylor L, Sheppard L, et al.** NICE guidance on long-term sickness and incapacity. *Br J Gen Pract* 2011;**61**:e118–24.

36. **Vargas-Prada S, Demou E, Lalloo D, et al.** Effectiveness of very early workplace interventions to reduce sickness absence: a systematic review of the literature and meta-analysis. *Scand J Work Environ Health* 2016;**42**:261–72.

37. **Smedley J, Harris EC, Cox V, Ntani G, Coggon D.** Evaluation of a case management service to reduce sickness absence. *Occup Med* 2013;**63**:89–95.

38. **Brown J, Mackay D, Demou E, Craig J, Frank J, Macdonald EB.** The EASY (Early Access to Support for You) sickness absence service: a four-year evaluation of the impact on absenteeism. *Scand J Work Environ Health* 2015;**41**:204–15.

39. **Black C.** *Working for a Healthier Tomorrow.* London: The Stationery Office; 2008.

40. **Health and Work Development Unit.** *Implementing NICE Public Health Guidance for the Workplace: A National Organisational Audit of NHS Trusts in England.* London: Royal College of Physicians; 2011.

41. **Health and Work Development Unit.** *Depression Detection and Management of Staff on Long-Term Sickness Absence—Occupational Health Practice in the NHS in England: A National Clinical Audit— Round 2.* London: Royal College of Physicians; 2010.

42. **Addley K, Hannah I, McQuillan P.** Occupational health reports: top 10 tips. *Occup Health* 2009;**61**:28.

43. **Clayton M, Verow P.** A retrospective study of return to work following surgery. *Occup Med* 2007;**57**:525–31.

44. **Jensen LD, Maribo T, Schiøttz-Christensen B, et al.** Counselling low-back-pain patients in secondary healthcare: a randomised trial addressing experienced workplace barriers and physical activity. *Occup Environ Med* 2012;**69**:21–8.

45. **Schaafsma F, Verbeek J, Hulshof C, van Dijk F.** Caution required when relying on a colleague's advice; a comparison between professional advice and evidence from the literature. *BMC Health Serv Res* 2005;**5**:59.

46. **Waddell G, Burton AK, Kendall NAS.** *Vocational Rehabilitation: What Works, for Whom, and When?* London: The Stationery Office; 2008.

47. **Hanson MA, Burton K, Kendall NAS, Lancaster RJ, Pilkington A.** *The Costs and Benefits of Active Case Management and Rehabilitation for Musculoskeletal Disorders* (RR493). London: Health and Safety Executive; 2006.

48. **Cooper C, Dewe P.** Well-being—absenteeism, presenteeism, costs and challenges. *Occup Med* 2008;**58**:522–4.

49. **Preece R.** Is health and productivity an issue for all employers? *J Occup Environ Med* 2009;**51**:989.

50. **Roelen CAM, Groothoff JW.** Rigorous management of sickness absence provokes sickness presenteeism. *Occup Med* 2010;**60**:244–6.

51. **Preece R.** Effective absence management *Occup Med* 2010;**60**:575.

Chapter 10

Rehabilitation and return to work

Danny Wong

Introduction

Levels of disability and health-related work absence continue to increase. Coincidentally, there is a pressing need to identify and address psychological and societal obstacles to recovery and a return to work. The interaction between health and work, the economic impact of work loss, and the influence of long-term sickness absence on health and social inequality have been covered in Chapter 1. This chapter will look at models of disability that influence the approach to work rehabilitation, the various experts who might advise or inform occupational rehabilitation, the assessment of functional capacity, psychosocial factors, availability of support services, and other aspects that might guide a rehabilitation plan. It outlines for occupational health professionals and other experts in the rehabilitation field the approaches to managing barriers to return to work and adjustments that may assist people with serious or long-term disability in acquiring, returning to, or retaining work.

Models of disability

Models are a practical approach to moving from theory to reality and a means of aiding understanding, research, and management. There are strengths and limitations in adopting the traditional 'medical model' when considering work. Social models and the role of personal and psychological factors provide a better understanding of sickness and disability. They also impact capacity for work and developing interventions aimed at facilitating return to optimal function, including work. A *biopsychosocial model* of human illness that takes account of the person, their health problems, and their social context has profound implications for healthcare, workplace management, and social policy.

The medical model

The medical model may be summarized as a mechanistic view of the body, in which illness is simply a fault in the machine that should be fixed. The medical model remains deeply entrenched in the way that most people think about symptoms, disability, and healthcare. Common health problems are erroneously seen as medical problems that are a matter for healthcare, often caused by 'injury' and often work related. Moreover, symptoms are taken to imply incapacity, so sickness absence is considered necessary and justified until full recovery and complete relief of symptoms. The weakness of the medical model is that it fails to take account of the patient or their human qualities and subjective experiences, and encourages passivity. The patient's accounts of illness are reduced to a set of simplistic symptoms and signs of disease. Focusing on disease and its *treatment* can lead to neglect of the person and the *management* of the health problem.

The social model

The most powerful determinants of ill health are social gradients[1] and the linked problem of regional deprivation. The social model rests on the personal experience and views of disabled people and thereby has considerable social and political acceptance and represents reality. This approach necessitates change in the work environment and thus in the attitudes and behaviour of employers, line managers, and other workers. Individuals may be empowered to adapt the work environment to meet their needs and other stakeholders also require education.

The holistic model

To help us understand barriers to fitness to work we need to understand the concepts of behaviour. The trilogy of illness, disease, and sickness described by Twaddle in 1968[2] can be broken down into:

1. illness—which is defined as the ill health the person identifies themselves with, often based on self-reported mental or physical symptoms varying in severity—a subjective approach

2. disease—which is defined as a condition that is diagnosed by a clinician with known management plans—an objective approach.

3. sickness—which is a social role a person with illness or disease takes on or is given in society.

These three concepts often coexist: when a person feels unwell, they see a physician; they are diagnosed with a health problem and if they are off work they are on sick leave. However, these stages are not always sequential, and all stages may not present each time. An individual can be on sick leave even though they haven't been diagnosed, or an individual who is ill, and has a diagnosed disease may still not accept their sick role and want to remain in work (sometimes against medical advice). This leads us to the issue of presenteeism or attending work while ill[3] which can cause additional problems with poor productivity and poor health.

Occupational health (OH) practitioners will frequently see individuals who are off work for no medical reason and, in contrast, individuals who have health problems affecting their fitness to work but who still wish to remain at work.

The triaxial model of physical, psychological, and social factors was proposed by the Royal College of General Practitioners (RCGP) in 1972.[4] It states that a doctor should be encouraged to extend their thinking and practice beyond the purely organic approach to patients. They need to consider the patient's emotional, family, social, and environmental circumstances, all of which can have a profound effect on health. This mirrors the constitution of the World Health Organization's principle of health as 'a state of complete physical, psychological and social well-being'.

The biopsychosocial model thus suggests a holistic approach assessing the biological, psychological, and social dimensions of the patient.

The biopsychosocial model

From the time of Aristotle, the main determinants of health and sickness were considered to be lifestyle, healthy behaviour, and the social and physical environment, rather than biological status or healthcare. A public health perspective suggests that this remains true today.[5,6] Empirically, the biopsychosocial model is an interactive and individual-centred approach that considers the person, their health problems, *and* their social/occupational context. The factors that influence the process of disablement and recovery, and their relative importance, vary over time. Self-perceptions fluctuate, and individuals move between being disabled or not, and between working and varying degrees of incapacity.[7] Duration of sickness absence is fundamental to this process.[8] Multiple interventions at several levels may be required. This is characteristic of many health and social policy interventions.

A biopsychosocial approach demands a more egalitarian patient–doctor relationship. Patients want to be 'cured', but at the same time expect more human healthcare. This is not an impossible goal: it is a major part of modern medical training.[9] The goal is to treat the person as well as their health condition: to strike the right balance between providing the most effective care and achieving the best social and occupational outcomes. Above all, patients need to be reassured that the biopsychosocial approach is an extension of standard healthcare and makes no assumptions about original causes.

The right balance must be struck between treatment, the focus on work as a health outcome, and all providers of advice and support working together. That *is* a biopsychosocial approach. The concept of early intervention is central: the longer someone is off work, the greater the obstacles to return to work and the more difficult vocational rehabilitation becomes. It is simpler, more effective, and less expensive to prevent people going on to long-term sickness absence (Figure 10.1).

Each dimension involves a different set of expectations, behaviours, and social interactions. The outcome of any intervention may differ at different stages, so the timing of healthcare, rehabilitation, and social interventions is critical. All successful rehabilitation programmes include some form of active exercise or graded activity component. The key element is activity per se, with the immediate goal of overcoming functional barriers/limitations and improving capability; the ultimate goal is to increase participation and restore social and physical functioning. These principles are equally applicable to mental health conditions, where increased physical activity has been shown to reduce depression and improve general mental health.[10]

In principle, there should be steady increments of activity level, which are time dependent rather than symptom dependent. Properly implemented, a programme of

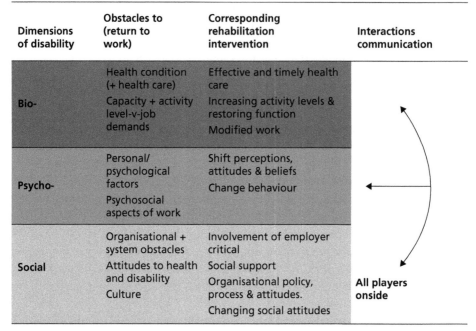

Dimensions of disability	Obstacles to (return to work)	Corresponding rehabilitation intervention	Interactions communication
Bio-	Health condition (+ health care)	Effective and timely health care	
	Capacity + activity level-v-job demands	Increasing activity levels & restoring function	
		Modified work	
Psycho-	Personal/ psychological factors	Shift perceptions, attitudes & beliefs	
		Change behaviour	
	Psychosocial aspects of work		
Social	Organisational + system obstacles	Involvement of employer critical	
	Attitudes to health and disability	Social support	
	Culture	Organisational policy, process & attitudes.	**All players onside**
		Changing social attitudes	

Figure 10.1 Biopsychosocial obstacles to return to work with corresponding rehabilitation interventions.

Reproduced from Waddell, G. and Burton, AK. (2014) *Concepts of rehabilitation for the management of common health problems*. London, UK: The Stationery Office. © Crown Copyright 2004.

increasing activity will increase a sense of well-being, confidence, and self-efficacy, which in turn will promote adherence.

The 2016 National Institute for Health and Care Excellence (NICE) guidance on back pain recognizes this approach.[11] Unlike previous guidance on the management of persistent low back pain between 6 weeks and 12 months which classifies back pain as 'acute, sub-acute and chronic', the latest guidance considers risk of poor outcome at any time point which is almost always more important than the duration of symptoms.

Psychosocial flags system

Clinical flags are common to many areas of clinical practice. Red flags indicate the possibility of serious pathology for which immediate medical intervention should be sought. For instance, red flags in low back pain include urinary or bowel dysfunction indicating possible cauda equina syndrome.

Psychosocial flags offer a holistic approach to identify an individual's susceptibility to prolonged illness or sickness absence which is summarized in Box 10.1.[12,13]

Early identification of these flags is very important in OH and rehabilitation consultations to either change the outcome or as a predictor of poor outcome. This will enable

Box 10.1 The flags system

'Yellow flags'

Psychosocial barriers (e.g. self-perception, beliefs, ideas, concerns, and expectations). Normally unrelated to the workplace.

- Beliefs about pain and injury.
- Unhelpful coping strategies.
- Psychological distress.
- Adopting the sick role.
- Passive role in recovery.

Potentially changeable behaviour during consultations with the patient. For example, reassurance to the patient that in mechanical back pain, keeping active is good for their recovery.

'Blue flags'

Workplace barriers:

- Low social support at work.
- Unpleasant work.
- Low job satisfaction.
- Excessive demands compared to the same individual with same job role.

Employee and workplace barriers which are potentially changeable with early input from OH and vocational rehabilitation. For example, early advice around stress risk assessment and modifiable workplace factors.

'Black flags'

Normally affected by financial situation:

- Company policy on rehabilitation.
- Threats to financial security.
- Litigation.
- Qualification criteria for compensation.
- Poor or lack of communication with the employer, either human resources or manager.

More difficult to address and strong predictor of poor return to work.

(continued)

Box 10.1 Continued

'Chequered flags'

Social factors:

- ◆ Carer at home for dependant, for example, for young, old, or disabled.
- ◆ Social responsibilities outside of work.
- ◆ Other commitments outside of work.

Early identification helps consider alternative employment options (e.g. flexible working, career breaks).

---

future discussions on employability and use of appropriate tools to help identify modifiable risk factors in certain cases.[14]

Cognitive behavioural, mindfulness, and talking therapies

Attitudes, beliefs, and behaviour can aggravate and perpetuate symptoms and disability, so addressing these issues is an essential part of rehabilitation management. This principle seems to apply generally across all rehabilitation for physical and mental symptoms, stress, distress, and disability.

Discussions with patients about behaviour change are integral to healthcare practice, for example, smoking cessation, weight reduction, and diabetes management. Behaviour change methods are now also applied to managing rehabilitation and return to work. For general practitioners (GPs), there is now specific training and e-learning programmes that address work and health and the management of the fitness for work consultation.[15]

Most psychological and behavioural approaches now combine *cognitive behavioural* principles[10]:

- ◆ Cognitive approaches focus on changing how patients think about and deal with their symptoms; they teach patients to rethink their beliefs about their symptoms, and what they do about them, building confidence in their own abilities and skills.
- ◆ Behavioural approaches focus on changing patients' illness behaviour. They try to extinguish symptom-driven behaviours by withdrawal of reinforcements such as medication, sympathetic attention, rest, and release from duties and to encourage healthy behaviour by positive reinforcement.
- ◆ Cognitive behavioural approaches try to address all psychological and behavioural aspects of the illness experience, in order to change beliefs, change behaviour, and improve functioning.

Evidence is accumulating for the applicability of the cognitive behavioural approach to all common health complaints.[16] For people experiencing common mental health problems at work brief (up to 8 weeks), individual therapy has been shown to be effective and cognitive behavioural therapy (CBT) to be highly effective in work retention.[17]

Engagement with therapy is important and influenced by ambivalence and motivation. Understanding how motivation enhanced behavioural change within the alcohol and addiction field was the basis for the development of motivational interviewing. Motivational interviewing is now recognized as an important method for engagement and compliance across many areas of healthcare.[18] Similar principles are applied in problem-solving, a technique that encourages self-directed goal setting in a journey to increase activity including work.[19]

CBT has also been shown to improve pain outcomes in some studies.[20] A Cochrane review of CBT treatment for subacute and chronic neck pain concluded that CBT was more effective for short-term pain reduction only when compared to no treatment. The quality of the evidence review was moderate and more trials are required.[21]

Mindfulness has become more popular with recent NICE [22] guidance recommending mindfulness-based cognitive therapy for people with recurring depression. Mindfulness focuses on knowing directly what is going on inside and outside of the individual, moment by moment. The concept is to help the individual take notice of their thoughts, feelings, body sensations, and the world around them.

Rehabilitation

Sickness absence management, assisting return to work, and promoting rehabilitation are matters of good practice, good OH management, and good business sense.[23] The *Oxford Dictionary of English* defines rehabilitation as 'The action of restoring someone to health or normal life through training and therapy after illness'.[24] The 'World Report on Disability', defines rehabilitation as enabling people with disabilities whose functions are limited to remain in or return to their home or community, live independently, and participate in education, the labour market, and civic life.[25]

Vocational rehabilitation

Vocational rehabilitation professionals assist those who have difficulties in entering the workforce, those having difficulties with their current jobs, and those who are out of work but seeking help to re-enter employment. They have knowledge and experience of the employment world as well as medical knowledge in an array of medical specialities. Vocational rehabilitation is *whatever helps someone with a health condition or disability to stay in, return to, or move into work.*[26] It is an idea and an approach, as much as an intervention or a service. Vocational rehabilitation is not a matter of healthcare alone: employers also have a key role. The traditional approach to rehabilitation is a secondary intervention after medical treatment is complete but the patient is left with permanent impairment. It accepts that impairment is irremediable, and attempts to overcome, adapt, or compensate for it by developing to the maximum extent the patient's (residual) physical, mental, and social functioning. Where appropriate, patients may be helped to return to their previous or modified work. That approach remains valid for some severe medical conditions.

Vocational rehabilitation professionals may be from a variety of backgrounds, including (among others) physiotherapy, occupational therapy, psychology, and ergonomics. They work within (or allied to) clinical NHS services, or in the private or third sectors. Access or funding may be provided by insurance companies, government, or employers. Relevant professional groups include the Royal College of Occupational Therapists, the Association of Chartered Physiotherapists in Occupational Health and Ergonomics, the British Psychological Society, the Case Management Society of the UK, and the Vocational Rehabilitation Association. Regardless of professional background, the Certified Disability Management Professional (CDMP) designation, supported by the International Disability Management Standards Council UK & Ireland, has become a desired qualification for those working in vocational rehabilitation. Those who achieve this internationally recognized designation have demonstrated the benefits of their interventions to employers, insurance companies, the legal profession, but most especially employees in enabling return to work successfully (see 'Useful websites').

With common health problems, the approach to rehabilitation should be different. Recovery is generally to be expected, even if with some persisting or recurrent symptoms. Given the right opportunities, support, and encouragement, most people with these conditions have remaining capacity for some work. The question is therefore not 'What makes some people develop long-term incapacity?' but 'Why do some people with common health problems not recover as expected?'

Biopsychosocial factors aggravate and perpetuate sickness and disability; crucially, these factors can continue to act as obstacles to recovery and return to work. The logic of rehabilitation then shifts from dealing with residual impairment to addressing the biopsychosocial obstacles that delay or prevent expected recovery and return to work. Mental ill health, particularly anxiety and depression, can be an effect as well as a cause of prolonged absence from work. It is important to consider mental health in managing rehabilitation irrespective of whether it is the primary reason for absence.

Rehabilitation medicine

Rehabilitation medicine is concerned with the prevention, diagnosis, treatment, and rehabilitation management of people with disabling medical conditions. Rehabilitation medicine covers a large number of disabling conditions and is broadly divided into four main areas:

◆ Neurological rehabilitation.
◆ Spinal cord injury rehabilitation.
◆ Limb loss or deficiency rehabilitation and prosthetics.
◆ Musculoskeletal rehabilitation.

Workplace management

Healthcare (primary, secondary, and tertiary) also has a key role in common health complaints but treatment by itself has little impact on work outcomes.[27] In fact, healthcare interventions delivered in isolation can remove individuals from the workplace and act as a barrier to successful rehabilitation. Work is an important outcome of health interventions in people of working age. However, employers also have a key role if rehabilitation is to be successful.

There is evidence that a proactive approach from employers to attendance management that includes temporary provision of modified work and adjustments is effective and cost-effective.[28] Modified work may take the form of temporary individual adaptations to reduce demand, or changes to work organization, the primary goal being to facilitate a timely return to sustained regular work. A review of 29 empirical studies demonstrated the success of modified work as an intervention that halved the number of work days lost and the number of injured workers who went on to chronic disability.[29] A recent randomized controlled trial of adding telephone follow-up to an occupational rehabilitation programme showed an increase in work participation.[30]

There is also evidence that for rehabilitation to be effective, both work-focused healthcare *and* accommodating workplaces are required.[31] Lower levels of organizational performance are associated with higher levels of sickness absence[32] and poor line manager support. The line manager can be thought of as 'the prism in which the organization is perceived'.[33] The line manager–employee relationship has a major impact on employee well-being[34] and therefore interventions must focus on both health professionals and line managers if change is to be successful. Communication is an absolute prerequisite for a coordinated intervention.[35]

Training and organizational approaches that increase participation in decision-making and problem-solving, and improved communication have been found to be most effective at reducing work-related psychological ill health and sickness absence.[36]

Policies and procedures to improve line management have been developed. However, the challenge of undertaking return to work conversations for line managers should not be underestimated. Being valued by the line manager and the organization are of great importance for employees and influences their attendance behaviours.

The 'fit note' introduced in April 2010 following Dame Carol Black's report (2008), provides a vehicle for communication with employers.[37] It also tries to address an important misconception held by both healthcare workers and employers that an individual must be 100% fit to return to work. This has been attempted by offering the option 'may be fit for work taking into account the following advice'. The note also allows doctors to recommend in the comments box that evaluation by OH specialists in complex cases should be sought.

In addition to the 'fit note', allied health professionals have also developed the Allied Health Professions (AHP) fitness report (see 'Useful websites'), a tool which works alongside medical advice to support both physical and mental well-being in the workplace. The information contained within this report is intended to provide practical modifications to enable maintained engagement with work or return to work.

A structured return-to-work programme provides a transparent pathway for employee and employer. It helps provide clarity, manage expectations, and integrate process with attendance management. Addressing psychosocial and inter-personal issues around return to work may be as important as modifying physical demands and should be central to any return-to-work programme. Building work experience is important in the transition between education and work, and for those who are remote from employment because of their disability (have never worked or not for a long time). Both these groups are likely to benefit from supported employment placements, either on a voluntary basis or as part of an apprenticeship scheme. Important features of return to work programmes include the following:

1. Communication between employee and employer soon after the onset of sickness absence.

2. Contact between the employee and line manager, continuing throughout the spell of absence.

3. The line manager should (with the employee's consent and where appropriate) inform co-workers of the absence and its likely duration.

4. The line manager should undertake a discussion with the employee on returning to work, to explore appropriate adjustments including modified work and psychosocial interventions.

5. Co-workers should be made fully aware of adjustments that are agreed (within the bounds of confidentiality and with the returning employee's consent).

Social and occupational interventions: services to assist return to work

Government strategy

In November 2017, following public consultation on an earlier green paper,[31] the UK government Department for Work and Pensions (DWP) and Department of Health (DH) published 'Improving Lives: The Future of Work, Health and Disability'.[38] The Faculty of Occupational Medicine (FOM) and the Society of Occupational Medicine jointly responded to the consultation.[39]

The government's vision is 'A society where everyone is ambitious for disabled people and people with long-term health conditions, and where people understand and act positively upon the important relationship between health, work and disability'. 'Improving Lives' sets out a 10-year plan as to how this vision will be realized and to see 1 million more disabled people in work over the next 10 years. The document states that it is important for action to be taken as the prevalence of disability among people of working-age has risen and is likely to rise further with an ageing workforce.

Key initiatives include establishment of a Working-Age Policy Research Unit. The strategy aims to bring about transformation change and address three questions:

◆ How to personalize and tailor employment support in the welfare system, with improved assessments for financial support.

◆ How to achieve the appropriate balance of incentives and expectations of employers of all sizes to recruit and retain disabled people and people with long-term health conditions, and create healthy workplaces where people can thrive.

◆ How to shape, fund, and deliver effective OH services that can support all in work; and options for fit note reform.

Two significant independent reviews published in 2017[40,41] have highlighted employer practices that particularly affect employees, and have recommended improvements. Lord Stevenson and Paul Farmer's review, 'Thriving at Work', acknowledges that all employees' mental health should be taken care of in the workplace.[40]

In studies, about three-quarters of those people in receipt of incapacity benefits say they would like to work.[10] The following services are available to assist return to work at the time of writing. However, a review of the provision of employment-related support for people with disabilities in the UK is underway following the white paper mentioned previously. Therefore this is an area likely to see extensive re-organization during the next 5 years (2018–2023).

Jobcentre Plus

Jobcentre Plus is a brand name of the Department for Work and Pensions (DWP) and provides services to those attempting to find employment and to those requiring working age benefits.[42] A government website named Universal Jobmatch has also been launched where jobseekers can search for employment and employers can upload and manage their own vacancies while searching for prospective employees. Services are provided in the first instance via in-house job-advisors and advisors contacted via telephony. Advisors have a specific focus on helping people with a health condition or a disability to work. The role of Jobcentre Plus is currently under government review.[38]

Access to Work

Access to Work is a DWP programme, accessible by self-referral, that aims to help people who have a disability or long-term health condition start or stay in work.[43] There are two main types of Access to Work provision: 'Assessments' and 'Elements'. Assessments involve exploring workplace-related barriers to employment and making recommendations on how these can be overcome. Elements are intended to supplement the reasonable adjustments that employers are required to make under the Equality Act 2010 and can include, for example:

◆ communication support for interviews

◆ special aids and equipment

◆ adaptations to premises and vehicles

◆ help with travel costs

◆ support workers

◆ a mental health support service.

In 2016/2017, Access to Work provision was approved for 25,000 people, assessments were approved for 13,000 people, and elements for 24,000 people. The most frequent elements approved were special aids and equipment (12,450), support worker (8450), travel to work (5750), and mental health support services (1780) (source: Access to Work statistics, data for April 2007 to March 2017; DWP).[44]

Access to Work is not available in Northern Ireland, where a different system of government support operates (Access to Work (NI)) (see 'Useful websites').

Disability organizations

A large number of organizations exist in the UK with the aim of assisting rehabilitation or providing employment services for those with disability (see 'Useful websites'). Many disease or condition-based charities provide guidance on work rehabilitation or adjustments to work (see 'Useful websites').

Remploy is one organization which provides employment placement services for disabled people (see 'Useful websites') and is described as a major welfare-to-work provider, delivering a range of contracts and employment programmes, for people with substantial barriers to work. Remploy was originally established under the terms of the Disabled Persons (Employment) Act 1944, to directly employ disabled persons in specialized factories and at one point had a network of 83 factories across the UK making a wide variety of products. In recent years, Remploy has undergone a major change to its operation and branched out into providing general employment assistance for disabled people, and others with barriers to employment. After the closure of most Remploy factories, the provision of these assistance services became Remploy's principal purpose. Remploy is now owned privately and by its employees. Between 2009 and 2014, Remploy found 100,000 jobs for disabled people.

The Shaw Trust is a national charitable organization that provides employment opportunities for disabled people, and skills development opportunities. They deliver services on behalf of DWP and other government departments that are aiming to support employment in groups with poor access to work and a high prevalence of health issues, such as HM Prison and Probation services.

Specialist employability support

Jobcentre Plus specialist employability support (SES) programmes focus on helping disabled people who may need support to either enter work or move closer to work. There are currently two strands to the SES programme following an initial assessment based on how long support is likely to be needed:

1. The SES Start Back Provision, which provides intensive support and training for up to 6 months.

2. The SES Main Provision, which provides longer-term support and training for an agreed length of time (usually 12 months).

The SES programme will end in 2018. The Work and Health programme is an employment support programme commissioned by the UK government on a regional basis. It aims to provide specialist employment support to people with disabilities and long-term unemployed people. Pilot schemes in North West England and Wales have informed a planned roll out to other regions in 2018.

Additional organizations that can offer employment support include third-sector organizations, for example, the Shaw Trust, Kennedy Scott, British Society for Supported Employment, and the Royal National College for the Blind.

There is a growing recognition of the importance of work in reducing health and social inequalities, and pilot schemes to devolve joint commissioning in health and social care are ongoing in London and Manchester. These are likely to include work and health as a theme and to promote access to work for those with ill health and disability. For example, the Greater Manchester Combined Authority includes partnership working across the health and social care network—and includes employers as important partners.

Occupational health

OH, or occupational medicine, is a branch of medicine focusing on maintenance of health in the workplace, including prevention and management of ill health in the workplace.[44] OH professionals must have a wide knowledge of clinical medicine and be competent in a range of areas. OH can evaluate ill health in the context of work and OH advice can bring about a beneficial outcome for the employee and employer from an impartial perspective. Provision varies from in-house to outsourced services. Commonly in the UK, small and medium-sized employers have poor access to OH.

The OH specialist may be involved with the employee in their journey through their entire career. Starting with pre-placement, annual health surveillance, sickness absence, short-term absences, management concerns, workplace assessments, and ending in ill health retirement.

Working directly with the employer and having also an understanding of the workplace puts the OH specialist in a unique position and advantageous perspective to advise on fitness to work.

There is a recognition that many people in the UK do not have access to OH services, and this is an area for active review and development following the white paper 'Improving Lives: The Future of Work, Health and Disability'.[38]

Important professional groups in OH and their resources (including the FOM, Society of Occupational Medicine, Faculty of Occupational Health Nursing, and the Council for Work and Health) are signposted under 'Useful websites'.

Recent strategic interventions

Patients and some doctors fail to consider the likely implications of long-term certification, including potential loss of employment. Fit notes, initially issued for acute illness or common health complaints, may then label people as sick and disabled, and thus unintentionally promote long-term incapacity.

GPs find sickness certification and work-related consultations challenging.[45,46] Many GPs also have strongly held beliefs that the management of certification, rehabilitation, and return to work lies outside their remit.

There is a pressing need to shift attitudes to health and work and in this context healthcare professionals should strongly challenge three incorrect assumptions:

- First, that work will be harmful—current evidence suggests that work is generally good for physical and mental health.[10,47]
- Second, that rest from work is part of treatment. On the contrary, modern approaches to clinical management stress the importance of continuing ordinary activities and early return to work as an essential ingredient of treatment.[10,31]
- Third, that patients should be fully fit before considering a return to work.

GPs as non-OH specialists nonetheless have a key role in relation to fitness for work advice. Most doctors who issue fit notes and advise about work and health have historically not been adequately trained in this area. For the majority of patients who return to work rapidly, this may not matter, but for those who receive repeated and long-term certification there is now compelling evidence that this may impact their health and well-being.

The 'fit note'

Dame Carol Black in her 2008 report highlighted the need for a more proactive approach to rehabilitation.[28] The government response, *Improving Health and Work: Changing Lives* (2008),[37] recommended several initiatives to improve practice among GPs and other health professionals. One major outcome of the government's response was the introduction of the new Statement of Fitness for Work, the 'fit note'.

The fit note, introduced in April 2010, was designed to switch the focus to what people are capable of doing, rather than signing patients 'off sick' altogether. It was also hoped this would improve communication between employers, employees, and GPs. Besides declaring a person to be fit or unfit for work, the fit note allows GPs to indicate that a person may be fit for some aspects of work. GPs may suggest approaches to facilitate a return to work including phased return, altered work hours, amended duties, and workplace adaptations.

Initial research evaluating GPs' attitudes to the fit note was positive. A study using experimental vignettes carried out prior to the introduction indicated that a statement of fitness for work may reduce the number of patients advised to refrain from work and surveys eliciting GPs views post introduction suggested that it improved consultations and outcomes for patients. Other work, however, found it may increase tension within the doctor–patient relationship. A study commissioned by the DWP collecting fit note data over a 12-month period found that 12% of fit notes issued to patients had some form of 'may be fit for work' advice; however, this study was not able to assess whether the fit note had impacted on reducing the proportion of cases that were signed off as unfit for work.[48]

An Institution of Occupational Safety and Health report in 2015 suggested that the fit note may be misunderstood by employers and GPs and suggested more training and investment is needed.[49]

The role of the fit note was reviewed in the government paper 'Improving Lives: The Future of Work, Health and Disability' (2017),[38] and there may be changes in its operation. This may include using the AHP fitness report, integrating fit note training into medical education, changing the way GPs complete fit notes, and extending fit note certification powers to other health professionals (other than doctors).

The Black report[28] also led to the development of e-learning modules for GPs and secondary care doctors, decision aids, as well as more easily accessible information, leaflets, and guidance for all heath and work issues. These initiatives sit on a single website, Healthy Working UK (managed by the RCGP). Other royal colleges and specialist societies have linked to this website prioritizing awareness of the importance of health and work in the patients they care for. Medical schools also have access to a wide range of resources to embed this training in their curricula via the FOM website.

The 'Fit for Work' service

The Fit for Work scheme was set up in December 2014 following an independent review of the sickness absence system in Great Britain published in 2011.[50] It was closed in 2018. The service was intended to offer health and workplace advice to employees, employers, and GPs. The service offered OH assessments for employees at risk of long-term sickness absence, but failed to get as many referrals by employers and GPs as the DWP had expected. There were just 650 referrals a month in England and Wales, compared with the original forecast of 34,000.

The service was not intended to replace in-house OH services, but to work alongside these. The initiative was able to offer OH provision to a wider audience of employers who did not previously have access. The Fit for Work online and phone services will still offer general health and work advice.

Functional capacity

Measurement of functional capacity is a process which should include using both standardized tools and clinical expertise/judgement to determine a person's physical and cognitive/mental ability. There are a variety of functional capability assessment protocols available in the marketplace, and with the appropriate training and experience many health professionals can support this way back to work (see 'Useful websites').

In order to support remaining in work, a successful return to work, or entry into work, it is important to understand a person's capability to perform a variety of common functional postures and activities, along with measuring strength, endurance, coordination, and tolerance to activity. By gathering objective information about safe functional ability and then comparing this with the physical and psychological requirements of a job, a pathway to safe productivity can be developed; whether that be in returning to a pre-existing job role, or in search of alternative work. By identifying both physical and psychological barriers, appropriate modifications (as described within the following section) can be implemented.

Adjustments to enable return to work

OH specialists have a unique opportunity of working impartially with both the employer and the employee to try to achieve a successful outcome. This triad of OH, employee, and employer ensures all parties can contribute to a return to work outcome or exit strategies as deemed appropriate. An OH service should have knowledge of the workplace and after full assessment of an individual can advise on adjustments to enable and assist an individual returning to work after a period of sickness.

Current practice and evidence[51-54] suggests adjustments can be broadly divided into hours, duties, environment, and support. These adjustments can either be short term to allow an employee time to recover, or long term if health conditions and functional limitations are permanent.

1. Hours of work:
   - Phased returns—for example, reduced time working for a period of time with a gradual increase to substantive hours.
   - Flexibility in working hour—later starts, earlier finishes.
   - Time to attend healthcare appointments—for example, flexibility around working schedule to attend for counselling/physiotherapy appointments.
   - More breaks during the day, for example, four breaks instead of three, or hourly 'mini-breaks'.
   - An area to de-stress or rest should there be an exacerbation of the individual's health condition—for example, relaxation lounge.
   - More time to carry out duties, for example, reduced task volume or pace of work.
   - Alteration in working hours—for example, reduction in hours.
2. Work duties:
   - Additional supervision—more guidance, one to ones.
   - Mentorship; buddying.
   - Training—training courses, enhanced skills.
   - Coaching support—peer-to-peer support.
   - Review scheduling of tasks—provision of other tasks if restricted, for example, unable to work from heights, adjusted duties to ensure more ground work instead.
   - Reassignment of tasks.
   - Delegating tasks—delegating the work to another member of staff.

3. Environment:

- Adjustment to work equipment—for example, work station assessments, voice-activated software.
- Altering place of work—for example, working on ground floor if reduced mobility.
- Incorporating home working.
- Setting up an early intervention programme to help maintenance at work such as a Wellness Action Plan (WAP)[55]—for example, should a mental health condition be exacerbated, early detection can provide temporary workload adjustments to enable an individual to stay at work to allow time for recovery without resorting to sick leave.
- Workplace risk assessments—for example, individuals who may be at risk of seizures to ensure safe working and timely access to first aid.

4. Support:

- Referral to 'Access to Work' or other vocational rehabilitation service—allowing a workplace assessment, so equipment or changes can be identified to enable return to work.
- Timely referral and reviews with OH—support from OH, may allow access to in-house services such as counselling, physiotherapy, and other therapies earlier than through the NHS.
- Referral to employee assistance programmes where available.
- Referral to counsellor or CBT practitioner for mental health conditions.
- Referral to physiotherapists for musculoskeletal problems.
- A management decision for redeployment to an alternative role, if adjustments are not possible in the current role. If such a role exists within the company and is available, allow earlier opportunity to apply for this role with guidance from OH or vocational rehabilitation services to advise on fitness to work and necessary adjustments.

Further guidance and examples of adjustments are published by a variety of organizations (see 'Useful websites').

The Equality Act 2010 places an additional legal duty on the employer to make reasonable adjustments if the employer is aware or should be aware that the employee has a disability (see Chapter 3). Through working with OH and/or a vocational rehabilitation specialist service, specialist advice should enable the employer and the employee to comply with legal requirements. Where continued employment is not possible, an employer may want to consider termination of employment through a capability process. In this situation, ill health retirement should be considered if the employee is contributing to an occupational pension scheme (see Chapter 12).

Key points

- Prolonged absence from normal activities, including work, is often detrimental to a person's mental, physical, and social well-being. Conversely, appropriately and supported return to work benefits the worker and their family by enhancing recovery and reducing disability.
- Mental health and musculoskeletal problems are the most common presentations of work-related ill health.
- An approach to rehabilitation based upon a biopsychosocial model and flag system is necessary to identify and address the obstacles to recovery and barriers to return to work. It should also meet the needs of those with common health problems who do not recover in a timely fashion.
- A patient's return to function and work as soon as possible after an illness or injury should be encouraged and supported by employers, health professionals, fellow employees, and occupational health and rehabilitation service providers with the use of reasonable adjustments as necessary.
- A safe and timely return to work preserves a skilled and stable workforce and reduces demands on health and social services.

Useful websites

Faculty of Occupational Medicine	http://fom.ac.uk/
Society of Occupational Medicine	https://www.som.org.uk/
Council for Work and Health	http://www.councilforworkandhealth.org.uk/
Access to Work	https://www.gov.uk/access-to-work/overview
Access to Work (NI)	https://www.nidirect.gov.uk/articles/access-work-practical-help-work
UK Citizens Advice. Benefits	https://www.citizensadvice.org.uk/benefits/
Gov.uk. Universal Credit	https://www.gov.uk/universal-credit/
British Society of Rehabilitation Medicine	http://www.bsrm.org.uk/
Vocational Rehabilitation Association	https://vrassociationuk.com/
Case Management Society UK	https://www.cmsuk.org/
Royal College of Occupational Therapists	https://www.rcot.co.uk/
Association of Chartered Physiotherapists in Occupational Health and Ergonomics (APCOHE)	http://www.acpohe.org.uk/

British Psychological Society	https://www.bps.org.uk/
Royal College of General Practitioners	http://www.rcgp.org.uk/
Remploy	https://www.remploy.co.uk
Shaw Trust	https://www.shaw-trust.org.uk
Scope	https://www.scope.org.uk/support/disabled-people/work/access-to-work
British Society for Supported Employment	https://www.base-uk.org/about-british-association-supported-employment
British Dyslexia Association. 'Reasonable adjustments'	http://www.bdadyslexia.org.uk/employer/reasonable-adjustments
Department of Health. 'Advice for employers on workplace adjustments for mental health conditions'	http://www.nhshealthatwork.co.uk/images/library/files/Government%20policy/Mental_Health_Adjustments_Guidance_May_2012.pdf
Royal College of Psychiatrists. 'Developing and putting in place 'reasonable adjustments"	https://www.rcpsych.ac.uk/usefulresources/workandmentalhealth/clinician/2workingtogethertosupport/developingandputtinginplac.aspx
Allied Health Professionals Federation. 'AHP Advisory Fitness for Work Report'	http://www.ahpf.org.uk/AHP_Advisory_Fitness_for_Work_Report.htm
International Disability Management Standards Council UK & Ireland	https://www.idmsc-uk-ireland.org/about/
Obair. 'UKFCE Certification Training'	http://www.weareobair.com/UKFCE-certification-training.html
Healthy Work. 'Functional Capacity Evaluation (Physical Ability Assessment)'	https://healthywork.org.uk/occupational-health-services/functional-capacity-assessment/

Acknowledgements

The author gratefully acknowledges the contribution of Shirley Morrison-Glancy on vocational rehabilitation and functional assessment, as well as the contribution of Paul Williams to this chapter.

References

1. **Marmot M.** *Status Syndrome.* London: Bloomsbury, 2004.
2. **Twaddle A.** *Influence and Illness: Definitions and Definers of Illness Behaviour Among Older Males in Providence, Rhode Island.* PhD dissertation, Brown University, Providence, RI, 1968.

3. **Johns G.** Presenteeism in the workplace: a review and research agenda. *J Organ Behav* 2010;**31**:519–42.

4. **Working Party of the Royal College of General Practitioners.** *The Triaxial Model of the Consultation.* London: Royal College of General Practitioners; 1972.

5. **Aylward M.** Beliefs: clinical and vocational interventions—tackling psychological and social determinants of illness and disability. In: Halligan PW, Aylward M (eds), *The Power of Belief*, pp. xxvii–xxxvii. Oxford: Oxford University Press; 2006.

6. **Marmot M** (Chair). Fair Society, Healthy Lives. A Strategic Review of Health Inequalities in England post-2010 (The Marmot Review). London: The Marmot Review; 2010. Available at: http://www.instituteofhealthequity.org/projects/fair-society-healthy-lives-the-marmot-review/fair-society-healthy-lives-full-report.

7. **Burchardt T.** The dynamics of being disabled. *J Social Policy* 2000;**29**:645–68.

8. **Waddell G, Burton AK.** *Concepts of Rehabilitation for the Management of Common Health Problems.* London: The Stationery Office; 2004.

9. **Buck R, Barnes MC, Cohen D, et al.** Common health problems, yellow flags and functioning in a community setting. *J Occup Rehab* 2010;**20**:235–46.

10. **Waddell G, Aylward M.** *Models of Sickness and Disability: Applied to Common Health Problems.* London: Royal Society of Medicine Press; 2010.

11. **National Institute for Health and Care Excellence.** Low back pain and sciatica in over 16s: assessment and management. NICE guideline [NG59]. Available at: https://www.nice.org.uk/guidance/NG59.

12. **Kendall N, Linton SJ, Main CJ.** *Guide to Assessing Psychosocial Yellow Flags in Acute Low Back Pain: Risk Factors for Long Term Disability and Work Loss.* Wellington, New Zealand: Accident rehabilitation and Compensation Insurance of New Zealand and the National Health Committee; 1997.

13. **Mayou R, Main CJ, Auty A.** *The IUA/ABI Rehabilitation Working Party – Psychology, Personal Injury and Rehabilitation.* London: International Underwriting Association of London.

14. **Keele University.** STarT Back Tool. 2017. Available from: https://www.keele.ac.uk/sbst/startbacktool/

15. **Chang D, Irving A.** *Evaluation of the GP Education Pilot: Health and Work in General Practice.* London: Department for Work and Pensions, 2008.

16. **Von Korff M.** Fear and depression as remediable causes of disability in common medical conditions in primary care. In: White P (ed), *Biopsychosocial Medicine*, pp. 117–32. Oxford: Oxford University Press; 2005.

17. **British Occupational Health Research Foundation.** *Workplace Interventions for People with Common Mental Health Problems: Evidence Review and Recommendations.* London: British Occupational Health Research Foundation, Sainsbury Centre; 2005.

18. **Miller W, Rollnick S.** *Motivational Interviewing: Preparing People to Change*, 2nd edn. New York: Guilford Press; 2002.

19. **Mynors-Wallis L.** Problem solving treatment in general psychiatric practice. *Adv Psychiatric Treat* 2001;**7**:417–25.

20. **Till SR, Wahl HN, As-Sanie S.** The role of nonpharmacologic therapies in management of chronic pelvic pain: what to do when surgery fails. *Curr Opin Obstet Gynecol* 2017;**29**:231–9.

21. **Monticone M, Cedraschi C, Ambrosini E, et al.** Cognitive-behavioural treatment for subacute and chronic neck pain. *Cochrane Database Syst Rev* 2015;**5**:CD010664.

22. **National Institute for Health and Care Excellence.** Depression in adults: recognition and management. Clinical guideline [CG90]. Available at: https://www.nice.org.uk/guidance/cg90/chapter/1-Guidance#continuation-and-relapse-prevention.

23. **Health and Safety Executive (HSE)**. *Managing Sickness Absence and Return to Work—An Employers' and Managers' Guide*. London: HSE; 2004.

24. **Rehabilitation**. In: *Oxford Dictionary of English*, 3rd edn. 2017. Available at: https://en.oxforddictionaries.com/definition/rehabilitation.

25. **World Health Organization**. World report on disability. 2011. http://www.who.int/disabilities/world_report/2011/en/.

26. **Trades Union Congress (TUC)**. *Consultation Document on Rehabilitation. Getting Better at Getting Back*. London: TUC; 2000.

27. **Waddell G, Burton K, Kendall N.** *Vocational Rehabilitation. What Works, for Whom, and When?* London: Vocational Rehabilitation Task Group; 2009.

28. **Black C.** *Working for a Healthier Tomorrow: Review of the Health of Britain's Working Age Population*. London: The Stationery Office; 2008.

29. **Krause N, Frank JW, Dasinger LK, et al.** Determinants of duration of disability and return to work after work-related injury and illness: challenges for future research. *Am J Ind Med* 2001;**40**:464–84.

30. **Vogel N, Schandelmaier S, Zumbrunn T, et al.** Return-to-work coordination programmes for improving return to work in workers on sick leave. *Cochrane Database Syst Rev* 2017;**3**: CD011618.

31. **Secretary of State for Work and Pensions and the Secretary of State for Health.** Improving Lives: The Work, Health and Disability Green Paper. 2016. Available at: https://assets.publishing.service.gov.uk/government/uploads/system/uploads/attachment_data/file/564038/work-and-health-green-paper-improving-lives.pdf.

32. **Ashby K, Mahdon M.** *Why Do Employees Come to Work When Ill? An Investigation into Sickness Presence in the Workplace*. London: AXA PPP Healthcare; 2010.

33. **Aylward M.** *What Are the Outcomes of Low Back Pain and How Do They Relate?* Boston, MA: Boston International Forum Primary Care Research on Low Back Pain, Harvard School of Public Health; 2009.

34. **Pransky G, Shaw WS, Loisel P, et al.** Development and validation of competencies for return to work coordinators. *J Occup Rehab* 2009;**20**:41–8.

35. **Sawney P, Challenor J.** Poor communication between health professionals is a barrier to rehabilitation. *Occup Med* 2003;**53**:246–8.

36. **Michie S, Williams S.** Reducing work related psychological ill health and sickness absence: a systematic literature review. *Occup Environ Med* 2003;**60**:3–9.

37. **Department for Work and Pensions, Department of Health.** *Improving Health and Work: Changing Lives. The Government's Response to Dame Carol Black's Review of the Health of Britain's Working-Age Population*. London: The Stationery Office; 2008.

38. **Department of Health, Department for Work and Pensions.** Improving Lives: The Future of Work, Health and Disability. 2017. Available at: https://www.gov.uk/government/publications/improving-lives-the-future-of-work-health-and-disability

39. **Kenyon L.** FOM/SOM Response to Improving Lives: the Work, Health and Disability Green Paper. Association of Occupational Health Nurse Practitioners. 2017. Available at: http://aohnp.co.uk/fom-som-response-to-improving-lives-the-work-health-and-disability-green-paper/.

40. **Department for Work and Pensions and Department of Health and Social Care.** Thriving at work: the Stevenson/Farmer review of mental health and employers. 2017. Available at: https://www.gov.uk/government/publications/thriving-at-work-a-review-of-mental-health-and-employers Good work.

41. **Department for Business, Energy & Industrial Strategy.** Good work: the Taylor review of modern working practices. 2017. Available at: https://www.gov.uk/government/publications/good-work-the-taylor-review-of-modern-working-practices.

42. **Job Centre Guide**. Guide to JobCentre Plus, job hunting and claiming benefits. 2017. Available at: http://www.jobcentreguide.org/.

43. **Gov.uk**. Access to work: overview. 2017. Available at: https://www.gov.uk/access-to-work/overview.

44. **Faculty of Occupational Medicine**. Homepage. Available at: http://www.fom.ac.uk/.

45. **Money A, Hussey L, Thorley K, et al.** Work-related sickness absence negotiations: GPs' qualitative perspectives. *Br J Gen Pract* 2010;**60**:721–8.

46. **Fylan B, Fylan F, Caveney L.** *An Evaluation of the Statement of Fitness for Work: Qualitative Research with General Practitioners.* London: Department for Work and Pensions; 2011.

47. **Waddell G, Burton AK.** *Is Work Good for Your Health and Well-Being?* London: The Stationery Office; 2006.

48. **Hussey L, Money A, Gittins M, Agius R.** Has the fit note reduced general practice sickness certification rates? *Occup Med* 2015;**65**:182–9.

49. **Coole C, Drummon A, Watson P, Nouri F, Potgieter I.** *Getting the Best from the Fit Note: Investigating the Use of the Statement of Fitness for Work.* Leicestershire: Institution of Occupational Safety and Health, University of Nottingham; 2015.

50. **Black C, Frost, D.** *Health at Work: An Independent Review of Sickness Absence.* London: Department for Work and Pensions; 2011.

51. **Thomson L, Neathey F, Rick J.** *Best Practice in Rehabilitating Employees Following Absence Due to Work-Related Stress.* London: Health & Safety Executive; 2003.

52. **Mills M.** *Phased Return to Work: The Evidence Base and a Survey of Occupational Physicians' Current Practice.* Manchester: The University of Manchester, 2008.

53. **Saunders C.** A healthy return: good practice guide to rehabilitating people at work. Institution of Occupational Safety and Health. 2015. Available at: http://www.iosh.co.uk/healthyreturn.

54. **Wynne-Jones G, Artus M, Bishop A, et al.** Does the addition of a vocational advice service to best current primary care improve work outcomes in patients with musculoskeletal pain? The Study of Work and Pain (Swap) Cluster Randomized Trial (ISRCTN 52269669), *Rheumatology* 2016;**55**(Suppl. 1):i50.

55. **MIND.** Guide to Wellness Action Plans (WAPs). 2017. Available at: https://www.mind.org.uk/media/1593680/guide-to-waps.pdf.

Chapter 11

Fitness for work after surgery or critical illness

Tony Williams and Neil Pearce

Introduction

Occupational health (OH) professionals frequently advise about return to work after surgery. Providing advice can be challenging, and considerable misunderstanding exists among patients and clinicians. One patient may return to work 1 week after a hysterectomy while another is absent for 5 months. Medical issues are often confounded by inconsistent advice, inappropriate beliefs and unhelpful motivators. There is a recognized limitation in the evidence base. However, consensus is available from a number of guidelines drawn up by various expert bodies, which are covered in this chapter.

Advice on time to return to work following surgery

A study of 100 general surgeons and 90 general practitioners (GPs), who recommended time off work for patients with various ages and jobs, found wide variation in advice.[1] After unilateral inguinal hernia repair in a 25-year-old returning to heavy manual work, surgeons' recommendations varied from 1 to 12 weeks, and GPs' from 2 to 13 weeks. Trainee surgeons within the UK are neither specifically trained nor assessed on their knowledge about fitness for work following surgery. Nonetheless, with the introduction of 'fit notes', surgical teams are expected to advise (at the point of discharge) on anticipated time to partial or full working ability.

An expert working group, in developing guidelines for the Royal College of Obstetricians and Gynaecologists (RCOG), found no empirical evidence about the risk of heavy lifting following vaginal hysterectomy. However, the group recommended (by consensus) a 4-week restriction from heavy work—a substantial shift from the 12 weeks that was often recommended previously.

Non-evidence-based advice

An example of a procedure where there is no obvious reason for a delay in return to work is a simple discectomy, which results in a stable spine with minimal disruption to surrounding tissues. Many doctors advise months off work, but without any objective justification. Carragee et al.[2] studied a group of 45 worker volunteers undergoing discectomies, and urged them to return to full activities as soon as possible. The patients worked in various roles from sedentary work to heavy manual labour. Eleven patients returned to work on the next available working day. Many returned to adjusted duties initially. The mean time to return to full duties was 2.5 weeks for light manual work and 5.8 weeks for heavy manual work.

This small study suggests that most clinicians are giving overly cautious advice and that patients who are motivated can return faster than clinicians expect. Factors such as sick pay schemes have a major impact on return to work times (see Chapter 9).

After carpal tunnel release, some patients return to work very quickly while others remain absent for many weeks. Ratzon et al.[3] followed 50 consecutive patients operated on by five surgeons, assessing them before and after for severity of symptoms. They found that the surgeons' recommendations for return to work varied from 1 to 36 days, and the time to return to work varied from 1 to 88 days. The surgeons appeared to relate their advice to the type of work, but this was not highly predictive. The duration of sickness absence was not related to the severity of symptoms before or after surgery. The surgeon's recommendation had the strongest influence on duration of absence.

The fact that patients follow their surgeon's advice is not surprising. It becomes a problem if the surgeon's advice is not evidence based and a much longer period of absence than necessary is recommended. This is particularly so if long rest periods are recommended, as this can lead to substantial deconditioning. In older patients, it can be extremely difficult to regain fitness and pre-surgery weight.

The evidence base

There is substantial evidence concerning the principles of surgical recovery. A great deal is known about wound healing, complications during recovery, and the impact of concurrent factors such as diabetes, age, and smoking. There is also good evidence regarding long-term recovery from various surgical procedures, but almost none for the relatively brief recovery period between the operation and a return to work. So, while it is possible to predict what someone might be able to do when they have fully recovered from a total hip replacement, there is little or no documented evidence on how long it will be before they can safely squat, walk a mile, or lift a bag of shopping or cement. Until studies produce direct evidence, we should rely on our knowledge of the principles of healing and recovery to assess scope for return to work after surgery.

What do we mean by 'fit for work'?

There are three main fitness issues to consider after an operation. The first is capability: can the person physically cope with any or some work? The second is safety: will they be harmed or potentially cause harm to others by going to work, and by doing any particular activity at work? The third is motivation: how well do they cope with pain, do they want to return, or are they seeking time away from work? All are relevant.

A person may be safe returning to heavy lifting within a few hours of a mesh repair of an inguinal hernia, but as the anaesthetic wears off they may experience substantial pain. Is it reasonable to expect them to return if they will be in pain? How much pain or discomfort is it reasonable to expect an employee to endure? How can their account of pain be verified, or its severity adjudged? If driving is involved, can the patient safely execute an emergency stop? Does the patient trust the hernia repair or the new hip? Do they trust their employer to make adjustments for them at work? Do they trust the OH professional who advises them that they will not be harmed?

These issues need to be explored with each patient to determine what they can do, what they believe they can do, and what they want to do. Care should be taken not to be judgemental in this process, but there is a need to address obvious motivational barriers.

Evidence from wound healing studies

The rate at which wounds heal plays a part in the decision about return to work. Healing can be delayed by infection, ischaemia, malignancy, poor nutrition, the presence of a haematoma or foreign body, diabetes mellitus, jaundice, uraemia, use of irradiation and treatment with oral steroids, immunosuppressive drugs, and chemotherapeutic agents.

The time course for healing also depends on the tissue involved. For skin and mucosal-lined organs, the stages of wound healing are relatively constant. By 5 days, granulation tissue has formed, new vessels start to proliferate, and collagen fibres start to bridge the wound. Remodelling starts at 2 weeks and by 4–6 weeks the wound has strengthened, the inflammatory response disappeared, and the wound appears healed.

The process and timescale is different for bone, which depends on osteoblast activity producing woven bone. After 3 weeks, the mass of healing tissue is maximal although has little strength and is unsuitable for weight bearing, but the newly formed cartilage starts to ossify and new bone starts to bridge the fracture gap. While pain lessens substantially at this point, full strength is not usually reached until 10–12 weeks, often longer for the tibia and femur.

Evidence from use of different closure methods and internal support

How a wound is closed and the technique and materials used may also influence recovery. A balance needs to be struck between absorbable sutures that minimize the foreign body irritation and non-absorbable sutures that can provide permanent strength to a wound. For abdominal closure, most surgeons now use a long-lasting absorbable suture material that maintains its tensile strength for about 8 weeks. Mass absorption takes about 6 months. Where prolonged approximation of tissues is required (e.g. the repair of an incisional hernia), a non-absorbable suture material or mesh of such material as polypropylene may be used. Skin closure adds very little to a wound's strength. There is no reason why a patient may not return to sedentary work even with skin sutures still *in situ*, but it would be unwise for a patient to undertake heavy manual labour or for the wound to be exposed to water, dust, or abrasive contact.

Factors affecting recovery

Diabetes

Significant postoperative complications are seen in patients with diabetes, reflecting a variety of specific physiological problems. These include elevated glucose, failure of mobilization of endothelial cells leading to failure of revascularization (essential in successful wound healing), and reduced clearance of dead cells (efferocytosis) within wound sites due to dysfunctional macrophages. The result is continued exposure of the healing wound to the toxic contents of dead and dying cells, resulting in persistent inflammation and delayed wound healing.[4]

Obesity

Obesity is associated with a state of chronic low-level inflammation, impaired antibody responses,[5] and an increased risk of chest infections with delayed mobilization. Patients who have had bariatric surgery also have a higher complication rate.[6]

Smoking

Smoking reduces oxygen in the blood and high nicotine levels impair angiogenesis and reduce the blood supply to the healing wound. Smoking may also impair collagen production and maintenance, weakening any scar formation. The result is a significant delay in healing and a weaker scar. High nicotine levels can be associated with e-cigarettes, so a change to e-cigarette use prior to and after surgery may not improve wound healing although there has been no published research yet.

Other studies have shown that smokers have significantly worse cosmetic results following surgery,[7] impaired wound healing (which improves in those who quit even quite late),[8] and a fourfold higher incidence of incisional hernia.[9] This may also be related to raised intra-abdominal pressure secondary to coughing and an increased incidence of postoperative respiratory tract infection. Smoking is also a major factor in delayed fracture healing[10]; in one study, vertebral fusion failed in 40% of smokers but only 8% of non-smokers.[11]

Age

The effects of age alone are minimal. One study found patients over 65 took on average 1.9 days longer to heal than those aged under 65.[12] Older patients may have more co-morbidities and less motivation to engage with rehabilitation.[13] However younger patients may push too hard during the initial recovery phase leading to surgical complications (e.g. after anterior cruciate ligament repair[14]).

The nature of the operation

It is important that the OH professional understands the exact nature of the surgical procedure before giving advice. Two procedures seen frequently in OH clinics illustrate how the nature of the procedure is influential.

Subacromial decompression may involve just debridement of excess acromial bone with an expected return to work within a week, and only minor discomfort. More frequently, the thickened synovium will also need debridement, leaving a very sore joint that takes 4–6 weeks to recover sufficiently for light manual handling. If the rotator cuff needs repair, the patient may be able to return to light administrative duties wearing an abductor brace after a couple of weeks. But they are unlikely to be fit for significant light manual handling duties for around 12 weeks, or heavy manual handling for 6–9 months. This is a particular problem if a poor vascular supply to the healing muscle delays recovery.

Bunions may represent just a little extra bone over the medial aspect of the first metatarsal head, or significant lateral displacement of the proximal phalanx with substantial degenerative changes in the metatarsophalangeal joint. Surgery may involve distal osteotomy of the metatarsal, proximal osteotomy of the metatarsal, or even surgery to the adjacent tarsal bones. Distal surgery is usually managed with a walking plaster at 2 weeks and early mobilization to avoid stiffening, while proximal surgery may require non-weight bearing for 6 weeks. So, some patients may be fit to return to most duties within a few weeks and may even be running after a couple of months, while others will take substantially longer to recover. While sedentary duties may be an option for some, care should be taken to find out exactly what procedure was undertaken before advising on a suitable return to work date and work duties.

Psychology and surgery

Any surgical procedure is likely to be a significant event in someone's life. Expectations and beliefs about recovery and safety of activities will vary between patients, sometimes reinforced by misguided clinicians. In general, patients can be reassured following most surgical procedures that normal activity will be safe, and they should be encouraged to carry out exercise activity such as walking as quickly as possible. OH professionals should be alert for yellow flags. These are an important predictor of outcome, indicating a higher risk of extended absence and the subsequent deconditioning that can make return to work more difficult. It can be important to note how the patient arrives in the consulting room. Attendance in a wheelchair or on two crutches, or wearing splints or braces that are not expected so long after a surgical procedure, should prompt supportive enquiry and emphasis of the need to develop confidence without the use of support.

Enhanced recovery after surgery programmes

Enhanced recovery programmes have been introduced for many types of surgery in recent years, with the aim of reducing the length of hospital stay for specific operations. These programmes typically select 70% of patients preoperatively who are mentally and physically fit with satisfactory social circumstances, who are therefore more likely to be suitable for rapid recovery. As well as standardized medical and nursing care, the programmes include a psychological element whereby the patient is given an expectation of a relatively rapid recovery and specific goals for mobilization, nutrition, and return of function. Patients are encouraged to be proactive in their recovery and increasingly are given post-discharge goals, which in turn can support faster return to work. Patients receive written information including these goals prior to surgery and are thus well informed and hopefully engaged in their recovery.

Time to return to work following surgery

The following sections provide guidelines on typical return to work times following common surgical procedures. In the absence of direct evidence, these guidelines have been compiled from a number of sources including the Royal College of Surgeons of England (RCS), and the RCOG who have both developed consensus-based guidelines for a number of common procedures, with downloadable leaflets (see 'Useful websites'). Use has also been made of two unpublished studies of surgeons working in the South West of England and Greater Glasgow. Surgeons were asked about advice given on timescales for return to work. In terms of consensus, there was good agreement between orthopaedic surgeons. General surgeons, gynaecologists, and urologists had moderate agreement on return to work timescales. But among breast surgeons, agreement was only fair. There are also many guidelines available on the Internet (see 'Useful websites').

Consensus guidelines should prevent large variation in recommendations and can help achieve standardization. They should also help employers predict the amount of time off, allowing alternative arrangements for cover if necessary. Some patients may be able to return without harm significantly sooner than suggested, while others may develop complications or may just take longer to adjust to recovery. Nevertheless, these are useful tools to help plan a phased return to work.

Walking immediately after these procedures will not be harmful and it should be encouraged. This is particularly important for conditions where traditionally many patients have been encouraged to rest. Such an approach can result in substantial loss of fitness and weight gain, perhaps never to be reversed. Employers may allow several months off to recover, but the employee should be encouraged to use this time to regain full physical fitness and if possible to adopt a new, healthier lifestyle following treatment of their underlying problem.

Advice to employees

Ideally employees should be advised about their procedure and, where available, shown web-based resources *before* surgery, so they know what to expect and can prepare to return to work in the recommended timelines. This can be a useful role of the OH service and is an opportunity to reinforce the significant benefits of exercise both before surgery and during the recovery period. There may be value in directing the employer to the web-based resources too, so there is a good understanding between employee and employer over what to expect and what support will be needed when the employee returns.

Fitness to drive after surgery

Many surgical procedures affect the ability to drive but very few have explicit restrictions in the Driver and Vehicle Licensing Agency (DVLA) guidelines (see 'Useful websites').

Some are provided below, but in general, it is up to the patient to decide when they feel able to drive safely. This includes the ability to control and stop the vehicle, and concentrate. Recovery from a general anaesthetic is usually only a matter of hours, so advice not to drive the same or following day would be sensible. Consideration should also be given to medication taken following surgery, particularly medication known to affect concentration. Following eye surgery, there may be a delay before new spectacles can be made, and those who do not meet the DVLA eyesight standards must not drive in the interim pending corrected acuity with glasses or contact lenses. The surgeon will usually advise patients on when it should be safe for them to drive.

Specific operation sites and procedures

Abdominal surgery

Laparoscopic surgery

The role of minimally invasive surgery has expanded in all specialties including general surgery, gynaecology, and urology. Large, painful surgical wounds have been replaced with small, relatively painless, 'keyhole' incisions, facilitating more rapid postoperative recovery for many patients. As well as laparoscopic surgery, further advances of the minimal access approach include robotic surgery, single incision laparoscopic surgery (SILS) and natural orifice totally endoscopic surgery (NOTES) (endoscopic access to intraperitoneal structures via endoscopic transgastric, transvaginal or transcolonic approaches). These have largely cosmetic advantages over the more conventional, multiple port site, laparoscopic approach. They may also lead to less pain and potentially a psychological advantage with improved recovery rate due to the lack of visible wounds. The small laparoscopic wounds are also less prone to complications such as wound infection and incisional hernia. Furthermore, the handling of the intestine and the fluid loss involved in abdominal procedures is largely avoided and postoperative ileus and pulmonary and thromboembolic complications are less frequent. Laparoscopic techniques thus promote early recovery and enable quicker return to work. Other minimally invasive procedures such as arthroscopy and thoracoscopy similarly contribute to earlier recovery after orthopaedic and chest surgery respectively (Table 11.1).

Laparotomy

Standard open abdominal wounds are still required when a laparoscopic procedure proves technically impossible or dangerous, including major abdominal operations where good visibility is required (e.g. certain procedures on the pancreas, those for abdominal aortic aneurysms when endovascular surgery is unsuitable, and some colorectal resections). Major abdominal wounds are a cause of considerable postoperative pain and morbidity.

Most abdominal wounds are now closed with non-absorbable or slowly absorbable materials rather than the rapidly absorbed cat gut used in the past. As a result of improved suture techniques, the incidence of wound dehiscence is reduced and early return to

Table 11.1 Suggested return to work times following abdominal surgery

Procedure	Sedentary admin	Sedentary light manual	Active light manual	Heavy manual	Physically demanding
Inguinal, small umbilical, femoral, epigastric or incisional hernia, laparoscopic repair	3–5 days	3–5 days	3–14 days	2–4 weeks	4 weeks
Inguinal, small umbilical, femoral, epigastric or incisional hernia, open repair	3–7 days	1–2 weeks	1–2 weeks	2–6 weeks	2–6 weeks
Large umbilical or incisional hernia laparoscopic repair	2–3 weeks	2–3 weeks	2–3 weeks	4–6 weeks	6 weeks+
Large umbilical or incisional hernia open repair	2–4 weeks	3–5 weeks	3–5 weeks	4–6 weeks	6–12 weeks
Hiatus hernia repair (open)	2–3 weeks	2–3 weeks	2–3 weeks	4–6 weeks	4–6 weeks
Hiatus hernia repair (laparoscopic)	10–14 days	10–14 days	2–3 weeks	3–4 weeks	3–4 weeks
Cholecystectomy laparoscopic	3–14 days	3–14 days	3–14 days	2–3 weeks	3 weeks+
Cholecystectomy open	1–2 weeks	1–2 weeks	2–3 weeks	3–4 weeks	4–6 weeks
Laparoscopic fundoplication	10–14 days	10–14 days	2–3 weeks	3–4 weeks	3–4 weeks
Major laparotomy	2–4 weeks	2–4 weeks	4–6 weeks	6–8 weeks	6–8 weeks
Gastrectomy or oesophago-gastrectomy for malignancy	8–12 weeks	8–12 weeks	12 weeks+	Unlikely	No
Duodenotomy for ulceration	4–6 weeks	4–6 weeks	4–6 weeks	6–8 weeks	6–8 weeks
Appendicectomy laparoscopic	1 week	1 week	1–2 weeks	2–3 weeks	3 weeks+
Appendicectomy open	2 weeks	2 weeks	2–3 weeks	4–6 weeks	6 weeks+
Right hemicolectomy with end-to-end anastomosis	3–6 weeks	3–6 weeks	4–8 weeks	6–12 weeks	6–12 weeks
Left hemicolectomy or anterior resection of rectum	6–12 weeks	6–12 weeks	6–12 weeks	12–16 weeks	16–26 weeks

(continued)

Table 11.1 Continued

Procedure	Sedentary admin	Sedentary light manual	Active light manual	Heavy manual	Physically demanding
Defunctioning stoma closure	3–4 weeks	3–4 weeks	3–4 weeks	4–6 weeks	4–6 weeks
Abdominoperineal excision of rectum with permanent colostomy	8–12 weeks	8–12 weeks	8–12 weeks	12–16 weeks	When and if compatible with stoma
Anal verge haematoma	When able to sit	When able to sit	1–3 days	1–7 days	1–7 days
Thrombosed internal haemorrhoids	When able to sit	When able to sit	1–2 weeks	2–3 weeks	2–3 weeks
Haemorrhoidectomy (sclerotherapy/ banding/ligation/ cryotherapy)	1–7 days	1–7 days	1–14 days	1–14 days	1–14 days
Haemorrhoidectomy (surgical)	When able to sit	When able to sit	2–3 weeks	3–6 weeks	3–6 weeks
Anal fissure— lateral internal sphincterotomy	1–2 days	1–2 days	1–2 days	4–6 weeks	4–6 weeks
Pilonidal sinus primary suture	1–3 weeks	1–3 weeks	2–4 weeks	3–6 weeks	3–6 weeks
Pilonidal sinus secondary intention	3 weeks+	3 weeks+	3–6 weeks	6–8 weeks	6–8 weeks
Anal fistula—small, little dressing required	1 week	1 week	1 week	2–3 weeks	2–4 weeks
Anal fistula—large, dressing changed by district nurse	When able to sit	When able to sit	Variable, when comfortable	Variable, when fully healed	Variable, when fully healed
Abdominoplasty	2–3 weeks	2–3 weeks	4–8 weeks	8–12 weeks	8–12 weeks
Gastric banding	2–4 weeks	2–4 weeks	3–6 weeks	12 weeks+	12 weeks+
Gastric bypass surgery	2–6 weeks	2–6 weeks	4–6 weeks	12 weeks+	12 weeks+

non-manual work should not increase the risk of incisional hernia. Heavy manual work, however, will not normally be undertaken for 6–8 weeks after a major laparotomy. The length of convalescence after laparotomy will be affected not only by the type and size of wound but also by the indication for surgery, the procedure performed, the occurrence of postoperative complications, and the nature of the patient's occupation. A patient undergoing appendicectomy for a perforated gangrenous appendix, with four-quadrant peritonitis and systemic sepsis, will require prolonged intravenous antibiotics and possibly intensive care, even though the surgical procedure may be little different from an early-stage appendectomy. The former may require 1 or 2 weeks in hospital and be substantially debilitated by the underlying inflammatory process, while the latter patient may be discharged within 2 days and able to return to sedentary occupation after 1 week. Perforation, generalized peritonitis, or septicaemia prior to any abdominal surgery indicates that the patient will be slow to recover and likely to require additional time off work, proportionate to their length of time in hospital.

A subcostal incision for removal of the gall bladder (if laparoscopic access has been unsuccessful) is less traumatic than the full-length vertical abdominal incision that is commonly needed for colonic or vascular procedures. The former may result in a hospital stay of 2–5 days and a quick return to work. In contrast, patients with a long vertical abdominal wound may remain in hospital for 1–2 weeks if there are no procedural or wound-related complications, and thus absence from work may be longer.

Complications of laparotomy wounds include infection and dehiscence and, later, the development of an incisional hernia. Occasional consequences of laparotomy, for whatever cause, include small bowel obstruction due to ileus in the immediate postoperative period or later due to adhesions. Following bowel surgery, including creating a stoma, return of fitness for non-manual work often takes 8–12 weeks. A significant manual role will be delayed until the patient is confident in managing the stoma (see 'Stomas'). Often other factors are involved, such as adjuvant therapy following surgery for malignancy or 'dumping' following gastrectomy. Adjustment to a new diet after bariatric surgery can take 2 or 3 months. There may be difficulty swallowing solid food for up to 3 months after oesophageal or gastric surgery, but this should not delay a return to work. The complications of chronic intra-abdominal sepsis, fistula formation, and collections may occur after any digestive tract surgery, resulting in severe and prolonged debility even after apparently straightforward surgery. They are particularly common after pancreatic or colonic surgery and occasionally may present after discharge from hospital; these complications should be suspected by the OH professional, in any patient who is deviating significantly from the expected trajectory of recovery after surgery of this nature.

Hernia repair

Current methods of hernia repair, using tension-free mesh and sutures,[15] give a very strong structural repair, so the patient is unlikely to be harmed by any activity as soon as they recover from the anaesthetic. Studies have shown that open prosthetic mesh repair can withstand any degree of stress immediately[16] and postoperative activity need not be restricted at all.[17] Patients should be encouraged to walk on the first day postoperatively. Despite less discomfort, lower risk of wound infection, and a smaller wound after laparoscopy, the overall recovery times do not vary greatly between laparoscopic and open repairs. The main issues affecting return to work are discomfort and complications such as wound infection. Recurrent hernia repair is associated with significantly more local tissue damage, slower healing, and greater discomfort over longer periods. The timelines before returning to work are therefore maximal estimates, and most employees would return before the times suggested. The RCS recommends 6 weeks to heavy manual work after inguinal hernia repair, and a return to playing football after 8 weeks and rugby after 12 weeks. These are all conservative recommendations. The key message is to allow employees to return as soon as they want to after hernia repair.

Haemorrhoids

There is no absolute clinical need for patients to remain off sick after thrombosed internal haemorrhoids although discomfort is likely to prevent many from working for a week or two. Surgical haemorrhoidectomy leads to significant discomfort and initial discharge. However, there is no need to wait until full healing has taken place before returning to work. Some employees may return after 2–3 weeks, although full healing may take 5–6 weeks. The majority of haemorrhoids can be managed without formal haemorrhoidectomy, by minor outpatient or day case procedures involving banding of the pile or haemorrhoidal artery ligation. Nonetheless, discomfort is common and advice is to avoid straining or heavy lifting for 2 weeks to reduce the risk of postoperative haemorrhage.

Anal fissure, pilonidal sinus, and anal fistula

Employees will be safe working at any stage after treatment for anal fissure, pilonidal sinus, or anal fistula but the discomfort and logistics of dressing changes may prevent a return until healing is near complete. Adjustments to working hours to allow dressings changes and the use of shaped cushions to aid comfortable sitting at work may facilitate earlier return. A lateral internal sphincterotomy causes little external disruption, so a return after a day or two can be expected. Where healing is delayed, the employee may have no option but to wait several months until the wound has healed sufficiently to allow them to sit at work.

Stomas

Stomas may be created with ileum or colon, including an ileal conduit for a urostomy. A temporary colostomy or ileostomy facilitates distal anastomotic healing before stoma closure in 3–6 months, or the stoma may be permanent. All stomas require some means to collect waste, and the design and process can vary significantly. Some patients with distal colostomies are able to manage the stoma by irrigation to stimulate emptying, so no collection bag is required. The stoma can be covered with a cap or plug allowing substantial freedom of movement and activity. Irrigation typically takes 45–60 minutes and ideally is required once every 48 hours—otherwise patients are likely to prefer the convenience of a bag which can be easily changed. Stoma bags can be drainable or may separate from a base plate to allow changing. The base plate is generally left attached for 3–5 days. Most patients are able to undertake all physical activities, including swimming and non-contact sports, with a stoma. More vigorous activities will require the use of a protective belt or shield. Patients have returned to work and coped well as prison and police officers, including 'control and restraint' duties.

Stomas have a number of potential complications. Failure of flatus escape through the integral filter leads to ballooning and requires early pouch change. Parastomal hernias are common, but not all are symptomatic and there is no evidence that regular exercise and heavy manual handling cause parastomal hernia provided that a support belt is worn. Problems may arise where the stoma is close to a scar or skin fold, affecting adhesion of the pouch plate. Leakage is unusual, but may be problematic at work. Ileostomies tend to fill more often with more fluid contents and are more likely to produce odours.

Most people can return to full employment with a stoma and usually only require minimal adjustments. There are only a few roles where difficulties arise, such as employees working overseas, away from normal toilet facilities, or those working outside with limited access to toilet facilities (e.g. postwomen, forestry workers, and linesmen). Occasionally, complications or significant psychological issues with a stoma undermine confidence or ability to cope in the workplace. All patients with stomas should be supported by a stoma nurse and have good access to advice and support. A useful source of support is the Colostomy Association (see 'Useful websites').

Reconstructive bowel surgery

As an alternative to a stoma, the surgeon may fashion a pouch from small bowel to replace the rectum and colon. Although the anal sphincters are retained, the patient may need to use a catheter several times a day to empty the pouch. The combination of recovery from surgery and adaptation to the new anatomy can delay return to work by several months. Appropriate toilet arrangements may be necessary, with a supportive phased return to work aimed initially at rebuilding confidence.

Invasive cardiology, cardiothoracic, and vascular surgery

Many patients having cardiothoracic surgery will have substantial co-morbidity that will affect recovery. Various access routes may be used, with route having a major effect on recovery times (see Table 11.2). Cardiology and cardiothoracic surgery have seen some significant developments in minimally invasive techniques including percutaneous transcatheter aortic valve implantation (TAVI) procedures, percutaneous coronary interventions, and radiofrequency ablation.

Thoracoscopic procedures

Thoracoscopy has significantly reduced morbidity relative to thoracotomy, allowing a much quicker return to work. Typically, this method is used for cervical sympathectomy, pulmonary resection, and surgery for pneumothorax. Robotic surgery has similar benefits.

Thoracotomy

A full thoracotomy is required for major lung and heart surgery. After a full pneumonectomy, a return to non-manual work may be possible after 2–3 months. Manual work may be problematic if there is substantially reduced exercise tolerance, which may be exacerbated by lifestyle issues (particularly smoking). However, many people, particularly if younger and fitter, can have effectively normal function despite removal of a lung.

Table 11.2 Suggested return to work times following cardiothoracic and vascular surgery

Procedure	Sedentary admin	Sedentary light manual	Active light manual	Heavy manual	Physically demanding
Thoracoscopy with cervical sympathectomy, pulmonary resection, and pneumothorax surgery	1–2 weeks	1–2 weeks	2–4 weeks	4 weeks+	4 weeks+
Thoracotomy with partial pneumonectomy	6 weeks	6 weeks	6 weeks	12 weeks	12 weeks
Thoracotomy with pneumonectomy	8–12 weeks	8–12 weeks	8–12 weeks	Unlikely	Unlikely
Spontaneous pneumothorax	1–7 days	1–7 days	1–7 days	4–6 weeks	4–6 weeks
Surgery for recurrent pneumothorax	2–3 weeks	2–3 weeks	2–3 weeks	6 weeks+	6 weeks+
Oesophagectomy	6–12 weeks	6–12 weeks	8–12 weeks	8–16 weeks	8–16 weeks
CABG, aortic or mitral valve replacement, TAVI	6 weeks	6 weeks	8–12 weeks	12–39 weeks	26–39 weeks
Angioplasty or coronary stents for stenosis[a]	3–7 days	3–7 days	1 week	2–4 weeks	6 weeks
Angioplasty, thrombectomy or coronary stents for myocardial infarction[a]	2–6 weeks	2–6 weeks	4–6 weeks	6–12 weeks+	12 weeks+
Aortic aneurysm open abdominal repair	8–12 weeks	8–12 weeks	8–12 weeks	4–6 months but unlikely	4–6 months but unlikely
Aortic aneurysm percutaneous endovascular grafting	1 week	1 week	1–2 weeks	2–4 weeks	4 weeks+
Femoro-popliteal bypass	4 weeks	4 weeks	4–8 weeks	12 weeks	12 weeks
Carotid endarterectomy	2–3 weeks	2–3 weeks	2–5 weeks	4–8 weeks	4–8 weeks
Radiofrequency ablation[b]	1–2 days	1–2 days	1–2 days	2 weeks	6 weeks
Varicose veins stripping	1–2 weeks	1–2 weeks	1–2 weeks	2–3 weeks	2–3 weeks

(continued)

Table 11.2 Continued

Procedure	Sedentary admin	Sedentary light manual	Active light manual	Heavy manual	Physically demanding
Varicose veins sclerotherapy	2–3 days	2–3 days	3–5 days	3–5 days	1 week
Varicose veins endovenous laser therapy	2–3 days	2–3 days	1–2 weeks	2–4 weeks	2–4 weeks

[a] No driving for 1 week, no large goods vehicle or passenger carrying vehicle driving for 6 weeks.
[b] No driving for 2 days, no large goods vehicle or passenger carrying vehicle driving for 6 weeks.

Lifestyle change is encouraged after coronary artery bypass grafting (CABG) more so than the prolonged rest often encouraged after other surgical procedures. Consequently, recovery rates often seem substantially faster than for other less invasive surgical procedures. The main delay in return to manual work is healing of the chest wall, as rib and sternal pain may persist for several months after surgery. Heavy upper body exercise should be avoided for the first 3 months to allow full healing of the sternum. Light upper body activity is encouraged to avoid extensive scarring and restricted mobility. Patients are unlikely to be harmed by working in a manual role after 3 months, even if they get unusual sensations or discomfort in the chest wall. It is important to encourage exercise in a controlled environment, as this will help the patient regain confidence as well as fitness.

Oesophagectomy is usually only used for malignancy, and although this is the mainstay of treatment, adjuvant chemotherapy may be used after surgery. If neoadjuvant chemotherapy or radiotherapy is given prior to surgery, there should be no delay to recovery from the surgery. A jejunostomy may be used for feeding, and the tube is usually removed 3–6 weeks after surgery, well before returning to work. Most oesophagectomy is performed by the minimally invasive approach; although this speeds postoperative recovery, it makes relatively little difference to time to return to work. The poor prognosis in most cases often means that the patient opts for ill health retirement.

Spontaneous pneumothorax

After spontaneous pneumothorax, an employee should be safe to return to a non-manual role without significant delay once they have left hospital, but may need several weeks to enable healing before returning to a heavy manual job. Chest discomfort is common after pleurodesis, and this is the main reason for the slower return to non-manual work.

Coronary stents and angioplasty

A quick recovery can be expected after elective coronary stents or angioplasty. Light exercise is usually safe immediately after the procedure, although allowing 3 days for stabilization of the coronary vessels and catheter site would be reasonable. Care is needed to avoid trauma to the catheter access site when undertaking heavy manual work. It is important to liaise with the treating cardiologist if the patient plans to return to high levels of physical activity. This should be included in a rehabilitation plan for the underlying ischaemic heart disease, particularly if this has been done as an acute percutaneous coronary intervention for myocardial infarction.

Patients often require high-dose dual antiplatelet therapy following percutaneous coronary intervention. Patients with metallic cardiac valves also require anticoagulation. The increased risk of prolonged haemorrhage should be taken into consideration for those whose occupation includes a significant risk of injury in remote locations (e.g. forestry workers, farmers, and trawlermen) or head injury, particularly from control and restraint procedures.

Vascular surgery

Aortic aneurysm

Healing after open abdominal surgery for aortic aneurysm grafting would be expected to enable a return to non-manual work after 2–3 months, but multiple co-morbidities are likely and these could extend the recovery time significantly (see Table 11.2). Treatment by percutaneous endovascular grafting would be expected to lead to a much more rapid recovery.

Arterial graft, angioplasty, and reconstructive surgery

Vascular reconstruction of the abdominal and lower limb arterial system is now generally a treatment of last resort. Patients are likely to have major co-morbidities including cardiac problems and diabetes and they are more likely to be older workers if still working. These issues are likely to play a major role in any decision on fitness to return to work. Faster healing would be expected for femoro-popliteal bypass (see Table 11.2). Recovery after carotid endarterectomy can be affected by psychological issues. Peripheral angioplasty when undertaken electively, with or without stenting, allows a relatively swift return to work.

Varicose veins

Fewer patients have the traditional stripping and tying varicose veins, and recovery may take a little longer after bilateral vein treatment, while laser ablation should allow a faster recovery. Bandages are usually replaced with thromboembolic deterrent stockings after a day, with stockings worn for 2 weeks. Many surgeons now use foam sclerotherapy, and early activity is encouraged after this treatment as prolonged inactivity can be harmful. Patients are typically advised to walk every day from the day following surgery.

Head, neck, and ear, nose, and throat (ENT) surgery

Many head, neck, and ENT procedures are undertaken for malignancy, and there may be significant co-morbidity where the thyroid or parathyroid glands are involved. This will inevitably affect return to work times. Patients requiring radical head and neck dissection

Table 11.3 Suggested return to work times in weeks following head and neck surgery

Procedure	Sedentary admin	Sedentary light manual	Active light manual	Heavy manual	Physically demanding
Hemi-thyroidectomy	1–2 weeks	1–2 weeks	1–4 weeks	2–8 weeks	3–8 weeks
Subtotal thyroidectomy	1–3 weeks	1–3 weeks	1–4 weeks	2–8 weeks	3–8 weeks
Total thyroidectomy	2–3 weeks	2–3 weeks	2–4 weeks	2–8 weeks	3–8 weeks
Parotid gland removal	2 weeks	2 weeks	2 weeks	2–4 weeks	2–4 weeks
Submandibular gland removal	1–2 weeks	1–2 weeks	1–2 weeks	2–3 weeks	2–4 weeks
Wisdom teeth removal	1–3 days	1–3 days	1–3 days	3–4 days	3–4 days
Nasal septoplasty	3–7 days	3–7 days	3–7 days	7–14 days	6–12 weeks

for carcinoma of the larynx or upper airways also often require major plastic surgical reconstruction as well as perioperative radiotherapy. The patients often have significant other co-morbidity in addition to the poor prognosis of their disease. Laryngectomy leads to significant long-term communication issues which will make return to work challenging for many patients and many occupations. An actively engaged speech and language therapy specialist is essential to ensure that communication skills are maximized, but many workers will require changes to their roles if clear verbal communication is a prerequisite (Table 11.3).

Thyroidectomy

Hemithyroidectomy for a solitary thyroid nodule is a relatively minor procedure. Subtotal or total thyroidectomy is significantly more traumatic and may be associated with alteration in thyroid function and disorders of calcium metabolism if the parathyroid glands are removed or injured.

Parotid and submandibular glands

The good vascular supply around the head and neck generally allows a quick return to work where the submandibular gland is involved, longer after surgery on the parotid gland. Removal of a stone from the submandibular duct is a simple procedure and a return to work can be expected in 1–2 days.

Nasal septoplasty

Nasal septoplasty is a common procedure in young fit workers. Once the packing is removed on the following day, the main symptom is stuffiness and mouth breathing for up to a week. A return to non-manual work in 3–7 days will not harm the employee, but slightly longer times are usual, with around a week suggested by the RCS. Hard physical exercise may cause nosebleeds within the first 7–10 days, and a return to manual work can be expected in the second or third week. A delay of around 6 weeks would be expected before undertaking 'control and restraint' activities at work.

Wisdom teeth extraction

This is a common procedure in young employees and there is no need for long periods of recovery after extraction. The RCS suggests that most people can expect to return to non-manual work in 1–3 days and it is reasonable to wait a day or so longer before heavy physical activity. Although employees are unlikely to be harmed, attempting hard physical activity the day after surgery is unwise, particularly if a general anaesthetic has been used. A return to contact sports and work involving control and restraint is contraindicated for a week, a second week may be needed for inflammation and discomfort to settle.

Urological surgery

The most common urological procedures are cystoscopy and vasectomy, and prostate surgery in older men. Most patients will return to work the day after a cystoscopy. Many will return to non-manual work the day after a vasectomy, although 2 weeks may be required before heavy manual activity (see Table 11.4). Longer would be required after vasectomy reversal; a week is suggested before returning to non-manual work. Two weeks off would be reasonable after an orchidectomy, assuming this involves entering the abdomen to retrieve the testis. A faster return would be expected following scrotal surgery.

Prostatectomy

The main issue after prostatectomy is regaining urinary continence, rather than recovering from the surgery itself; this can be delayed after surgery via the transurethral route. Radical prostatectomy usually involves robotic surgery, with longer recovery times and up to 8 weeks before return to manual work.

Table 11.4 Suggested return to work times following urological surgery

Procedure	Sedentary admin	Sedentary light manual	Active light manual	Heavy manual	Physically demanding
Prostatectomy—transurethral	1–3 weeks			3–4 weeks	
Prostatectomy—retropubic, suprapubic, or perineal	2–4 weeks	2–4 weeks	2–4 weeks	4–8 weeks	4–8 weeks
Prostatectomy—radical	4–6 weeks	4–6 weeks	4–6 weeks	6–12 weeks	6–12 weeks
Renal lithotripsy	1–2 weeks	1–2 weeks	1–2 weeks	1–2 weeks	2 weeks
Vasectomy	1–7 days	1–7 days	1–7 days	2 weeks	2 weeks
Vasectomy reversal	1 week	1 week	1 week	2 weeks	2 weeks
Orchidectomy	2 weeks	2 weeks	2 weeks	2 weeks	2 weeks
Renal transplant	4–6 weeks	4–6 weeks	4–6 weeks	6–12 weeks	12 weeks[a]
Laparoscopic nephrectomy	2–4 weeks	2–4 weeks	2–4 weeks	4–6 weeks	6–12 weeks
Cystoscopy	0–1 day	0–1 day	0–1 day	0–1 day	0–1 day

[a] Ask surgeon for advice for contact sports and for control and restraint.

Renal surgery

Return to any work should be possible within 2 weeks following lithotripsy and within 6–8 weeks following renal transplant (see Table 11.4).

Breast surgery

Breast surgery is common, but the underlying reasons may have a major impact on an individual's ability and motivation to work. A return after a couple of days would be expected after a simple procedure, for example, non-manual work within 1 week after a benign lumpectomy and manual work after 2 weeks. Factors including the size of the scar, the amount of internal disruption, and the breast size will all affect discomfort and therefore return to work times (see Table 11.5).

Cosmetic breast surgery

The surrounding tissues need to settle and heal after breast enlargement surgery, and women will usually be advised to remain off work for 2 weeks and avoid significant arm or chest exercise, with no heavy lifting for 4 weeks after surgery. If the implant is placed under the muscle, up to 6 weeks may be needed before resuming full activities. Similar guidelines apply for breast reduction surgery.

Lumpectomy and mastectomy

Most breast surgery for malignancy will involve a wide local excision and sentinel node biopsy initially, and the RCS recommend a return to non-manual work in 2 weeks or to manual work in 6 weeks. There is little difference in tissue disruption or healing with wide local excision and axillary clearance as compared with mastectomy, so the RCS recommends the same timelines.

Surgery may be followed by radiotherapy and chemotherapy. Some women choose to continue working part-time during this period or between cycles of treatment. The main side effect of fatigue may not arise until towards the end of treatment, typically continuing for a month or two afterwards. Herceptin may cause significant flu-like symptoms, nausea, and diarrhoea within a day or two of the first few treatment cycles.

Gynaecological surgery

The RCOG website provides excellent patient information leaflets covering eight common procedures and sensible advice about expected timescales and activity during the recovery period. They emphasize the need to regain physical fitness and promote walking immediately after surgery. Traditionally, there has often been an expectation of much longer recovery periods of 3 or more months following gynaecological procedures and some websites continue to recommend prolonged periods of inactivity. This can be counterproductive and is only rarely necessary. Employers should be advised regarding this and encouraged to refer employees either preoperatively for advice and counselling or early following surgery where there is an expectation or risk of extended absence. Some guidelines on indicative return to work times are given in Table 11.5. Also see Chapter 8.

Table 11.5 Suggested return to work times in weeks following breast and gynaecological surgery

Procedure	Sedentary admin	Sedentary light manual	Active light manual	Heavy manual	Physically demanding
Benign lumpectomy	1–2 days	1–2 days	1 week	2 weeks	2 weeks
Breast cancer wide local excision and sentinel node biopsy	1–2 weeks	1–2 weeks	1–3 weeks	3–6 weeks	4–6 weeks
Breast cancer wide local excision or mastectomy and axillary clearance	2–3 weeks	2–3 weeks	3–6 weeks	6–12 weeks	12 weeks+
Breast cancer with radiotherapy and endocrine therapy	2–12 weeks	2–12 weeks	4–12 weeks	12 weeks+	12 weeks+
Breast cancer with chemotherapy, radiotherapy, endocrine therapy and Herceptin	2–39 weeks	2–39 weeks	26–39 weeks	26–52 weeks	26–52 weeks
Breast implant	2 weeks	2 weeks	4 weeks	6 weeks	6 weeks
Abdominal laparoscopy—minimal intervention	1–3 days	1–3 days	2–7 days	1–2 weeks	1–2 weeks
Myomectomy—laparoscopic	2–3 days	2–3 days	2–7 days	1–3 weeks	1–3 weeks
Endometrial ablation	1–2 days	1–2 days	2–5 days	2–5 days	2–5 days
Hysterectomy—abdominal	2–4 weeks	2–4 weeks	2–4 weeks	6–8 weeks	6–8 weeks
Hysterectomy—laparoscopic	2–4 weeks	2–4 weeks	2–4 weeks	4–6 weeks	4–6 weeks
Hysterectomy—vaginal	2–4 weeks	2–4 weeks	2–4 weeks	4–6 weeks	4–6 weeks
Mid-urethral sling	3–4 days	3–4 days	1–2 weeks	2–3 weeks	6 weeks
Miscarriage D&C	1–2 days	1–2 days	1–2 days	1–7 days	1–7 days
Pelvic floor repair	2–3 weeks	2–3 weeks	3–4 weeks	6–8 weeks	6–8 weeks

Laparoscopy

Gynaecological laparoscopy may be exploratory with little active surgery. Longer absence would be expected after procedures such as removal of an ovarian cyst.

Endometrial ablation

Some cramping abdominal pain may be experienced for 48 hours after endometrial ablation, but the RCOG recommends that most women can return to work within 2–5 days. It would be reasonable to limit manual handling within the first week.

Hysterectomy

There are three different approaches to hysterectomy, the classical abdominal route (now reserved for a large bulky uterus), or the less invasive laparoscopic/vaginal hysterectomy or vaginal hysterectomy for the smaller uterus. When discussing the potential risks, the RCOG working group acknowledged the lack of research evidence, but expressed a view on potential risk to internal structures if the patient attempts heavy lifting within the first 4 weeks after hysterectomy. Accordingly, a guide time of 2–4 weeks before returning to non-manual work was recommended for all three types of operation, with 4–6 weeks before returning to manual work for the less invasive procedures and 6–8 weeks before returning to manual work after abdominal hysterectomy. Many women get back to work well within this timescale. The main reason for delay in returning to work is obesity with wound infection. Provided the infection clears up within the first 2 weeks, little or no delay would be expected in returning to work.

Many women see hysterectomy as a life-changing procedure and this may be an opportunity to consider major lifestyle changes at the same time, including stopping smoking and doing more exercise. Motivational interviewing techniques[18] can be very useful when approaching these matters, using the RCOG leaflets and guidance on early walking as part of the approach.

Mid-urethral sling

Sling or tape support for the urethra was a common procedure for stress incontinence. However, this may only rarely be used in future. Pain may persist in the thighs for 2 weeks or more after a transobturator tape procedure and although women will not be harmed by working through this, some will not wish to do so.

Pelvic floor repair

Pelvic floor repairs may involve stitching or (now rarely) mesh support. Where mesh is used this may require access through the inner thighs for an anterior vaginal repair and through the buttocks for a posterior repair. Subsequent discomfort may prevent driving for at least 2 weeks, with a delay in returning to work related more to the discomfort than to any risks from working. Many women develop pelvic floor problems from a combination of obesity and major physical deconditioning. Both factors are likely to result in surgical complications and delay healing and recovery. Lifestyle change prior to surgery can mitigate this and in many cases, make surgery unnecessary.

Dilation and curettage

A dilation and curettage (D&C) is usually a straightforward day case procedure following which there is no physical need for delay in returning to work. The RCOG suggests 1–2 days for return to any work but the psychological issues surrounding a miscarriage may require further support and advice from OH if it results in extended absence.

Orthopaedic surgery

Many orthopaedic procedures are carried out on people of working age, often with widely varying recommendations about returning to work (Table 11.6). It is particularly

Table 11.6 Suggested return to work times in weeks following orthopaedic surgery

Procedure	Sedentary admin	Sedentary light manual	Active light manual	Heavy manual	Physically demanding
Discectomy via laminotomy or foraminotomy	1–2 weeks	2 weeks	2–4 weeks	4–6 weeks	6–12 weeks
Discectomy via laminectomy	4 weeks	4 weeks	6–8 weeks	6–12 weeks	12 weeks
Spinal decompression and fusion	6–12 weeks	8–12 weeks	12 weeks	3–6 months	6–12 months
Carpal tunnel release	1–2 weeks	2–4 weeks	2–4 weeks	6–10 weeks	6–10 weeks
Cubital tunnel release	1–7 days	1–7 days	1–7 days	1–4 weeks	4–6 weeks
De Quervain's release	1–2 weeks	2–4 weeks	2–4 weeks	6–10 weeks	6–10 weeks
Dupuytren's collagenase injection	1 week	1 week	1 week	2 weeks	2 weeks
Dupuytren's fasciectomy	2–3 weeks	3–4 weeks	3–4 weeks	8–12 weeks	8–12 weeks
Finger arthroplasty	4–6 weeks	6–8 weeks	6–8 weeks	12 weeks	12 weeks[a]
Fractured clavicle	2–6 weeks	2–6 weeks	6–10 weeks	10–12 weeks	12 weeks
Fractured finger	0–6 weeks[b]	0–6 weeks[b]	0–6 weeks[b]	12 weeks	12 weeks
Fractured radial head, uncomplicated	1–2 weeks	1–2 weeks	2–6 weeks	6–12 weeks	12 weeks
Fractured scaphoid open reduction and fixation	4–6 weeks	4–6 weeks	8–12 weeks	After union	After union
Fractured wrist non-dominant	1 week	1 week	8–10 weeks	12 weeks	12 weeks
Fractured wrist dominant, assuming hand is required for writing, mouse use, etc.	8–10 weeks	8–10 weeks	8–10 weeks	12 weeks	12 weeks
Finger fusion	1–6 weeks[b]	1–6 weeks[b]	1–6 weeks[b]	12 weeks	12 weeks
Ganglion surgery	3–7 days	1 week	1–2 weeks	4–6 weeks	4–8 weeks
Hand tendon repair (assuming some manual activity such as writing, mouse use etc.)	6–8 weeks	8 weeks	8–10 weeks	12 weeks	12 weeks
Metacarpophalangeal joint arthroplasty	4 weeks	4–8 weeks	4–8 weeks	12 weeks[c]	Unlikely
Pisiformectomy	2–3 weeks	3–4 weeks	3–4 weeks	6–12 weeks	8–12 weeks

Table 11.6 Continued

Procedure	Sedentary admin	Sedentary light manual	Active light manual	Heavy manual	Physically demanding
Scaphoid non-union bone graft and open reduction and internal fixation[d]	6 weeks	6–12 weeks	6–12 weeks	12 weeks+	12 weeks+
Scapholunate ligament reconstruction	6 weeks	6 weeks	8–12 weeks	12 weeks	12–26 weeks
Shoulder arthroscopy (no additional procedures)	3–7 days	3–7 days	3–7 days	1–2 weeks	1–2 weeks
Shoulder subacromial decompression	1–3 weeks	2–6 weeks	4–8 weeks	6–12 weeks	6–12 weeks
Shoulder subacromial decompression with debridement	4–6 weeks	4–6 weeks	6–8 weeks	8–12 weeks	8–12 weeks
Shoulder rotator cuff repair	2–12 weeks	4–12 weeks	12 weeks	3–6 months	6–9 months
Shoulder biceps tendonotomy[e]	1–2 weeks	1–2 weeks	4–8 weeks	6–12 weeks	6–12 weeks
Shoulder acromioclavicular joint excision[f]	1–3 weeks	3–6 weeks	3–12 weeks	12 weeks	12–26 weeks
Tennis elbow surgery	1–2 weeks	1–4 weeks	2–6 weeks	6–26 weeks	12–26 weeks
Trapeziectomy[d]	4–6 weeks	4–6 weeks	6–8 weeks	12–26 weeks	12–26 weeks
Trapeziometacarpal fusion[d]	6 weeks	6 weeks	6–8 weeks	12–26 weeks	12–26 weeks
Trigger finger surgery	1–3 days	1–3 days	3–5 days	2–4 weeks	4 weeks
Ulnar head excision[d]	2 weeks	2 weeks	4–6 weeks	12–26 weeks	12–26 weeks
Ulnar osteotomy[d]	6 weeks	6 weeks	6 weeks	12–16 weeks	12–16 weeks
Wrist arthroscopy (no additional procedures)	1–3 days	1–3 days	3–7 days	7 days+	7 days+
Wrist fusion	6–10 weeks	6–10 weeks	10–12 weeks	12–16 weeks	Unlikely
Total hip replacement	2–8 weeks	4–8 weeks	6–8 weeks	12–16 weeks	12 weeks+
Hip arthroscopy for femoroacetabular impingement	1–2 weeks	1–2 weeks	1–2 weeks	6 weeks	12–26 weeks
Knee arthroscopy	2–14 days	2–14 days	2–4 weeks	2–4 weeks	2–4 weeks
Knee arthroscopic meniscectomy	1–2 weeks	1–2 weeks	2–4 weeks	2–6 weeks	4–6 weeks

(continued)

Table 11.6 Continued

Procedure	Sedentary admin	Sedentary light manual	Active light manual	Heavy manual	Physically demanding
Knee arthroscopic cartilage regeneration	2–4 weeks	2–4 weeks	12 weeks +	12–26 weeks	26 weeks[g]
Knee anterior cruciate ligament reconstruction	2–4 weeks	2–4 weeks	3–6 months	3–9 months	6–12 months
Total knee replacement	4–6 weeks	4–6 weeks	6–8 weeks	12–26 weeks[g]	26 weeks[g]
Achilles tendon repair	2–4 weeks	2–4 weeks	12 weeks	26 weeks	26 weeks+
Bunionectomy—distal osteotomy	2 weeks	2 weeks	2–6 weeks	8–12 weeks	12 weeks+
Bunionectomy— proximal osteotomy	2–6 weeks	2–6 weeks	6–8 weeks	12 weeks+	12 weeks+
First metatarsophalangeal joint fusion	2–4 weeks	2–4 weeks	6–12 weeks	12–24 weeks	12–24 weeks
Other toe fusion	Up to 2 weeks	Up to 2 weeks	1–4 weeks	4–6 weeks	6 weeks+
Cheilectomy	1–2 weeks	1–2 weeks	2–6 weeks	6–12 weeks	12 weeks
Ingrowing toenail removal of nailbed	2 days	2 days	1–2 weeks	2 weeks	2 weeks
Lower limb amputation	6–12 weeks	6–12 weeks	12–26 weeks	26 weeks	26 weeks+

[a] Return to physically demanding work may not be possible.

[b] Depending on which finger.

[c] Return to heavy and physically demanding work unlikely unless the remainder of the hand is functioning normally.

[d] For dominant hand use.

[e] Long head of biceps is cut to release worn tendon, may create 'Popeye' appearance. No requirement for immobilization.

[f] May be safe to drive after 1 week, work above shoulder height after 3 weeks, sustained overhead activities after 3 months, breast stroke as soon as comfortable, front crawl after 3 months.

[g] Unlikely to return

important to identify those where there is a substantial risk of harm if the person returns too soon to active work, particularly heavy manual handling. On the other hand, many individuals can return on crutches or with a sling to sedentary administrative work within a week or two of surgery without adverse effects. As noted earlier, it is important to find out exactly what procedure was undertaken and as with any other condition, motivation is an important influence on timescales to return to work.

Preoperative rehabilitation, 'prehabilitation', providing physiotherapy prior to surgery, may slightly improve early postoperative pain and function, but a systematic review found the effects were too small and short term to be considered clinically important.[19] Particular issues in relation to return to work are outlined below. Also see Chapter 22.

Shoulder surgery

The most common shoulder procedure is arthroscopic subacromial decompression. Patients may return to non-manual work within a week if this only involves debridement of the acromion, but where the bursa is debrided, the discomfort usually prevents significant use of the arm for 4–6 weeks (although the patient won't be harmed by working at any stage after surgery).

Rotator cuff repairs often involve completely severing and reattaching the tendon using staples, so the patient must keep the arm immobilized for at least 3 weeks and care needs to be taken using the arm for the first 6 weeks. The tendon is often significantly damaged by prolonged wear and tear, with a compromised vascular supply and extensive scarring and this can delay healing by several months. A return to non-manual duties may be accommodated with the arm in a sling. Many patients can use a keyboard and mouse with the sling in place after 2 weeks, but a return to manual work may take substantially longer (3–6 months).

Patients may have had substantial discomfort and limited use of the arm for a year or more prior to surgery, with significant psychological impact and deconditioning. Recovery can be prolonged where lack of engagement with rehabilitation leads to stiffness with a need for manipulation under anaesthetic, or where loss of muscle bulk from deconditioning results in a prolonged period before regaining full use of the arm.

Wrist surgery

Carpal tunnel release is usually a simple procedure with minimal damage to surrounding structures. There is no need to delay a return to work as the patient is unlikely to be harmed and some people return within a few days. It may be sensible to discourage heavy manual work for a week or two while the wrist heals. Around 1–3 weeks is recommended,[3] although the RCS suggests longer return to work times.

Total hip replacement

Better surgical technique is now allowing much earlier mobilization and weight bearing after hip replacement, with patients walking out of hospital after 3 or 4 days on a cemented prosthesis with only two sticks for support. Cementless prostheses require a period of partial weight bearing, often 6 weeks, to allow bone ingrowth.

There is a significant risk of posterior dislocation within the first 6 weeks of surgery, particularly following a posterior approach, and patients may be advised to take care to avoid flexing beyond 90 degrees and rotating more than 45 degrees internally or externally. This advice does, however, affect recovery time. In one randomized study, patients who were given no advice to restrict activity early in the recovery period returned to work after an average of 6.5 weeks as compared with 9.5 weeks in those advised to restrict activity.[20]

There seems to be little evidence against early return to work, with early activity seeming beneficial, and a review found that where surgeons gave advice, this tended to delay both recovery and return to work without apparent benefit.[21]

There is little evidence for and against particular work activities after hip replacement, but there is good guidance from the 1999 American Hip Society Survey[22] on return to sport. Activities such as stationary cycling, doubles tennis, and swimming are recommended or allowed. Canoeing and horse riding are allowed with experience. But jogging, squash, and football are not recommended. Climbing ladders should be safe after 6 weeks.

Knee surgery

Arthroscopy does not disrupt the knee significantly so many patients can return to work within 2–3 days of surgery, although prolonged sitting may be uncomfortable in the early stages and lead to stiffness. The RCS suggests an average of 10–14 days before returning to non-manual work and 2–6 weeks for manual work after arthroscopic partial meniscectomy, although many patients return sooner. Some develop chronic pain that may persist for months, although work during this period is unlikely to cause harm. Where the problem is altered central pain sensitivity, early activity will speed recovery.

Recovery times after total knee replacement can be very variable, often related more to weight and fitness rather than to the surgery itself. Some patients cope with part-time sedentary work after a couple of weeks. The most common longer-term problem is stiffness and reduced flexion, and encouraging an early return to work may help regain flexion with a better long-term outcome.

Advice on returning to heavy manual handling, sporting activities (see American Hip Society Survey[22] in 'Total hip replacement'), or control and restraint duties, after total knee replacement varies substantially. There is no clear evidence for or against. The main issue preventing control and restraint is limited flexion, which in turn prevents kneeling or squatting. There is no absolute contraindication to resuming work as a prison officer or police officer after total knee replacement, but many will either be unable to cope with the fitness test and control and restraint or will choose an alternative career.

Risk of deep vein thrombosis after joint replacement surgery

After hip and knee replacement, flying carries a substantially increased risk of deep vein thrombosis. Employees should avoid all flying until around 6 weeks after surgery and avoid flights exceeding 3 hours until 12 weeks after surgery.

Foot surgery

After bunion surgery, a return to sedentary work can be expected within a couple of weeks, and where the extent of surgery is limited, early mobilization is encouraged, with a return to manual work in around 6 weeks. If non-weight bearing is recommended for the first few weeks, a return to manual work will not be feasible until around 12 weeks. A study of emergency brake response time after first metatarsal osteotomy found that 25% of patients were fit to drive at 2 weeks and all were safe after 6 weeks.[23]

After Achilles tendon rupture, return to work times are little influenced by whether the tendon is repaired surgically or treated conservatively. The patient may be able to cope with non-manual work within a few weeks while wearing a support boot, with some mobility after 3 months but no significant manual work until 6 months after rupture.

Spinal surgery

Return to work after orthopaedic operations on the spine is covered in Chapter 21.

Neurosurgery

Patients may be safe to return to work within a week or two of craniotomy; however, their overall ability to work will depend greatly on the underlying pathology, the procedure undertaken, and nature of work. Any skull defect will represent vulnerability particularly for those involved in control and restraint, or where even minor head trauma (e.g. from working in a confined space) may be likely. There may be an increased risk of epilepsy, poor concentration or communication, loss of dexterity, or sensory change. All must be taken into account when advising on return to work times and adjustments at work. Long delays in returning to work are not usually needed; a study of suboccipital decompression for Chiari malformation showed return to work times of 4–12 weeks, median 6 weeks, with 76% returning to work.[24]

Complex regional pain syndrome

Around 7% of patients will develop complex regional pain syndrome (CRPS) following trauma or surgery, particularly to a limb. There is a substantial body of research around this subject. Although a peripheral trigger may be present, a significant part of the problem is central pain sensitization, which may result from pain-avoidance behaviour, catastrophization, and hypervigilance. The natural history of CRPS suggests that it may be very common in the acute form, but resolves (undiagnosed) within a few months in most patients. One study showed that 26 of 30 patients with post-traumatic CRPS recovered fully without intervention over an average of 13 months. Recovery from well-established CRPS is less common, with around 30% of patients recovering fully in 6 years.[25]

Poor recovery rates may reflect poor recognition and understanding, along with limited access to evidence-based treatment. The National Centre for CRPS at the Royal National Hospital for Rheumatic Diseases in Bath leads in research and treatment, with great success from treatments including mirror visual feedback, sensory re-education, and graded motor imagery as well as the more traditional cognitive behavioural approach combined with medication and physiotherapy. OH professionals can play a significant role in identifying patients who may be developing CRPS, and encouraging graded activity in a controlled environment to avoid chronicity.

Returning to work after critical care treatment

The term 'critical care' encompasses care on intensive care units (ICUs), intensive therapy units, and high-dependency care. Many patients are admitted to critical care as a precaution after injury or surgery for a period of enhanced care, observation, and invasive monitoring before discharge to a general ward after 1–2 days. The time in critical care does not therefore reflect any complications in treatment or a severe underlying pathology. Extended periods of time in critical care with organ system support (e.g. ventilation, haemofiltration, and inotropes) are required for serious illness or serious complications of treatment. Recovery is affected both by the underlying pathology and by a period of complete inactivity, often promoted by a combination of sedatives, analgesics, and physical constraints. Psychological issues are common (see 'Psychological effects') and social issues often impact immediate family, with loss of income, and potential future changes in lifestyle. Prolonged periods of critical care are often associated with widespread vascular and metabolic problems resulting from sepsis, shock, or systemic inflammatory response leading to organ hypoxia and organ failure. Damage may be permanent, or recovery may be very slow, leaving the patient very weak and fatigued. Post-intensive care syndrome (PICS) is the term now used to describe new or worsening problems in physical, cognitive, or mental health status arising after a critical illness and persisting beyond acute care hospitalization.[26] While the term PICS has now been adopted and recognized as a major issue, research into early rehabilitation interventions and the long-term management of PICS is still awaited.[27,28] This may be an evolving topic that substantially impacts primary care and OH, as many patients needing support will have left hospital and may be looking to rehabilitate back to work without secondary care support.

The National Institute for Health and Clinical Excellence has developed a guideline for rehabilitation after critical illness,[29] which emphasizes the importance of identifying patients at risk and starting rehabilitation early within a structured programme involving frequent follow-up. As a result, patients can expect to be referred to follow-up clinics for critical care rehabilitation, which may include a self-directed rehabilitation manual.[30]

Physical effects

A prolonged period of complete inactivity may lead to massive loss of muscle bulk and strength through a combination of atrophy and catabolism. A patient may leave hospital with functioning organs but so little strength that they struggle to walk more than a few steps and cannot cope with stairs. Loss of bone mass may also be seen.[31]

Some groups of employees are at risk of complete inactivity in non-medical settings, including astronauts,[32] submariners, and special forces personnel.[33,34] While only a small number of OH professionals will be involved directly in these groups, the principles of prolonged inactivity can apply widely to patients recovering from prolonged ill health (including chronic fatigue and/or chronic pain) or trauma, or just those who have lived very sedentary lives for a prolonged period. Research has included the process and timeline of deconditioning, and guidelines for minimizing or avoiding significant morbidity. Where an employee can exercise while recovering they may be able to substantially reduce the impact of long-term deconditioning and return to useful employment much sooner. OH professionals need to be able to assess activity levels and advise on appropriate simple exercise routines and nutrition.

Deconditioning

Deconditioning occurs independent of disease and healthy subjects who are confined to bed or become inactive show the same deconditioning effects as those who become inactive because of disease or injury.[35] Studies show changes in cardiovascular response including changes in blood volume, blood physiology, and heart function, loss of muscle volume and changes in muscle physiology, loss of bone strength, thermoregulatory changes, neuroendocrine changes, and immune response changes.

The initial loss of aerobic capacity is rapid and occurs in parallel with loss of plasma volume. Just 3 days of bed rest can have substantial effects, with endurance athletes showing a decrease of 17% in VO_{2peak} and sedentary individuals showing a 10% decrease.[36] Thereafter, the reduction in aerobic capacity is slower and is influenced by both central and peripheral adaptation. Cardiovascular changes, both central and peripheral, are all significant over the first 4 weeks including a 20% reduction in ventricular mass.[37] A 20% decrease in muscle strength was noted in 5 weeks.[38] This loss of force is mostly explained by muscle atrophy and decrease in myosin content which can be fully restored after resistance training.[39] Recovery rates follow similar timelines, although there is little specific objective evidence to determine expected time from baseline to pre-illness/injury levels. Military experience shows that it takes on average 5 weeks of exercise-specific training for a recruit to recover from a stress fracture and return to military training.[40]

The deconditioning effects of bedrest can be countered by regular exercise. A number of studies ranging from 2 to 8 weeks of bed rest have shown consistently that exercise such as supine cycling or use of a rowing ergometer can preserve cardiac function.[41,42] Exercise does not have to be daily, but at least 3 days per week of intense exercise (interval style, and near maximal) with orthostatic stress.[36] The use of these protocols for long-duration international space station flights has demonstrated considerable success, with an initial decrease in VO_{2peak} after 5 days recovering to preflight levels by day 30.[43]

General problems experienced after critical care

Besides the physiological deconditioning from immobility, critical care patients also experience problems from joint immobility, nerve damage both central and peripheral, and muscle contractures from vascular compromise.

Two months after discharge from an ICU, almost half of survivors still cannot manage stairs or have difficulty climbing more than a few steps, and one-third are still using a wheelchair outside the house.[44] Fatigue may persist, with 63% of men and 60% of women reporting fatigue at 3 months and 32% of men and 38% of women reporting fatigue at 1 year.[45] Acute axonal neuropathy related to sepsis may play a part in muscle atrophy, and can lead to permanent muscle weakness with quadriplegia.[46]

Neurophysiological tests should help distinguish those with myopathy, who may recover strength, from those with severe neuropathy, who have a poor prognosis. Immobility and associated vascular compromise may lead to muscle contractures particularly affecting the ankles, fingers, and neck. Neck and shoulder pain are other recognized problems associated with prolonged periods of ventilation in the prone position. Joint immobility affects 5–10% of patients, and immobility of the large joints, weakness, and fatigue, are common reasons for failing to return to work.[47]

Respiratory effects

Acute lung injury may be associated with widespread inflammation, leading to acute respiratory distress syndrome (ARDS). As the inflammatory process resolves, there may be permanent residual fibrotic changes. In the long term, the restrictive pattern seen on lung function testing is usually mild, and spirometric values are usually within 80% of normal by 6 months. Persistent breathlessness is usually muscular in origin, rather than pulmonary. Only a small proportion of patients will have long-term lung injury and some may require domiciliary supplemental oxygen. Tracheostomy may lead to long-term tracheal stenosis in 2–5% of surviving patients, but tracheal compromise can usually be corrected surgically.

Psychological effects

The trauma of severe illness or injury commonly leads to post-traumatic stress disorder (PTSD) and associated psychiatric morbidities; the incidence of PTSD in patients following ARDS was 27%.[48] Younger patients seem more vulnerable, possibly because they metabolize or clear sedative drugs more rapidly and have a better memory of distressing events during their illness. Prolonged treatment and the slow recovery may cause affective disorders, half of survivors having clinically significant anxiety and depression.[49] Physical damage to the brain, either from trauma or oxygen deficit, may lead to cognitive impairment, a common sequel to sepsis-related encephalopathy.[50] A year after hospital discharge, three-quarters of survivors of ARDS have impaired memory, attention, concentration, and processing speed, and a quarter still have mild cognitive impairment 6 years later. Side effects of opiates, sedatives, and other medications, lack of sleep, and circadian disruption can also be problematic. Substantial weight loss and the effects of trauma may affect appearance, alopecia being surprisingly common (seen in 47% of women and 8% of men, although it normally resolves by 6 months).

Returning to work

A review by the Intensive Care National Audit and Research Council (ICNARC) found that of those who had been working prior to ICU admission, 42% were still absent 6 months later, most (79%) for health reasons. Of those who had returned to work, 23% stated that their health was affecting their work. An Australian study found that only half of patients admitted to ICU for more than 48 hours had returned to work at 6-month follow-up.[51] Any patient who has spent more than 48 hours on ICU may develop the complications outlined above. OH professionals need to be alert to this, to check for sequelae and be prepared to recommend prolonged and comprehensive rehabilitation programmes as necessary, liaising with treating physicians to ensure that all parties are working in concert to rebuild the patient's confidence and achieve fitness to return to work.

Key points

- Recovery times after surgery are poorly understood with little evidence base and most clinicians recommend longer times than necessary.
- Delayed return can be as harmful as returning too early.
- Advice on returning to work after surgery should be based on knowledge of tissue healing processes, along with adverse effects of smoking and obesity, perioperative infection, and co-morbidity.
- Significant periods of critical care substantially delay recovery and often include significant psychological sequelae.
- Prolonged rest for any reason leads to substantial physical deconditioning. Early rehabilitation will also reduce deconditioning effects.

Useful websites

DVLA	http://www.gov.uk/government/publications/assessing-fitness-to-drive-a-guide-for-medical-professionals
Royal College of Surgeons	http://www.rcseng.ac.uk/patient-care/recovering-from-surgery
Royal College of Obstetricians and Gynaecologists	https://www.rcog.org.uk/en/patients/patient-leaflets/
Working Fit	http://www.workingfit.com
MDGuidelines. Subscription service with return to work times based on industry experience	http://www.mdguidelines.com
Colostomy Association	http://www.colostomyuk.org/

References

1. **Majeed AW, Brown S, Williams N, Hannay DR, Johnson AG.** Variations in medical attitudes to postoperative recovery period. *BMJ* 1995;**311**:296.
2. **Carragee EJ, Han MY, Yang B, Kim DH, Kraemer H, Billys J.** Activity restrictions after posterior lumbar discectomy. A prospective study of outcomes in 152 cases with no postoperative restrictions. *Spine* 1999;**24**:2346–51.
3. **Ratzon N, Schejter-Margalit T, Froom P.** Time to return to work and surgeons' recommendations after carpal tunnel release. *Occup Med (Lond)* 2006;**56**:46–50.
4. **Khanna S, Biswas S, Shang Y, et al.** Macrophage dysfunction impairs resolution of inflammation in the wounds of diabetic mice. *PLoS One* 2010;**5**:e9539.
5. **Marti A, Marcos A, Martinez JA.** Obesity and immune function relationships. *Obes Rev* 2001;**2**:131–40.

6. **Nickel BT, Klement MR, Penrose CT, Green CL, Seyler TM, Bolognesi MP.** Lingering risk: bariatric surgery before total knee arthroplasty. *J Arthroplasty* 2016;**31**(9 Suppl):207–11.

7. **Siana JE, Rex S, Gottrup F.** The effect of cigarette smoking on wound healing. *Scand J Plast Reconstr Surg Hand Surg* 1989;**23**:207–9.

8. **Kuri M, Nakagawa M, Tanaka H, Hasuo S, Kishi Y.** Determination of the duration of preoperative smoking cessation to improve wound healing after head and neck surgery. *Anesthesiology* 2005;**102**:892–6.

9. **Sorensen LT, Hemmingsen UB, Kirkeby LT, Kallehave F, Jorgensen LN.** Smoking is a risk factor for incisional hernia. *Arch Surg* 2005;**140**:119–23.

10. **Sloan A, Hussain I, Maqsood M, Eremin O, El-Sheemy M.** The effects of smoking on fracture healing. *Surgeon* 2010;**8**:111–6.

11. **Brown CW, Orme TJ, Richardson HD.** The rate of pseudarthrosis (surgical nonunion) in patients who are smokers and patients who are nonsmokers: a comparison study. *Spine* 1986;**11**:942–3.

12. **Holt DR, Kirk SJ, Regan MC, Hurson M, Lindblad WJ, Barbul A.** Effect of age on wound healing in healthy human beings. *Surgery* 1992;**112**:293–7.

13. **Toogood PA, Abdel MP, Spear JA, Cook SM, Cook DJ, Taunton MJ.** The monitoring of activity at home after total hip arthroplasty. *Bone Joint J* 2016;**98B**:1450–4.

14. **Henle P, Bieri KS, Brand M, et al.** Patient and surgical characteristics that affect revision risk in dynamic intraligamentary stabilization of the anterior cruciate ligament. *Knee Surg Sports Traumatol Arthrosc* 2018;**26**:1182–9.

15. **Stoker DL, Spiegelhalter DJ, Singh R, Wellwood JM.** Laparoscopic versus open inguinal hernia repair: randomised prospective trial. *Lancet* 1994;**343**:1243–5.

16. **Amid PK, Shulman AG, Lichtenstein IL.** Critical scrutiny of the open 'tension-free' hernioplasty. *Am J Surg* 1993;**165**:369–71.

17. **Shulman AG, Amid PK, Lichtenstein IL.** The safety of mesh repair for primary inguinal hernias: results of 3,019 operations from five diverse surgical sources. *Am Surg* 1992;**58**:255–7.

18. **Miller WR, Rollnick S.** *Motivational Interviewing: Preparing People for Change.* New York: Guilford Press; 2002.

19. **Wang L, Lee M, Zhang Z, Moodie J, Cheng D, Martin J.** Does preoperative rehabilitation for patients planning to undergo joint replacement surgery improve outcomes? A systematic review and meta-analysis of randomised controlled trials. *BMJ Open* 2016;**6**:e009857.

20. **Peak EL, Parvizi J, Ciminiello M, et al.** The role of patient restrictions in reducing the prevalence of early dislocation following total hip arthroplasty. A randomized, prospective study. *J Bone Joint Surg Am* 2005;**87**:247–53.

21. **Kuijer PP, de Beer MJ, Houdijk JH, Frings-Dresen MH.** Beneficial and limiting factors affecting return to work after total knee and hip arthroplasty: a systematic review. *J Occup Rehabil* 2009;**19**:375–81.

22. **Golant A, Christoforou DC, Slover JD, Zuckerman JD.** Athletic participation after hip and knee arthroplasty. *Bull NYU Hosp Jt Dis* 2010;**68**:76–83.

23. **Holt G, Kay M, McGrory R, Kumar CS.** Emergency brake response time after first metatarsal osteotomy. *J Bone Joint Surg Am* 2008;**90**:1660–4.

24. **Parker SL, Godil SS, Zuckerman SL, et al.** Comprehensive assessment of 1-year outcomes and determination of minimum clinically important difference in pain, disability, and quality of life after suboccipital decompression for Chiari malformation I in adults. *Neurosurgery* 2013;**73**:569–81.

25. **Bruehl S.** Complex regional pain syndrome. *BMJ* 2015;**351**:h2730.

26. **Needham DM, Davidson J, Cohen H, et al.** Improving long-term outcomes after discharge from intensive care unit: report from a stakeholders' conference. *Crit Care Med* 2012;**40**:502–9.

27. **Kondo Y, Fuke R, Hifumi T, et al.** Early rehabilitation for the prevention of postintensive care syndrome in critically ill patients: a study protocol for a systematic review and meta-analysis. *BMJ Open* 2017;7:e013828.

28. **Ohtake PJ, Coffey Scott J, Hinman RS, Lee AC, Smith JM.** Impairments, activity limitations and participation restrictions experienced in the first year following a critical illness: protocol for a systematic review. *BMJ Open* 2017;7:e013847.

29. **National Institute for Health and Care Excellence.** *Rehabilitation after Critical Illness.* London: National Institute of Health and Clinical Excellence; 2009.

30. **Jones C, Skirrow P, Griffiths RD, et al.** Rehabilitation after critical illness: a randomized, controlled trial. *Crit Care Med* 2003;31:2456–61.

31. **Ferrando AA, Lane HW, Stuart CA, Davis-Street J, Wolfe RR.** Prolonged bed rest decreases skeletal muscle and whole body protein synthesis. *Am J Physiol* 1996;270:E627–33.

32. **Convertino VA, Bloomfield SA, Greenleaf JE.** An overview of the issues: physiological effects of bed rest and restricted physical activity. *Med Sci Sports Exerc* 1997;29:187–90.

33. **Fothergill DM, Sims JR.** Aerobic performance of Special Operations Forces personnel after a prolonged submarine deployment. *Ergonomics* 2000;43:1489–500.

34. **Luria T, Matsliah Y, Adir Y, et al.** Effects of a prolonged submersion on bone strength and metabolism in young healthy submariners. *Calcif Tissue Int* 2010;86:8–13.

35. **Smorawinski J, Nazar K, Kaciuba-Uscilko H, et al.** Effects of 3-day bed rest on physiological responses to graded exercise in athletes and sedentary men. *J Appl Physiol (1985)* 2001;91:249–57.

36. **Lee SM, Moore AD, Everett ME, Stenger MB, Platts SH.** Aerobic exercise deconditioning and countermeasures during bed rest. *Aviat Space Environ Med* 2010;81:52–63.

37. **Martin WH, 3rd, Coyle EF, Bloomfield SA, Ehsani AA.** Effects of physical deconditioning after intense endurance training on left ventricular dimensions and stroke volume. *J Am Coll Cardiol* 1986;7:982–9.

38. **Berg HE, Eiken O, Miklavcic L, Mekjavic IB.** Hip, thigh and calf muscle atrophy and bone loss after 5-week bedrest inactivity. *Eur J Appl Physiol* 2007;99:283–9.

39. **Campbell EL, Seynnes OR, Bottinelli R, et al.** Skeletal muscle adaptations to physical inactivity and subsequent retraining in young men. *Biogerontology* 2013;14:247–59.

40. **Wood AM, Hales R, Keenan A, et al.** Incidence and time to return to training for stress fractures during military basic training. *J Sports Med (Hindawi Publ Corp)* 2014;2014:282980.

41. **Shibata S, Perhonen M, Levine BD.** Supine cycling plus volume loading prevent cardiovascular deconditioning during bed rest. *J Appl Physiol (1985)* 2010;108:1177–86.

42. **Hastings JL, Krainski F, Snell PG, et al.** Effect of rowing ergometry and oral volume loading on cardiovascular structure and function during bed rest. *J Appl Physiol (1985)* 2012;112:1735–43.

43. **Moore AD, Lynn PA, Feiveson AH.** The first 10 years of aerobic exercise responses to long-duration ISS flights. *Aerosp Med Hum Perform* 2015;86(12 Suppl):A78–86.

44. **Jones C, Griffiths RD.** Identifying post intensive care patients who may need physical rehabilitation. *Clin Intens Care* 2000;11:35–8.

45. **Eddleston JM, White P, Guthrie E.** Survival, morbidity, and quality of life after discharge from intensive care. *Crit Care Med* 2000;28:2293–9.

46. **de Seze M, Petit H, Wiart L, et al.** Critical illness polyneuropathy. A 2-year follow-up study in 19 severe cases. *Eur Neurol* 2000;43:61–9.

47. **Herridge MS, Cheung AM, Tansey CM, et al.** One-year outcomes in survivors of the acute respiratory distress syndrome. *N Engl J Med* 2003;348:683–93.

48. **Stoll C, Schelling G, Goetz AE, et al.** Health-related quality of life and post-traumatic stress disorder in patients after cardiac surgery and intensive care treatment. *J Thorac Cardiovasc Surg* 2000;120:505–12.

49. **Scragg P, Jones A, Fauvel N.** Psychological problems following ICU treatment. *Anaesthesia* 2001;**56**:9–14.
50. **Gordon SM, Jackson JC, Ely EW, Burger C, Hopkins RO.** Clinical identification of cognitive impairment in ICU survivors: insights for intensivists. *Intens Care Med* 2004;**30**:1997–2008.
51. **Dennis DM, Hebden-Todd TK, Marsh LJ, Cipriano LJ, Parsons RW.** How do Australian ICU survivors fare functionally 6 months after admission? *Crit Care Resusc* 2011;**13**:9–16.

Chapter 12

Ill health retirement

Jon Poole and Glyn Evans

Introduction

This chapter gives advice to doctors who provide reports for pension schemes about the merits of a patient's application for ill health retirement (IHR). This is a challenging area of practice in which the structure and wording of the report is important if difficulties are to be reduced. An overview of pension provision in the UK is included as well as advice contained in determinations by the Pensions Ombudsman. Rates of IHR for national schemes are shown against which doctors should audit their practice. In general, a retiree's perceived health status tends to improve after retirement, although the improvement will attenuate over time. Heavy manual workers are more likely to retire on the grounds of ill health than non-manual workers, which has been attributed to their poorer health and less favourable working conditions.

The chapter advises on how to prepare a report for an occupational pension scheme, and gives examples of common difficulties and ways these can be avoided. Problems for the doctor can be minimized by approaching cases in a consistent way. A standard structure for a report should be used which makes reference to the regulations or pension scheme rules, the job, and the evidence that has been reviewed. It is advised that doctors are transparent about inferences they make and about the existence of any differing medical opinions. The role of the doctor is to examine the patient, gather the relevant medical information, weigh the evidence, write a report, and where necessary complete a certificate for the scheme's administrators or trustees, who will make the decision as to whether the applicant has, on a balance of probability, met the eligibility criteria.

Demographics

In the UK, the number of people of pensionable age has been rising as life expectancy has increased and fecundity has fallen. The number of workers to the number of retirees, which is known as the support ratio, is falling in most developed counties. In the UK, the crude ratio was 4.3 in the 1970s, but fell to 3.6 in 2010 and is expected to fall to 3.0 in 2025. Pension schemes are addressing the problem of a falling support ratio by increasing the retirement age, increasing contribution rates, and moving from 'defined benefit' to 'defined contribution' schemes.

During the 1980s, early retirement due to ill health rapidly increased, with rates of 10–25/1000 contributing members in several public sector schemes.[1] The reason for this high rate of retirement is unknown, but was probably influenced by changes to working practices and some employers' desire to use the pension scheme for workforce management. Currently, only a small proportion of people work after the age of 65, but this is likely to increase with the removal of default retirement ages, changes to the normal pensionable age, relaxation of tax rules on the receipt of pension benefits while continuing to work, and lifting of the maximum number of pensionable years of service.

Wide variations in rates of early retirement have been reported between employers and even within different parts of the same organization.[1] While some variation is to be expected, such as a higher rate in jobs that require high levels of physical fitness, or in an older workforce, most variation is inexplicable on medical grounds alone. For example, a concurrence of modes of IHR with an enhancement in benefits can only be explained by the influence of non-medical factors on decisions to retire. There is no medical reason why increases of ill health (mainly in the form of minor psychiatric and musculoskeletal disorders) should occur at these times. It is reasonable to assume that other reasons, such as lack of motivation to remain with a particular employer and an exaggerated declaration of incapability, have been contributory factors.

In general, rates of retirement due to ill health, rather like sickness absence, are higher in the public than the private sector. The reasons are likely to be multifactorial, but probably include a sharper focus by the latter on performance and attendance, with greater readiness to dismiss on incapability grounds. However, in response to the Treasury's review of IHR in the public sector,[2] pension schemes have tightened up their processes and eligibility criteria for granting early pensions. Occupational physicians are now more likely to be involved in the decision-making process and conflicts of interest for other doctors have been reduced. Rates of IHR have fallen. For example, the Home Office estimated that it saved £42 million in pension payments to firemen between 2005 and 2010 (personal communication).

But is retirement good for your health? Early studies suggested that retirement led to a doubling of the risk of myocardial infarction,[3] but mental health was likely to improve, particularly for those with high socioeconomic status.[4] More recent longitudinal studies, which have controlled better for health selection effects prior to retirement, have shown that mortality after retirement depends on the health of the retiree and not on early retirement per se.[5,6] For most people, retirement makes no difference to their health, although some will feel better. Longitudinal analysis has shown that perceived health status tends to improve after retirement, although the improvement will attenuate over time.[7] Self-perceived health, higher employment grade, and job dissatisfaction have been shown to be independent predictors of early retirement[8] with heavy manual workers having twice the risk of IHR as upper-grade non-manual workers. This has been attributed to poorer health and inferior working conditions for the manual workers.[9]

Types of pension schemes

State pensions

The state scheme in the UK is two tiered, consisting of a basic pension and an additional state pension known as the State Second Pension (previously SERPS). Individuals may opt out of this additional scheme in favour of an occupational, stakeholder, or personal pension. It is funded directly from National Insurance contributions from both the employer and the employee. The state pension will be payable to both men and women from age 65 in 2018. The pensionable age for both sexes will then move to 66 in 2020 and to 68 in 2046. The state pension cannot be taken early (other than for bereaved spouses), but can be deferred until age 70, with a 1% increase for every 5 weeks of deferment.

Occupational and personal pensions

Occupational pension schemes in the UK have traditionally been offered by the larger and longer established employers. Since 2012, employers have been required to enrol their workers into 'qualifying pension schemes' to which both the employer and the employee contribute. Occupational pension schemes are generally funded by investment, though some large public sector schemes are funded from taxation. They are generally run by representatives of the employer in the form of trustees, with the help of administrators, investment managers, and external consultants such as auditors. The trustees should include representatives from staff and pensioners. Occupational and personal pension schemes tend to be more flexible than the state scheme, with the possibility of taking benefits early, such as age 35 for sportsmen, or later, up to age 75. Trustees have discretionary powers over eligibility to an early pension and in the case of ill health will base their decision on information submitted by the member and from independent doctors. Pension schemes must have a formal internal dispute resolution procedure for complaints and appeals. These are usually divided into two stages, firstly at the level of the employer and secondly at the level of the pension scheme's administrators.

Defined benefit and defined contribution schemes

The model for most occupational pension schemes through the twentieth century was that of defined benefits or final salary schemes. Characteristically each year of service with the organization would qualify the individual for a proportion (e.g. 1/80 or 1/60) of their final salary at retirement as a pension. There are also schemes where benefits are based on average career earnings. The main alternative model is the defined contribution scheme or money purchase scheme. Here, individuals and employers pay a proportion of salary into a fund of which each member has a share dependent upon their contribution. Upon retirement, the individual is free to use the sum accumulated to purchase an annuity that will provide an income. UK employers in the private sector are moving towards defined contribution pension schemes and such a move has been recommended for the public sector as well.[10] Most schemes include a provision for compensating members who have to give up work early because of ill health or injury. They typically pay a pension immediately, rather than at the normal retirement age, without actuarial reduction of benefits and often with an enhancement to the pensionable years of service.

The Pensions Advisory Service and Ombudsman Service

Advice about pensions can be obtained in the UK from the Pensions Advisory Service, an independent organization that is grant aided by the Department for Work and Pensions. Complaints or appeals which cannot be resolved by an internal dispute resolution procedure can be referred to them, who may in turn refer the case to the Pensions Ombudsman (PO). Individuals may complain directly to the PO who receives 30–40 complaints per year about IHR, mostly disputing the non-permanence of their incapacity.

Criteria for ill health retirement

Eligibility for an early and enhanced pension is dependent on the member meeting criteria set out by the trustees or regulators of the pension scheme. Criteria vary between schemes, but most require the applicant to be permanently incapable of undertaking their job, or any work, as a consequence of ill health, illness, or injury. It is essential for the doctor to understand the precise criteria for the scheme on which they are advising and the interpretation that is applied to the wording. For example, permanence is usually defined as until the scheme's normal pensionable age, which can vary by scheme, date of joining, length of service, and job. Most pension schemes allow for flexible retirement whereby members can draw an occupational pension while continuing to work for the same employer. The removal of the default retirement age does not affect a pension scheme's normal pensionable age, which is likely to be the same for both men and women and some patients may need to have this explained to them.

A number of pension schemes in both the private and public sectors have more than one tier of eligibility criteria for IHR. Characteristically, the lower tier (lower benefits) requires evidence of incapacity to undertake the job for which the member is employed and the upper tier (higher benefits) requires evidence of incapacity to undertake any gainful employment. The job may be defined in various ways, for example, for NHS staff as their contracted duties for that employing trust, for teachers as teaching in any school (including part-time), and for police officers as the ordinary duties of an officer in any force (not just the one for which they are employed).

In general, incapacity for all work from a medical perspective is more clear cut than incapacity for a specific job. Furthermore, in most schemes, capability to undertake a job other than the contracted one need not be restricted to one of similar earning capacity, for example, a patient may not be capable of working as a director, but if they are capable of working as an administrator or driver this would make them ineligible for a higher-tier pension. Determining incapacity from an individual's own job requires the advising doctor to have a good knowledge of the functional requirements of the job, working practices, and the sort of adjustments that can reasonably be accommodated by the employer.

The terms ill health or infirmity of body or mind are rarely defined in regulations so doctors are advised to become familiar with any explanatory guidance of the scheme, or any circulars sent out in the light of recent case law. Conditions that are not contained within the current International Classification of Diseases,[11] such as stress or burnout, should not be accepted as medical illnesses for the purpose of IHR. Words not defined in guidance should assume their everyday meaning and as given in the *Oxford English Dictionary*, such as 'gainful' which is defined as 'serving to increase wealth or resources'.

Care should also be taken to ensure that there is a direct causal link between any incapacity and ill health. Some applicants will declare incapability for carrying out tasks for which they are employed and a long-standing coexisting illness may be convenient for terminating employment on favourable terms funded by the pension scheme. An area of difficulty is that of secondary ill health. Employees with performance, attendance, or disciplinary problems may absent themselves from work citing 'stress', anxiety, or depression and choose to pursue IHR as the solution to their employment problems. Some schemes insist that the ill health qualifying for a pension must be primary (i.e. unrelated to any effects of a reasonable employment process), rather than secondary, and require that issues related to employment such as a grievance or investigation for misconduct be resolved before eligibility to a pension is considered. In any case, reactive ill health is unlikely to be permanently incapacitating unless it occurs shortly before the normal pension age.

Evidence

The optimum means of determining whether an individual is likely to meet the criteria for IHR will vary by case. However, it will be usual for evidence to include an assessment of capability, matched to the requirements of the job, as well as medical evidence about the illness or injury that allows the formulation of a diagnosis and prognosis. In most cases, sufficient medical evidence can be gleaned by examining the patient and from the patient's medical records, but where this is deficient, an independent examination or additional investigations may be needed to provide the necessary quality of evidence. When requesting a report it should be made clear that it is information on diagnosis, treatment, and prognosis which is being sought, and not a view on employment issues or entitlement to a pension, the terms of which may not be known to the treating doctor. Where the illness is terminal, prognosis should be ascertained as pension benefits may be commuted (replacement of monthly payments with an augmented lump sum) when life expectancy is less than 12 months.

It is a matter of professional judgement as to whether the doctor who is advising the pension scheme examines the applicant before giving an opinion. Pension decisions and the advice provided should be made on a balance of probabilities, that is, more likely than not. In the doctor's report, it is important that he or she does not give the impression that they are setting a higher standard, for example, by saying they cannot be certain that the applicant will not respond to treatment. Words like 'possible' should be avoided as they convey no indication of the likely outcome. For this reason, inclusion of

> ### Box 12.1 Principles to follow when making recommendations for IHR
>
> 1. Have only relevant and no irrelevant matters been taken into account?
> 2. Have the correct questions been addressed?
> 3. Have the regulations or rules been correctly interpreted?
> 4. Has a perverse decision been made, which is a decision that no reasonable decision-maker properly directing themselves could arrive at in the circumstances?

the words 'likely' or 'unlikely' are recommended. Recommendations should follow the principles summarized in the case of *Bewley* v. *Gateshead Council and South Tyneside Council.* See Box 12.1.

The PO will look at the way in which a decision was reached, but will not set it aside purely because they disagree with the decision. Most pension schemes require a certificate to be completed by the independent doctor but it is essential to also include a report, so that at any subsequent appeal the evidence on which the doctor's inferences were made and the reasons for subsequent recommendations about IHR are clear.

Where there is uncertainty over diagnosis, the PO has stated in the case of *Hussain* v. *Birmingham City Council* that a lack of a definite diagnosis should not automatically be a bar to IHR. The doctor should consider the course of the applicant's illness to date, whether the illness is likely to be treatable, and if so, whether the individual is likely to benefit from treatment and over what period of time. To this we would add that a failure to respond to treatment should be for medical reasons and not, for example, because of a failure to engage or agree to reasonable treatment.

Where there is uncertainty over prognosis, the PO has indicated in the case of *Williams* v. *The Trustees of the TRW Pension Scheme* that the doctor should answer three questions:

1. Is the applicant currently incapable of the work in question?
2. In the absence of future treatment, is the incapacity likely to be permanent?
3. Is future treatment likely to alter this?

It is good practice for the doctor to make explicit statements in the report about these three questions and whether an improvement in health is likely to occur before the scheme's normal pension age. It may be acceptable for the doctor to recommend that a decision is deferred pending further information. However, to say that it would be premature to make a decision has been interpreted by the PO as 'ducking the decision'.

When faced with divergent views, the doctor should acknowledge that they exist. If they do not, then it could be argued that the doctor has failed to take relevant information into account. This risk is reduced by referring to the divergent view in the report. This does not mean that the doctor is bound by the divergent view. The general principle is that

Table 12.1 Elements of a report and the rationale for their inclusion

Elements of report	Rationale for inclusion
Refer to the relevant scheme regulations, rules, and/or the questions to be answered	Demonstrates an understanding of the eligibility criteria and that the right questions have been addressed
A brief description of the job and any adjustments that may have been made by the employer	Demonstrates familiarity with the job and the Equality Act 2010
The materially relevant evidence that has been considered should be listed	Demonstrates the types of relevant information that have been taken into account and not irrelevant information
The diagnosis, treatment, and prognosis in relation to the applicant's age and their normal occupational pension age	Demonstrates the relevant medical information that has been taken into account and not irrelevant medical information. Do not refer to irrelevant information
From the history and examination, the functional abilities of the applicant in work and outside work	Demonstrates that incapability to do the job and/or other work has been considered and not just ill health
Inferences, recommendation, and justification	Demonstrates the understandings that have been made about the applicant, the evidence that has been used to formulate an opinion, and provides a robust rationale for the decision-maker

it is for the person making the decision or recommendation to decide how much weight to give to a particular piece of evidence. The doctor must say, however, why they preferred a particular opinion. The expertise and familiarity with the individual and the job of the person providing the opinion should be taken into consideration, as should any conflicts of interest or inconsistency in the evidence (see Table 12.1).

Conflicts of interest

Those charged with advising a pension scheme about eligibility to IHR must remember that they have a contractual duty to the trustees of the scheme or the taxpayer, but not to the individual scheme member or to the employer. Advice must be objective and evidence based. Factors such as expediency or social circumstances should be disregarded. Doctors who may be involved in the treatment of the patient, or are the patient's general practitioner, should not advise the pension scheme about eligibility because of the inherent potential for a conflict of interests. Such a doctor should, with consent, provide factual information about the patient's health, treatment, and prognosis. In larger pension schemes, it is usual to separate occupational health advice to the employer from advice to the pension scheme. Smaller schemes may have to rely on the employer's medical adviser as the only source of competent advice on health related to employment, so those undertaking such a role must be assiduous in acting impartially. For this reason, it is good practice for two or more doctors to be involved in the process of IHR and for those doctors not to be colleagues.

Sometimes when providing a professional opinion when a patient wishes to avoid work or to gain a pension or injury award, this may be problematic for the doctor. This is because the relationship between doctor and patient is not a normal therapeutic one, but is for the purposes of providing specific advice to a third party. Guidance on the ethical issues for doctors with such a dual responsibility has been published by the General Medical Council and the Faculty of Occupational Medicine. While it is the duty of all doctors to put the care of the patient first, this should be for medical and not economic purposes. In the process of the examination the doctor may identify inconsistencies in the history or examination, abnormal illness behaviour, entrenched beliefs or views about prognosis, undiagnosed psychological ill health, or illness deception. Such findings should be documented and taken into account when formulating a professional opinion. The patient should be given an opportunity to comment on a draft.

Competence

Advice on eligibility for IHR must be given only by doctors who have sufficient knowledge of the job and working environment. Many pension schemes require their medical advisers to have a qualification in occupational medicine. The minimum qualification varies between schemes but is usually not less than the Diploma in Occupational Medicine, supplemented by training in the application of the scheme criteria. Such doctors should be overseen by an accredited specialist (i.e. a Member or Fellow of the Faculty of Occupational Medicine in the UK, or equivalent qualification issued by a competent authority in a European Economic Area State). An appeal against an initial decision should be considered by an accredited specialist in occupational medicine. In the case of *Aspinall v. Department for Education and Teachers' Pensions*, the PO has accepted that an occupational physician is the most appropriate person to give an opinion about ability to work and the treating specialist is the most appropriate person to provide a diagnosis.

Appeals and complaints

All IHR assessment processes should have an appeal mechanism. The scheme member should be advised of the grounds for the original decision and have an opportunity to appeal with or without further medical evidence. The appeal may be considered by a doctor or panel of doctors who should include an accredited specialist in occupational medicine with sufficient knowledge and experience to judge the issues. Some schemes require appellants to present for medical examination, but most appeals are conducted on a 'papers only' basis, partly for logistical reasons, but also because further examination may not provide new objective evidence.

Assessment of eligibility for IHR can result in a complaint by the patient against the doctor. This is most likely to occur if the application has been unsuccessful. It is essential not only to have a robust complaints procedure running alongside the appeal procedure but also one which identifies potentially vexatious or vindictive complaints. Requests to remove factually relevant material that is not supportive of the patient's case should be resisted, as should requests to assess a case without medical reports unfavourable to the appellant, or without sight of the previous doctor's rationale for their opinion. A request not to send a report because it does not support an appellant's case should be resisted and if asked to remove relevant clinical information, the doctor should make it clear in the report where such information has been deleted. Difficulties of this nature for doctors with dual responsibilities is understood by most employers and regulatory bodies and seen as an occupational hazard for the doctor.

General guidance

Where possible, the true functional ability of the applicant should be ascertained. If the doctor believes that the true functional ability of the patient has not been obtained, despite reasonable efforts, or the degree of disability declared by the patient is more than would be normally expected for that illness or injury, it is recommended that the doctor bases their advice on what would normally be expected by way of function or prognosis in a patient with the same diagnosis but who is not seeking early retirement.

Reasonable adjustments, aids, or workplace adaptations should have been tried to accommodate the patient's incapacity, as well as exploring opportunities for redeployment before a decision is made about IHR. Adjustments might include adaptive technology, involvement of the Access to Work team, and 'permitted' or 'supported' employment. IHR is also a dismissal in law, so a failure to make reasonable adjustments may constitute grounds for a claim of unfair dismissal. Workplaces and the people who work in them are in constant flux, so refusal by an employee to return to a particular workplace should not merit IHR unless there is a demonstrable inability to do so because of permanent incapacity for medical reasons.

Advice should, whenever possible, be based on objective medical evidence. Non-medical factors contributing to the patient's ill health (e.g. anger, embitterment, or disaffection with the employer, or a lack of motivation to return to work) should generally be disregarded. Illnesses that are the most difficult to assess objectively are those that rely entirely on subjective complaints (e.g. chronic fatigue syndrome, fibromyalgia, and some mental health disorders). Advice on these illnesses in relation to IHR is given elsewhere.[12]

Audit

The additional cost to the pension scheme of IHR has been estimated at about £50,000/case.[2] Great variability in IHR decisions has been shown,[1] which is disconcerting for scheme trustees, administrators, and patients, and indicates the need for audit. This can be done by comparing a doctor's rate of recommended IHR relative to the national rate of IHR for that scheme, or if this information is unavailable, with other schemes with similar criteria. Figure 12.1 shows the distribution of IHR by 216 trusts in the NHS and by 85 administering authorities in local government for 2015–2016. Tiers of IHR were combined so the rate is all retirements by ill health per 1000 employees. The median

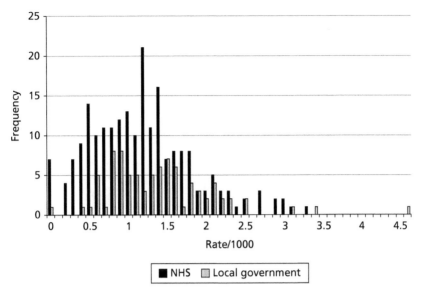

Figure 12.1 Distribution of rates of ill health retirement by NHS trusts and local government administering authorities 2016–2017.

and 5th–95th percentiles for the NHS was 1.2 (0.3–2.4) and for local government 1.3 (0.6–2.45). The distribution by tier for the NHS was 64% tier 2 and 36% tier 1 (tier 2 being incapable of all work). For local government it was 75% tier 1, 8% tier 2, and 17% tier 3 (tier 1 being incapable of all work). By square rooting their rate/1000, doctors can see where they and the employer fall in a normal distribution (Figure 12.2). Where their rate of IHR lies more than two standard deviations outside the mean, they (or ideally someone else) should audit a sample of their cases against published diagnostically specific guidance on IHR.[12]

Medico-legal aspects

Employees and managers often view IHR as an alternative to resignation, redundancy, or dismissal. In fact it is not an employment issue but rather a process for paying pension benefits once a decision to terminate an employee's contract has been made. Even if the individual applies for the benefit, the employer must be satisfied that all decisions relating to employment have been made fairly and according to due process, otherwise a case for unfair dismissal may be justified. The Equality Act 2010 applies equally at the end of employment as it does at recruitment and during employment. Examples of employers being found to have unlawfully discriminated against an employee by giving them IHR can be found in case law such as *Kerrigan* v. *Rover Group Ltd* (1997) and *Meikle* v. *Nottinghamshire County Council* (2004). Dismissing an employee with illness or injury without making reasonable adjustments or offering opportunities for redeployment, with or without an IHR pension, or not considering eligibility to a pension, may be grounds for

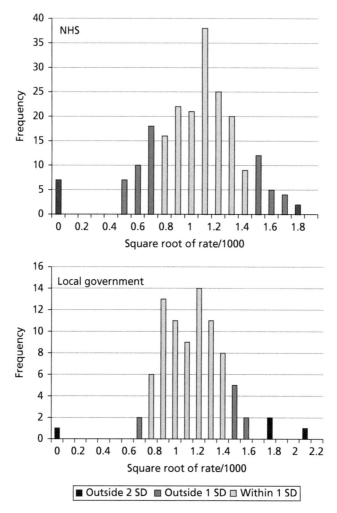

Figure 12.2 Distribution of normalized rates of ill health retirement with standard deviations (SD) by NHS trusts and local government administering authorities 2016–2017.

unfair dismissal. In these circumstances, a doctor should be wary of recommending IHR, or of not making a comment about eligibility to a pension.

Limited life expectancy

Most pension schemes allow for commutation of benefits for members in employment (but not usually for deferred members) with a life expectancy of less than 12 months. Trustees or administrators may apply this discretion if it is within the scope of their scheme, but it is also governed by tax rules. The Inland Revenue has stated that such commutation is intended for the benefit of the scheme member rather than their dependents or estate. Consequently, well-intentioned efforts to secure commutation for individuals who are terminally ill are potentially unlawful and, if repeated across several cases, could result in the withdrawal of the concession by the Inland Revenue for that scheme. Unfortunately, the patient or a relative has the task of requesting commutation, which creates difficulty if they are unaware of or are sensitive about the prognosis. A doctor will need to confirm the prognosis in writing. Most schemes offer some form of death benefit for the dependents of members employed at the time of death.

Key points

◆ Doctors who advise on the merits of a patient's application for a pension should be familiar with the eligibility criteria of the pension scheme and not be in a position of conflicts of interest.

◆ A doctor's report about the merits of a patient's case for IHR should include the four principles outlined in this chapter.

◆ Sometimes the patient will see the doctor as an obstacle to them obtaining their entitlement and seek to discredit the doctor or the report.

◆ A doctor who advises a pension scheme should audit their rate of IHR against national rates.

◆ Mortality after retirement depends on the health of the retiree and not on early retirement per se.

References

1. **Poole CJM.** Retirement on grounds of ill health: cross sectional survey in six organisations in United Kingdom. *BMJ* 1997;**314**:929–32.
2. **HM Treasury.** *Review of Ill Health Retirement in the Public Sector.* London: HM Treasury; 2000.
3. **Casscells W, Evans D, DeSilva RA, et al.** Retirement and coronary mortality. *Lancet* 1980;**315**:1288–9.
4. **Mein G, Martikainen P, Hemingway H, Marmot M.** Is retirement good or bad for mental and physical health functioning? Whitehall II longitudinal study of civil servants. *J Epidemiol Community Health* 2003;**57**:46–9.
5. **Brockmann H, Muller R, Helmert U.** Time to retire – time to die? A prospective study of the effects of early retirement on long-term survival. *Soc Sci Med* 2009;**69**:160–4.
6. **Hult C, Stattin M, Janlert U, Jarvholm B.** Time of retirement and mortality – a cohort study of Swedish construction workers. *Soc Sci Med* 2010;**70**:1480–6.
7. **Jokela M, Ferrie JE, Gimeno D, et al.** From midlife to early old age: health trajectories associated with retirement. *Epidemiology* 2010;**21**:284–90.
8. **Mein G, Martikainen P, Stansfeld SA, et al.** Predictors of early retirement in British civil servants. *Age Ageing* 2000;**29**:529–36.
9. **Polvinen A, Gould R, Lahelma E, Martikainen P.** Socioeconomic differences in disability retirement in Finland: the contribution of ill health, health behaviours and working conditions. *Scand J Public Health* 2013;**41**:470–8.

10. **Hutton J.** *Independent Public Service Pensions Commission: Final Report.* London: Pensions Commission; 2011.

11. **World Health Organization.** *The International Statistical Classification of Diseases and Related Health Problems,* 11th revision. Geneva: World Health Organization; 2010.

12. **Poole CJM, Bass CM, Sorrell JE, Thompson ME, Harrison JR, Archer AD.** Ill health retirement: national rates and updated guidance for occupational physicians. *Occup Med* 2005;55:345–8.

Chapter 13

Medication and employment

Caroline Swales and Peter McDowall

Introduction

Medication allows many people with long-term health conditions to pursue productive employment when they would otherwise be unable to work safely and effectively. However, both short-term and long-term pharmacological treatments can have implications for work. The number of medications taken by individuals has increased; the risk of harm increasing with polypharmacy. The Internet has transformed communications, and practitioners have greater accessibility to updated clinical data with increased communication between specialists, but easier access to data on medication and health conditions for employees has both positive and negative influences. High-profile road traffic fatalities have raised public concerns about the potential adverse effects of medication and of employees not reporting or managing conditions effectively. Occupational health (OH) professionals are not regular prescribers. However, they can help to monitor safe use of medications, by observing and recording compliance and adverse effects in relation to workplace health and safety. Greater involvement in employees' medication management, with onward communication of problems to treating physicians, is required to enable OH to participate in medicines optimization.[1]

Epidemiology of medication use

NHS Digital is the national provider of information, data and IT systems, previously known as the Health and Social Care Information Centre. iView provides prescribing data for Clinical Commissioning Groups in England (Box 13.1).[2–6]

Figures for England from 2016 show that those aged between 19 and 65 years account for 35% of all prescription items and on average were prescribed 12.7 items each year.[7] Prescribing patterns have also changed, and the use of prescription-only medicines (PoMs) increases with age, whereas over-the-counter (OTC) purchases reduce.

Data on prescription medication abuse in the workforce is available but there are little recent data about prescription medication usage in UK workforces. Evidence indicates that some employers are concerned about the hazards as opposed to the benefits of medication to maintain fitness and function. Research and education to progress this issue are essential.

Box 13.1 Prescriptions

NHS Digital reported that the number of antidepressant items has more than doubled in the last decade.[2]

	Prescriptions 2016	Prescription items per head
England	1.1 billion (0.51 billion in 2000–2001)	20
Scotland	103 million	19
Wales	80 million	26
Northern Ireland		20

Source: data from NHS Digital, Prescriptions Dispensed in the Community, Statistics for England - 2006–2016 https://digital.nhs.uk/data-and-information/publications/statistical/ prescriptions-dispensed-in-the-community/prescriptions-dispensed-in-the-community- statistics-for-england-2006-2016-pas. The NHS Information Centre, Prescribing Support Unit, Lloyd D. *General pharmaceutical services in England 2000–01 to 2009–10.* Version 1.0. London: NHS Information Centre, 2010; and Scottish Government Information Services Division, Prescribing and medicines: dispenser payments and prescription cost analysis 2016/ 2017 https://www.isdscotland.org/Health-Topics/Prescribing-and-Medicines/Publications/2017- 08-29/2017-08-29-Dispenser-Payments-and-Prescription-Cost-Analysis-Summary.pdf; and Welsh Government, Prescriptions dispensed in the Community (http://gov.wales/docs/statistics/ 2017/170524-prescriptions-dispensed-community-2016-en.pdf); and Health and Social Care Information Centre (HSCIC). Office of Health Economics. Health services data. http://www.ohe. org/page/health-statistics/access-the-data/health-service/data.cfm.

Medicines optimization

It is estimated that between 30% and 50% of medicines prescribed for long-term conditions are not taken as intended. Medicines optimization is a person-centred approach to safe and effective medicines use in the NHS, through improved collaboration of health and social care practitioners and greater patient engagement. The Royal Pharmaceutical Society (RPS) supports medicines optimization and suggests four guiding principles[1] (Box 13.2). Although medicines optimization is solely related to patient care, OH assessments provide opportunities to improve the management of medication and associated

Box 13.2 RPS principles for optimization of medicines

- ◆ Aim to understand the patient's experience.
- ◆ Evidence-based choice of medicines.
- ◆ Ensure medicines use is as safe as possible.
- ◆ Make medicines optimization part of routine practice.

risks in employees. There is little evidence of OH participation in managing medicines, apart from for some safety-critical industries. Despite challenges (e.g. ethical issues arising with data access), the variability of employers, and different operating practices, there is benefit in including OH in the optimizing medication agenda.

Classification of medications

There are three legitimate ways of obtaining licensed medicines in the UK, defined in the Medicines Act 1968 (Box 13.3).

Reclassification of many PoMs to pharmacy use in the 1980s led to easier accessibility to some drugs, with potentially hazardous effects.[8] The RPS advised accredited training for counter staff.[9,10] Prescribing now includes medical apps, for example, a smartphone app, GDm-health, focusing on gestational diabetes, enabling women to send blood glucose results to their specialist clinician.

New technology and advances in knowledge influence both the choice of medication and the priority of medication versus non-pharmacological interventions. For example, greater understanding of pain pathways has focused on non-medication management, such as cognitive behavioural therapy. In theory, this assists in reducing long-term analgesia, although patient preference may still be an important driver of chronic polypharmacy.

Online medication

Changes in healthcare delivery have enabled better access to prescribed drugs via online medical consultations. Moreover, in the UK more than 2 million people buy medication regularly from online pharmacies. Illegal Internet pharmacies often sell outdated or counterfeit medications without normal safeguards. Since 2005, it has been legal for pharmacies to complete NHS prescriptions over the Internet. In April 2016, there were 46 registered online pharmacies in England. Since 2008, a green cross Internet pharmacy logo has helped to identify accredited online pharmacies.[11,12] Since 2015, the Medicines Healthcare products Regulatory Agency (MHRA) require online sellers to

---

Box 13.3 Ways of obtaining licensed medicines in the UK

1. PoM: prescription-only medicines from qualified prescribers (doctors, dentists, nurse, or pharmacist independent prescribers, or supplementary prescribers).

2. P: pharmacy-only medicines, obtained without a prescription from, or under the supervision of, a qualified pharmacist.

3. GSL: general sales list medicines, obtained without a prescription from, for example, a pharmacy or a supermarket.

P and GSL (over-the-counter) medicines can also be prescribed.

adopt an European Union-wide logo and maintain an entry in the MHRA medicines sellers registry.[13]

Classification of adverse drug reactions

Harm from medications can be categorized as adverse effects (physiological or pathological effects at the molecular, cellular, or tissue levels) and adverse reactions (the resulting signs and symptoms). The classifications of adverse outcomes called EIDOS and DoTS involve descriptions of the mechanisms by which they occur, their clinical features, their uses in pharmacovigilance, planning, risk management, and prevention of adverse reactions.[14]

Unwanted reactions may also result from interactions with other drugs, herbal medicines, foods, alcohol, recreational drugs, performance-enhancing drugs, specific chemicals at work, and some medical devices. The effects of such reactions on performance are of particular concern in safety-critical jobs.

Harm from medications

Harm from medications that are trivial for non-workers can affect employee safety. Common reasons for adverse events are listed in Box 13.4.

The Department of Health found that 5–8% of unplanned hospital admissions were due to medication issues[15] including lack of knowledge, failure to follow systems and protocols, interruptions during prescribing, administration, or dispensing. Medicines optimization aims to minimize these preventable risks.

The Yellow Card Scheme, for reporting side effects to medicines, now has over 600,000 UK Yellow Cards received, with integral reporting online. In 2014, NHS England launched the National Patient Safety Alerting System (NPSAS) for improved dissemination of urgent patient safety alerts to healthcare providers.

Box 13.4 Common reasons for adverse events

◆ Medication taken at an incorrect time or inappropriately.

◆ Intercurrent illness (e.g. diarrhoea and vomiting).

◆ Incorrect dosage regimen or changes to dosages.

◆ Introduction of a new medication.

◆ Incomplete identification of previous reactions or polypharmacy.

◆ Self-prescribing or unsupervised dosage manipulation.

◆ Illegal medication obtained without prescription.

◆ Interaction with alcohol.

Frequencies of adverse drug reactions in the workplace

In 1999, 11% of a study population had adverse reactions that they felt could have affected their safety.[16] Of these, 30% were working in high-risk occupations and 25% in moderate-risk occupations. For men, the most frequent adverse reactions were drowsiness (29%), poor concentration (18%), and dizziness (12%). Among women, visual deterioration was the most common. Of those with adverse reactions, only 40% informed any medical personnel, and only 23% informed OH. Such reactions may be minimized by better understanding of their mechanisms, better reporting by employees, and improved guidance on using over-the-counter (OTC) medicines.

Patient information

European Commission Directive 92/97 requires information, including a description of possible adverse reactions, to be provided for the consumer, either in a leaflet or on the packaging, for all medicines licensed by the MHRA including PoM, P, and GSL medicines. However, these are often lengthy and list such a variety of side effects that it can be difficult to differentiate medication-related symptoms from other causes.

In a study of PoMs used by employees in a chemical plant,[16] 74% of employees reported having read and understood advisory information, 17% had not understood, and 6% had not consulted the information; 75% reported that their general practitioner (GP) had not warned them about possible adverse reactions that could affect safety at work; of these, 43% were taking medications with potentially disabling adverse effects. In 1999, 30% of employees taking OTC medications had not read the information provided, of whom 57% were taking OTCs that could have caused adverse reactions.[16]

Clinical pharmacology relevant to harm

Drug elimination

Drugs are eliminated by the kidneys and liver and in the lungs, saliva, sweat, and breast milk. Many drugs are inactivated by hepatic detoxification and the metabolites are primarily excreted via the bile and kidneys. Hepatic and renal impairment can reduce the elimination of drugs. Therefore, doses should be altered accordingly and guidance can be found in the *British National Formulary (BNF)*.

Drug interactions

Drug interactions occur when one drug (the precipitant or perpetrator drug) alters the disposition or actions of another (the object or victim drug). Certain foods can also be precipitants (Box 13.5). Drug interactions are detailed in the appendix of the *BNF*, and online checking tools are available for prescribers via *BNF* online (see 'Useful websites').

Box 13.5 Examples of drug interactions

- Erythromycin is a hepatic enzyme inhibitor, increasing the effects of other medication. It is also one of many medications that have the potential to prolong the QT interval.

- Non-steroidal anti-inflammatory drugs (NSAIDs) increase the risk of gastrointestinal ulceration, but also potentiate the anticoagulant effect of warfarin (by competing for protein binding sites), giving rise to a serious bleeding risk.

- Diuretics, such as furosemide, can cause hyponatraemia and hypokalaemia and potentiate the actions of lithium and digoxin respectively.

- Grapefruit inhibits gut and liver enzymes, reducing the metabolism of many medications, including statins, ciclosporin, and carbamazepine.

- Milk or antacids reduce absorption of antibiotics, such as tetracycline and ciprofloxacin.

- Alcohol has an additive effect with other central nervous system (CNS) depressants, such as benzodiazepines, opioids, and gabapentinoids. Alcohol can cause a disulphiram-like drug reaction with metronidazole.

Influence of legislation/guidance

The Health and Safety at Work etc. Act 1974 and the Management of Health and Safety at Work Regulations 1999 require employees to take reasonable care of their own health and safety and that of any other person who may be affected by their actions or omissions at work. These provisions encompass medications and their effects.

The Equality Act 2010

The Equality Act 2010 (see Chapter 3) prohibits discrimination and requires employers to make reasonable adjustments to enable qualifying employees to remain at work. Such adjustments may relate to the actions of medications. The Equality Act 2010 applies if the employee would be substantially impaired in day-to-day activities in the absence of treatment. Drug addiction is normally excluded, but any addiction that was originally the result of medically prescribed treatment is covered. The Equality Act 2010 prohibits health enquiry before offering employment, but those who apply for safety-critical roles should have a pre-placement assessment, and discussion of prescription medications. Standardized/national guidance specifies screening for some employment, increasing the likelihood of recognizing the impact of medications.

Effects of medications on performance

Performance testing involves measurement of the effects of drugs on psychomotor function or on activities of everyday life (e.g. driving). There is much evidence that laboratory tests of psychomotor function can reliably demonstrate the effects of drugs on cognitive information processing, short-term memory and learning, motor functions, and activities involving sensory, central, and motor abilities. In theory, such approaches could be used to screen workers taking long-term medication, such as anticonvulsants, in safety-critical roles. However, marked variability in individual responses reduces the precision of these tests. Testing of a safe level of function for an employee is often best done by a simulated assessment in the work area. Functional capacity assessment provides a comprehensive summary of an employee's function related to their health conditions in a safe protected manner before a trial of adjusted duties in the workplace.

Circadian rhythms

Medication compliance can be affected by shift working and travel across time zones. While adaptation occurs within 2 weeks, employees are often required to work shortly after arrival. Additional health effects can occur through poor control of a health condition, because of altered timing of medication, or other factors (e.g. mealtimes in insulin-controlled diabetes).

Circadian rhythms can influence the efficacy, toxicity, and metabolism of some medications,[17] for example, serum amitriptyline concentrations are higher after a morning dose than an evening dose.[18] Epidemiological data and clinical trials are starting to show that timing medications to the body's internal clock could improve their effectiveness and reduce side effects (chronotherapy). This might have implications for shift and night work that should be considered on a specific case basis.

Occupational exposures and medication

Work environments that can influence prescribed medications include extremes of temperature (e.g. relating to cardiovascular medications), or unexpected or unknown exposure to CNS depressants (e.g. solvents). Many environmental chemicals are also enzyme inducers, including polycyclic aromatic hydrocarbons, organochlorines, and organophosphorus compounds. Workers engaged in pesticide manufacture may have enzyme induction.[19]

Cytotoxic chemotherapy is potentially carcinogenic, mutagenic, and is hazardous as defined by the Control of Substances Hazardous to Health Regulations 2002. Chemotherapy treatment must be prescribed, dispensed, supplied, and administered in accordance with the Medicines Act 1968. Employees working in the manufacture of pharmaceuticals and staff handing cytotoxic drugs require safety measures to control exposure.[20-22] Such medication is handled in a range of healthcare settings including specialist oncology units and hospices but also by community staff and in veterinary clinics.

Medication and occupation

Medication is usually positive for employment by controlling underlying health conditions. However, it may also impair safety or function at work through an impact on cognition, mobility, and dexterity, or distraction by side effects such as nausea, fatigue, malaise, tremor, or gastrointestinal or urinary upset. For some occupations (e.g. diving), medication management is focused on the prevention of harm to the individual. For others (e.g. safety-critical drivers), the priority is control of risk to employees or members of the public. Such occupations often work to specific regulations and guidance, an outline of which is provided here with comprehensive guidance in specific, other chapters. Some industries have in-house guidance for particular occupations or work environments, but OH may provide guidance in other roles, whether safety critical or not.

Drivers

Driving is a highly complex skill including the ability to interact simultaneously with both the vehicle and the external environment.

OH professionals should assume that most employees drive, some of whom will drive specifically for work. Drowsiness is a major cause of road traffic accidents and may be aggravated or caused by medication. In addition, loss of attention or slowing of reactions may occur. Sedation caused by benzodiazepines results in compromised steering, road positioning, and reaction times in both laboratory and road tests.[23] A study in Dundee,[24] showed a significant increase in the risk of road traffic accidents among those taking anxiolytic benzodiazepines and the short-acting hypnotic zopiclone. The authors suggested that anyone taking long half-life anxiolytic benzodiazepines or zopiclone should be advised not to drive. Users of hypnotic benzodiazepines were not at increased risk while zopiclone displayed residual effects that impaired driving, despite a relatively short half-life (5 hours).

Driving when under the influence of drink or drugs, whether illicit or prescribed drugs, is an offence under Section 4 of the Road Traffic Act 1991. The UK Driver and Vehicle Licensing Agency (DVLA) provides guidance on fitness to drive for group 1 or group 2 licences for medical practitioners (see 'Useful websites'). Doctors have a duty of care to advise patients of the potential dangers of adverse reactions from medications and interactions with other substances, especially alcohol. The guidance includes advice on the potential risks of medication (Box 13.6). Drivers with psychiatric illnesses are often safer when well and taking regular psychotropic medications than when ill.

DVLA group 2 drivers

Stricter criteria apply to certain drivers (group 2), since they drive for longer hours and are at greater risks of the effects of adverse drug reactions or interactions.

All drivers with diabetes must follow 'Information for drivers with diabetes', Appendix D (see 'Useful websites'). Drivers taking insulin should check their blood glucose (using a monitor with a memory function) within 2 hours of starting driving, every 2 hours while driving, and at least twice daily even when not driving. Monitoring may also be necessary for drivers taking oral medication with a risk of hypoglycaemia.

Shift workers

Sixteen per cent of all UK employees work shifts. Shift working itself can cause sleepiness. Additive effects on somnolence can occur from sedative medications because of adverse

---

Box 13.6 Common adverse effects of medications

- Opioids: reduced cognitive performance before neuroadaptation is established; impairment is possible due to the miotic effects on vision. All CNS-active drugs can impair alertness, concentration, and driving performance, particularly within the first month of starting or when increasing dose.
- Benzodiazepines: these are the most likely psychotropic drugs to impair driving performance, particularly the long-acting compounds. Alcohol potentiates their effects.
- Antipsychotic drugs, including depot formulations: motor or extrapyramidal effects, sedation, poor concentration.
- Older tricyclic antidepressants: can impair driving by pronounced anticholinergic and antihistaminic effects.

---

or hangover effects. Employees may deliberately omit doses, with an adverse impact on the underlying condition. Shift patterns and changes to them should be discussed with the prescribing physician and OH. The Working Time Regulations 1998 require employers to carry out periodic health assessments for night workers, which should take account of medications and their effects.

Management of clinical conditions

Management of a condition with prescribed medication has to be balanced against the risk of adverse reactions. Patients may be impaired by both the medication and the disease. Medicines that affect performance in the initial stages may be well tolerated after a period of time and dose adjustment. Medicines may alleviate the effects of illness that may otherwise cause impairment at work, for example, pain or mood disturbance. Particular attention should be paid to psychological medication, strong analgesics, insulin, and cardiovascular medication.

The following summarizes specific medication effects for some of the more common disorders. General employment is covered in these paragraphs. However, a few safety-critical roles have special considerations in respect of prescribed medication, particularly those in the transport industry, or seafaring. These aspects are covered in Chapter 15 and Chapter 16, respectively.

Central nervous system drugs

For mental health conditions, maintaining employment depends on the effectiveness of treatment in reducing behavioural aspects of a condition while trying to limit adverse drug reactions. This is often best achieved by non-pharmacological interventions, for example, talking therapies or 'e-therapies' (with access via message boards, instant messenger with therapists, or via live platforms, such as Skype). E-therapies show considerable clinical benefits, especially in the treatment of depression and anxiety, and are recommended by the National Institute for Health and Care Excellence (NICE).

Antidepressants

The commonly prescribed antidepressants are the selective serotonin reuptake inhibitors (SSRIs), the serotonin–noradrenaline (norepinephrine) reuptake inhibitors (SNRIs), trazodone, and mirtazapine. The SSRIs, such as fluoxetine and paroxetine, and the SNRIs, such as venlafaxine, do not usually produce sedation and appear to have little effect on performance. However, they can cause heightened anxiety and gastrointestinal upset in the early weeks of treatment. Tricyclics are now less frequently used for depression, but often still have a role in chronic pain management, or may be used in treatment-resistant depression. Many tricyclics produce sedation, especially at the start of treatment, which is markedly potentiated by alcohol. Tricyclic antidepressants with anticholinergic effects produce blurring of near vision, and can cause a tremor, potentially affecting work performance. Hyponatraemia due to inappropriate secretion of antidiuretic hormone has been associated with all antidepressants, but is more common with SSRIs.

Hypnotics and sedatives

Hypnotics and sedatives are CNS depressants and most can inhibit psychomotor function, delay responsiveness, and impair motor skills and coordination. As such, they may affect ability for safety-critical roles. The duration of effect depends on the half-life of the drug, but most hypnotics produce residual effects the following morning. Effects persist during long-term administration and tolerance or habituation occurs; they are more marked in elderly patients and are potentiated by alcohol and other sedative medication. NICE recommends that people on long-term benzodiazepines should be advised to stop. Benzodiazepine withdrawal should be controlled as otherwise it can produce seizures and a characteristic syndrome, including anxiety, sleeplessness, perceptual disturbances, and depersonalization.

Benzodiazepines are the most commonly used hypnotics for the short-term relief of severe or disabling anxiety. Individual benzodiazepines differ in their effects on psychomotor performance; as hypnotics, short-acting drugs, such as temazepam, are less likely than nitrazepam to have hangover effects; as anxiolytics, clobazam appears to have less effect on performance, particularly memory, than lorazepam and diazepam. Benzodiazepines and newer hypnotics and anxiolytics, such as zaleplon (the 'Z drugs') can cause dizziness, light-headedness, confusion, and visual disturbances.

Antipsychotic drugs

Antipsychotic drugs are used mainly for schizophrenia and bipolar disorder but can also be used in severe anxiety or depression and acute psychosis from any cause. The older or 'typical' medications such as the phenothiazines (e.g. chlorpromazine) and the butyrophenones (e.g. haloperidol) act by blocking the action of dopamine. Side effects include extrapyramidal symptoms, such as parkinsonian effects which can interfere significantly with performance for which anticholinergic drugs can be effective; tardive dyskinesis affects about 1 in 20 people every year. Interference with hypothalamic temperature regulation and cholinergic control of sweating can occur in extreme temperatures, leading to hypo- or hyperthermia. Other potential effects on function include slowness of thinking and akathisia. Chlorpromazine can cause blurred vision with corneal and lens opacities possible with chronic high-dose therapy. Thioridazine can cause a pigmentary retinopathy and reduced visual acuity.

The 'atypical drugs' have less of a dopamine-blocking effect but some additional effects of neurotransmitters such as serotonin. They include clozapine, olanzapine, risperidone, and quetiapine. They are also used for depression in combination with an antidepressant. Compared to the older drugs, they are less likely to cause parkinsonian effects or tardive dyskinesis but more likely to raise the risk of cardiovascular disease, diabetes, and weight gain. Clozapine appears more effective with reduced common side effects but it can affect the bone marrow, reducing white cell count, so isn't the first line of treatment.

Flupentixol is mainly prescribed as a depot injection. It has a predominantly alerting effect and hence less effect on performance than the more sedative phenothiazines.

Lithium

Lithium is used in the prophylaxis and treatment of mania, hypomania, and depression in bipolar disorder and recurrent unipolar depression. It is also used as an augmenter in treatment-resistant depression. Careful monitoring is required due to its narrow therapeutic/toxic ratio. Toxicity is aggravated by hyponatraemia so diuretics and dietary changes that might alter sodium intake should be avoided and adequate fluid intake maintained. Postural hypotension can cause problems, particularly in hot environments. Lithium can also cause polyuria and polydipsia, resulting in further toxicity. Lithium can cause tremor that can persist after stopping the drug. It is associated with only mild cognitive and memory impairment during long-term use. Reduced performance, increased morbidity, and sickness absence can result because of adverse reactions.

Antiepileptic drugs

Antiepileptic drugs (AEDs) allow normal careers for most epilepsy sufferers, usually by long-term monotherapy. For some, occupation will be affected, particularly with combination therapy and those performing safety-critical roles (see Chapter 24). Safety-critical roles should be restricted during dosage adjustment. The wide range of AEDs increases the likelihood of achieving successful treatment without significant side effects. Combination therapy is considered when treatment with two first-line AEDs has failed or improved control occurs when two medications are taken simultaneously during a planned withdrawal.

The clinical classification of epilepsy, the risk of adverse effects, and interactions are key in determining initial monotherapy for each patient. Lamotrigine is commonly prescribed for focal-onset seizures, with carbamazepine and levetiracetam as alternatives. Lamotrigine is also licensed for use as a mood stabilizer.

Any decision to cease long-term therapy after a number of years of being symptom free usually involves a period of driving cessation under DVLA regulations. This can be a discouragement to discontinuation, particularly for those in safety-critical roles.

Chronic anticonvulsant therapy is associated with impairment of cognition and concentration, which is greater with polytherapy, and with phenytoin. There is evidence to suggest that some of the newer AEDs (e.g. lamotrigine) are better tolerated with fewer cognitive effects.

Useful dose–response and dose–toxicity relationships support monitoring for carbamazepine and phenytoin but not for sodium valproate or any of the newer AEDs.

Antihistamines

Antihistamines are available in a variety of formulations and GSL medications. Most older compounds are short-acting and associated with sedation, dry mouth, and blurred vision, and potentiate the actions of alcohol. The newer, first-line antihistamines, such as cetirizine and fexofenadine, are non-sedating. They cause less sedation and psychomotor impairment and do not impair fitness to drive or operate machinery.

Antimigraine drugs

The 5-hydroxytryptamine type 1 agonists (such as naratriptan and sumatriptan), used for acute migraine, can cause drowsiness and should be used with care in patients with cardiac disease. Other drugs, used as prevention, such as pizotifen, are associated with dizziness and postural hypotension.

Drugs for Parkinson's disease

Parkinson's disease is the second commonest neurodegenerative disorder; 40% of those affected are under 65 years and 5–10% under 45 years. With an increasing working age, a greater proportion of employees experience dysfunction. Symptoms often predate diagnosis, including fatigue, reduced concentration, and sleep disturbance. Co-morbid depression affects 60% of patients. Levodopa, the mainstay of medication treatment, improves motor function by its dopaminergic effects; it is used in conjunction with carbidopa. Dopamine agonists such as rotigotine can be used alongside dopamine but may cause confusion or hallucinations. Dopamine dysregulation syndrome occurs in 10% of patients. It causes erratic risk-taking behaviour change that can have important implications for work (including excessive drug taking, alcohol use, sexual promiscuity, and gambling), especially at the start of treatment and times of dosage change.

Hypotensive reactions can occur during the initial days of treatment with dopamine receptor agonists, levodopa, and selegiline, when care should be taken when driving or operating machinery. Blurred vision can complicate the use of most anti-Parkinsonism drugs.

Medications for multiple sclerosis

Multiple sclerosis is the commonest neurological condition in young adults (see Chapter 23). Natalizumab, an intravenous monoclonal antibody, reduces the relapse rate by 80%, allowing increased function and return to work; it is associated with a 1:1000 risk of progressive multifocal encephalopathy, a fatal viral infection of the brain. Fingolimod, a sphingosine-1-phosphate receptor modulator, is claimed to reduce relapse rates by 60%, can be taken orally, and has not been associated with progressive multifocal encephalopathy. Employers may need to consider adjustments to allow attendance for injection-administered treatment and absences secondary to side effects (e.g. flu-like symptoms with interferon). Duloxetine is beneficial in addressing coexistent depression and painful peripheral neuropathy.

In January 2018, ocrelizumab was approved by the European Medicines Agency for both relapsing and primary progressive multiple sclerosis. It is given by intravenous infusion and was well tolerated during research trials.

Autonomic nervous system

Antimuscarinic medications (such as oxybutynin and pilocarpine) can cause blurred vision, which can affect night driving. Mydriatic eye drops, such as homatropine and cyclopentolate, paralyse accommodation and produce blurred vision.

Anaesthetics

The effect of anaesthesia on fitness for work relates to recovery time from general anaesthesia. For in-patient anaesthesia, the symptoms of the condition usually necessitate sickness absence until after the anaesthetic effects have abated. Following general anaesthesia for day surgery, patients should not drive or operate machinery for 24 hours. A greater number of procedures are now performed under local anaesthesia. Nerve root blocks reduce the short-term effects of the anaesthetic as well as the risk of negative effects particularly in those with multimorbidities.

Cardiovascular medication

Adverse reactions from cardiovascular medication are relatively common and some are disabling. It is advisable to start such medication or to have dose increments on rest days. Visual disturbances may occur with disopyramide, flecainide, propafenone, and the lipid-regulating agent, gemfibrozil, and most patients taking amiodarone develop corneal microdeposits, sometimes with night glare. Fibrates, statins, and dipyridamole can cause myalgia or myositis, which can affect physical performance.

Antihypertensive drugs

Antihypertensive treatment is common in working populations. All antihypertensive drugs have the potential to cause hypotension, such as alpha blockers and beta blockers with vasodilatory properties, such as carvedilol and labetalol. Diuretics increase the risk of dehydration at high temperatures and are not the antihypertensive drugs of choice for employees working in hot environments. Antihypertensive drugs such as low-dose thiazides, calcium channel blockers, and angiotensin-converting enzyme inhibitors do not have important central effects and do not appear to affect performance.

Beta blockers, especially the more lipophilic agents, such as propranolol, can affect psychomotor functions, which return to normal after about 3 weeks. Aircrew are permitted by the Civil Aviation Authority to take specified beta blockers, but only after careful specialist evaluation and simulation testing with a period of ground duties necessary after starting treatment. Reduced exercise tolerance has been reported with all beta blockers, without significant differences between cardioselective drugs and non-selective drugs. Both types significantly increase the sense of fatigue during exercise, and a given workload appears subjectively more difficult to achieve. Beta blockers can produce bronchospasm in susceptible people which should be considered when prescribing for employees working in irritant atmospheres. Exacerbation of Raynaud's phenomenon and cold intolerance is important in cold working environments.

Anticoagulants

Workers requiring long-term anticoagulation need careful risk assessment in terms of potential injuries at work and ensuring regular therapeutic monitoring.

Multiple anticoagulants exist on the market, including warfarin and direct oral anticoagulants (DOACs; e.g. dabigatran, rivaroxaban, and apixaban). Common indications include atrial fibrillation, venous thromboembolism, valvular heart disease, and thrombotic disorders. Bleeding risk increases during the initial phase of warfarin treatment and during intercurrent illnesses that may affect warfarin intake absorption or metabolism (e.g. diarrhoea, fever, heart, and liver failure). Other cautions include alcohol intake, previous cardiovascular and gastrointestinal disorders, age, history of bleeding, and polypharmacy. The intracranial bleeding risk with DOACs is lower than with warfarin.

Anticoagulation point of care testing and self-monitoring is increasing in use. In cases of warfarin-related bleeding, management (active reversal) depends on the international normalized ratio. DOACs do not require such regular monitoring and have fewer restrictions on lifestyle such as alcohol intake. However, only dabigatran has a reversal agent if bleeding occurs.

Combining clinical assessment alongside individual risk assessments of the workplace and of the individual's job role will guide OH advice. Those in heavy physical roles, or work associated with injury (e.g. sharp equipment, working at height, confined spaces, and safety-critical roles) may need work adjustments, personal protective equipment, or reassignment of job roles. Employees working with moving machinery and sharps should be trained, supervised, and use appropriate safety equipment. Furthermore, safety guards alongside jigs, holders, and push sticks can be used to prevent access to dangerous parts. Machinery maintenance, good record-keeping, and regular risk assessments can reduce the risk. In certain occupations (e.g. firefighting), the use of anticoagulants may be considered a contraindication to operational roles.

Analgesics and non-steroidal anti-inflammatory drugs

Both short- and long-term use of analgesics and NSAIDs can have side effects, including marked sedation and cognitive impairment (particularly for opioids, e.g. morphine). Risk assessments are required for employees in safety-critical roles. Codeine and dihydrocodeine can affect driving-related skills and have implications for drug screening (see Chapter 14). The effects vary between employees, doses, and formulations. Alcohol potentiates the effects of all opioid analgesics. Indomethacin impairs laboratory tests of driving-related skills. NSAIDs, even the cyclooxygenase-2 inhibitors, can cause gastro-intestinal irritation and sometimes gastric bleeding, renal impairment (with long-term use), and increased cardiovascular risk. High doses of salicylates can be ototoxic and in-crease the harmful effects of noise exposure.

Of the disease-modifying antirheumatic drugs, methotrexate, a drug initially intro-duced for its antiproliferative effects, is used in much lower doses in rheumatoid arthritis, psoriasis, and autoimmune inflammatory conditions (e.g. sarcoidosis). While significant side effects may occur (e.g. bone marrow suppression, hepatotoxicity, and pulmonary fibrosis), this drug lessens the requirement for high-dose steroids and their associated debilitating side effects. Despite successfully managing the inflammatory effects, common side effects of malaise and nausea can limit function during the 24 hours following the weekly dose, with potential effects on attendance and performance. Even if taken at week-ends, these effects can continue into the working week. Good education can assist the employer with appropriate adjustments, including variation of working hours or duties to support safety and function. For patients with significant side effects from oral medica-tion, subcutaneous administration or increasing oral folic acid rescue to daily rather than weekly can be effective at reducing side effects.

Hypoglycaemic drugs

Hypoglycaemia, especially in the absence of warning signs, is one of the most incapacitating effects of treatment for diabetes mellitus (see Chapter 25). Insulin-dependent workers are most affected, but also those taking sulphonylureas (e.g. gliclazide). Many road acci-dents caused by hypoglycaemia occur because drivers continue driving despite warning symptoms of hypoglycaemia. Assessment of an employee's degree of glycaemic control is essential, especially for safety-critical roles. Care is needed to ensure that employees recognize the warning signs and act accordingly. Where hypoglycaemic awareness has been lost, driving may be restricted. Beta blockers can also blunt the peripheral effects of hypoglycaemia, apart from sweating. The use of insulin pump technology and continuous glycaemic monitoring is resulting in significant improvements for diabetic workers, espe-cially if shift or safety-critical work is required.

Further guidance on driving and diabetes is provided in Chapter 15 and Chapter 25, respectively.

Anticancer medications

Many employees continue working while undergoing chemotherapy, assisted by flexible working arrangements. Oral (rather than intravenous) treatment options are increasingly available and preferred by patients. The nature of employment and safety-critical work influence the need for restrictions. Employees who travel oversees are often unable to work during treatment. Side effects from chemotherapy can affect employees during immediate treatment (see Chapter 35). Chemoprevention can result in common side effects (e.g. hot flushes and sweating with tamoxifen), as well as the less common visual disturbances (corneal opacities, cataracts, and retinopathy) and an increased risk of thromboembolism.

Anti-infective agents

Gastrointestinal symptoms are common, although they rarely affect function significantly. Serious diarrhoea with *Clostridium difficile* is associated with broad-spectrum antibiotic use. The fluoroquinolones, such as ciprofloxacin, can affect performance of skilled tasks, such as driving, enhance the effects of alcohol, and elevate the risk of Achilles tendon rupture. The risk of convulsions is increased, particularly if they are used with NSAIDs. Many antimicrobials, for example, the cephalosporins, can cause dizziness. The antituberculosis drug ethambutol can cause reduced visual acuity and colour blindness; immediate discontinuation of therapy is required in such circumstances. Ototoxic drugs, such as gentamicin, can cause vestibular damage, increasing the harmful effects of noise exposure. QT prolongation can occur, especially with co-treatment with macrolides, fluoroquinolones, antimalarials, pentamidine, and azole antifungals.

Malaria prophylaxis

Side effects of antimalarials should be considered in occupational travellers. Chloroquine can be associated with visual disturbances. Mefloquine causes frequent mild dizziness or disturbed balance, but is associated with significant transient neuropsychiatric reactions (the frequency is 1 in 13,000 during prophylactic use, and 1 in 215 with therapeutic use). Symptoms include disorientation, mental confusion, hallucinations, agitation, and reduced consciousness. Unpredictable reactions can be provoked by concomitant use of CNS-active drugs and alcohol. To determine tolerance and to establish habit, prophylaxis should generally be started 2–3 weeks before travel with mefloquine, 1 week with Malarone®, and 1–2 days before travel for doxycycline.

Steroids

Steroids are used for a wide range of medical conditions, in high doses for acute inflammation and lower doses for maintenance. Prolonged use can cause causes osteoporosis, diabetes, and psychiatric reactions. Higher doses of steroids are often used while other treatment is established, such as methotrexate in rheumatoid arthritis. Temporary absence is sometimes required at such times. Function can be affected by adverse effects, such as general malaise, weight gain, and effects on mood and appetite.

Impact of prescribed medication on fitness for specific work

Good occupational health practice

It is essential to assess the benefits of medication and to support employees taking medication to reduce the risk of harm (Box 13.7). Most employees take their responsibilities seriously, but some fail to report poorly controlled illnesses or adverse drug reactions. For safety and to comply with legislation, employers should have procedures to control the risks associated with medication use:

♦ Access to expert advice concerning the effects of medicines.

♦ Provision of training and information for managers and employees.

♦ A requirement for employees to report the use of medication to a responsible person.

♦ A process for risk assessing duties for individuals who report safety effects.

In OH, self-report is the main source of information about prescribed medication. OH professionals may review workers with health problems, and identify positive or untoward medication effects opportunistically. Occupational physicians practise with the understanding of not being the patient's treating physician but have the same priority to actively consider therapeutic efficacy. Communication across specialties including occupational medicine is encouraged as part of medicines optimization to share data about medication effects and potential non-compliance.

Use of medications by the self-employed and employees without access to OH requires particular consideration, if employees work in safety-critical roles.

Box 13.7 Measures to encourage safer use of medications

♦ Clear supportive methods to report medication concerns.

♦ Encourage employees to report new or long-term treatment, or changes to medications or dosages.

♦ Specific enquiry about employees' medications, including GSL medicines.

♦ Educate employees about possible adverse reactions.

♦ Educate employees about the potential risks of online pharmacies.

♦ Advice on alternative GSL medication with fewer adverse reactions.

♦ Improve links with prescribers, including enquiry about medications in requests for reports from treating physicians.

♦ Encourage employers to maintain self-referral options.

Box 13.8 Practical measures for medication management

- Highlight medication times with instructions on the person, at the workstation, by personal alarm, or use of pill-dispensing containers.
- Flexible work routines to accommodate medication needs.
- Advise the employer, with the employee's consent, of the risk of serious drug reactions.
- Employee education about potential hazards of operating machinery or vehicles with drowsiness related to new medication or dose changes.
- Encourage employers to provide safe, secure storage for medication, including fridges, sharps containers, and private space for administration of medications.

Workplace solutions and adjustments

Practical measures for medication management are listed in Box 13.8.

Prescribing in occupational health

Prescribing is required less in OH than in other specialties. However, knowledge about the benefits and potential harms of medication is essential. Common types of prescriptions in occupational medicine are listed in Box 13.9; guidance on prescription writing is provided in the *BNF*.

The General Medical Council's 'Good practice in prescribing and managing medicines and devices' (2013) outlines the responsibilities for prescribing physicians and incorporates 'Remote prescribing via telephone, video-link or online' (2012). Practitioners should also refer to 'Good Occupational Medical Practice' from the Faculty of Occupational Medicine. Practitioners are advised to adopt electronic and other systems to improve the safety of prescribing. Patient group directions are often used in OH to enable nurse practitioners to carry out limited drug administration and immunization under physician signed responsibility (Box 13.10).

Box 13.9 Practitioner responsibilities

- Prescribe treatment with adequate knowledge of the patient's health and when satisfied that the treatment serves the patient's needs.
- Provide effective treatments based on the best available evidence and proper assessments of the benefit-to-harm balance.
- Keep clear, accurate, and legible records of any prescribed drugs.
- Inform primary care physicians of prescriptions.

Box 13.10 Common prescriptions in occupational health

- Vaccinations for healthcare workers, for example, measles, mumps, and rubella (MMR), and hepatitis B.
- Vaccinations for travel overseas, and antimalarial drugs.
- Mantoux test/Bacillus Calmette–Guérin (BCG) inoculation.
- Post-exposure prophylaxis for high-risk, needle-stick injuries.
- Treatment for work-related infections (mainly in healthcare), for example, scabies or methicillin-resistant *Staphylococcus aureus*.

Robust policies for sourcing post-exposure prophylaxis are essential, especially out of hours, as early treatment is vital.

Resources

Good communication with pharmacists and specialist clinical teams encourages good compliance with prescribing policies. It is good practice to keep abreast of the more commonly used prescription medications and to have reference resources, such as the *BNF*, readily available (see Box 13.11). Practitioners are encouraged to use digital versions of resources for the most recently updated information. For sources of travel health guidance online, see 'Useful websites'.

Suspected adverse reactions should be reported directly under the Yellow Card Scheme (see 'Useful websites'). The MHRA's interactive Drug Analysis Profiles (iDAPs) on the Yellow Card Scheme website are provided for all licensed drugs for which reports have been received about suspected adverse reactions.

Box 13.11 *British National Formulary*

The *BNF* is a joint publication of the British Medical Association and the Royal Pharmaceutical Society, published biannually under the authority of a Joint Formulary Committee. Online access to the full publication with regular newsletters is available, with free access for UK-based individuals undertaking work (or training) for the NHS; there is also access via software applications. The *BNF* includes key information on the selection, prescribing, dispensing, and administration of medicines in the UK. Information is drawn from manufacturers' product literature, medical and pharmaceutical literature, UK health departments, regulatory authorities, and professional bodies. The *BNF* also takes account of authoritative national guidance and guidelines and emerging safety concerns.

Key points

◆ Medication may be necessary to maintain health and thus employability, productivity, safety, and effectiveness in the workplace.

◆ OH can significantly influence the safe management of medications and enquiry about medications should be a standard part of OH practice.

◆ For workers without access to OH, their prescribing doctor should consider the implications of treatment for work.

◆ Inclusion of medication enquiries within the audit of OH records could improve practice surrounding medication management in employees.

◆ Continued development of links between OH and prescribers is required, including a greater recognition and involvement of OH as a specialty in medicines optimization.

Useful websites

British National Formulary	http://www.bnf.org
Medicines and Healthcare products Regulatory Agency. 'Yellow Card Scheme'	http://www.mhra.gov.uk/yellowcard
DVLA. 'Assessing Fitness to Drive: A Guide for Medical Professionals'	https://www.gov.uk/guidance/assessing-fitness-to-drive-a-guide-for-medical-professionals
General Medical Council. 'Good practice in prescribing and managing medicines and devices'	https://www.gmc-uk.org/ethical-guidance/ethical-guidance-for-doctors/prescribing-and-managing-medicines-and-devices
Faculty of Occupational Medicine. 'Good Occupational Medical Practice'	http://www.fom.ac.uk/gomp/gomp-2017
Travel abroad	
Medical Advisory Service for Travellers Abroad (MASTA)	http://masta-travel-health.com
National Travel Health Network and Centre (NaTHNaC)	http://www.nathnac.net
NHS	http://www.travax.nhs.uk

References

1. **Royal Pharmaceutical Society**. Medicines optimisation: helping patients to make the most of medicines. Good practice guidance for healthcare professionals in England. 2013. Available at: https://www.rpharms.com/Portals.

2. **NHS Digital**. Prescriptions dispensed in the community, statistics for England – 2006–2016. Available at: https://digital.nhs.uk/data-and-information/publications/statistical/prescriptions-dispensed-in-the-community/prescriptions-dispensed-in-the-community-statistics-for-england-2006-2016-pas.

3. **The NHS Information Centre, Prescribing Support Unit, Lloyd D.** *General Pharmaceutical Services in England 2000–01 to 2009–10.* Version 1.0. London: NHS Information Centre; 2010.

4. **Information Services Division Scotland**. Prescribing and medicines: dispenser payments and prescription cost analysis 2016/2017. Available at: https://www.isdscotland.org/Health-Topics/Prescribing-and-Medicines/Publications/2017-08-29/2017-08-29-Dispenser-Payments-and-Prescription-Cost-Analysis-Summary.pdf.

5. **Welsh Government**. Prescriptions dispensed in the community. Available at: http://gov.wales/docs/statistics/2017/170524-prescriptions-dispensed-community-2016-en.pdf.

6. **Health and Social Care Information Centre (HSCIC), Office of Health Economics**. Health services data. Available at: http://www.ohe.org/page/health-statistics/access-the-data/health-service/data.cfm.

7. **NHS Digital**. Prescriptions dispensed in the community England 2006 to 2016. 2017. Available at: https://files.digital.nhs.uk/publication/s/o/pres-disp-com-eng-2006-16-rep.pdf.

8. **Aronson JK.** From prescription-only to over-the-counter medicines ('PoM to P'): time for an intermediate category. *Br Med Bull* 2009;**90**:63–9.

9. **Hargie ODW, Morrow NC.** Introducing interpersonal skill training into the pharmaceutical curriculum. *Int Pharm J* 1987;**1**:175–8.

10. **Moclair A, Evans D.** Vocational qualifications for pharmacy support staff. *Pharm J* 1994;**252**:631.

11. **Pharmaceutical Services Negotiating Committee**. Distance selling pharmacies. Available at: https://psnc.org.uk/contract-it/market-entry-regulations/distance-selling-pharmacies/.

12. **General Pharmaceutical Council**. Internet pharmacy. Available at: https://www.pharmacyregulation.org/registration/internet-pharmacy.

13. **Medicines and Healthcare products Regulatory Agency**. New mandatory logo for selling medicines online. Available at: https://www.gov.uk/government/news/new-mandatory-logo-for-selling-medicines-online.

14. **Aronson JK.** Adverse drug reactions: history, terminology, classification, causality, frequency, preventability. In: Talbot J, Aronson JK (eds), *Stephens' Detection and Evaluation of Adverse Drug Reactions: Principles and Practice*, 6th edn, pp. 1–119. Oxford: Wiley-Blackwell, 2011.

15. **Frontier Economics**. *The Department of Health, Exploring the Costs of Unsafe Care in the NHS: A Report Prepared for the Department of Health.* London: Frontier Economics Ltd; 2014.

16. **Swales CL.** *A Study to Determine the Prevalence of Adverse Side Effects Arising from the Use of Prescription and Non-Prescription Medication on a Chemical Manufacturing Site.* MFOM Dissertation, Royal College of Physicians, Faculty of Occupational Medicine, 1999.

17. **Nicholson AN, Stone BM.** Disturbance of circadian rhythms and sleep. *Proc R Soc Edin Sect B Biol Sci* 1985;**82B**:135–9.

18. **Nakano S.** Time of day effect on psychotherapeutic drug response and kinetics in man. In: Takahashi R, Holberg F, Walker CA (eds), *Towards Chronopharmacology*, pp. 51–9. Oxford: Pergamon Press; 1982.

19. **Hunter J, Maxwell JD, Stewart DA, et al.** Increased hepatic microsomal enzyme activity from occupational exposure to certain organochlorine pesticides. *Nature* 1972;**237**:399–401.

20. **The Scottish Government**. (Revised) guidance for the safe delivery of systemic anti-cancer therapy. CEL30. 2012. Available at: http://www.sehd.scot.nhs.uk/mels/CEL2012_30.pdf.

21. **Health and Safety Executive**. Handling cytotoxic drugs in isolators in NHS pharmacies. MS37. 2015. Available at: http://www.hse.gov.uk/pubns/ms37.htm.

22. **Health and Safety Executive**. 2017. Safe handling of cytotoxic drugs in the workplace. Available at: http://www.hse.gov.uk/healthservices/safe-use-cytotoxic-drugs.htm.

23. **Hindmarch I.** Psychomotor function and psychoactive drugs. *Br J Clin Pharmacol* 1980;10: 189–209.

24. **Barbone F, McMahon AD, Davey PG, et al.** Association of road-traffic accidents with benzodiazepine use. *Lancet* 1998;352:1331–6.

Chapter 14

Drugs and alcohol in the workplace

David Brown and David Rhinds

Introduction

Drug and alcohol misuse is present at all levels of society and throughout the world although the patterns of use, the substances involved, and the prevailing attitudes vary widely. However it presents, drug and alcohol misuse is a particularly challenging issue for employers, managers, and occupational health (OH) professionals. This includes the effects of drugs and alcohol on health and well-being and the direct and indirect impact on output, performance, and behaviour at work. There are legal implications if employees are under the influence of alcohol or drugs or in possession of illegal drugs where there may be a degree of vicarious liability for the employer. A lack of under-standing and stigmatization may lead to limited tolerance towards such individuals, and there may be significant issues regarding public confidence towards those working in safety-critical industries. While awareness of alcohol-related problems in society and the workplace appears to be increasing, the distinction between what is social drinking and problematic drinking is often blurred.

Prevalence

Alcohol

Alcohol is 'Britain's favourite drug' and most adults drink sensibly. However, over 7% of adults regularly drink over the Chief Medical Officer's low-risk guidelines and 2.5 million people report drinking over 14 units on their heaviest drinking days. About 28.9 million people in Great Britain (58% of the population) report drinking alcohol in the previous week.[1]

Drugs

According to the 2015/2016 Crime Survey for England and Wales, 8.4% of adults aged 16–59 had used illicit drugs (almost 2.7 million people) and 3% had used a class A drug in the last year (just under 1 million people). These estimates were similar to the 2014/2015 survey; however, they are statistically significantly lower than a decade ago.[2]

Alcohol-related harm

Drinking is associated with more physical, psychological, and social harm than any other drug, including tobacco. In the UK in 2015, there were 8758 alcohol-related deaths with the highest morbidity rates in the 55–64 years age group.[3] Alcohol harms are estimated to cost the NHS around £3.5 billion annually. In 2014/2015, there were 1.1 million estimated admissions where an alcohol-related disease, injury, or condition was the primary reason for admission or a secondary diagnosis. This is 30% more than 2013/2014.[1] There are an estimated 704,000 incidents per year of alcohol-related violence and despite over 30 years of drink–drive education and enforcement, over 70,000 cases of drink-driving.[1]

Occupation

According to the 2011 General Lifestyle Survey, men and women aged 16–64 years and in employment were more likely to have drunk alcohol in the previous week compared to individuals who were unemployed or economically inactive.[4] The type of occupation also has an impact on drinking patterns and levels of consumption. Occupations known to have a high risk of morbidity and mortality from alcohol-related disease include publicans, bar staff, male caterers, cooks, kitchen porters, and seafarers.[5] Men whose jobs are classified as 'routine', such as van drivers and labourers, face a 3.5 times higher risk of dying from an alcohol-related disease than those in higher managerial and professional jobs. Women in 'routine' jobs, such as cleaners and sewing machinists, face a 5.7 times higher chance of dying from an alcohol-related disease than women in higher professional jobs such as doctors and lawyers.[4]

Recent data quoted by the Chartered Institute of Personnel and Development (CIPD) from Crossland Employment Solutions in 2016 suggests that one in five UK employees admits to regularly taking drugs and one-third suspect a colleague may have a drug problem.[6]

Impact of substance misuse in the workplace

In 2009, work-related alcohol misuse was estimated to cost the UK economy up to £6.4 billion per year and in 2010, the UK government estimated that there were up to 17 million working days lost annually in the UK from alcohol misuse.[7] The taking of drugs and alcohol at work has a negative impact on productivity as well as on the quality of work produced.[8] This may impact cognitive performance, affecting performance and safety at work. The implications for safety and its cost are more difficult to quantify.

Driving and work-related incidents

Many people in employment will drive, either to get to work or as part of their job. Drugs and alcohol are significant factors in road traffic accidents. OH professionals and employers should be aware of the Driver and Vehicle Licensing Agency (DVLA) guidelines (see 'Useful websites') and the need for the employee to inform the DVLA should they have a drug or alcohol problem and to be aware that they will not be insured should they have an accident. OH professionals should also be aware of General Medical Council guidelines about breaching confidentiality should the patient continue to drive despite being advised not to (see 'Useful websites').

Driving and alcohol

After consuming alcohol, the risk of causing a driving accident increases 3-, 10-, and 40-fold if the blood alcohol concentration (BAC) exceeds 80, 100, or 150 mg/100 mL, respectively. Driving at levels below the prescribed BAC introduced in the Road Traffic Act 1967 (80 mg/100 mL) is not free from hazards.[9] Even 'safe' levels of alcohol may be associated with significant impairment of driving ability. Drivers who have consumed moderate doses of alcohol and have BACs of 30–60 mg/100 mL have an impaired ability to negotiate a test course with artificial hazards. There is a body of evidence which shows that all of the drugs listed in the new drug-driving law (see 'Drug-driving'), prescription and illicit, result in a significantly greater road safety risk when taken in combination with alcohol, even in small amounts.

Drug-driving

On 2 March 2015, eight prescription and eight illicit drugs were added into new regulations that came into force in England and Wales. Regulations on amphetamine came into force on 14 April 2015.[10] These related to a new offence in regard to driving with a specific controlled drug in the body above that drug's accepted limit. The aim was to reduce expense, effort, and time wasted from prosecutions that failed because of difficulties proving that a particular drug impaired a driver. Limits were set at a level where any claims of accidental exposure can be ruled out. A risk-based approach was adopted for eight drugs associated with medical use, with that for amphetamine balanced between medical use and abuse (Table 14.1).

Table 14.1 Drugs defined in UK driving regulations

Prescription drugs	Illicit drugs
Clonazepam	Benzoylecgonine
Diazepam	Cocaine
Flunitrazepam	Cannabis
Lorazepam	Ketamine
Methadone	LSD
Morphine and opiates	Methylamphetamine
Temazepam	MDMA
Oxazepam	Heroin

Drugs in the workplace

The evidence base of how drug impairment affects safety in the workplace remains relatively small. In practice, many OH professionals will be able to cite specific cases of the noxious impact of drug use by an employee on both work performance and safety, but this experience is not yet supported by published well-designed studies.

Cannabis

Cannabis is the most used illicit drug in the UK.[2] Over the last 15 years, increasingly potent forms have become available including 'skunk', a selective breed of cannabis with two or three times the tetrahydrocannabinol content of normal cannabis weed. Cannabis can have an adverse effect on any complex learnt psychomotor tasks involving memory, judgement, skill, concentration, sense of time, orientation in three-dimensional space, and on the performance of multiple complex tasks. Psychophysiological activities impaired by cannabis include tracking ability, complex reaction time, hand steadiness, complicated signal interpretation, and attention span. Therefore, work requiring a high level of cognitive integration is adversely affected. Among the consequences of using cannabis is a dose-related memory impairment effect and even moderate cannabis use is associated with selective short-term memory deficits that persist despite weeks of abstinence. A single 'joint' of cannabis can cause measurable impairment of skills for more than 10 hours due to its half-life of 36 hours. Cannabis has a particularly deleterious effect on pilots who have to orientate themselves in three-dimensional space which is particularly crucial for flying a helicopter.[11,12] A review for the UK Department for Transport concluded that the actual effect of cannabis on real driving performance rather than the effects measured in the laboratory were not as pronounced as predicted.[13] While 4–12% of accident fatalities have levels of cannabis detected, the majority of these cases also have detectable levels of alcohol. There is insufficient knowledge concerning detectable levels of cannabis in non-fatal cases to identify a baseline for comparison. However, the combination of alcohol and cannabis increases impairment, accident rate, and accident responsibility.

Prescription-only medications and over-the-counter medications

There are no authoritative data on the number of people affected by dependence and withdrawal. Evidence submitted to the British Medical Association (BMA) estimated that there are over 1 million long-term users of benzodiazepines in the UK, and up to 4 million people taking antidepressants at any one time. These figures need to be treated with caution in the absence of robust data and further research.[14–16]

Further information about prescription-only medication and over-the-counter medication is given in Chapter 13.

Novel or new psychoactive substances

Over the last 10 years, there has been increasing use of club drugs and novel or new psychoactive substances (NPS), formerly called 'legal highs'. Due to the increasing number of NPS obtained both legally and illegally via the Internet, it is not possible to discuss these within the scope of this chapter. However, these drugs may be classified mainly due to whether they are depressant, stimulant, or hallucinogenic. One group of NPS is synthetic cannabinoid receptor agonists (SCRAs) which do not fit neatly into either one of these categories. Currently, hundreds of these compounds are available with street names such as 'black mamba', 'spice', and 'annihilation'. Further information is available from the Novel Psychoactive Treatment UK Network (see 'Useful websites').[17]

Accidents

In the US, there were several critical accidents involving drugs or alcohol during the 1980s and early 1990s, which are thought to have played a part in the introduction of workplace drug and alcohol testing in safety-critical industries.[18]

Data from the UK Marine Accident Investigation Bureau shows that between 2005 and 2014 there were 124 incidents reported involving shipping around the UK where alcohol was a factor, with 11 fatalities and 84 injuries to crew, passengers, and others on board. There were 11 groundings.[19]

Absenteeism

There is strong evidence that alcohol problems affect absenteeism.[1] Problem drinkers have a rate of absence between two and eight times higher than non-problem drinkers.[20] The Whitehall II study found that alcohol consumption, even at moderate levels, led to increased risk for absence due to injury, but with a much weaker relationship to all other absences.[21]

The research evidence may be limited, but the belief that there are clear-cut deleterious effects of drugs and alcohol on work is very strongly held. Many employers consider that both alcohol and drug use are major causes of absenteeism (Box 14.1).[22]

Box 14.1 Drug misuse in the workplace according to employers

- 27% reported problems of some kind.
- 31% reported a negative impact on attendance.
- 27% reported poor employee performance.
- 3% reported damage to their business.
- 3% reported accidents at work.

Source: data from CIPD. (2007) *Managing drug and alcohol misuse at work*. London, UK: CIPD. Copyright © 2007 CIPD.

Presenteeism

Presenteeism is impaired workplace performance resulting from deterioration in quantity and quality of work, impaired judgement and decision-making, reduced reaction times and efficiency, and increased error rates. It can be an after-effect of drinking alcohol, such as a hangover, even though there may be no residual alcohol in the body, and is often associated with sleep deprivation and dehydration. Logically, it should also apply to the after-effects of drugs although the evidence base is small. In an Australian study of 78,000 workers, drug and alcohol use was found to increase the risk of presenteeism by 2.6-fold and 8.6-fold when compounded with the use of psychotropic drugs.[23]

Drug and alcohol at work policies

All employers should have a drug and alcohol policy (Box 14.2).

Overall, health and safety is the predominant reason for introducing drug and alcohol testing in all employment sectors, but particularly safety-critical organizations. Non-safety-critical organizations are more likely to identify employee health as the reason, but there still may be business-critical reasons (e.g. a financier entrusted with investing millions of pounds). A survey of 505 human resources managers in 2007 in the UK showed that about 60% of their companies had policies in place for drug and alcohol problems.[22] These policies included rules concerning the possession of drugs and alcohol on the premises and alcohol consumption during working time. A quarter of respondents used a capability procedure as part of their approach.

Even if there is no formal policy, there is a need for clarity as there is huge variation in what is tolerated at work. Using alcohol as an example, attitudes range from permitting alcohol to be consumed at work through to a zero tolerance policy that expects employees to have no alcohol in their system during working hours. Some employers may ban alcohol at work, but be tolerant of people coming to work regularly with a hangover. The employer may have a differential policy according to the type of work that

---

Box 14.2 Reasons to introduce drugs and alcohol policies

- Mitigate health and safety risks.
- Promote employee health.
- Reduce accident levels.
- Limit employee absence.
- Respond consistently to alcohol/drug-related disciplinary offences.
- Protect organizational reputation.
- Enhance employee performance.
- Protect against the risks from poor decision-making.

the employee does. For example, employees in a large company who work closely with the media or who entertain clients may be permitted to drink while involved in this type of work, whereas employees involved in work that has an impact on safe working or product safety may not be permitted to drink at work at all. Where safety is of paramount importance to the organization, it is not uncommon for a zero alcohol policy to be in place, at least for those directly involved in activities which may affect safe working or product safety. There may, however, be difficulty in differentiating between groups of workers and the policy must avoid any impression of deliberate targeting of individuals (Box 14.3).

Box 14.3 Elements of a drug and alcohol at work policy

+ An explanation of why there is a policy.
+ The scope of the policy—to whom it applies, including whether or not it applies to contractors, consultants, and agencies.
+ The required code of conduct. This is likely to cover:
  • consumption of alcohol while at work or during meal breaks
  • consumption, possession, and storage of drugs at work
  • consumption of alcohol while in uniform.
  • arrival to work when under the influence of drugs/alcohol (zero alcohol, hangovers).
+ An alcohol and drugs testing programme, if used; whether random or routine, and reference to the action that will be taken when an employee has a positive test.
+ The consequences if the policy is breached.
+ Any support that the company offers to someone prepared to address an alcohol problem.
+ The responsibilities of all relevant parties.
+ A requirement not to bring the company into disrepute by being involved in activities related to drugs at work.
+ A requirement to find out about the side effects of prescription-only and over-the-counter medications and declare the medication to the OH professional (or manager) if the side effects could affect performance, safety, safety of others, or quality of the product.
+ Any security considerations, for example, the reporting of positive results in the nuclear industry to the Office for Nuclear Regulation or the need for regulatory bodies (responsible medical officer, General Medical Council, Nursing and Midwifery Council) to be informed in the case of healthcare professionals.

The policy may also contain reference to the use of alcohol in relation to company cars and the procedure for employees who have been banned from driving due to alcohol. The Faculty of Occupational Medicine and the BMA Occupational Medicine Committee have produced guidance on the contents of a drugs and alcohol policy.[24,25]

Implementation of a new policy

Implementation of a new drug and alcohol policy requires a careful prior assessment of the financial and other implications, and clear agreement on who will be responsible for drawing it up. The workforce should be educated about the content and the implementation of the policy, which should be carefully monitored and reviewed. In setting up company drug and alcohol policies, it is essential that wide consultation is held at the draft stages, particularly with staff associations or trade unions. Their acceptance and co-operation is crucial to success.

Training for managers

It is useful if training and information on awareness of drug and alcohol-related issues is included as part of people management training. This would usually include information about the company's policy, how to recognize potential problems (see Box 14.4), how to arrange testing if this is available, and what support is available. Guidance should also be provided on how to handle those smelling of alcohol at work. Unfortunately, surveys have shown that only 33% of managers have received training in handling drug and alcohol misuse at work.[20]

Box 14.4 Possible signs of drug and alcohol misuse

- Short-term sickness absence, especially recurrent Mondays.
- Lateness.
- Unkempt appearance.
- Involvement in accidents and assaults.
- Inappropriately aggressive behaviour.
- Worsening performance.
- Unreliability in someone previously reliable.
- Smelling of alcohol.
- Shaking/tremor/sweating.
- Pinpoint or very large pupils.
- Inability to concentrate.

Referral to occupational health

This section assumes that the manager has access to OH advice, although this is not always the case. Ideally managers will identify the warning signs described previously, discuss their concerns with the individual, and refer them for assessment by OH. It is common for managers who suspect a problem to find it difficult to discuss these openly and honestly with the person concerned. Most OH professionals will be familiar with the scenario in which a manager contacts them, describes behaviour that is strongly suggestive of a problem, and then suggests that they refer the person to OH 'so that you can just ask about drug or alcohol use in passing'. This is a recipe for an unsuccessful consultation and the manager should be advised that these issues cannot be assessed unless the employee has been made aware of the manager's concerns.

In some companies there is a contractual requirement for employees to attend the OH department if their managers refer them. In such companies it is essential for the manager to explain to the individual what they have observed and why they are making a referral, and then confirm this in writing. Even where this occurs in an unequivocal way, the employee may deny it and state that they have no idea why they have been referred. If the manager requests that the employee attend OH, and the employee refuses, the manager will need to document this and then take action without the benefit of an OH assessment.

Drug and alcohol assessment

The assessment is twofold. The first part is to identify whether the employee has a significant drug or alcohol problem and if so, the nature and severity of it as well as the individual's willingness to address the issue.

The second part is to advise the employee and their manager on whether they are fit to work and if so, whether adjustments are needed. These assessments are among the most challenging in OH practice. Underreporting is often a prominent feature for those with substance misuse, but the employee may have concerns that disclosing the full extent of their substance misuse might negatively impact their career. One of the aims of the initial session is to help the employee to understand that this is an opportunity to finally address an issue that in many cases may be long-standing, often with significant existing negative repercussions on family and personal quality of life.

The assessment by the OH professional should include taking a full history of drug or alcohol use, examination, and appropriate investigations. A variety of questionnaires may be useful and those available for the identification of alcohol misuse include the Alcohol Use Disorders Identification Test (AUDIT-C)[26] or the Severity of Alcohol Dependence Questionnaire (SADQ).[27] For alcohol, blood tests may assist (gamma-glutamyl transferase, alanine transferase, mean corpuscular volume, carbohydrate deficient transferrin) but are rarely diagnostic on their own and in some cases, may be normal in employees who subsequently admit to a serious problem.[28] However, a combination of raised test results and a corroborative history and examination increases predictive value. The use of near patient testing (breathalyser for alcohol and dipsticks for drugs) can give immediate feedback.

In one OH centre that employs addiction specialists, assessment is undertaken over a period of 3 weeks, using questionnaires, assessment in a series of groups and through one-to-one enquiry, liver function blood tests, and breath or urine testing for alcohol and/ or drugs. This is an unusually thorough provision and is unfortunately becoming rarer in the UK due to the reduction in addiction specialists, but gives an idea of the complexity of this area of diagnosis. Treatment should be tailored according to the severity of the addiction problem as the degree of drug and alcohol use and misuse lies on a spectrum, from social use not associated with harm, through to harmful use, and to dependence.

Dependence syndrome

The dependence syndrome is at the severe end of the spectrum for substance use disorder and not all hazardous or harmful drinkers will become dependent. According to the tenth revision of the International Classification of Diseases (ICD-10) classification, the dependence syndrome is a cluster of behavioural, cognitive, and physiological phenomena that develop after repeated substance use. The dependence syndrome is diagnosed if three or more features have occurred together for the last year (Box 14.5).

In cases of harmful use, an initial brief intervention may be all that is necessary to avoid further misuse of substances, but for most people whose drug and alcohol use is detected at work, the issues may well be far greater, as their use will have likely escalated from recreational use at weekends to daily. For the majority of cases, referral or self-referral to a local addiction service should be instigated and information on local mutual aid groups such as Alcoholics Anonymous, Narcotics Anonymous, or SMART Recovery should be provided (see 'Useful websites'). Harm minimization advice should also be given making dependent drinkers aware that they should not stop drinking alcohol abruptly due to risk of seizures, but to keep drink diaries and to try to gradually reduce their drinking

Box 14.5 Features of the dependence syndrome

- A strong desire or compulsion to take the substance.
- Impaired capacity to control substance use.
- Physiological withdrawal state on stopping or reduction of substance use.
- Evidence of tolerance, that is, increased amounts of the substance are required to produce the same effects.
- Preoccupation with substance misuse resulting in neglect of other interests.
- Persistent substance use despite clear evidence of harmful consequences.

Source: data from ICD-10, Available at: http://apps.who.int/classifications/icd10/browse/2010/en.

in amounts of 1–2 units a day. Thiamine (100 mg twice daily) and multivitamins should be prescribed for prophylaxis of Wernicke's encephalopathy. Patients addicted to opioids and other medications such a gabapentinoids should be made aware of the potential risk of overdose.

Features of under-reporting minimizing drinking and drug-taking behaviour

Patients with drug and alcohol problems often minimize the nature or extent of their problems, especially when first raised by their manager. Such underreporting should be dealt with firmly, but sensitively, as it is rarely productive to engage in directly confrontational arguments about whether or not someone is addicted. However, a carefully considered history and examination encouraging curious discussion by an experienced clinician can be helpful. The clinical interview should focus on the evidence available, and on the realities of the workplace. Thus, to say 'the problem is that you have lost 12 hours' work over the last month due to lateness on Monday mornings' is preferable to 'the problem is that you are obviously an alcoholic'. The former can lead to constructive discussion, which may eventually lead to admission of the underlying cause of the problem. The latter is likely to lead to outright denial, anger, and breakdown of trust. If motivational interviewing techniques are used to explore ambivalence in a non-threatening way, the patient may experience some discomfort or cognitive dissonance, when they realize that their beliefs do not match their behaviours. For example, a patient may believe that drinking alcohol prior to giving a presentation at work may make them confident when in fact the audience are aware that they are slightly disinhibited and slurring their words.

Assessment of fitness to work

It may not be possible for the OH professional to come to a conclusion on initial assessment. A corroborative history is often required and discussion with the employee's general practitioner (GP) is essential. Referral to an addiction specialist in cases of diagnostic uncertainty or due to the need for specialist intervention should be considered. Where the employee admits a problem and believes that they can address it, a return to full or adjusted duties may be appropriate under regular review. If the employee works in a safety-critical or business-critical role, it may be necessary for them to be placed in a non-critical role or even to take sickness absence for the duration of assessment and treatment if it is provided. These decisions involve an assessment of risk, and the involvement of the manager and a health and safety adviser will assist the process. The permission of the individual is, of course, required to reveal the nature of the risk, but will usually be given if it means they are likely to get back to work. Assessment of immediate fitness to work when the individual is suspected or known to have taken drugs and alcohol is an equally challenging area. It is best addressed by clear guidance in the local drug and alcohol policy.

Although the Equality Act 2010 specifically excludes addiction to or dependence on alcohol or any substance (other than the consequences of that substance being legally prescribed), it does cover long-term health effects of alcohol dependency such as liver disease.

Treatment of dependence

Principles of treatment are initially stabilization, detoxification, followed by relapse prevention. Detoxification will be unsuccessful unless there is adequate preparation and aftercare in place. It is unlikely that individuals suffering from dependence will be able to achieve abstinence without support from agencies with addiction expertise.

A reducing regimen of chlordiazepoxide (Librium®) is the most commonly used for alcohol detoxification. When the patient is dependent, it is not safe to stop drinking suddenly as this may lead to withdrawal seizures and in extreme cases even death. Detoxification in the community is possible for people who are mildly dependent, who have no severe physical or mental health problems, and no history of seizures. They should have significant support (e.g. spouse/partner living with them) and can be reviewed daily by the treatment provider.

Detoxification for substance dependence varies depending on the drug. Treatment should be tailored according to the substance taken and the individual. It is not uncommon for individuals to be poly-drug takers and to take a combination of stimulant and depressant drugs including cocaine, heroin, and alcohol. Requesting expert advice from an addiction specialist has to be a priority if dependence, rather than harmful use, is the problem.

Return to work and relapse prevention

The '12-step' philosophy of Alcoholics Anonymous and Narcotics Anonymous is the basis of many non-statutory treatment programmes. This is based on abstinence and the ongoing support of peers, through mutual help groups. However, this is not the only approach available, and is more prevalent in North America than in the UK. Professional treatment programmes, based upon psychological and medical approaches to treatment, are also available and should be considered as potentially valuable alternative resources. Matching individual patients to particular treatment philosophies is a controversial subject and research evidence provides little information upon which to base such decisions. Patient preference, and availability of treatment programmes with demonstrable results such as outcome data at 3, 6, and 9 months post treatment, should therefore dictate the choice. Support to engage in community recovery and peer-based recovery support should be offered. Community day programmes, residential treatment, and therapeutic communities may be considered.[28] Relapse rates are variable and depend on the substance taken, individual factors, and societal factors. For example, a patient suffering from co-morbid anxiety and depression with little family support is more likely to relapse than a patient with no mental health problems and a good supportive network.

It is often possible to support an employee in their return to work after treatment for addiction. In safety-related jobs, this may need ongoing testing, at least for an agreed period of time. A signed 'contract' between the manager and the employee can be useful, giving written details of expected behaviour. The manager is usually in a position to identify signs of relapse. There are good success rates from such an approach. A report by the Health and Safety Laboratory (HSL) cites a Civil Aviation Authority estimate that about 85% of professional pilots whose medical certification of fitness has been withdrawn for drug and alcohol problems and have undergone treatment and rehabilitation could be returned to flying.[29]

Drug and alcohol testing at work

Drug and alcohol testing in the workplace is becoming more common in the UK. The 2007 CIPD survey showed that 22% of respondent organizations carried out some form of testing (compared to 18% in 2001) with a further 9% who were planning to introduce testing.[22] A comprehensive review of the issues is given in the Independent Inquiry into Drug Testing at Work (IIDTW) published in 2004.[20] Studies in the US have reported that 40–50% of organizations use some type of testing with 85% of major firms doing so.[29] In the US, there is a government body, the Substance Abuse and Mental Health Services Administration (SAMHSA), which provides guidance and regulation for the drug testing of federal employees. In Europe, there is a European Workplace Drug Testing Society (EWDTS). In the UK, there is the UK Workplace Drug Testing Forum, which currently has a membership almost exclusively of laboratories who undertake drug testing.

Drug and alcohol testing should always form a part of a workplace drug and alcohol policy, rather than being in lieu of a policy. It follows that the decision to test, and then how to test, should be made following a risk analysis, looking at the company in question, its activities, and any legislation that may apply.

Organizations must be clear about why they wish to test. The Information Commissioners Employment Practice Code (Data Protection) 2011 states that the collection of information through drug or alcohol testing is unlikely to be justified unless it is for health and safety reasons, and that employers should confine information gathered through testing to those employed in 'safety-critical activities'.[30] The Human Rights Act 1988 confers a right to privacy and has been cited to support objections to testing; however, case law suggests that justifiable safety grounds will not violate the Act. There may also be a risk of breaching guidelines for good employment practice as recommended in the Data Protection Act 1998. Nevertheless there are obligations on employers and employees with regard to the risk posed by those who might be under the influence of drugs or alcohol while at work. These responsibilities are defined within the Health and Safety at Work Act 1974, the Road Traffic Act 1988, the Transport and Works Act 1992, the Compressed Air Regulations 1996, and the Diving at Work Regulations 1997.

All testing will require appropriate consent and those people carrying out testing should be appropriately trained in the techniques. Technology for remote alcohol testing has recently been developed and although at present it is only used in the criminal justice system, it may be eventually used for monitoring in the workplace in high-risk professions (e.g. the Secure Continuous Remote Alcohol Monitoring® system (SCRAM®)).

Evidence that testing is effective

The effectiveness of drug testing programmes depends on why they are being implemented. In general, the evidence of benefit is inconclusive, but negative studies have often been criticized as being poorly designed. Those studies with very positive findings have been reviewed by Francis et al.[31] These include a review of the US construction industry which concluded that companies undertaking testing were able to reduce injury rates by 50% over a 10-year period and that for the average company this reduction was achieved within 2 years of introducing the testing programme. In the US military between 1980 and 1990, the 1-month prevalence of reported drug use fell from 28% to 5% and the proportion of positive drug tests fell from 48% to 3% as a result of introducing a drug testing programme.

When to test?

Possible timings for testing are summarized in Box 14.6.

Each type of testing has its own practical and ethical issues which need to be considered in the light of the company's overall drug and alcohol policy.

Random testing

This is commonly used in safety-critical industries, but is the most expensive and difficult testing schedule to organize. No prior warning is given to the individuals who are tested.

Box 14.6 Drug and alcohol testing

- Pre-placement.
- Induction.
- Post accident or incident.
- Prior to promotion or transfer. This is usual in safety-critical industries when employees are first promoted or transferred into jobs with a safety-critical element.
- At random and without announcement.
- For cause or due cause, that is, where the manager has reason to suspect that drugs or alcohol may be affecting performance or safety, or after an accident or incident at work.
- Voluntary testing can give an employee the opportunity to clear their name or confirm a problem for which help and support could be offered.
- As part of an employee's rehabilitation programme, in order to monitor their recovery and/or identify otherwise undisclosed relapse to drug use.

Ideally testing is undertaken at the worksite. It usually requires a visit by a person or team acting as the collecting agent. One option is to test everyone in the workplace but it is more usual to test a sample of the workforce. This requires careful advanced planning, to ensure that the right facilities are available and it is clear who is to be tested. Usually at least one manager needs to be involved. Both staff and managers should be well informed of the procedures. An impartial method of selecting those to be tested is required. This type of testing is often known as 'random' testing, but in fact it may be semi-random, opportunistic, or systematic. Where there is a geographically dispersed workforce or it is too difficult to organize the testing on site, the employee may be advised to attend a centre and may be given a period of notice.

Types of test

Tests can either be point of contact (near field/on site) which is used to give an immediate result or via a laboratory, or a combination of the two. With the exception of alcohol, when drugs are detected on a near-field test, the results are normally referred to as 'non-negative' and a further sample is sent under 'chain of custody' to an accredited laboratory for full analysis. If the employee is involved in safety-critical work, the management may decide to remove or suspend him or her from such duties; however, any further action should await the laboratory report and medical review officer (MRO) confirmation. Depending on the medium sampled, the test may give a direct reading of the substance present in the body at the time of the test (e.g. blood, breath) or a historic reading from past exposure (urine, hair).

Alcohol screening

This can be conducted in various biological media.

Breath

This methodology is similar to that used for roadside testing of drivers by the police, and uses validated instruments. The breath measurements can be directly related to blood measurements, which themselves can be directly related to the likely degree of impairment of performance. If the first sample is positive, testing laboratories normally recommend taking a second sample after 20 minutes: a rising total indicates very recent drinking.

Saliva (or oral fluid)

Saliva testing involves a real-time read-out, based on absorption of saliva on to a pad, with level indications from a change of colour. It relates directly 1:1 to blood alcohol levels and can be regarded as more sensitive than breath testing. It is not widely used in the UK.

Urine

Urine testing for alcohol is sometimes used for convenience if drug testing is also undertaken on a urine sample. The disadvantage is that it does not directly reflect the level of alcohol in the blood at the time of testing, but the delayed excretion of alcohol through the renal system. In order to be more representative of blood alcohol, urine from a second void needs to be analysed.

Blood

This represents the definitive measure of alcohol level and can be directly related to the likely degree of impairment of performance. It is not usually used in a workplace context though, as it is too invasive.

It is possible to backtrack from alcohol readings using standard rates of metabolism of alcohol to determine whether an individual was over the limit after starting work and some companies use this approach. However, there may be difficulties if faced with a legal challenge when a positive reading results in loss of employment.

Drug testing

Urine is the most common form of sample collection in the UK but other approaches may be less intrusive and may be indicated depending on the purpose of the test. These include saliva, hair, and sweat testing. Table 14.2 summarizes the key types of drug testing and provides details of detection times and reliability. A review of drug

Table 14.2 Types of drug testing with detection times (length of time test remains positive following drug use) and reliability

Type of test	Detection time	Reliability
Urine	2/3 days	Most researched; has been around for 20 years; best test for cannabis use; sample needs to be stored and preserved properly; most open to fraud (substitution of samples); positive result needs laboratory confirmation
Saliva	24 hours	Good for recent drug use (cannabis and opiates in particular) but a mouthwash would defeat on-site detection; samples may need refrigeration; dipsticks can be used for on-site results (e.g. can test saliva at the road side); positive tests need to be confirmed. The range of substances that can be detected by near-field tests is smaller than with urine
Sweat	24 hours to 2–3 days	Drug patches used mainly for monitoring; when worn, can detect up to a week; drug swipes can detect other use (last 24 hours) but not very reliable
Blood	Up to 31 hours	Sample needs careful storage and preservation; needs laboratory analysis; on-site results not available
Hair	1 week to 18 months	Expensive; ethyl glucuronide testing now available for alcohol. Requires collection by trained collection officer and analysis is generally slower; however, can give historic picture of drug taking and is more difficult to falsify. It has been known for some patients to shave off their body hair prior to being seen for testing

Source: data from *DrugLink*. March/April 2004; 19(2). Copyright © 2004 DrugScope.

testing methods, undertaken for the Railway Safety and Standards Board by HSL, concluded that in addition to urine testing there is a justifiable case for testing oral fluids and hair.[29] The choice of test depends on convenience, cost, and the aim of the testing programme.

What to test for

Testing programmes in the UK usually cover amphetamines, benzodiazepines, cannabis, cocaine, methadone, and opiates. A metabolite of heroin, 6-mono-acetyl-morphine is present if heroin has been taken. Due to increasing use of NPS, especially SCRAs and gabapentinoids (pregabalin and gabapentin), near-patient immunoassay test kits are available for these compounds, but detection of the majority will require laboratory analysis. More sophisticated analytical tests are in development. The specific profile should be reviewed regularly to reflect drugs in local use. Testing laboratories and toxicologists with an interest in drug misuse can provide useful advice (Table 14.3).

Cut-off levels

The cut-off levels for positivity differ between international authorities. For example, in the US, SAMHSA has set a much higher cut-off level for opiates in urine (2000 ng/mL) than is set in Europe (300 ng/mL). This is to allow for the possibility of poppy seed in the diet. The prevalence of poppy seeds in health foods and particularly seeded bread and cakes, has led to an increasing proportion of non-negative tests for opioids on instant testing. Laboratory testing is normally able to demonstrate that poppy seeds are the cause of the non-negative rather than illegal drugs through the presence of the metabolite thebaine. Similarly, the increasing use of combination opioid over-the-counter medications and prescription opioids has led to some near-field testing kits having higher cut-off levels in order to help to discriminate between legitimate and illicit drug use.

Table 14.3 Time for which drugs remain present

Drug	Saliva	Urine	Hair
Cannabis	Up to 18 hours	2–8 days Up to 28 days if heavy user	7 days onwards
Cocaine	Up to 18 hours	1–3 days	7 days onwards
Amphetamines including ecstasy	Up to 18 hours	2–4 days	7 days onwards
Opiates	Up to 18 hours	2–4 days Heroin metabolites 8–20 hours	7 days onwards
Buprenorphine	Up to 18 hours	1–5 days	7 days onwards
Methadone	Up to 18 hours	1–3 days	7 days onwards
Benzodiazepines	Up to 18 hours	2–8 days but can be 42 days if prolonged use	7 days onwards.

Chain of custody

One key aspect of drug testing is to maintain the 'chain of custody'. This is a process that ensures results can indisputably be connected with the person who produced the test sample. It includes the requirement for secure storage of samples. The procedures are based on those used for handling forensic samples. A second sample is held by the collection laboratory and available to be tested independently if the individual disputes the result. This process can either be used as the primary process or following a non-negative near-field test. In the latter instance, the laboratory performing the test should use the same media as the near-field test, so that the same substances are tested for. If urine is used for laboratory testing following a non-negative saliva near-field test, it is recommended a urine near-field test is taken at the same time as the laboratory sample.

Samples which are non-negative on near-field testing can be found to be negative on laboratory testing. It is important that no formal disciplinary action takes place until the results have been confirmed although there may be a requirement to suspend an individual from safety-critical work temporarily.

There are many examples of individuals trying to tamper with their biological samples. This commonly involves passing off someone else's sample as their own or dilution. This can be prevented by strict collection protocols, monitoring of the temperature of urine, and laboratory assessment (including creatinine levels).

Refusal of test

The drug and alcohol policy must include the action to be taken in the event of refusal of a worker to provide a sample or more commonly absenting themselves from testing once selected. Normally refusal or evidence of adulteration should be regarded as a 'non-negative' or positive sample and appropriate action taken.

Medical review officer

The MRO is a health professional, normally a doctor or forensic pathologist, who can issue a negative report for a positive analytical result. Where a drug test is classified as positive following laboratory analysis, good practice requires that medical review is arranged. The purpose of this is to tell the individual the test result and confirm that the positive result came from a drug, usually an illicit drug, which was not prescribed by the GP or other specialist. This advice is based on consultation with the individual, their GP, the laboratory toxicologist, and any information provided at the time the test was undertaken. This stage is an important check. Codeine use, for example, often results in a positive analytical test but a negative report following MRO review.

The experience, skills, and knowledge to undertake the MRO role are covered by US guidelines; as yet, these are not well defined in Europe. Training courses on medical review are available in the UK. The company occupational physician is well placed to be the MRO, particularly where individual interviews are concerned, but must avoid giving medical advice when in this role.

Interpretation of results

The interpretation of results for drug tests cannot usually be taken further than confirmation that the drug was taken. Unlike alcohol, it is not usually possible to relate the result to a quantitative estimate of the degree of impairment of performance at the time at which testing was conducted. A positive result may indicate a large dose taken some time ago or a small dose taken recently, and often it is not possible to establish which one of these is the case. One of the underlying objections to the use of drug testing in the workplace is the problem of interpretation. One of the arguments for using oral fluid testing for drugs, rather than urine testing, is that the tests remain positive for a much shorter time and are therefore more likely to be associated with actual impairment in the workplace.

Management of a positive result

The consequences of a positive result, confirmed by the MRO, will depend on the policy of the employer. It can range from no action being taken, through the provision of assistance in addressing a drug or alcohol problem, to disciplinary action leading to loss of job. It is important that the employer has decided and communicated to employees the consequences of a positive drug test before drug testing is introduced.

Role of occupational health departments in a drug and alcohol testing programme

There are differences of opinion as to the involvement of OH teams in drug and alcohol testing in the workplace, which is a balance between avoiding a perception of acting in a policing capacity and maintaining the trust of the workforce, with the potential for a conflict of interest particularly in random and 'for cause' testing. Consideration should be given to utilizing an external provider unless there is a sufficient volume of testing to justify this being carried out internally with OH staff well practised and trained. This is likely to be limited to a few safety-critical industries (e.g. nuclear). If the OH team is involved, they must not assist in determining who is tested (including sampling) or have any part in the disciplinary process as this will compromise their professional relationship with employees. There is a requirement for medical involvement in drug screening programmes and there are benefits in maintaining an in-house MRO.

In pre-placement screening, which can be done at the same time as the standard new entrant medical assessment, the drug screening process should be regarded as a management responsibility, delegated to the OH department. Separation of function can be achieved by separately reporting results so that the drug screening test is not perceived as part of the clinical procedure. It is possible to delegate collection of samples for random testing and 'for cause' testing to an external company which might avoid any concerns over separation of policing and rehabilitation roles. If this is the case, the OH professional should be involved in selection of the company and agreeing the necessary procedures.

Testing for impairment

Breathalyser/alcometer testing for alcohol can be related to impaired performance, but the same is not true of the results of most other types of testing for drugs in the workplace. Direct tests of impairment would be more acceptable, and could be followed up with a drug test if impairment were demonstrated. Although there is potential for this in the future and various tests have been trialled in the US, within the UK it is only possible to say whether drugs are present rather than what their effect is.

Key points

- The management of problematic drug and alcohol use in the workplace requires careful consideration, a high level of people management skills, and up-to-date knowledge of what is good practice.
- It is an area where even the most experienced managers, OH specialists, and addiction specialists sometimes struggle.
- Due to inconsistencies in history taking, objective testing is essential. This includes breathalyser readings, urine drug screening, saliva, blood, or hair testing
- It is important that processes are carefully developed and then regularly reviewed with full involvement of all stakeholders.
- Close liaison with local specialist addiction services is essential.

Useful websites

Driving and Vehicle Licensing Agency. Fitness to drive	https://www.gov.uk/guidance/assessing-fitness-to-drive-for-medical-professionals
General Medical Council. Good medical practice (2013) and reporting concerns about patients to the DVLA	http://www.gmc-uk.org/guidance
Novel Psychoactive Treatment UK Network	http://www.neptune-clinical-guidance.co.uk
Alcoholics Anonymous	http://www.alcoholics-anonymous.co.uk/
Narcotics Anonymous	http://ukna.org/
SMART: Self-Management and Recovery Training	https://www.smartrecovery.org/uk
Alcohol Concern	http://www.alcoholconcern.org.uk
Drugs Meter. Self-help resource	http://www.drugsmeter.com
DrugWise. Promoting evidence-based information on drugs, alcohol, and tobacco	http://www.drugscope.org.uk

European Workplace Drug Testing Forum	http://www.ewdts.org
Health and Safety Executive. Information and resources on drugs and alcohol at work	http://www.hse.gov.uk
International Labour Organization. An international perspective	http://www.ilo.org
FRANK. Resources on recognizing effects and risks of drugs and alcohol	http://www.talktofrank.com

References

1. **Alcohol Concern: Alcohol Statistics June 2016**. Available at: https://www.alcoholconcern.org.uk/alcohol-statistics.
2. **Home Office**. Drug misuse: findings from the 2016/2017 Crime Survey for England and Wales. 2017. Available at: https://www.gov.uk/government/statistics/drug-misuse-findings-from-the-2016-to-2017-csew.
3. **Office for National Statistics**. Alcohol-related deaths in the UK: registered in 2015. 2017. Available at: https://www.ons.gov.uk/peoplepopulationandcommunity/healthandsocialcare/causesofdeath/bulletins/alcoholrelateddeathsintheunitedkingdom/registeredin2015.
4. **Office for National Statistics**. *General Lifestyle Survey Overview – A Report on the 2011 General Lifestyle Survey*. Newport: Office for National Statistics; 2013.
5. **Coggon D, Harris EC, Brown T, et al.** *Occupational Mortality in England and Wales, 1991–2000*. London: Office for National Statistics; 2009.
6. **Calnan M.** One in five employees 'regularly' uses drugs. People Management, April 2016. Available at: https://www.peoplemanagement.co.uk/.
7. **National Institute for Health and Care Excellence**. Alcohol-use disorders: prevention. Public health guideline [PH24]. 2010. Available at: https://www.nice.org.uk/guidance/ph24.
8. **HM Government**. *Drug Strategy 2010*. London: Home Office; 2010.
9. **Davenport M, Harris D.** The effect of low blood alcohol levels on pilot performance in a series of simulated approach and landing trials. *Int J Aviat Psychol* 1992;**2**:271–80.
10. **Department for Transport**. *Guidance for Healthcare Professionals on Drug Driving*. London: Department for Transport; 2014.
11. **Calder IM, Ramsey J.** A survey of cannabis use in offshore rig workers. *Br J Addict* 1987;**82**:159–61.
12. **Yesavage JA, Leirer VO, Denari M, et al.** Carry-over effects of marijuana intoxication on aircraft pilot performance: a preliminary report. *Am J Psychiatry* 1985;**142**:1325–9.
13. **Department for Transport**. *Cannabis and Driving: A Review of the Literature and Commentary*. London: Department for Transport Report; 2003. Available at: http://www.dft.gov.uk.
14. **NHS Digital**. *Prescriptions Dispensed in the Community, Statistics for England–2005–2015*. Leeds: NHS Digital.
15. **NHS National Services Scotland**. *Prescription Cost Analysis 2016*. Edinburgh: NHS National Services Scotland; 2016.
16. **NHS Wales Shared Services Partnership**. Prescriptions dispensed in the community in Wales, 2016. Welsh Government; 2016. Available at: https://gov.wales/docs/statistics/2017/170524-prescriptions-dispensed-community-2016-en.pdf.

17. **Abdulrahim D, Bowden-Jones O, NEPTUNE Expert Group**. *Guidance on the Management of Acute and Chronic Harms of Club Drugs and Novel Psychoactive Substances*. London: Novel Psychoactive Treatment UK Network (NEPTUNE); 2015. Available at: http://www.neptune-clinical-guidance.com.

18. **Department of Environment**. *Railway Accident Report on Collision at Glasgow Central Station on 29 March 1974*. London: Department of Environment; 1975.

19. **Marine Accident Investigation Branch**. Accident Investigation Report No. 25/2014. Available at: https://www.gov.uk/maib-reports.

20. **Joseph Rowntree Foundation, Drug and Alcohol Research Programme**. *Drug Testing in the Workplace: The Report of the Independent Inquiry into Drug Testing at Work*. York: York Publishing Services Ltd; 2004.

21. **Head J, Martikainen P, Kumari M, et al**. *Work Environment, Alcohol Consumption and Ill-Health. The Whitehall II Study*. Norwich: HSE Books; 2002.

22. **Chartered Institute of Personnel and Development**. *Managing Drug and Alcohol Misuse at Work*. London: Chartered Institute of Personnel and Development; 2007.

23. **Holden L, Scuffham PA, Hilton MF, et al**. Health-related productivity losses increase when the health condition is co-morbid with psychological distress: findings from a large cross-sectional sample of working Australians. *BMC Public Health* 2011;**11**:417–26.

24. **British Medical Association**. Alcohol, drugs and the workplace - the role of medical professionals. 2016. Available at: https://www.bma.org.uk/advice/employment/occupational-health/alcohol-drugs-and-the-workplace.

25. **Faculty of Occupational Medicine**. *Guidance on Drug and Alcohol Misuse in the Workplace*. London: Faculty of Occupational Medicine, 2006.

26. **Babor TF, de la Fuente JR, Saunders J, et al**. *AUDIT: The Alcohol Use Disorders Identification Test. Guidelines for use in primary health care*. Geneva: World Health Organization.

27. **Stockwell T, Murphy D, Hodgson R**. The severity of alcohol dependence questionnaire: its use, reliability and validity. *Br J Addict* 1983;**78**:45–156.

28. **Clinical Guidelines on Drug Misuse and Dependence Update 2017 Independent Expert Working Group**. *Drug Misuse and Dependence: UK Guidelines on Clinical Management*. London: Department of Health; 2017.

29. **Akrill P, Mason H**. *Review of Drug Testing Methodologies, Prepared for Railway Safety and Standards Board*. London: Health and Safety Laboratory; 2005.

30. **Information Commissioner**. *Quick Guide to Employment Practice Codes*. Wilmslow: Information Commissioner; 2011.

31. **Francis P, Hanley N, Wray D**. *A Literature Review on the International State of Knowledge of Drug Testing at Work, with Particular Reference to the US*. Newcastle: University of Northumbria; 2003.

Chapter 15

Transport

Tim Carter, Rae-Wen Chang, Andrew Colvin,
and Robbert Hermanns

Introduction

Fitness to work in all modes of transport is an area of public concern. Air and rail are the safest modes of transport by distance travelled; both hold a risk of less than 0.01 deaths per 100 million passenger-kilometres, compared to motorcycle and car: 83 and 1.6 per 1000 million passenger-kilometres respectively.[1] This chapter considers fitness to drive, and to work in the rail or aviation industries, including the statutory frameworks in each mode of transport. Although they have much in common, each has its own pattern of performance and fitness standards.

Decisions on fitness are frequently taken not for the benefit of the person examined but to safeguard those at risk as a consequence of their performance deficits or incapacitation. Hence, standards for medical aspects of fitness are often formal and published. They are usually applied by physicians acting on behalf of regulatory authorities, and have associated review or appeal mechanisms. Standards necessarily balance public risk against potential loss of employment, with the former predominating.

The evidence base for current standards is of variable quality and this is often a cause of contention. Patient groups and equal opportunities organizations may find it difficult to accept standards based on epidemiological estimates of risk. Equality legislation may encourage applicants to demand individual risk assessment and job adaptations, but often this is impossible.

Long-term health problems are usually covered by formal standards, but transport workers may also have short-term impairments from injury, minor illness, or medication. In some areas (e.g. aviation), even short-term decreases in medical fitness are subject to national or international regulation.

Safety-critical tasks

The term 'safety-critical task' usually means that personal impairment can put other people at risk. Driving provides a good example of a complex 'safety-critical' transport task:

- Information about the vehicle, other road users, and the road are perceived, mainly using vision.

- This is processed cognitively against a learned background of skills and intentions.
- Based on this, the vehicle speed, direction, and signalling are determined by hand and foot controls.
- The results of these actions are, in turn, processed to determine subsequent control requirements.

Lack of experience, inattention, behavioural traits such as risk-taking, and impairment, including medical impairment, may interfere with this loop, potentially increasing the risk of error and accident.

A similar perceptual, cognitive, and motor loop pertains to rail drivers and aircraft pilots. However, the visual and auditory environment, sensory inputs, response to control actions, and safety support systems vary greatly (e.g. presence of an aircraft co-pilot or protective railway signalling).

Health-related impairment does not appear to be a major direct contributor to transport accidents, although there is no recent definitive study on this. Other forms of impairment such as fatigue and alcohol, and driver inexperience or risk-taking behaviour, are much more significant. These behavioural aspects are much more important in adverse events than the condition of either the vehicle or the road.[2,3]

Performance decrement may be permanent (e.g. amputated limb or reduced visual acuity) or episodic (e.g. seizure, cardiac event, or hypoglycaemia). Many conditions present with a mix of characteristics, for example, the fluctuating impairments of multiple sclerosis or progression of a malignancy or motor neurone disease. Treatments frequently reduce risk, but some, such as insulin or psychoactive medications, can create new risks.

The approaches to static and to episodic conditions are different. With static conditions, it is possible to include the impact of corrective appliances or treatments (e.g. spectacles or modified controls) in an individual capability assessment, but measures of impairment often cannot be precisely linked to accident risk.[4] Therefore, practical assessment of performance may be the most useful and acceptable arbiter of safety, although its predictive value has not been formally evaluated.

With episodic impairments, individual assessment of performance is less feasible, and the best approach is a valid estimate of the future risk of recurrence derived from relevant epidemiological data. Good information on recurrence rates for seizures and for cardiac events are useful for stratification. Assessment is more difficult where disease management is subject to variable individual control, as with the risk of hypoglycaemia from insulin treatment or adherence to continuous positive airway pressure (CPAP) treatment in obstructive sleep apnoea (OSA).

Critical features of an episodic condition include the time taken to become incapacitated, the level of awareness, and the ability to take action during this time. Whereas a seizure may instantly incapacitate without warning, cardiac events are sometimes associated with a warning period that is sufficient for drivers to pull over and stop. Where an incapacitating episode is not perceived, either through lack of awareness of the prodromal symptoms or because cognition is clouded, as with hypoglycaemia or substantial hyper-glycaemia, then driving may continue as incapacitation increases.

Occupational driving: public highways

There is great diversity in the risks and performance requirements for occupational driving tasks. In the UK, 25–33% of all fatal and serious accidents on public roads are attributed to work-related driving. This amounts to around 500–600 road fatalities per annum and thus is the major cause of work-related fatal accidents.

The implications of employment on responsibilities for meeting standards are complex. This is addressed in several ways. For road transport in Great Britain, the Driver and Vehicle Licensing Agency (DVLA) makes no statutory distinction between drivers at work and other road users. Differential standards are based on vehicle size, structure, and use. Vehicle definitions and associated medical fitness requirements for drivers are standardized across the European Union (EU).[5] More stringent fitness levels apply to drivers of group 2 vehicles: those weighing over 3.5 tonnes or with more than eight passenger seats. The rationale is good evidence of higher consequential damage from such vehicles, and with large numbers of passengers, more fatalities. These statutory minimum standards are supplemented by a local licensing system for taxis, for which the more stringent group 2 standards may be applied. In the past, it was found that approximately half of local authorities applied group 2 standards. In recent years, many employers have developed their own enhanced driver medical standards, in particular the emergency services. For all other drivers, the less stringent, group 1, medical licensing standards apply.

The basis for control in all cases is by the issue, revocation, or restriction of the person's driving licence. Restriction is either of duration of licence period or in terms of required vehicle adaptations (occasionally both duration and adaptation are required). This is only applicable to longer-term health conditions. Avoidance of driving with short-term impairment is the responsibility of an individual driver, and some find this duty challenging if their livelihood is threatened. Hence, some employers have established corporate driving risk-reduction programmes that include provision for declaration of short-term incapacity and temporary cessation of driving without penalty.[6]

Occupational driving: off-road

Many workers drive vehicles off the public roads. These include farmers, dock-workers, and crane or forklift truck drivers. Highly specialized vehicles used, for instance, in mines, quarries, airports, and at container ports may involve operation in close proximity to workers or members of the public.

Where vehicles are operated occupationally, but not on the public highway, there is often confusion about the application of medical fitness standards. The legal requirement of the Health and Safety at Work etc. Act 1974 is that the employer has a safe system of work. This applies to all those who drive at work, whether on highways or off-road. Although there is no specific legal requirement for medical assessment, there is a clear implication that medical fitness may be a prerequisite of a safe system. Health and safety law is applicable to all workplaces. The employer will normally require the advice and assistance of a competent person, in this case an occupational health (OH) professional, for both the setting of appropriate medical fitness standards and their implementation.

If part or all of the driving activity takes place on the public highway, then the DVLA standards generally apply, but with some limited exemptions for agricultural vehicles. In setting standards for occupational drivers who are not using the public highway, it is often beneficial to use the DVLA group 1 and 2 standards as initial benchmarks and then to deviate from them based on a task-specific risk assessment.[7] Despite the lack of DVLA jurisdiction on private property, these standards are evidence based and familiar to doctors, This approach is advisable, as direct application of DVLA medical standards may not be suitable, resulting in challenges under the Equality Act 2010.

Medical aspects of licensing

For road drivers, licensing is formally a responsibility of the Secretary of State for Transport. In practice, in Britain it is delegated to the DVLA, where assessment of the medical aspects is the responsibility of the Drivers' Medical Group. Northern Ireland has a comparable agency. The legal basis for the standards and for their enforcement lies in the Road Traffic Act 1988.[8] This specifies certain disabilities, known as 'relevant disabilities', which bar a person from driving, and 'prospective disabilities', which may require regular medical licensing review. In both instances, the fact of the disability places an obligation on the driver to notify the DVLA of the medical condition, its nature, and extent. The standards are aligned with the EU driver licensing directives, but there are national variations in application and enforcement. The UK has a single driver licensing centre, with its own medical staff who make decisions based on clinical information obtained from drivers, clinicians, and sometimes from commissioned investigations and examinations. Around 130,000 new enquiries are received each year, growing annually by 10%. Nearly 20% of cases now arise from licence renewal in those aged 70 or over. Complex cases are assessed by the DVLA doctors, who are also available to health professionals by telephone and letter to discuss individual cases (see 'Useful websites').

Medical standards are published in *Assessing Fitness to Drive: A Guide for Health Professionals* which is revised twice a year (see 'Useful websites'). The DVLA is advised by six expert honorary medical panels covering the range of adult medical practice relevant to safe driving: vision, heart disease, diabetes, neurology, psychiatric illness, and the effects of drug and alcohol misuse and standard setting is supported by in-house or external reviews and research (see 'Useful websites').

New applicants for a group 1 licence have a legal obligation to declare any relevant medical conditions. Basic visual performance is assessed at the practical driving test (reading a car number plate at 20 metres). The licence terms require declaration to the DVLA of any arising relevant medical conditions. This remains the licence holder's personal responsibility, but the General Medical Council (GMC) recommends a process for a doctor to follow if a patient fails to notify the DVLA despite advice to do so (see 'Useful websites'). The group 1 licence expires at the age of 70, with subsequent 3 year renewal subject to new medical declaration.

Declaration of a relevant medical condition on application, during the currency of a licence, or one found during group 2 medical assessment will trigger a medical enquiry. For group 1 this usually involves questionnaires to both driver and treating doctor(s). Specialist referral may be required, particularly for group 2 licences. The DVLA Drivers Medical Group will reach a licensing decision. Options include issuing or continuing a full licence, issuing one for a shorter period with review, restricting a licence to the use of certain vehicles or use of vehicle adaptations, refusing a licence application, or revoking the existing licence. Appeals against licensing decisions are rare.

The Glasgow 'bin lorry' fatal accident

This Fatal Accident Inquiry (December 2015) examined the cause of a serious accident resulting in the deaths of six pedestrians and serious injury to many others in Glasgow city centre on 22 December 2014.[9] The driver of a bin lorry suffered sudden neurocardiogenic syncope and temporarily lost consciousness, causing his uncontrolled vehicle to mount the pavement on a busy main street. A previous incident had occurred in 2010 when he was driving a passenger bus. On that occasion, he was assessed by a company occupational physician before it was concluded, after a GP medical report, that he had suffered a simple faint and was allowed to return to vocational driving.

The driver subsequently failed to provide a true and accurate medical history when completing OH questionnaires for fitness to drive group 2 vehicles over several years.

The Sherriff made 19 recommendations and three matters for consideration in the report.

Summary of main recommendations relevant to occupational health

◆ Doctors should ensure that medical notes are made and kept in such a way as to maximize their ability to identify repeated episodes of loss of consciousness, or altered awareness, in patients who are or may become drivers.

◆ When a doctor is advising an organization following a medical incident while driving, that organization should provide all available information about the incident to the doctor and the doctor should insist on having it prior to giving advice to the organization and the driver.

◆ Employers should carry out an internal review of its employment processes to improve checking medical and sickness absence information provided by applicants, for example, by having focused health questions within reference requests for drivers and obtaining medical reports in relation to health-related driving issues from applicants' GPs.

- The DVLA should satisfy itself as to precisely what the categorization is intended to mean and to achieve in the loss of consciousness/altered awareness section of *Assessing Fitness to Drive: A Guide for Medical Professionals.*
- The DVLA should then ensure that the meaning is made clear to those who apply the guidance in practice.
- The Secretary of State for Transport should instigate a consultation on whether it is appropriate that doctors should be given greater freedom, by the GMC, or an obligation, by Parliament, to report fitness to drive concerns directly to the DVLA.

Matters for consideration

- OH doctors performing examinations on group 2 drivers and providing advice to employers on applicant drivers, and employers of drivers who facilitate their staff applying for renewal of group 2 licences without the involvement of GPs, should consider whether to require the applicant to sign a consent form permitting release by any GP of relevant medical records to the OH doctor.
- The DVLA, the Crown Prosecution Service, and the Crown Office and Procurator Fiscal Service should review whether there are policies in place which prevent or discourage prosecution for breaches of sections 94 and 174 of the Road Traffic Act 1988. If there are such policies, consideration should be given to whether they are appropriate where the current fitness to drive regime is a self-reporting system which is vulnerable to the withholding and concealing of relevant information by applicants.
- The DVLA and the Department for Transport should consider how best to increase public awareness of the impact of medical conditions on fitness to drive and the notification obligations in that regard.

Specific medical conditions

Details of the standards are in the DVLA publication *Assessing Fitness to Drive: A Guide for Health Professionals,* which is available online. The evidence linking medical conditions to accidents has been reviewed in detail and summarized in a guide for health professionals.[10,11] Other chapters of this book discuss most of the conditions of concern. The following are standards where there are important features specific to driving, and to a varying extent, to other modes of transport. The detail around the assessment of syncope has significantly tightened in response to the Glasgow 'bin lorry' inquiry report published in 2015.

Cardiac events and strokes

Arterial disease poses a risk of both progressive impairment and relatively sudden incapacity. Standards are based on current capabilities and especially on likelihood of recurrence. For group 1 drivers, a period without driving after satisfactory recovery from an event is required but for group 2 drivers, the additional probability of recurrence must be stratified, based on the Bruce protocol exercise electrocardiogram or other equivalent functional test. Driving may resume if this is satisfactorily completed, though it is then subject to periodic review.

A cautious approach has been adopted to implanted defibrillators in any driver because they may discharge without warning. Their internal memories can be used to determine the frequency of discharge and if this is very low it may allow group 1 driving. The need for an implanted defibrillator is at present a bar to group 2 entitlement.

Seizures

Good evidence about the probability of a repeat seizure at various times after the last one, both with and without medication, enables standards based on a quantitative risk of recurrence. The level used is a probability of less than 20% in the next year for group 1 and less than 2% for group 2. The difference reflects the time likely to be spent at the wheel and the consequential damage likely if an accident occurs.[12] (See Chapter 24.)

Diabetes

The major risk is from insulin-induced hypoglycaemia, although sulphonylureas and glinides may also cause comparable risk.[13] Each year the DVLA receives around 300 police notifications of presumed impairment from this cause while driving, some leading to serious accidents. This is an area of considerable concern as any threat of a restriction on driving (particularly if vocational) may lead to less than optimal treatment of the disease to avoid the risk of 'hypos'.

The DVLA has allowed diabetics treated with insulin to drive group 2 vehicles subject to strict medical criteria since November 2011. The DVLA has issued detailed guidance on diabetic control and driver education on recognition and prevention of severe hypoglycaemia with appropriate personal preventative measures for group 2 drivers including annual health checks and monitoring of blood glucose level and it may be sensible to adapt these guidelines for all vocational drivers or within a company safe system of driving. The risk and type of hypoglycaemic episodes (defined as 'mild' or 'severe' under the current EU directive and related UK legislation) requires careful assessment for all diabetic drivers. The medical requirements advised by the DVLA have also tightened for group 1 drivers since 2011.

Vision

Vision and the use of visual information is a multistage process. Current assessments are limited to acuity and visual fields, for which there are few clear correlations between degree of impairment and accident risk. For on-road driving there is good evidence that colour vision is not a requirement; conversely, impairments of twilight vision, contrast sensitivity, and glare may have greater relevance but, as yet, cannot easily be assessed nor standards defined. One of the most contentious areas is visual field loss, associated with stroke, glaucoma, and certain retinopathies. Here decisions have to be taken on a wide variety of defects, each of which can be mapped in detail but for which the consequences in terms of current risk and progression are not predictable.

Sleep disorders

The majority of sleep-related road accidents are in those with sleep deficits that do not have a medical cause. However, three medical conditions, OSA, narcolepsy, and cataplexy, are important. OSA is particularly prevalent in the overweight, middle-aged male and is reliably associated with an excess risk of road crashes. The detection of undiagnosed OSA in professional drivers is important and can be improved by driver education and its recognition by company managers and medical advisers. Treatment with CPAP during sleep is acceptable and has been shown to reduce the risk of accidents.[14] The British Thoracic Society has published a position statement on driving and OSA which provides a useful summary and reference on best and required practice.[15]

The severity of narcolepsy may be reduced by medication; where satisfactory control can be objectively demonstrated (e.g. by the Osler wakefulness test), driving may be permitted.

Psychiatric illness

Severe psychoses are normally a bar to driving but for less severe illness there may be other potentially debarring issues, which relate to the side effects of the medication used as much as to the risks from the disease. There are no good correlations between non-psychotic mental illness and road accidents.

Drugs and alcohol

In England and Wales, it is illegal for an individual to drive if they are either:

◆ unfit to do so because they are on legal or illegal drugs
◆ have certain levels of illegal drugs in their blood (even if they haven't affected driving)
◆ have certain levels of some legal/prescribed drugs unless they have a medical defence.

In England and Wales, the police now routinely conduct a 'field impairment assessment' and perform roadside checks using a roadside drug kit (saliva checks). This provides an immediate test result for commonly abused recreational drugs including cannabis or cocaine. If drivers are thought to be unfit to drive because of taking drugs, they will be arrested and have to provide a blood or urine sample at a police station.

In recent years, attention on the impairment of road drivers caused by some prescribed medications has also been highlighted in the UK and abroad.[16] This has led to restrictions on the blood levels of some commonly prescribed medications in England and Wales since March 2015 unless the driver has discussed fitness for driving with their GP or treating specialist and has been medically advised that there is no driver safety risk and they are not impaired to drive. Drivers can also be prosecuted if they drive with certain levels of these drugs without medical prescription. This law doesn't currently cover Northern Ireland and Scotland but drivers there can still be arrested if found to be unfit to drive.

The assessment of longer-term dependency and misuse arises as a medical issue and there are provisions for certain classes of driving offences in 'high-risk offenders' to require medical clearance before returning to driving.

The legal alcohol limit in Scotland is 50 mg in every 100 mL of blood (equivalent to a breath alcohol of 22 micrograms of alcohol per 100 mL of breath) but elsewhere in the UK is from 80 mg per 100 mL of blood.

Fixed disabilities

People with fixed disabilities such as paralysis, cerebral palsy, spina bifida, and amputations can often drive safely once they have been trained to use a modified vehicle. Assessments and advice on vehicle adaptations are provided by a network of Driving Mobility centres (see 'Useful websites'). Any clinician can arrange a referral.

The role of the occupational health professional

Any organization that employs occupational drivers should develop policies on driving at work. Health risk management requires OH advice both to set policies and to manage decisions on fitness.

Where OH professionals are determining medical fitness standards for vocational or business driving, these should consider job-specific factors as part of a risk assessment, while benchmarking against DVLA medical standards. Professional or vocational drivers may work shifts or have to meet tight delivery deadlines ('driving against the clock'). They may complete high annual mileages, drive at higher speeds, have limited opportunity for planned breaks, or be driving in adverse weather conditions or on unknown roads. The vocational or company driver cannot always 'self-limit' driving activities especially if these are scheduled and there is perceived self-generated or operational pressures at play. The company safety culture or specific operational circumstances such as dangerous loads or the need for non-driving role-related tasks such as manual handling of loads on delivery, may also dictate that DVLA medical standards are not appropriate for direct application to all company or professional driver roles. In practice, companies may have medical fitness standards for vocational or business drivers based on their specific health and safety risk assessments that are more stringent than DVLA standards. Many larger companies will include the development of such driver medical standards and their effective implementation by managers across the business within a road safety strategy or 'Management of Road Risk Policy' with the intention to ensure safe driving for all while engaged on company activities.

Checks on return to work after illness and surveillance to detect new health problems, to check vision, and to ensure that existing medical conditions are controlled are commonly used by companies to reduce driving risks. Adherence with therapy and self-management are important aspects of risk reduction. It is now possible to record objective information about the quality of self-management from data-logging devices such as blood glucose monitors and CPAP machines. This can improve the quality of risk assessment in occupational drivers.

It is important to ensure that health risk management includes both long-term conditions and short-term impairment from acute illness, injury, or the use of impairing medications. This requires rapid access to OH advice.

Treating clinicians often see a conflict between their patient's interests and fitness to drive advice that may limit work and mobility, and may have limited knowledge of fitness standards. OH professionals should be aware of this, and communicate with treating clinicians to obtain a full and up-to-date clinical picture that supports valid advice and relevant job adaptations if there is a limitation on fitness to drive.

In any OH setting where groups of doctors are assessing drivers to company or DVLA medical standards, there is an opportunity for periodic group discussion of the relevant standards, specific driver cases, sharing of clinical practice, and examination technique. Such meetings should form part of continuous professional development and clinical governance procedures for all OH staff.

Rail

Regulatory and advisory framework

Currently, many different train operating companies (TOCs) are in existence in the UK, together with some heritage railways. This fragmentation impacts OH provision, with differences in approach between TOCs and their OH providers. In the future, computerization, automation, the rise of driverless transport systems, and the development of artificial intelligence will impact rail systems.

The regulator for the railways in the UK is the Office of Rail and Road (ORR). The key legislation is The Railways and Other Guided Transport Systems (Safety) Regulations 2006 (see 'Useful websites'). They are based partly on The Railways (Safety Critical Work) Regulations 1994, which transpose the 2004 European Railway Safety Directive into UK law. They contain the terms 'safety critical work' which the regulations define as certain activities that require specific competencies and fitness from those carrying them out (Regulations 23 and 24). The concept of safety-critical tasks is an important foundation for the railways' primary requirement for OH provision. The ORR provides guidance regarding the type of jobs or tasks that are considered safety critical (see 'Useful websites'). They include train driving and other operational train safety duties (conductors), train dispatch, signalling operations, maintenance activities in depots, training delivery, and supervision of the training for safety-critical tasks. Consequently, a wide range of jobs and tasks in the rail industry require pre-placement, routine periodic assessments, and/or other medical assessments, such as after sickness absence prior to a return to work or when prescribed medications could affect alertness and concentration. For mainline train drivers, the requirements were further codified in an EU Directive transposed in the UK Train Driving Licenses and Certificates Regulations 2010 (see ORR website in 'Useful websites'). These regulations came into full effect from October 2018.

The Rail Standards and Safety Board (RSSB) is a trade organization with members from the rail industry and aims, 'through research, risk modelling and analysis to help the rail industry' and 'to provide knowledge, skills and expertise ... independent of any commercial interests' (see 'Useful websites'). It operates a large number of specialist working groups and expert forums, including the health and well-being policy and human factors groups. The RSSB recognizes that no single body provides expert (health) guidance and input into railway health and well-being standards.

OH support generally appears to focus on sickness absence management, fitness for role, and prevention of occupational diseases through systematic health surveillance under general health and safety law or other health interventions. OH provision for the UK rail industry is largely provided to the various TOCs and Network Rail by external OH providers. There are plans to develop a specific accredited railway medicine course for physicians who want to work in the rail industry. The recognized gap in the development and adoption of agreed and widely supported health guidance across the industry at a strategic level makes it difficult for TOCs to judge what level of quality and OH expertise they should procure.

The Association of Rail Industry Occupational Health Practitioners (ARIOPS) is a voluntary group of OH professionals interested in rail (see 'Useful websites'). It aims to promote and disseminate rail industry-relevant health and medical information, through its website and through an annual conference, covering rail-relevant health topics.

Union International des Chemin de Fer (UIC) is a worldwide railway organization that has produced guidelines for medical fitness of railway personnel in safety-critical functions (see 'Useful websites'). It differentiates two classes of risk. Group A (characterized by high risk, dependent on one person, and not entirely compensated for by technical and other systems) covers train drivers and probably also train conductors. The guidance, in addition to a pan-European acceptance of minimum standards, now also incorporates guidance from Canada and Australia. It provides a framework to assess fitness for safety-critical roles based on accepted medical standards for hearing, vision, cognitive function, and physical capabilities. This includes judgement about the possible risk of sudden incapacitation from disease and the effect of prescribed medication.

The Rail Accident Investigation Branch (RAIB) is an investigative branch of the Department for Transport but acts independently. It investigates railway accidents to identify lessons learned, without apportioning blame or prosecuting organizations or individuals. It publishes its findings via its website (see 'Useful websites'). Since 2005, it has investigated at least 12 accidents where fatigue played a role, a challenge of particular concern for train drivers.

Specific health challenges

Obesity

In addition to safely operating their train, drivers may need to be physically active for various reasons. They must be able to protect their train from oncoming traffic, perform other emergency duties, climb in and out of the cabin onto the track (vertical ladder), and walk on uneven ground/ballast for more than a mile in good time. A body mass index of 32 or higher, increases the risk of lower limb injuries when walking on rough ground, even in highly fit individuals.

Formal fitness requirements for aerobic capacity and physical agility do not currently exist in the UK. They could in future provide a more rational basis for fitness assessment.

Obstructive sleep apnoea

OSA can lead to excessive daytime sleepiness and cause drivers to fall asleep. There is a strong relationship between OSA and obesity, hypertension, metabolic syndrome, diabetes, and cardiovascular complications and high road traffic accident risk. Significant central obesity, as measured by abdominal girth, perhaps in combination with heartburn, with or without its medication, or hoarseness may be a significant warning flag for OSA.[17]

A study of Australian rail workers, published in 2016, investigated the use of the Epworth sleepiness scale (ESS) compared to health risk markers (body mass index, presence of hypertension, and type 2 diabetes).[18] The study found the prevalence of OSA in the study population had increased from 2% in 2009 when screening with the ESS to 7% in 2016 after risk-based referral for sleep study. No worker reported an elevated ESS and the study suggests that job bias can make screening instruments that are developed for clinical practice unreliable in safety-critical work settings.

Diabetes

The over-riding concern in safety-critical activity such as train driving is the avoidance of hypoglycaemia in diabetes controlled with insulin or other medications. In the past, people with diabetes controlled with insulin were not passed fit for safety-critical tasks, but in line with decisions taken on the risks in road vehicle driving, this is being relaxed by some TOCs. The adherence to the standards set for driving by the DVLA including the use of frequent blood glucose monitoring has been essential. This can represent a challenge in the UK, where blood glucose meters are not always readily available unless a significant risk of hypoglycaemia exists.

All diabetics may be at risk of experiencing high blood sugar levels. For the purpose of undertaking safety-critical work, blood glucose levels above 15 mmol/L are thought to lengthen reaction time, interfere with the observation and processing of information (signals), impair decision-taking (executive function), and cause frontal lobe dysfunction and mood disturbance.[19, 20] All of this may become more pronounced and relevant in a highly dynamic and multitasking environment such as train driving.

NHS treatment guidelines are not aimed at ensuring fitness for safety-critical work. The National Institute for Health and Care Excellence guidelines refer to (road) driving, hypoglycaemia, and blood glucose monitoring but not the risk from hyperglycaemia (see 'Useful websites'). For the diabetic patient to understand the effect of food intake, physical exercise, and the timing of any medication on their blood glucose levels they have to measure blood glucose. Glycated haemoglobin (HbA1c) measurements are important as a marker for the long-term risk of complications for the purpose of assessing fitness for a safety-critical role but do not capture significant acute changes in blood sugar that could be relevant for safety-critical work.

Signal passed at danger and OH review

A signal passed at danger (SPAD) is a very serious occurrence, both for the TOC and the train driver. A SPAD constitutes a critical incident and has the potential of terminating a driver's career. The purpose of the OH consultation is to explore, in collaboration with the driver, if there were any contributory medical circumstances or issues that could reasonably have contributed to the SPAD. This can include general health issues, either not yet detected or known, or broader issues such as shift rota leading to fatigue and personal pressures.

Any OH consultation in such a context is naturally fraught with tension. Potential contributory issues should be explored sensitively once initial rapport has been established.

Shift work

Fatigue has been found to be a contributing factor to accidents and is considered a major risk factor in the rail and other safety-critical industries. Shift durations of 10 or 12 hours which are common in the UK rail industry can lead to a doubling of the risk of fatigue, impairing attention, memory, and reaction time. The effects of such an extended period of wakefulness have been equated to the same impairment seen when blood alcohol concentrations reach approximately 0.1%. Fatigue can also occur on returning after an extended leave period, when the wake–sleep rhythm has shifted more to a 'day-shift' cycle.[21] It is suggested that performance and alertness deteriorates steadily after cumulative sleep loss of as little as 2.5 hours per night for more than a week. Chronic sleep loss also appears to be an independent risk factor for obesity and diabetes, possibly by changes in insulin sensitivity and longer waking time, with more opportunity to eat.[22] Research and guidance on fatigue is available from the HSE, ORR, and RSSB.[23-25]

Mental health

Assessment of mental health is an important aspect of fitness to drive or to carry out safety-critical activity. Caution is required when using clinical mental health screening tools in safety-critical industries. Screening questionnaires do not diagnose or score severity of disease as such but rather provide a guide for diagnosis on balance of a collection of symptoms. A useful scale for screening for anxiety and depression is mentioned in the Australian Standards guidance (K10) together with a suggested interpretation of different scores.[26]

Train drivers and other transport workers may experience fatalities (suicides) on the line. These can have a significant impact on train driver mental health and lead to long-term absence.[27] TOCs should have procedures in place for responding to these incidents to include peer support and, where necessary, referral to OH or for specialized counselling or psychotherapy.

Aviation

Risk in aviation

Air transport safety has continued to improve over the past 50 years based on advances in technology and regulatory standards. Aviation organizations must develop safety management systems to consider operational hazards, assess risks, and provide effective mitigations.[28] A seminal paper considered flight crew as one of the 'systems' on the aircraft.[29] The concept was adopted by the UK Civil Aviation Authority (CAA), and led to a safety target for accidents from medical incapacitation of less than 1 in 1000 million flights. This risk target can be achieved by only certificating pilots with medical conditions that carry an incapacitation risk of 1% per year or less, and operating with two pilots. This has become known as the '1% rule'. With improvements in technical systems, it is possible that a standard of 2% per year could be applied without significant detriment to overall flight safety. Conversely, it is more difficult to identify, quantify, and mitigate risks from subtle incapacitation such as psychiatric illness or hypoglycaemia.

Medical standards

Internationally agreed medical standards for pilots are outlined in Annex 1 of the Convention on International Civil Aviation and associated guidance material.[30,31] A few (e.g. visual requirements) are specific, but many are couched in general terms. There is also a waiver clause, 'accredited medical conclusion', which allows a national authority to issue a medical certificate even if the standards are not fully met, if it believes it is safe to do so. The authority must take into account the relevant ability and skill of the applicant, operational conditions, and apply any special limitations that would allow safe performance. The application of case-based flexibility is in line with the tenets of occupational risk assessment.

In Europe, aviation regulations applying to all states and underpinned by EU law are necessary given the freedom of movement of citizens and aircraft crossing several international boundaries during one flight.[32] The European Aviation Safety Agency (EASA) was created in 2003 with the responsibility for setting common medical and licensing standards for pilots and air traffic controllers (ATCOs). These are implemented in each state by the national aviation authority. The aviation-related impact of the UK leaving the EU in 2019 is presently unknown.

Aviation legislation

The Equality Act 2010 does not apply to matters of disability employment on board a ship, aircraft, or hovercraft. Civil aviation legislation (The Civil Aviation Act 1982 and the Air Navigation Order 2016) specifies the requirements for licensed jobs. However, if a licence holder is no longer able to meet medical standards due to a disability, an employer should consider alternative roles within the company that could allow continued employment.

Awareness in the medical community

Many treating physicians are unaware of the specific requirements surrounding the assessment of fitness to fly or control. This can lead to situations where a licence holder is advised they may return to work with a 'minor' condition, but experiences symptoms that could impair their ability to carry out the role safely. An example is a pilot with a cold who is unable to equalize their ear pressure; on descent, this can lead to distracting pain, acute hearing loss, and potentially perforation. If this occurs during a critical phase of flight and distracts them from completing checklists or hinders communication, safety of crew and passengers is compromised. Similarly, medication may be prescribed by health professionals who are unaware of incompatibility with certification due to the condition itself or potential side effects (e.g. codeine for back pain). In cases where there may be a risk to public safety, such as alcohol-related disorders, treating doctors should refer to the GMC confidentiality guidance (see 'Useful websites') and consider if their duty to protect the public outweighs maintaining patient confidentiality. If so, they should inform the regulatory authority and advise the licence holder of the intended action, if safe and practicable.

Licence holders are responsible for ensuring they seek advice from aeromedical examiners (AMEs) in any decrease of medical fitness, injury or illness, or prescription of medication.[33,34] They must also inform their employer if they are unfit to fly or control. OH professionals who are asked for advice should refer the licence holder to their AME.

Role of the aeromedical examiner

An AME is a doctor with specialist training in aviation medicine.[28] Training incorporates an understanding of aerospace physiology, job tasks, and operating environment of pilots, ATCOs, and cabin crew to provide an objective assessment of fitness in accordance with regulatory standards. AMEs have a role in educating medical colleagues to consider the distinctive requirements of these safety-critical workers.

Case example: Germanwings Flight 4U9525, 24 March 2015

This accident[35] resulted in 150 deaths when the co-pilot locked the cockpit door, intentionally set the autopilot to descend, and crew were unable to prevent impact into mountainous terrain. The pilot had a past history of severe depression and symptoms of anxiety during the preceding several months. He was treated by several physicians with psychotropic medication and issued certificates of sickness absence. Neither the pilot nor treating physicians informed the AME, regulatory authority, or employer of his condition and treatment.

Recognizing the increasing proportion of workers experiencing mental compared to physical health conditions, the accident report and recent surveys recommended that the focus for assessment should shift to identifying subtly incapacitating psychiatric conditions, encouraging open reporting and peer support.[36]

Organizational factors pertinent to aviation include reliance on self-declaration, protracted periods of unfitness for work during episodes of mental ill-health affecting employability, financial costs of training, strict insurance policies, and ethical conflicts for doctors balancing patient confidentiality with a wider duty to protect the public.

Overview of occupational hazards

Pilots

Pilots are subject to physical hazards including aircraft noise, cosmic radiation, reduced atmospheric pressure, extremes of temperature especially in military operations, and whole body vibration in helicopters. Aircraft may not be designed ergonomically to cater for extremes in height or habitus, so individual risk assessment should ensure all cockpit controls can be accessed and emergency egress can be performed rapidly. In terms of medical standards, exposure to relative hypobaria and hypoxia require good cardiorespiratory function and freedom from conditions likely to be aggravated by sudden changes in pressure and volume, such as middle ear and sinus disorders, lung bullae, and bowel herniation.

Equally important are psychosocial hazards. A flight may be characterized by spikes of intense mental workload interspersed with periods of inactivity. Therefore, clear cognition, good communication, and team working skills are vital to flight safety. Many pilots are shift workers flying an irregular pattern. The International Civil Aviation Organization defines fatigue as 'a physiological state of reduced mental or physical performance capability, resulting from sleep loss or extended wakefulness, circadian phase or workload (mental and/or physical activity) that can impair a crew member's alertness and ability to safely operate an aircraft or perform safety-related duties'.[37] Fatigue risk in aviation is well recognized and requires careful management by the regulator, operator, and individual to minimize flight safety impacts. Consider secondary effects of shift work such as irregular eating patterns in a pilot managing diabetes, and sleep disturbance in a pilot with depression.

Medical standards for commercial pilots are rigorous and current guidance should be referred to.[31] Assessment of fitness to fly includes consideration of the condition itself and symptoms, the effect of any treatment including medication or surgery, and operational limitations that may allow a safe return to duty.

Air traffic controllers

Medical standards for ATCOs were originally derived from those applied to commercial pilots. However, the working environment and tasks performed by ATCOs vary significantly from pilots and case-based flexibility can be applied by the licensing authority when assessing fitness to control.

There is no exposure to hypoxic or hypobaric conditions in the ground-based environment. Tasks for aerodrome or tower-based ATCOs include clearing aircraft to take off and land within close proximity to the airport, and instructing aircraft and vehicles on the ground. ATCOs based in large operational area control centres may work in area, terminal, or oceanic control. They prevent collisions between aircraft in upper airspace or approaching airports, and maintain an orderly flow of air traffic over the UK's congested skies. Shift work may follow a more regular pattern than pilots; 2 mornings/2 afternoons/ 2 nights followed by 4 days off. Duty hours are strictly regulated.

Intensive use of colour-rich display screen equipment has led to EU colour vision standards requiring normal trichromacy, an exceptionally high bar. In the UK, this is modified to allow functionally normal trichromats to commence training.[38]

Cognitive requirements include the ability to process multiple sensory inputs, interpret information, safe decision-making, and handle emergency situations. This requires a level of psychological and emotional resilience reflected in intensive training. Commonly, ATCOs work in 'watches' where a cohort may work together for several years; this may be a protective factor with peer support and possibly lead to earlier detection of behavioural changes, compared to pilots who infrequently fly together. In 2016, harmonization of some ATCO and pilot medical standards allowed the use of selected antidepressants for maintenance treatment of depression for the first time in the UK.

Sudden incapacitation of an ATCO can pose a risk to flight safety that varies according to the speed of onset and seriousness of the illness event, speed of reaction of colleagues and supervisors, and the duration and circumstances of incomplete surveillance of the airspace. Research in the UK into risks and consequences of incapacitation suggests that fitness standards should vary between the differing ATCO roles.

Cabin crew

Although cabin crew do not hold licences, they play an important safety role on board an aircraft, and require competence in operating aircraft emergency systems. The EASA produced new medical requirements for cabin crew in 2014 that require periodic examination and/or assessment by either an AME or occupational physician and consideration of their operating environment.

Environmental and shift work exposures reflect those of pilots. Cabin crew are exposed to potential biological hazards from contact with passengers with infectious disease (including performing first aid), cleaning, and food handling. Ergonomic hazards working in confined galleys include reaching above shoulder height, pushing and manoeuvring heavy carts, risks of slips, trips, and spillage of hot liquids. There are psychological and physical challenges dealing with passengers who pose security risks or exhibit disruptive behaviour after consuming alcohol.

Flight engineers, flight navigators, and flight information service officers

With modernization of aircraft, there are fewer flight engineers and flight navigators. They assist in monitoring the actions of pilots as well as controlling aircraft systems, hence cognitive and physical function should be commensurate with their safety-related role. National medical standards are similar to those of pilots.

Flight information service officers are licensed by the CAA to provide information and instructions to pilots by radio. They must hold a medical declaration of fitness; the standards follow DVLA group 2 drivers, with specific requirements for vision, colour perception, and hearing.

Future challenges

The roles of pilots and ATCOs are evolving to interact more closely with technological tools, therefore selection and training should reflect the skillset required. As a workforce, numbers required to fly aircraft or look after vast tracts of airspace are likely to decrease and the cultural change will need to be handled carefully by operators. Remotely piloted aircraft systems are a reality, with specific occupational hazards for the ground-based pilots who may be exposed to visually traumatic scenes discordant with their physical location. There are opportunities for physicians in this field to work closely with specialists in human factors, vision science, psychologists, engineering, and ergonomics to continually improve aviation safety.

Key points

- The prime purpose of medical fitness assessments in transport is to reduce public safety risks.
- The evidence base on risk is limited and much of it is common to all modes of transport.
- Stable disabilities can best be assessed by tests that simulate the demands of work.
- Disabilities that are episodic are assessed in terms of the probability of recurrence.
- Many of the safety-critical tasks in transport are based on workstations (road and rail driving, flying, rail, and air traffic control). Some in addition involve other physically or mentally demanding routine or emergency duties.

Useful websites

DVLA. Drivers Medical Unit. *Assessing Fitness to Drive: A Guide for Health Professionals*	https://www.gov.uk/government/publications/assessing-fitness-to-drive-a-guide-for-medical-professionals
DVLA. Medical advisers email—see website for contact phone numbers	medadviser@dvla.gsi.gov.uk
Department for Transport	http://www.dft.gov.uk
Department for Transport. Agendas, minutes, and annual reports of the medical panels	http://www.dft.gov.uk/dvla/medical/medical_advisory_information/medicaladvisory_meetings/
General Medical Council.' Confidentiality: patients' fitness to drive and reporting concerns to the DVLA or DVA', 2017	https://www.gmc-uk.org/ethical-guidance/ethical-guidance-for-doctors/confidentiality---patients-fitness-to-drive-and-reporting-concerns-to-the-dvla-or-dva

Driving mobility. A network of centres which offer information, assessment and advice about mobility	https://www.drivingmobility.org.uk/
Office of Rail and Road (ORR)	http://orr.gov.uk/
ORR. Safety-critical tasks	http://orr.gov.uk/__data/assets/pdf_file/0014/2633/rsp004-rogs-crtcl_tasks.pdf
ORR. Train driver licensing	http://orr.gov.uk/__data/assets/pdf_file/0003/4998/train-driving-licences-regulations-guidance.pdf
Rail Standards and Safety Board (RSSB)	http://www.rssb.co.uk
Association of Rail Industry Occupational Health Practitioners (ARIOPS)	http://www.ariops.org.uk
Union International des Chemin de Fer (UIC)	http://www.uic.org
Rail Accident Investigation Board (RAIB)	https://www.gov.uk/government/organisations/rail-accident-investigation-branch
National Institute for Health and Care Excellence. Self-monitoring of blood glucose (section 1.6.13) when driving and at risk of hypoglycaemia	https://www.nice.org.uk/guidance/ng28/chapter/1-recommendations#blood-glucose-management-2
Civil Aviation Authority. Guidance for medical certification of professional pilots	http://www.caa.co.uk/Commercial-industry/Pilot-licences/Medical/Guidance-for-medical-certification-of-professional-pilots/

Acknowledgements

The editors gratefully acknowledge the contribution of Wyn Parry.

References

1 **Department for Transport**. Passenger casualty rates by mode: 2006–2015 (RAS 53001). Available at: https://www.gov.uk/government/statistical-data-sets/ras53-modal-comparisons.
2 **Taylor JF** (ed). *Medical Aspects of Fitness to Drive*. London: Medical Commission on Accident Prevention; 1995.
3 **Department for Transport**. Reported road casualties in Great Britain: main results 2015. Available at: https://assets.publishing.service.gov.uk/government/uploads/system/uploads/attachment_data/file/556396/rrcgb2015-01.pdf.
4. **Owsley C, McGwin Jr G.** Vision and driving. *Vis Res* 2010;50:2348–61.

5. **The European Parliament and the Council of the European Union**. European Union Directive on driving licences 2006/126/EC, from 19 January 2013. Available at: http://ec.europa.eu/transport/road_safety/behavior/driving_licence_en.htm

6. **Department for Transport, Health and Safety Executive**. Driving at work: managing work-related road safety. 2004. Available at: http://www.hse.gov.uk/pubns/indg382.pdf.

7. **Health and Safety Executive**. *Rider-Operated Lift Trucks: Operator Training and Safe Use. Approved Code of Practice and Guidance*. London: Health and Safety Executive; 2013.

8. **Road Traffic Act 1988 (Section 92). Motor Vehicles (Driving Licence) Regulations** 1999.

9. **Judiciary of Scotland**. Fatal accident inquiry: Glasgow bin lorry crash. Available at: http://www.scotland-judiciary.org.uk/10/1531/Fatal-Accident-Inquiry--Glasgow-bin-lorry-crash.

10. **Charlton J, Koppel SN, O'Hare MA, et al.** *Influence of Chronic Illness on Crash Involvement of Motor Vehicle Drivers*. Monash University Accident Research Centre Report 213. Clayton: Monash University Accident Research Centre; 2004. Available at: http://www.general.monash.edu.au/muarc.

11. **Carter T.** *Fitness to Drive: A Guide for Health Professionals*. London: RSM Press; 2006.

12. **Spencer MB, Carter T, Nicholson AN.** Limitations of risk analysis in the determination of medical factors in road vehicle accidents. *Clin Med* 2004;**4**:50–3.

13. **Driver and Vehicle Licensing Agency**. Diabetes mellitus: assessing fitness to drive. Advice for medical professionals to follow when assessing drivers with diabetes mellitus. 2016 (Last updated January 2018). Available at: https://www.gov.uk/guidance/diabetes-mellitus-assessing-fitness-to-drive.

14. **Carter T, Major H, Wetherall G, et al.** Excessive daytime sleepiness and driving: regulations for road safety. *Clin Med* 2004;**4**:454–6.

15. **British Thoracic Society**. Position statement: Driving and sleep apnoea (OSA) 2018. https://www.brit-thoracic.org.uk/document-library/about-bts/documents/position-statement-on-driving-and-obstructive-sleep-apnoea/.

16. **Rudisill TM, Zhu M, Kelley GA, Pilkerton C, Rudisill BR.** Medication use and the risk of motor vehicle collisions among licensed drivers: a systematic review. *Accid Anal Prev* 2016;**96**:255–70.

17. **Shepherd KL, Hillman D, Holloway R, Eastwood P.** Mechanisms of nocturnal gastroesophageal reflux events in obstructive sleep apnea. *Sleep Breath* 2011;**15**:561–70.

18. **Colquhoun CP, Casolin A.** Impact of rail medical standard on obstructive sleep apnoea prevalence. *Occup Med* 2016;**66**:62–8.

19. **Kodl CT, Seaquist ER.** Cognitive dysfunction and diabetes mellitus. *Endocr Rev* 2008;**29**:494–511.

20. **Roriz-Filho JS, Sá-Roriz TM, Rosset I, et al.** (Pre)diabetes, brain aging, and cognition. *Biochimica et Biophysica Acta* 2009;**1792**:432–43.

21. **Kandelaars K, Lamons N, Roach GD, et al.** The impact of extended leave on sleep and alertness in the Australian rail industry. *Ind Health* 2005;**43**:105–13.

22. **Knutsona KL, Van Cauter E.** Associations between sleep loss and increased risk of obesity and diabetes. *Ann N Y Acad Sci* 2008;**1129**:287–304.

23. **Office of Rail and Road**. Managing rail staff fatigue. 2012. Available at: http://orr.gov.uk/__data/assets/pdf_file/0005/2867/managing_rail_fatigue.pdf.

24. **Health and Safety Executive**. Fatigue management. Available at: http://www.hse.gov.uk/humanfactors/topics/fatigue.htm.

25. **Rail Standards and Safety Board**. Fatigue and its contribution to railway accidents. 2015. Available at: https://www.rssb.co.uk/Library/risk-analysis-and-safety-reporting/2015-02-str-fatigue-contribution-to-railway-incidents.pdf.

26. **National Transport Commission Australia**. *National Standard for Health Assessment of Rail Safety Workers*. Melbourne: National Transport Commission Australia; 2017. Available at: https://www.ntc.gov.au/rail/safety/national-standard-for-health-assessment-of-rail-safety-workers/.

27. **Chavda S.** Sickness absence of LU train drivers after track incidents. *Occup Med* 2016;**66**:571–5.

28. **UK Civil Aviation Authority**. CAP 795: Safety management systems – guidance to organisations. 2015. Available at: http://publicapps.caa.co.uk/modalapplication.aspx?appid=11&mode=detail &id=6616.

29. **Anderson IH.** *Prediction of the High Risk Airline Pilot.* Presented at the 44th Annual Scientific Meeting of the Aerospace Medical Association, Las Vegas, 7–10 May 1973.

30. **International Civil Aviation Organization**. *Annex 1 to the Convention on International Civil Aviation*, 11th edn. Amendment 172. Montreal: International Civil Aviation Organization; 2011.

31. **International Civil Aviation Organization**. *Manual of Civil Aviation Medicine*. Montreal: International Civil Aviation Organization; 2012. Available at: https://www.icao.int/ publications/pages/publication.aspx?docnum=8984.

32. **Evans ADB, Evans S, Harper G.** International regulation of medical standards. In: Gradwell DP, Rainford DR (eds), *Ernsting's Aviation and Space Medicine,* 5th edn, pp. 357–71. Boca Raton, FL: CRC Press; 2016.

33. **European Commission**. Commission Regulation (EU) No. 1178/2011. Aircrew Regulation – Annex IV Part-MED General Requirements. 2011. Available at: https://www.easa.europa.eu/document-library/regulations/commission-regulation-eu-no-11782011.

34. **European Commission**. Commission Regulation (EU) No. 2015/340. Aircrew Regulation – Annex IV Part ATCO.MED: Medical Requirements for Air Traffic Controllers. 2015. Available at: http:// eur-lex.europa.eu/legal-content/EN/TXT/PDF/?uri=OJ:JOL_2015_063_R_0001&from=EN.

35. **Bureau d'Enquêtes et d'Analyses**. Final Report: Accident on 24 March 2015 at Prads-Haute-Bléone to the Airbus A320-211 registered D-AIPX operated by Germanwings. 2016. Available at: https:// www.bea.aero/uploads/tx_elydbrapports/BEA2015-0125.en-LR.pdf.

36. **Mitchell S, Lillywhite M.** Medical cause fatal commercial air transport accidents: analysis of UK CAA worldwide accident database 1980-2011. *Aviat Space Environ Med* 2013;**84**:346.

37. **International Civil Aviation Organization**. *Doc 9966. Manual for the Oversight of Fatigue Management Approaches*, 2nd edn. Montreal: International Civil Aviation Organization; 2016. Available at: https://www.icao.int/safety/fatiguemanagement/FRMS%20Tools/9966_cons_en.pdf.

38. **UK Civil Aviation Authority**. UK CAA policy statement – ATCO colour vision v1.1 July. 2017. Available at: http://www.caa.co.uk/Aeromedical-Examiners/Connecting-with-the-CAA/ Documents-for-download/.

Chapter 16

Seafaring, offshore energy, and diving

Tim Carter, Sally Bell, Mike Doig,
Robbert Hermanns, and Phil Bryson

Introduction

Seafaring, work in the offshore energy sector, and commercial diving share a number of common features that are relevant to the assessment of fitness to work. Physically and mentally demanding tasks, many of which are considered safety critical, are performed, often in an unforgiving environment. Workplaces are commonly remote from onshore health and emergency services, necessitating the provision of emergency medical and incident (including fire) response on site. Employees must be trained and physically and mentally capable of performing these rare but demanding roles. The risks from a serious injury or illness are raised by the lack of full medical care facilities. Transfer to shore may be delayed and place rescue services in danger. Many employees live on board their workplace, often for weeks at a time. This means that work and leisure intertwine, sometimes in stressful ways. Safe and acceptable food and sleeping quarters are required and, as shift work or watchkeeping is usual, these must be available 24 hours a day. Travel to work may be lengthy and complex, involving fixed wing and helicopter flights. Work may commence immediately on arrival in a new time zone and there can be exposure to exotic infections and other risks while in transit.

Systems for medical assessment of fitness for work in these sectors address capacity for both routine and emergency duties and likelihood of serious medical incapacitation that compromises performance or puts the individual, workmates, or rescue services at increased risk as a result of their distance from medical facilities. In addition, there are opportunities for health promotion and data collection for disease prevention initiatives.

Many fitness criteria are necessarily task and location specific; criteria for a ship's officer with navigating duties on a coastal car ferry will differ from those applicable to a ship's cook working in the Antarctic. Employees on an offshore platform with emergency response functions must meet additional standards for physical capability. In diving, standards are influenced by diving depths and techniques. Time and distance from, and accessibility to, medical support are crucial in assessing the risk of serious medical incapacitation; even a relatively close offshore installation can be impossible to reach for days in poor weather conditions and decompressing from saturation working depth to normal atmospheric pressure can take 4–5 days or longer.

The evidence base for medical fitness criteria in these sectors is limited, and many derive from onshore population data or progressive modification of existing criteria with experience, changes in medical practice, or changing expectations about employment among those with disabilities.

The detailed arrangements for medical assessment vary. Seafaring has statutory national fitness standards set by governmental maritime authorities, and underpinned by international conventions agreed by United Nations agencies. Employers and their insurers sometimes set additional criteria with the aim of reducing their liabilities.

By contrast, the offshore energy sector in the UK and in some other countries relies on non-statutory fitness criteria that are set by the relevant trade association. A non-statutory system has the potential advantage of greater flexibility, but there is less public accountability and less influence on standard setting by employees, their representatives, and the medical profession.

Diving also has a statutory system for assessment of fitness. Diving medical assessors need a good understanding of the special demands and risks of diving work. They are required to have appropriate training and, in the UK, approval by the Health and Safety Executive (HSE). Approval for UK seafarer medical examiners is given by the Maritime and Coastguard Agency (MCA). The trade association Oil & Gas UK (OGUK) oversees the medical fitness assessment system for workers on fixed offshore platforms.

Seafaring, offshore work, and diving are all very international, with employees moving regularly between countries. Consequently, international bodies are actively moving to improve the compatibility of fitness criteria. However, not all recognize the importance of quality assurance systems to ensure consistent, valid decision-taking and good ethical practice in medical assessments.

Seafaring

Seafaring is a job and a way of life. As a job, it has both risks and performance requirements. As a lifestyle, the impact on diet, exercise, social interactions, distance from healthcare facilities, and worldwide travel are all important. The sector has complex international patterns of staffing, ownership of vessels, and employment contracts. Therefore, maritime countries have limited freedom to set their own policies and standards.

Work demands on seafarers vary widely. Service may be worldwide, inshore, or on inland waterways. Vessel types include bulk carriers, container ships, cruise liners, ferries, commercial yachts, and canal boats. Responsibilities differ between officers and ratings. Risks and performance requirements on the bridge, in the engine room, and in passenger service have little in common. In an emergency, physically and psychologically demanding tasks may be undertaken by all crewmembers, including firefighting in restricted spaces, launching and manning lifeboats, or rescuing casualties from the sea.

All seafarers are required to hold a statutory certificate of medical fitness issued in accordance with the requirements of the state where the ship is registered. Some employers and maritime insurers also require additional medical assessments, but these are not always properly validated or ethically justifiable.

Standard setting

Several major international organizations have a part to play in standard setting:

◆ The International Labour Organization (ILO), Maritime Labour Convention 2006 consolidates into a single instrument the requirements and recommendations on medical fitness certification, medical care at sea, many other aspects of working and living at sea, and seafarers' welfare. This has been ratified worldwide, with signatories introducing compatible laws and regulations. These include sanctions that can be applied to ships that fail to meet the convention's requirements.[1]

◆ The Maritime Labour Convention does not apply to fishing but the similar Work in Fishing Convention 2007 came into force in late 2017. National laws are being revised to make them compatible with it.[2]

◆ The International Maritime Organization (IMO) is concerned with vessel safety and the contribution to safety of human performance. Their amended Convention on Standards of Training, Certification and Watchkeeping for Seafarers (STCW), includes requirements for medical fitness in safety-critical jobs.[3] These have been adopted into national laws by most maritime nations.

◆ The ILO and IMO have jointly published detailed guidelines on the medical examination procedures and fitness criteria for the issue of statutory medical certificates.[4]

◆ The World Health Organization is important in relation to infection control, port health agreements, and emergency care of seafarers.[5]

◆ The European Union (EU) regulates working hours and emergency medical supplies carried on EU vessels.[6,7]

◆ There is also a wide range of internationally integrated employer, trade union, and professional bodies (see 'Useful websites').

Within each country, a maritime authority implements these standards and may also be concerned with their enforcement. In the UK, the responsibility for this is with the MCA, an agency of the Department for Transport. Medical standards for determining the fitness of seafarers are produced and updated regularly by the Agency.[8] These standards align with international requirements. Seafarers serving on UK-flagged ships must have a medical certificate, issued within the last 2 years, showing that they meet these standards. Certificates of certain other countries are accepted as equivalent.[9]

The standards have been developed over more than a century in the light of experience, changes in medical practice, and with a view to practicability and fairness in application. The rationale of the fitness criteria for each condition is specified and this is increasingly based on validated evidence of risk. There are two patterns of medical assessment against the standards, one for the majority of merchant seafarers who need to comply with international requirements and another for the masters of small commercial craft such as yachts, work-boats, and passenger vessels in inland and estuarial waters.[10]

Guidance for use of the same standards with respect to fishing is being developed to align with the ILO Work in Fishing Convention 2007.

Seafarer medicals

Merchant seafarer medicals are undertaken by doctors approved by the Agency. Approval is at the discretion of the MCA and is based on local need. There are about 240 approved doctors in the UK and overseas. Most are available to any seafarer but a few are approved only in relation to a single company or for a range of company contracts (see 'Useful websites' for a live list of MCA-approved doctors). Approved doctors are assisted by a procedural manual and have access to MCA administrative and medical staff for advice (see 'Useful websites'). Standards of work are monitored and the majority of doctors now have relevant occupational medical or maritime experience.

Over 50,000 merchant seafarer medicals are done each year. Of these, about 3000 lead to some form of restriction on service or to failure. Seafarers have the right to a review by an independent medical referee, of whom there are eight. About 40 seafarers seek review each year.

Those who work on local commercial boats and yachts may alternatively go to any doctor registered in the UK, but normally their general practitioner (GP), who will complete a medical screening form (ML5). If there are no positive findings, an MCA marine office or the Royal Yacht Association will, subject to other tests of knowledge and competency, issue a boatmasters' licence or commercial endorsement. If a possibly relevant medical condition is identified, an MCA-appointed medical assessor will review the available medical information. They may fail the applicant or may issue a full or restricted ML5 certificate, which can then be used to support the licence application.

For some conditions, fitness criteria are straightforward. Thus, in an environment where navigation lights are red, green, and white, anyone who cannot distinguish these colours cannot undertake lookout duties. Others may be very complex. A cardiac event may cause continuing impairment to physical or cognitive performance, either of which could affect capability for routine or emergency duties. An increased risk of sudden incapacity is critical when navigating the ship or working alone. Recurrence poses a greater risk to seafarers but also to others if evacuation is needed, and creates operational problems if other crew members need to provide care or the ship has to be diverted. Fitness decisions will depend on the person's duties and where the ship is operating.

As seafarers live in close quarters and food is prepared on board, infection risks (e.g. tuberculosis or foodborne illness) are important.

Formal standards are particularly contentious where they concern risk factors rather than disease; for instance, those concerned with future cardiac risk such as hypertension and obesity—two of the commonest reasons for restriction. Related lifestyle interventions concerned with diet and smoking may be difficult for the individual to implement at sea unless there is commitment from owners and masters.

As a consequence of the variety of job requirements, most standards depend on the job of the seafarer and on the part of the world in which the vessel sails.[11] Like any other statutory measure affecting employment and livelihood, the fitness assessment system must be demonstrably fair and credible, applied uniformly, and associated with an independent review procedure. The balance in standard settings is between public safety and individual employment opportunities.

Some maritime employers have additional fitness criteria but they may not go below the statutory minimum. Seafarers, to secure or maintain employment, sometimes fail to disclose health problems or may seek to avoid optimum treatment of conditions that require medications such as insulin or warfarin, which, because of their side effects, can be a bar to work at sea.

A wide range of health professionals can, from time to time, be involved in the care of seafarers and potential seafarers. In such situations, there are a number of considerations:

1. Young people who want to work at sea should be aware of the need to meet medical standards. It is helpful to advise anyone who is unlikely to meet these standards to reconsider their career options. Issues that commonly cause work limitation relate to vision, especially colour vision; asthma, which is usually better at sea but very dangerous in the event of a sudden exacerbation; congenital conditions, for instance, of the heart or limbs; seizures; and diabetes.

2. Immunizations and antimalarial prophylaxis may be needed. Seafarers should be advised of this and arrangements made for provision, usually by their employer, but they may seek advice or medications from others.[12]

3. Seafarers requiring elective surgery. Priority may be sought so that they can comply with medical standards and return to work (see Dreadnought Unit in 'Useful websites').

4. After a diagnosis of a significant illness such as heart disease, diabetes, or epilepsy, the seafarer will need to obtain a new medical certificate. They may have to wait until the condition is stabilized, and may find themselves restricted or declared unfit.

5. When continuing medication is needed, the acceptability of the person for sea service should be assessed. In some cases, the medication itself will dictate restricting duties or an unfit declaration.

6. If cardiac risk factors are poorly controlled, especially weight and blood pressure, the patient should be reminded that failure to achieve control may lead to termination of their sea career even in the absence of a cardiac event.

Offshore workers

Offshore oil and gas production is found in almost all the oceans of the world (shallow and deep water, arctic and tropical). Despite the increase in renewable energy, the quest to find and extract resources through exploration and development continues. The UK remains an important world oil producer. Total production in the UK peaked in 1999, but in 2016 the United Kingdom Continental Shelf (UKCS) still produced 45% of the UK's primary energy needs.[13] Fourteen UKCS fields ceased production in 2016 with a similar number expected in 2017 and a further 30–40 fields are expected to cease production before 2020.[14] Although decommissioning is the most rapidly increasing threat to the industry, it provides employment for 300,000 people in the UK with 28,000 directly employed by oil and gas companies. Following a number of fatal accidents, helicopter safety has been prominent in recent years—resulting in revised safety and medical standards for helicopter evacuation.

Offshore windfarms have become a major source of energy in the UK. While geographically proximal to the oil and gas industry, this industry has a unique set of health challenges associated with its isolation, tall structure and cramped working conditions.

Offshore installations

There are currently 261 fixed (rigid or floating) installations (143 manned, 118 unmanned) in the North Sea with a varying number of supporting mobile drilling and accommodation rigs.[15] They range in size from small exploration and drilling semisubmersibles to massive semi-permanent fixed-leg, or floating, oil production and export installations. Production installations are complex, requiring (in a limited space) an engineering plant to receive pressurized hot crude oil, and process and export it under pressure, through an undersea pipeline to onshore or an adjacent holding and discharge vessel. They are usually fixed-leg platforms, or floating moored facilities. In addition to the engineering infrastructure, there are accommodation and administration areas or modules for the workforce.

The offshore working environment

These complex, compact facilities pose a harsh and challenging working environment. Each offshore installation is a self-sufficient community in which people work and sleep for the full duration of their offshore tour—normally 3 weeks. Shift work is the norm and typically involves rotating 12-hour shifts. Living quarters offshore are modest but comfortable and usually shared, with two bunks per cabin. There are recreational facilities (e.g. gym or cinema). No alcohol is allowed. Smoking is restricted to a small smoking room. The use of nicotine vapour devices varies; OGUK recommends they are not permitted but some operators do allow use.[16]

Communication with the mainland can be fragile—radio or satellite links are subject to interference in bad weather. Logistic support is provided by helicopters for personnel movement, and supply vessels delivering food, water, and equipment. Depending on geographical location and weather, helicopter access can be impossible for several days. Supply vessel visits can also be disrupted by the weather, hampering supply of engineering tools, service supplies, fresh food, and water.

Constraints on manning and accommodation mean that sick or incapacitated staff may have to return onshore and be replaced by another worker. Emergency medical evacuations can be risky for a severely ill or injured person, expensive, and dangerous, particularly in inclement weather.

Range of functions

Typically a core crew of 50–250 undertakes a wide range of duties associated with a technically complex heavy engineering and oil production operation. Many of the tasks offshore are physically arduous. Regular heavy manual handling is required, and many large valves are still manually operated. Equipment needs regular maintenance and repair, often in a confined working space using heavy tools. The drilling team probably have the most arduous tasks. They regularly manhandle and connect pipe casings to form lengths of many kilometres that penetrate deep into the seabed. There are also specialized functions such as control room operators, chemists to test the oil and drill cuttings, health and safety professionals, geologists, caterers, stewards, cleaners, and importantly an offshore medic (see 'Health legislation').

Each installation falls under the authority of the offshore installation manager who is deemed, for legislative purposes, to be the on-site person in charge.

The provisions of the NHS do not extend offshore, so private health providers supply medical resources and health services mandated by legislation, industry standards, and best practice (Table 16.1).[17–21]

Table 16.1 Health legislation

The Continental Shelf Act 1964[17]	Extended petroleum exploration licensing arrangements to the offshore environment with provision for the safety, health, and welfare of persons employed on operations undertaken under the licence authority
The Management of Health and Safety at Work Act Control of Substances Hazardous to Health (COSHH) Working Time Directive	Extended to cover the offshore workforce
Safety Case Regulations (2005)[18]	Requires operators to have a safety case for fixed and mobile installations accepted by the HSE
Offshore Installations and Pipeworks (Management and Administration) Regulations 1995[19]	Requires provision of health surveillance and potable food and water
The Offshore Installations and Pipeline Works (First-Aid) Regulations 1989[20]	Requirements for the provision of healthcare facilities for everyone on an offshore installation and the responsibilities of the dedicated on-site medical provider: the offshore medic
The Offshore Installations (Prevention of Fire and Explosion, and Emergency Response) Regulations 1995 (PFEER)[21]	Set out requirements to plan an effective emergency response including that of the medical team in the event of serious incidents on an offshore installation

Industry guidance

Health and fitness standards in the oil industry are developed and published by the oil companies for internal application, and by external bodies representing the industry, that is, the Energy Institute through the Health Technical Committee and the Occupational Health and Hygiene Committee. They include the Physical Fitness Standards for the Oil Industry,[22,23] the Medical Standards of Fitness to Wear Respiratory Protective Equipment,[24] and Medical Aspects of Work for the Onshore Oil industry.[25] OGUK, the industry trade organization, also publishes the guidance for examining physicians for work offshore[26] using their own forum for expert input.

Because they are not defined by legislation, there is significant variation in published medical standards and a reluctance to universally adopt potentially restrictive standards such as capability assessments for physical tasks. However, in some cases these have already been implemented by the operating companies themselves.

Offshore survival training

Transport to offshore installations is normally by helicopter, in all but the most severe weather conditions. In a major emergency, rescue is likely to involve evacuation by lifeboat into the sea. Every employee offshore must hold a Certificate of Offshore Survival Training, approved by the Offshore Petroleum Industry Training Organisation (OPITO) and valid for 4 years.

This physically demanding Basic Offshore Safety Induction and Emergency Training (BOSIET) course[27] involves significant physical stressors such as water immersion, embarking a life raft from the water, and helicopter underwater escape training. Civil Aviation Authority (CAA) regulations[28] require helicopter passengers to be physically able to get out of their adjacent exit. A new emergency underwater breathing system (EBS) using pressurized air (category 1 EBS), which was introduced to aid escape from a helicopter, requires a specific survival training module. Successful completion of this course, as with a real emergency evacuation, requires a significant level of fitness, mobility, and psychological well-being as it can be stressful especially for non-swimmers. Candidates for this part of the course must have a specific fitness certificate signed by an OGUK-accredited physician. Refresher courses are required every 4 years. Recruits must also undergo Minimum Industry Safety Training (MIST).[29] This 2-day training programme promotes a common understanding of safety and awareness of the variety of tasks and safety risks on offshore installations: major accident hazards, workplace hazards and personal safety, risk management, control of work, and helicopter safety.

Offshore health facilities

All crewed offshore installations have a fully equipped medical clinic under the supervision of the offshore medic, usually comprising an examination area, a small one- or two-bedded ward, and the means to treat hypothermia.

Sickbay medical equipment is comprehensive. Basic recommended items, as defined in the industry first-aid and medical equipment guidelines, are often supplemented by sophisticated medical response and emergency equipment,[30] and drugs to cover most routine treatment and common emergencies.

The offshore medic

Offshore medics are usually trained nurses or armed services medical attendants who have passed the specific HSE-approved medic training course defined in the First-Aid Regulations.[30] This 4-week intensive course extends competency and skills to enable a first-line medical response for any sick or injured individual, including a wide range of medical interventions with no expectation of immediate medical back-up other than remote advice from an on-call physician. An on-board first-aid team can assist in extreme circumstances.

The medic's duties include the provision of primary medical care to personnel, emergency response, medical surveillance for occupationally related exposures, advising on hygiene, and health promotion. Normally a platform has one medic who is on call 24 hours per day.

A consulting onshore physician, 'the topside doctor', is available for 24-hour support for difficult cases. This may involve basic telemedicine techniques or lead to medical evacuation.

Medical screening

The examining physician should assess both fitness for duties and the likelihood of physical or mental illness offshore that could place the worker, their colleagues, or the emergency rescue services at undue risk (Box 16.1).

Box 16.1 Determinants of an individual's fitness for work offshore

- Diagnosis, aetiology, and prognosis of any medical conditions.
- Impact of current or planned treatment.
- Risk of relapse, or acute exacerbations that could require urgent medical intervention.
- Risk of any adverse effects that could be precipitated or exacerbated by the offshore environment.
- Significantly restricted and remote access to specialist medical support, facilities, and supplies.
- Match between physical ability to do the essential tasks and limited ability to modify work environment or job function.

Physicians who assess fitness to work offshore must be approved by the OGUK. The OGUK medical examination is biannual, with more frequent reviews for workers with significant ongoing pathology.

Workers for the Norwegian and Dutch sectors have separate certification to their country specific standards, NOG and NOGEPA respectively. OGUK, Norwegian, and Dutch medicals are mutually accepted.

Increasingly within the oil industry, functional capacity evaluations are recognized as an essential part of medical evaluations for jobs with significant physical elements. These determine, through simple physical tests such as muscular strength, stamina, aerobic capacity, and functional task simulation, capability to perform essential physical tasks safely.

Emergency response team

Offshore installations must have arrangements to provide an effective response in the event of an offshore emergency.[31] One element of this is a specifically trained emergency response team (ERT) with various specialized roles including the rescue of casualties and firefighting. ERT members have their normal full-time duties while on board, and ERT responsibilities are additional. The Energy Institute has published evidence-based guidelines for oil and gas workers, both onshore and offshore, including ERT members.[22,23] The OGUK Medical Guidelines[26] currently only stipulate task-related physical fitness guidelines for ERT members.

All ERT members undergo specific training at an OPITO-approved facility, see Box 16.2.

Medical fitness and disability

The Equality Act 2010 applies offshore and to offshore workers,[32] but it may be justifiable on safety grounds to exclude persons with significant disability that might reduce mobility in an emergency or impede the egress of others. The final decision on the fitness of anyone with a significant disability should always be made by an occupational physician who has a thorough knowledge of the offshore environment—usually with reference to the medical advisor of the operating oil company.

Box 16.2 ERT training tasks

- Use of multiple cylinder breathing apparatus.
- Repeated or prolonged manual casualty lifting and carrying.
- Firefighting including fire hose handling and moving foam barrels.
- Search and rescue in smoke filled/hot environments.
- Casualty rescue from platform legs or vessel holds.

Obesity and body size

In the absence of resultant disease, obesity is now managed offshore primarily as a safety issue. The practicalities of mobility, transport, and evacuation in an emergency are the restricting issues. Ability to physically escape from a ditched helicopter through the emergency exits and window openings has received CAA priority. It is recognized that the average weight of offshore workers has increased significantly over recent years, such that the HSE has issued guidelines on how to avoid exceeding design loads and seating space in lifeboats.

In order to ensure safe emergency exit from a helicopter, workers' bi-deltoid (shoulder) measurement is recorded in an offshore database (Vantage) and matched at heliport check-in to their allocated seating.

Occupational health

It is important in calculating exposure limits in the offshore environment to allow for the 12-hour shift pattern. Multiple exposures may be present with potential interaction and potentiation. Health surveillance is required by law where there is a known adverse health effect and a valid means of delivering it (Box 16.3). The Energy Institute publish comprehensive guidance on health surveillance applicable to the oil industry.[33]

Catering

Food safety is critical on an offshore installation. Each installation has a single catering facility for the whole workforce, which must observe the highest food hygiene standards and comply with the Offshore Environmental Health Guidelines.[34] Any significant episode of food poisoning could be catastrophic, both for the crew and the safe production.

Drilling

Drilling, whether exploratory or on established fields, is a high-risk activity with both physical and chemical hazards. Although highly mechanized, this part of the offshore operations is one of the most hazardous with respect to manual handling and

---

Box 16.3 Hazard and toxic exposures offshore

- Chemical: toxic, corrosive, irritant, sensitizing, and potentially carcinogenic agents.
- Physical: noise, vibration, radiation, and extremes of temperature.
- Biological: risk of food poisoning, and *Legionella*.
- Ergonomic: manual handling, computer workstations.
- Psychosocial: work overload, shift work, tour patterns, work relationships, travel, isolation from home and family.

musculoskeletal injuries. High-pressure drilling fluids that may contain toxic chemicals, and high levels of noise are also constant hazards.

Drugs and alcohol

Alcohol and drugs that may interfere with performance are not tolerated on safety grounds at any time. Operating companies have strictly enforced drug and alcohol policies monitored by random testing, searches at the heliport, and sometimes searches offshore. Sniffer dogs may be taken offshore to scan accommodation and living areas, and urine testing is used post incident or for random personal screening.

Infectious diseases

The close, and constantly changing, community of an offshore oil installation is the perfect environment for the spread of infectious diseases. The threat from pandemics or biological terrorism has identified offshore installations as potentially vulnerable. The industry has detailed infectious disease protocols that define the processes for liaison between companies, including the helicopter operators, and onshore NHS facilities to minimize the risk of the transfer of infectious agents in an outbreak or pandemic situation.

Mental well-being

The demands of this working environment including shift work, isolation, and separation from family and friends for weeks at a time can threaten mental well-being. The spouse or partner who is running the household during this period may also be under considerable pressure. Consequently, many operating and contracting companies have stress awareness programmes for offshore workers and their families. Employee assistance programmes are often provided by the major oil operators. These services support organizations with managing the stressful consequences of reorganization, redundancy, and traumatic incidents such as major accidents or workplace deaths.

Shift work

The 24-hour operation of an offshore installation requires that most workers are on shifts. Unmanaged circadian desynchrony can threaten safety through a fall in alertness and decreased reaction times. A number of recognized factors contribute to fatigue, see Box 16.4.

Following a shift change, it takes several days for circadian–chronological synchrony to occur, so workers on a new nightshift may not perform optimally for the first few nights. Some studies suggest that, for some, synchrony may not take place at all during the period of a nightshift. This can lead to sleep disturbance, fatigue, and reduced performance.[35] Good practice includes minimizing shift changes during an offshore rotation and optimizing sleeping conditions with good blackout and low noise. HSE guidance sets out specific advice related to working practices for managing shift work and fatigue offshore, see Box 16.5.[36]

Box 16.4 Hazards of shift-working offshore

- Early shifts starting before 6 a.m.
- Overtime in excess of the 12-hour shift.
- Call-outs when off duty.
- Being offshore too long without breaks.
- Long periods of attention.
- Failure to provide back-up crew for absences or no-shows.
- Tasks with low error tolerance combined with high consequences.
- Long journey times preceding travel offshore and immediately commencing night shift on arrival on the platform.

The ageing workforce

The offshore workforce shows a bimodal demographic distribution with the majority of the personnel in the younger age groups. The average age has remained static at 40.8 years, not increasing as was previously expected.[37] There are no age limits to working in the offshore environment. Workers are subject to the same age-related factors of any workforce: decreasing muscle mass and physical capacity, decreased endurance and earlier fatigue, decrements in coordination and balance, and an increase in pathological conditions that may affect performance.

Initiatives to combat the issues include programmes to optimize health and physical fitness, workplace design, better control of job content and task allocation, and importantly, functional capacity testing to match individual capability to task requirements.

Box 16.5 Recommended working practices for managing shift work and fatigue offshore

- Provide appropriate staff when and where required.
- Minimize physiological and psychological penalties associated with adjustment to shifts.
- Promote alertness over the working period.
- Minimize tiredness and fatigue.
- Recognize individual variability.
- Control occupational exposure.
- Avoid travel hazards for night workers in excess of those encountered by day workers.

Safety

Safety is the greatest concern to the offshore industry, with constant efforts to minimize work-related illness and injury. There is a focus on human factors and behavioural-based safety, exploring aspects of health and safety where operator decision-making, error, or violation of process is safety critical. Behavioural-based safety aims to change safety consciousness by creating a culture of modified health and safety-sensitive behaviours. In considering the interface of the individual, the job, and the organization, five main factors are important: fatigue, communication, risk perception, risk-taking behaviour, and the health and safety culture of the organization (see 'Useful websites').

Offshore windfarm workers

The UK now has 30 offshore windfarms with 1463 turbines generating over 5.1 GW of power (over 5% of UK needs). This is expected to grow to 20% by 2020.[38]

Wind turbines are immense structures (up to 200 m diameter propeller blade and 135 m pylon hub height). The heavy machinery of the propeller, gearbox, transmission, and generator are all housed within the nacelle at the top of the pylon. Workers, sometimes wearing survival gear and carrying their equipment, are transferred to the base of the wind turbine by boat and ascend inside the pylon to work in the confined space of the turbine housing. Although offshore wind turbines are fitted with lifts, many still involve a significant ladder climb requiring strength, agility, and endurance. The offshore windfarm industry, Global Offshore Wind Health and Safety Organisation (G+, formerly G9), has used the OGUK medical standards for offshore workers, with an added capability assessment, but is now discussing developing its own medical standards to reflect the unique workplace requirements.

Commercial diving

Commercial diving in the UK, including the UKCS, is regulated by the Diving at Work Regulations 1997 (DWR)[39] which are enforced by the HSE. Diving is considered commercial under the DWR when it is carried out for employment or reward. Commercial diving covers a large number of activities, ranging from mostly shallow police diving, training of recreational divers, and cleaning of aquariums, to scientific, media, and construction diving. Diving techniques range from the use of self-contained breathing apparatus ('scuba') to surface supply diving, where the diver is supplied from the surface through a hose (umbilical), and saturation diving at depths of several hundred metres.

In the commercial world, diving is just the way a diver 'commutes' to work. Specialist work activities in the workplace include non-destructive testing, inspection, construction or welding, use of power tools and cutting equipment, and media or scientific work. The HSE publishes the approved dive qualifications and five approved codes of practice applicable to different sectors of diving. These cover commercial diving projects offshore and inland/inshore, and media, recreational, and scientific and archaeological diving projects (see 'Useful websites').

Occupational health aspects of commercial diving

The fitness of any individual diver influences the risks to the entire dive team, making diving a safety-critical activity. Although the concept of safety-critical work activities is not clearly defined in law, except perhaps in the rail industry, many industries use and are familiar with this concept. It generally applies to situations where a failure (of a person or system of work) could have significant financial, safety, or health implications. It is usually accepted that the term applies where there is a risk of severe injuries or multiple injured parties. HSE-Approved Medical Examiners of Divers (AMEDs) must have a detailed appreciation of the diving environment and the relevant workplace risks in order to perform an appropriate medical examination, correctly interpret information, and form a sound judgement as to a diver's physical and mental fitness to dive.

The regulations do not stipulate a minimum age for commercial divers. However, the safety-critical nature of diving requires an adult attitude to learning and risk appreciation. In practice, training organizations and/or employers will only recruit people of 18 years or older, and working offshore is only permitted at this age threshold.

Saturation diving

While in saturation, divers are kept at working depth pressure during the entire dive project. They live in steel chambers on board specialized diving support vessels. They 'commute' to work by transferring from their living habitat on board the diving support vessel or ship into a small diving bell in which they are lowered into the water. Having reached working depth, they leave the bell to travel short distances to the work site. Divers are connected to the bell by an umbilical that provides the breathing gasses, communication, often video systems, and hot water for their dive suits.

Saturation diving allows for up to 8 hours of working per shift, including the time to lower and raise the bell. After a shift, divers will return to their pressurized living habitat without experiencing any significant change in pressure. The UK DWR allow up to a maximum of 28 days in saturation, but elsewhere in the world this limit is sometimes significantly exceeded. Depending on the working depth pressure, the gas pressure in the human tissue reaches equilibrium with the gas pressure in the living environment within hours to a few days. Consequently, to prevent decompression illness, decompression back to atmospheric pressure at the end of a work period can take 4–5 days or more. The breathing gas in the habitat depends on working depth and usually consists of variable gas mixtures of oxygen, nitrogen, and/or helium. Helium has a much greater ability to conduct heat than air. Consequently, the habitat temperature must be kept much higher (28–32°C) to maintain core body temperature. Environmental humidity can also be high. These conditions create ideal circumstances for bacterial contamination, with a raised risk of infections, despite attempts at habitat controls. Up to six people live together in a chamber for extended periods of time, relatively isolated from the outside world. In large diving vessels, several of these chambers can be connected. The largest diving systems now hold up to 24 divers at a time. While it is possible to introduce small medical instruments, equipment, and medication within a diving habitat, the provision of advanced medical care is severely limited, not least because medical personnel will usually need to be transported to the site by helicopter.

AMEDs should therefore always consider in their assessments the 'safety-critical' nature and isolation of saturation diving. These apply to all commercial diving operations to some degree.

Emergency escape

In 2017, emergency cold water survival training centres for the UK oil and gas offshore industry introduced the use of a short-term air supply system (see 'Offshore workers'). So that participants in offshore helicopter survival training do not require assessment by an AMED using the MA1 standards, an exemption from Regulation 12(1)(b) of the DWR has been granted for HUET training and shallow water training (maximum 0.7 m) using the compressed air emergency breathing system.

Diving medical examination and training of medical practitioners

Before medical practitioners can apply to the HSE for approval to conduct commercial diving medical examinations they must meet minimum training requirements in occupational medicine and attend a dedicated training course (see the HSE's diving website listed in 'Useful websites'). These also list the requirements to maintain competency and ensure ongoing approval.

Examination and diver fitness certification mechanism

Advice for AMEDs regarding the medical examination and assessment of commercial divers (MA1) is available from the HSE's website. This provides updated administrative advice and a framework for the fitness assessment. Even though it has the status of guidance, AMEDs should maintain detailed documentation and be able to justify their judgements and decisions. The latest guidance includes changed sections on obesity and exercise testing. The HSE also publishes AMED 'ebulletins' online.

A detailed examination is important, with particular emphasis on the cardiopulmonary, nervous, and musculoskeletal systems. The diver should receive a completed copy of the HSE MA2 and bring this to their next diving medical examination, failing which an AMED may refuse to examine the diver or treat such a medical as an initial examination. Continuity of information is essential.

A certificate of fitness to dive is valid for a maximum of 12 months and in order to continue to dive the diver must present to an AMED for another fitness assessment. It is strongly recommended that the AMED retains a copy of the diver's previous MA2 if they were examined elsewhere. Where a diver experiences an illness or injury, especially any pulmonary, cardiac, neurological, or otological disorder, including decompression illness, or has been off work for more than 14 days, a diver must undergo re-examination. This does not replace the annual review.

International context and reciprocity of medical certificates within Europe

The medical subcommittee of the European Diving Technology Committee, an international forum of medical practitioners interested in diving, has published 'Guidelines for Medical Assessment of Working Divers'.[40] The Diving Medical Advisory Committee (DMAC), under the secretarial umbrella of the International Marine Contractors Association, is a voluntary group of international medical practitioners which produces advice aimed at the diving industry. In 2009, the DMAC produced a position statement in collaboration with the European Diving Technology Committee regarding the required fitness expectations and suitable exercise framework for commercial divers.[41] Subsequent updates include guidance issued in November 2017 on the fitness to return to diving after decompression illness.

Examination: process considerations

The first examination of an aspiring diver should establish the medical history and fitness. Previous medical history must be confirmed by a health questionnaire signed by their GP. An example of the minimum dataset is provided on the HSE diving pages website (see 'Useful websites').

The MA1 guidance does not differentiate between the physical requirements and levels of fitness of male and female divers. In practice, this does not appear to cause a major problem considering that saturation, offshore, and inshore civil/construction diving are almost exclusively male domains, whereas in scientific, media, aquarium, shellfish/clam, or police/fire and rescue diving more female divers can be found.

Where an AMED is in doubt about the full ability for all possible diving activities, they can issue a dive certificate that is restricted to a particular category of diving. A restriction in diving depth is rarely justified. If second opinions are required, the HSE maintains a list of clinical specialists with an interest in diving.

The MA1 details a diver's right of appeal. For peer support and informal expert opinion and advice AMEDs can also consult the UK Diving Medical Committee and join its discussion forum: 'the UK Diving Medical Community' (UKDMC) (see 'Useful websites'). This is a voluntary affiliation of medical practitioners with an interest in recreational and/or commercial diving medicine.

Medical examination

The medical examination of divers follows the same template as any other medical examination. Given the safety-critical nature of diving and the fact that working under water can affect many organ systems, the examination has to be thorough and detailed. This should be appropriately reflected in the health questionnaire, the clinical examination, communication with other health professionals if required, the regular calibration of instruments, and in the auditable way in which the AMED reaches and document their judgement.

Investigations that are required as a minimum are detailed in the MA1. A full blood count is not required and a test for sickle cell disorders only on indication. A resting electrocardiogram (ECG) may be included by clinical indication, but is no longer advised as a matter of routine. However, experience has shown that, even considering the low yield of resting ECGs in general, pathology is occasionally found. Appropriate investigations can be performed outside of these minimum requirements as clinically indicated.

Routine radiology of the lungs and/or long bones has not proven to be of value and should only be undertaken when a clear clinical indication can be identified.

Obesity

Body weight should be assessed critically when determining fitness to dive. Body mass index (BMI) alone is a poor descriptor of body morphology and adiposity and the HSE recommends that an individual's BMI should be supplemented by waist circumference, because this provides a good measure of central obesity and hence general health risks. The MA1 provides a decision flow chart as a guide.

Physical fitness requirements of divers and other safety-critical work

Diving is an inherently dangerous activity where the margins for error are small. The fitness assessment of commercial divers aims to ascertain whether or not a diver has sufficient physical reserves to deal with emergency situations. The HSE MA1 requirement for an aerobic capacity of 45 mL/kg/min of oxygen consumption or more for young and fit divers appears to have been derived from early navy research. This remains the fitness level to encourage all divers to aim for, especially for saturation divers or when diving deeper than 50 m. However, the MA1 now incorporates a flow diagram that provides a more stepped approach to dealing with less aerobically fit divers. An aerobic capacity below 40 mL/kg/min would, however, likely require an unfit certificate and the provision of fitness advice.

Exercise testing

The HSE specifies the Chester step test as the preferred exercise test because it is repeatable, reasonably accurate, and suitable for monitoring changes. Exercise testing must be carried out safely and this requires up-to-date training in basic resuscitation, clear emergency response procedures, uncomplicated access/egress for emergency services, and the provision of an automated external defibrillator. A very large study reported 17 deaths and 96 severe complications during or subsequent to exercise testing among 700,000 patients but no incidents from exercise testing among a group of 350,000 sports people. The best predictor for conducting a safe exercise capacity test is ongoing regular exercise. The risks from testing have been estimated as 1 in 2500 to 1 in 10,000 cases of myocardial infarction or death in patients with coronary artery disease. Pre-exercise cardiac risk screening questionnaires have been criticized, given the possibility of biased reporting in the occupational setting, when continued work depends on receiving a fitness certificate.

The test validity depends significantly on accurate monitoring of the heart rate response during exercise, and standardized conditions (e.g. allowing a higher heart rate in heat). Exercise testing with a step test in occupational practice in the UK is rarely monitored with an ECG. To exclude post-exercise arrhythmias, AMEDs may wish to consider recording/repeating an ECG after the exercise test or capturing a single lead rhythm ECG afterwards.

Where other methods are used, such as a Bruce protocol on a treadmill, and the results may be reported in metabolic equivalents (METs), care must be taken in converting this to mL/kg/min aerobic capacity. Byrne et al. have shown that the accepted conversion of METs in VO_2 (1 MET ± 3.5 mL/kg/min O_2 consumption) may overestimate the actual resting VO_2 on average by 35% and that the greatest variance occurs in people with a high percentage of body fat.[42] In October 2018, IMCA issued guidance on Health, Fitness and Medical Issues in Diving Operations (D 061).

Effects of pressure on organ systems

Appreciation of the gas laws and the physiological changes caused by hydrostatic pressure and gas pressures is fundamental to understanding the effects of gas and water pressures on the different organ systems. These are part of the training of AMEDs and are explained in detail in relevant textbooks. Barotrauma effects can occur during descent and ascent, and hydrostatic pressure causes significant fluid shifts from the periphery into the body core with an associated rise in blood pressure and cardiac stroke volume. The gas laws (Boyle's inverse relationship between volume and absolute pressure) dictate that the most significant changes in gas expansion occur during the first and last 10 m of descending and surfacing respectively.

The AMED must communicate clearly with the consultant to whom the diver is referred. Most specialists do not work in the field of diving medicine and will not necessarily understand all the nuances.

Communicable diseases

The AMED should be satisfied that the diver is not suffering from an infectious disease. Where there is doubt, then further assessment and referral should be made to a medical microbiologist or specialist in infectious diseases. Ongoing communicable diseases would probably bar a worker from diving until resolution because good hygiene practices are more difficult in a diving environment.

Psychiatric assessment

Evidence of psychological states that might affect the safety of the diver or others in the water must be sought. Diving itself will impose a specific stress, depending upon the type of work, its location, and the operational risks involved. Living and working for significant periods of time (up to 1 month in the UK) in a saturation chamber system will also bring its own psychological pressures. Divers should be free from psychiatric illness and/or impairment of cognitive function.

Alcohol or drug dependence would normally be a bar from diving unless there has been a period of abstinence of at least 1 year for alcohol and 3 years for drugs, off medication, and without relapse while under continuous monitoring by a competent health professional. Detailed evidence from treatment facilities, and current psychological and/or psychiatric assessment, including ongoing drug screening, may be required before a return to commercial diving can be allowed.

A detailed referral for an opinion from a psychiatrist should be obtained in cases of doubt. This referral must explain the nature of the work involved.

Respiratory system

The integrity of the respiratory system is vital for diving. The British Thoracic Society has produced guidelines for the examination of fitness to dive.[43]

Any condition that might compromise gas exchange or exercise response must be sought. Any abnormality that may cause air trapping and could lead to barotrauma on ascent from depth should be investigated. Pulmonary barotrauma represents escape of air from the lung/alveoli into various other anatomical structures and can lead to pneumothorax, pneumomediastinum, or arterial gas embolism or any combination of these. Right-to-left shunting in the lung circulation, for instance, from arteriovenous malformations, can circumvent the normal filter function of the lung with the potential for increased risk of bubbles crossing from the right to the left circulation with an increased risk of decompression illness.

Clinical assessment of the chest and pulmonary function testing should also be normal. When variations from normal are found, AMEDs should, where necessary, clarify these with peers or arrange appropriate referral. However, the routine taking of chest X-rays seldom contributes to the detection of relevant pathology and should only be undertaken if justified on individual clinical grounds. The MA1 contains a table (see Table 16.1) that lists conditions that are an absolute contraindication to diving or require further assessment.

Approach to assessment of lung function

Routine spirometry is required. The target should be a forced expiratory volume in 1 second (FEV_1) of greater than 80% of predicted and greater than 70% of predicted FEV_1/forced vital capacity (FVC) ratio. If, after the exercise test, peak expiratory flow or FEV_1 drops by greater than 15% or if there is another suggestion of exercise-induced bronchoconstriction then consulting a respiratory physician with an interest in diving is recommended. Where required, the AMED could also consider more formal exercise testing, which may include testing in a cold environment to exclude cold-induced asthma.

Asthma

Safety to dive in those with asthma is controversial. There is no convincing evidence that asthma is a significant cause of pulmonary barotraumas, but careful initial assessment is necessary in a new candidate. Those with asthma induced by cold, exercise, or emotion are barred from diving. Diving may be permitted for asthmatics who are either at step 1 or step 2 of the British Thoracic Society Asthma Guidelines. GPs have recently started to implement step 3 of the British Thoracic Society's guidance, involving combination therapy of long-acting beta-2-agonists and anti-inflammatory medication, at a much earlier point in the patient's treatment. In this situation, if diving is still thought to be possible, it is recommended that AMEDs only take such a decision in consultation with the diver's GP and possibly a respiratory specialist with an interest in diving.

Cardiovascular system

This organ system is the one which is the most complex and which stimulates the most debate. The basic rules are outlined within the MA1, but the UKDMC forum is a useful place to debate the nuances of interpretation and to discuss each case individually.

A history, or finding on examination, of any type of heart disease including septal defects, cardiomyopathies, ischaemic heart disease, valvular disease, shunts, and dysrhythmias, except for sinus arrhythmia and infrequent ventricular extrasystoles not related to exercise, should lead to certification of unfitness for diving and the individual should be referred for a cardiological opinion assuming they wish to pursue diving. The cardiologist should have knowledge of diving medicine as per HSE's list of such specialists.

Patent foramen ovale and other causes of right-to-left shunting

Patent foramen ovale (PFO) is a common condition, affecting an estimated 25% of the population to some degree. Most lesions are small and appear not to introduce a significant risk of right-to-left shunting, relevant for paradoxical embolism and hence also for cross-over of bubbles during decompression in diving. The gold standard for detecting PFO is by transthoracic echocardiography, provided the correct protocol is followed by a well-trained investigator.

Screening for PFO is not routinely conducted in either the preliminary or annual medical assessments. However, where there is a history of unexplained neurological, cardiorespiratory, or cutaneous decompression illness (DCI), particularly if there is also a history of migraine with aura, then transthoracic echocardiography bubble testing should be performed under supervision of a cardiologist experienced in the procedure. The PFO can now be effectively repaired through a percutaneous approach, thereby reducing the risk of bubble transfer from the right-to-left circulation.[44] This procedure carries a 1–2% risk of life-threatening complications, even in experienced hands. Other conditions that permit intracardiac shunting from right to left, such as atrial septal defects, are contraindications to diving until repaired and deemed safe.

Blood pressure

Taking 24-hour readings during daily activities or blood pressure measurements under exercise load may need to be considered to exclude significant hypertension in certain situations. Hypertension and/or left ventricular diastolic dysfunction may constitute a risk factor for developing pulmonary oedema when diving and has in rare cases been reported along with other physical activities. If in any doubt, the advice of a cardiologist with an interest in diving medicine should be sought.

The central nervous system

Assessment of the central nervous system is extremely important initially and at subsequent intervals. AMEDs should consider documenting the detail of the diver's neurological examination. A diver must have no functional disturbance of motor power and sensation, coordination, level of consciousness or cognition, special senses and balance, bowel, or bladder.

Neurological symptoms of acute DCI may present with loss or alteration of sensation, or with muscular weakness. Thus, any neurological condition with these symptoms may mimic DCI and if present in a diver may greatly complicate its management.

Where there is doubt, an opinion must be sought from an appropriate specialist with an interest in diving.

Ear, nose, and throat system

A history of surgery of the ear is usually a contraindication to commercial diving, and individual advice should be sought from a specialist. Stapedectomy has previously been an absolute contraindication to diving; however, recent evidence indicates that this may be too strict and that each case should be judged individually.

Visual system

Any condition that leads to reduced vision or surgical procedure or injury that leads to secondary infection may pose a hazard in diving.

As the diver goes deeper, progressively less light from the surface arrives at depth. Only 20% of available surface light is perceived when at 10 metres of sea water (msw) and this can be made worse by backscatter from suspended silt and particles. Colour vision is also progressively lost; reds disappear at 10 msw and at 30 msw only blues and greens remain. Most commercial diving for inspection or construction purposes will, however, use artificial light to compensate for darkness at depth. The full-face mask or helmet reduces the visual field considerably and the air/mask interface causes distortion, such that objects appear about one-quarter nearer and are magnified by about one-third.

Corneal corrective surgery

Myopic correction may now be accomplished in a number of surgical ways. As these procedures are increasingly used, more is known about the effects of this type of surgery in terms of success rates, healing times, and complication rates. Communication between the AMED and treatment facility should clarify these details. The Divers Alert Network provides some relevant information.

Dental

Dental care is important. Scuba divers need to be able to retain a mouthpiece. Dental caries and periodontal disease need to be treated. Unattached dentures should be removed during diving. Changes in pressure can cause pain in teeth or exploding fillings, due to small pockets of air or gas being trapped within the tooth. It is therefore recommended that divers see a dentist every 6 months to maintain a high standard of dental health. Ideally they should be able to (and encouraged to) produce evidence of these consultations at each diving medical. If in doubt, the AMED should issue a temporary unfit dive certificate until a certificate of dental fitness is obtained.

Endocrine system

Most endocrine conditions are contraindications to professional diving. However, well-controlled hypothyroidism is acceptable. It is sensible to obtain evidence of this control and to ensure there are no secondary organ complications.

Diabetes mellitus of any type and controlled by any means has until recently been a contraindication to diving. Since the revision of the MA1 in 2005, there are possibilities for people with diabetes to gain work within the diving industry.

Diving under close supervision in a pool, aquarium, very sheltered inland waters, or even as a sport diving instructor (for example) may be acceptable in some cases. The AMED should discuss each potential case with an appropriate diving medical specialist with a specific interest in this area. Consultation with the diver's treating physician is required to ascertain the facts of each case. It is clearly appropriate to ensure that the potential diver's diabetic control and level of fitness have been good for some time and that there is no end-organ damage. Should the diver be passed fit with restrictions, his level of care and control must be monitored regularly. Ongoing consultation between the AMED, the diver's treating physician, and the diving medical specialist should occur regularly. Attention should be given to possible autonomic dysfunction and acute cognitive impairment from hypo- as well as hyperglycaemia. Suitable frequency of blood sugar measurements need to be in place, demonstrating good control at all times, likely in a similar ways as for the UK Driver and Vehicle Licensing Agency group 2 vehicle requirements.

Gastrointestinal system

Active peptic ulceration is not compatible with diving, but the relapse rate after a course of triple therapy is sufficiently low to allow return to air diving. However, objective evidence of ulcer healing and symptom resolution is required. Saturation diving, given its long periods of isolation and potentially stressful environment, is unlikely to be appropriate.

Asymptomatic cholelithiasis may not be problematic. However, saturation diving would be unsuitable and the same may apply to all types of diving depending on the remoteness of the location. Chronic hepatic disease requires specialist assessment.

Stomas need to be individually assessed and free draining ones are compatible with diving. 'Continent' stomas requiring a catheter to relieve pressure are not compatible with diving. However, stomas may not be suitable for saturation diving for social reasons, rather than medical ones, associated with living in confined spaces with other divers.

Dermatological system

Integrity of the skin is important for the diver. Immersion, use of diving suits and equipment, and raised temperature and humidity of saturation diving chambers can lead to skin damage and risk of secondary infection. Professional divers are at increased risk of infections of hands, ear canals, facial skin, and the most prevalent infection in saturation diving, *Pseudomonas aeruginosa*. The confined and easily contaminated living space, high temperature, high humidity, and a hyperoxic atmosphere significantly contribute to the risk of bacterial skin contamination. Fungal infections of the skin are not uncommon and may require repeated treatment.

Haematological system

Blood dyscrasias, even in remission, will usually be a cause for rejection and polycythaemia will increase the risk of acute DCI. Coagulation disorders are incompatible with diving. Divers who have had splenectomy are at an increased risk of overwhelming infection from *Pseudomonas* and are not fit for saturation diving.

Malignancy

After conclusion of treatment, cases of malignancy should be individually assessed for factors affecting in-water safety and fitness to dive. If involved in saturation diving, then suitability for an extended stay in an isolated environment needs to be assessed. Ongoing or intermittent chemotherapy, liable to compromise the immune system, would bar patients from working in saturation diving and possibly other types of diving. Fitness certificates and any restriction need to be carefully considered and documented. Regular and frequent reviews of the diver's fitness are required. Full involvement of the diver's treating physician is appropriate.

The disabled diver

The question of a disabled diver requiring an MA2 AMED examination is mostly raised within the context of recreational instruction diving, or following a return to work diving medical following a previous accident. In most instances, divers with obvious impairments would find it very difficult to gain employment in the wider dive industry. Although it is sometimes suggested that the Equality Act 2010 should also be considered, it seems unlikely that an employer would be able to make a 'reasonable adjustment' for an impairment if that could lead to an increase in risk for the rest of the dive team. In practice, the employer and the dive team will have to be able to compensate for any diminished work capacity of a disabled diver, including emergency egress. It is important to assess individuals in conjunction with their proposed work as divers. The assessment should include the individual's ability to look after themselves and others in the water and should also consider the overall safety of the dive team. Full details of the restriction regarding the type of diving and other safety considerations should be recorded on the diving medical certificate. Peer discussions before issuing a certificate of fitness to dive may be required.

Return to diving after acute decompression illness

This is well documented within the MA1 and is discussed in DMAC guidance. It is recommended that all cases of DCI in a diver are reviewed by the AMED and/or a diving medical specialist to consider the need to further assess the diver for potential predisposing causes.

Long-term health effects

There has been much consideration of long-term effects but so far the only proven and potentially disabling condition is dysbaric osteonecrosis. This can, in most cases, be prevented through safe diving practice in the now standard procedures for regulated professional diving. Magnetic resonance imaging scanning is the most sensitive method of investigation.

Aberdeen University has conducted a study called the 'Examination of the Long Term Health Impact of Diving' (ELTHI). Overall, the ELTHI study did not identify any long-term health effects associated with professional diving that amounted to clinical abnormality compared to matched offshore workers, although the complaint of 'forgetfulness or loss of concentration' was associated with significant impairment of health-related quality of life. The only factor that appeared to unexpectedly amplify any symptoms experienced by divers was the occupation of welding, albeit that the number of welders in the group was too small to draw definitive conclusions.

Hyperbaric chamber workers

The DWR covers the use of hyperbaric chambers within diving projects. People who may be routinely subjected to hyperbaric conditions need to have the same level of medical fitness. Hyperbaric chambers in hospitals are not covered by the DWR but the British Hyperbaric Association recommends that medical attendants working in such chambers undergo medical examinations and that the standards are similar to those for professional divers. As a general rule, employers should not examine their own staff for fitness to enter into the chamber. This could likely be taken as a potential conflict of interest and could introduce bias on behalf of both parties.

Key points

- The maritime, offshore, and diving sectors each have their own specific risks and fitness requirements. These have some features in common, as workers undertake safety-critical tasks at locations remote from care.
- Fitness standards may be statutory or set by industry bodies.
- The evidence underlying these standards is sometimes limited.
- Assessments need to be performed in a fair and ethical way, with access to appeal arrangements.
- Work is often international, as is the workforce. Fitness assessment needs to align with international conventions and recommendations.

Useful websites

Seafaring

International Labour Organisation (ILO)	www.ilo.org
International Marine Contractors Association	www.imca-int.com
International Maritime Organization	www.imo.org
International Shipping Federation	www.marisec.org
International Transport Workers' Federation	www.itf.org.uk
Nautilus International (the officers trade union)	www.nautilusint.org
International Maritime Health Association	www.imha.net
Marine and Coastguard Agency (MCA). Live list of approved doctors, UK and overseas	https://www.gov.uk/government/publications/mca-approved-doctors-uk-based https://www.gov.uk/government/publications/mca-approved-doctors-overseas
MCA. Approved doctor's manual: seafarer medical examinations.	https://www.gov.uk/government/publications/the-approved-doctors-manual
Dreadnought Unit, Guy's and St Thomas' Hospital (a service providing treatment for seafarers)	http://seahospital.org.uk/dreadnought-medical/

Offshore

Energy Institute. Safety behaviours	www.energyinst.org.uk/humanfactors

Diving

HSE. 'Approved Codes of Practice for the Diving at Work Regulations 1997'	http://www.hse.gov.uk/diving/acop.htm
HSE. Diving pages	http://www.hse.gov.uk/diving/index.htm
UK Diving Medical Community. Discussion forum for recreational examiners and AMEDs. Available via the secretariat for registered medical practitioner members only.	http://www.ukdmc.org

References

1. **International Labour Organization**. Maritime Labour Convention 2006. Available at: http://www.ilo.org.
2. **International Labour Organization**. Work in Fishing Convention 2007. Available at: http://www.ilo.org.

3. **International Maritime Organization**. International Convention on Standards of Training, Certification and Watchkeeping for Seafarers (STCW Convention) 1978 as amended. Available at: http://www.imo.org/en/OurWork/HumanElement/TrainingCertification/Pages/STCW-Convention.aspx.

4. **International Labour Organization (ILO), International Maritime Organization (IMO)**. *Guidelines on the Medical Examinations of Seafarers*. Geneva: ILO/IMO, 2011. Available at: http://www.ilo.org/wcmsp5/groups/public/---ed_dialogue/---sector/documents/normativeinstrument/wcms_174794.pdf

5. **World Health Organization**. *International Medical Guide for Ships*, 3nd edn. Geneva: World Health Organization; 2007.

6. **The Maritime Working Time Directive (1999/63/EC)**. Available at: www.europa.eu.int/eurlex/en/index.html

7. **Maritime and Coastguard Agency**. *Merchant Shipping Notice MSN 1768 (M+F). Ships' Medical Stores*. Southampton: Maritime and Coastguard Agency; 2003.

8. **Maritime and Coastguard Agency**. *Merchant Shipping Notice MSN 1839 (M) Maritime Labour Convention: Medical Certification* (and subsequent amendments). Southampton: Maritime and Coastguard Agency; 2016.

9. **Maritime and Coastguard Agency**. *Merchant Shipping Notice MSN 1815. Countries whose Seafarer Medical Certificates are Accepted as Equivalent to the UK Seafarer Medical Certificate (ENG1) from 1 July 2007*. Southampton: Maritime and Coastguard Agency; 2007.

10. **Maritime and Coastguard Agency**. Seafarer Medical Report Form (ML5) and ML5 Certificate (MSF 4112). 2014. Available at: https://www.gov.uk/government/publications/ml5-medical-report-form-and-certificate-msf-4112.

11. **Carter T**. The evidence base for maritime medical standards. *Int Maritime Health* 2002;53:1–4.

12. **Maritime and Coastguard Agency**. *Marine Guidance Note MGN 399. Prevention of Infectious Disease at Sea by Immunisations and Medication*. Southampton: Maritime and Coastguard Agency; 2009.

13. **Oil and Gas UK**. *Economic Report 2017*. London: United Kingdom Offshore Oil and Gas Industry Association Limited trading as Oil & Gas UK; 2017.

14. **Oil and Gas UK**. *Business Outlook 2017*. London: United Kingdom Offshore Oil and Gas Industry Association Limited trading as Oil & Gas UK; 2017.

15. **Oil and Gas Authority**. *Table of Current UKCS Installations*. London: Oil and Gas Authority Limited; 2016.

16. **Oil and Gas UK**. *Managing Nicotine Offshore*. London: United Kingdom Offshore Oil and Gas Industry Association Limited trading as Oil & Gas UK; 2015.

17. **Continental Shelf Act 1964**. Available at: http://www.legislation.gov.uk/ukpga/1964/29/contents.

18. **The Offshore Installations (Safety Case) Regulations SI 2005/311**. Available at: http://www.legislation.gov.uk/uksi/2005/3117/contents/made.

19. **Offshore Installations and Pipeline Works (Management and Administration) Regulations 1995**. Available at: https://www.legislation.gov.uk/uksi/1995/738/contents/made.

20. *The Offshore Installations and Pipeline Works (First-Aid) Regulations 1989 SI 1989/1671*. London: The Stationery Office, 1989.

21. *The Offshore Installations (prevention of Fire and Explosion, and Emergency Response) Regulations 1995*. Approved Code of Practice and Guidance L65. London: HSE Books, 1995.

22. **Energy Institute**. *A Recommended Fitness Standard for the Oil and Gas Industry*. London: Energy Institute; 2010.

23. **Energy Institute**. *Fitness Assessment Manual*. London: Energy Institute; 2011.

24. **Energy Institute**. *Medical Standards for Fitness to Wear Respiratory Protective Equipment*. London: Energy Institute; 2011.

25. **Energy Institute.** *Guidelines for the Medical Aspects of Work for the Onshore Oil Industry.* London: Energy Institute; 2011.

26. **Oil and Gas UK.** *Guidelines for Medical Aspects of Fitness for Offshore Workers.* Issue 6. London: Oil and Gas UK; 2008.

27. **Offshore Petroleum Industry Training Organisation.** *Basic Offshore Safety Induction and Emergency Training and Further Offshore Emergency Training.* Aberdeen: Offshore Petroleum Industry Training Organisation; 2003.

28. **UK Civil Aviation Authority.** Safety Review of Offshore Public Transport Helicopter Operations in Support of the Exploitation of Oil and Gas. CAP1145 report 20 February 2014. Available at: https://publicapps.caa.co.uk/modalapplication.aspx?appid=11&mode=detail&id=6088.

29. **Offshore Petroleum Industry Training Organisation.** *Minimum Industry Safety Training Standard (MIST) Revision 1 Amendment 2. Standard Code: 5301.* Aberdeen: Offshore Petroleum Industry Training Organisation; 2017.

30. **UK Offshore Operators Association.** *Industry Guidelines for First Aid and Medical Equipment on Offshore Installations.* London: UK Offshore Operators Association; 2000.

31. **Oil and Gas UK.** *The Management of Competence and Training in Emergency Response for Offshore Installations.* London: Oil and Gas UK; 2010.

32. **The Equality Act (Offshore Work) Order 2010.** Available at: http://www.legislation.gov.uk/uksi/2010/1835/contents/made.

33. **Energy Institute.** *Guidance on Health Surveillance.* London: Energy Institute; 2010.

34. **UK Offshore Operators Association.** *Environmental Health Guidelines for Offshore Installations,* Issue 3. London: UK Offshore Operators Association; 1996.

35. **Gibbs M, Hampton S, Morgan L, et al.** *Effect of Shift Schedule on Offshore Shiftworkers Circadian Rhythms and Health.* Research report 318. London: Health and Safety Executive; 2005.

36. **Health and Safety Executive.** *Guidance for Managing Fatigue and Shiftwork Offshore.* Offshore Information Sheet 7/2008. London: Health and Safety Executive; 2008.

37. **Oil and Gas UK.** *2015 UKCS Offshore Workforce Demographics Report.* London: United Kingdom Offshore Oil and Gas Association Limited trading as Oil & Gas UK; 2015.

38. **The Crown Estate.** *Offshore Wind Operational Report January – December 2016.* London: The Crown Estate, 2017.

39. **The Diving at Work Regulations (1997). Statutory Instrument 1997, no. 2776.** Available at: http://www.legislation.gov.uk/uksi/1997/2776/contents/made.

40. **The European Diving Technology Committee.** Fitness to dive standards. Guidelines for medical assessment of working divers. Available at: http://www.edtc.org/Fitness%20to%20dive.htm.

41. **The Diving Medical Advisory Committee.** DMAC Statement on Exercise Testing in Medical Assessment of Commercial Divers. October 2009. Available at: http://www.dmac-diving.org/guidance/DMAC-Statement-200910.pdf.

42. **Byrne NM, Hills AP, Hunter GR, et al.** Metabolic equivalent: one size does not fit all. *J Appl Physiol* 2005;**99**:1112–9.

43. **British Thoracic Society.** BTS guidelines on respiratory aspects of fitness for diving. 2003. Available at: https://www.brit-thoracic.org.uk/document-library/clinical-information/diving/diving-guideline/guidelines-on-respiratory-aspects-of-fitness-for-diving/.

44. **Smart D, Mitchell S, Wilmshurst P, et al.** Joint position statement on persistent foramen ovale (PFO) and diving. South Pacific Underwater Medical Society (SPUMS) and the United Kingdom Sports Diving Medical Committee (UKSDMC). *Diving Hyperb Med* 2015;**45**:129–31.

Chapter 17

International travel

Dipti Patel

Introduction

International travel is a common feature of employment, and accounts for 7 million UK trips (10% of all trips) overseas annually, with some residing overseas in the longer term.[1] Those who travel for work are a diverse group comprising a variety of professions ranging from short-term city-based business executives to long-term rural aid workers, and the preparation and support for an overseas assignment can be as diverse as the workers' occupational backgrounds.

Organizations that send employees overseas owe them a legal and moral duty of care regardless of where in the world they work. Additionally, employers have a vested interest in supporting their employees, ensuring that they are fit and adequately prepared for their overseas assignment, and that appropriate procedures are in place to take care of them if they become ill or injured. The financial costs of healthcare overseas, sickness absence, and, in extreme cases, repatriation, can be considerable.

However, it is important to note that many people are working abroad without any support from well-organized parent organizations. In these circumstances, the principles in this chapter still apply, but arrangements for the provision of medical care become even more important.

Epidemiology of travel-related health problems

International travellers are an epidemiologically important group due to their movement, the risk of adverse health outcomes abroad, and the possibility of importation or exportation of infectious diseases. They have a higher and well-recognized risk of illness and injury, and are exposed to a variety of new cultural, psychological, physical, physiological, environmental, and microbiological challenges. Their ability to adapt and cope with these challenges is affected by many variables including their pre-existing physical, psychological, immunological, and medical health, and their personality, experience, and behaviour while overseas.

Estimation of disease risk in travellers, however, has proved elusive, with difficulty ascertaining precise data on both numbers travelling to specific locations and incidence of illness. Despite their limitations, a consistent and coherent body of data has made it possible to obtain consensus on the type of illnesses and risks experienced by different groups of travellers. Frequently quoted studies show that a high proportion of travellers experience health problems, with the overall risk of morbidity from illness or injury being between 22% and 64%. While most illnesses tend to be self-limiting, approximately 5% of travellers will consult a doctor, 1% are hospitalized while abroad, and some require medical care on returning home.[2] Diarrhoea, respiratory infections, and skin disorders are the most commonly reported illnesses. Deaths abroad are rare, the main causes being a cardiovascular event, accidents, and injuries.[2,3]

Research on business travellers has produced similar results, although illness rates tend to be higher and psychological problems more prominent.[4] Extensive business travel has been found to be associated with poorer self-rated health, higher alcohol consumption, and lower confidence in keeping up with the pace of work.[5,6] In expatriates, in particular, illnesses, hospital admissions, injuries, violent episodes, and psychological problems are reported with higher frequency as a result of their longer stay overseas and cumulative exposure to country-related hazards.[4,7–11]

Fortunately, many travel-related health problems are preventable by taking sensible precautionary measures, by having the appropriate immunizations, and taking chemo-prophylactic medication.

Role of occupational health departments

Occupational health (OH) departments have a key role in supporting overseas workers. The degree of involvement will depend on the potential hazards associated with the overseas assignment and the organization's approach to international health and safety. The approach should be based on a suitable risk assessment; for example, the risks relevant to a charity sending staff to work on an aid project in Africa will differ from those for a financial service organization sending executives on short-term trips to Europe.

At a strategic level, OH can help ensure that clear processes and policies are in place to meet the OH needs of overseas workers, and the global nature of the organization. These could, for example, include assistance in developing a global health and safety policy, advice on disability-related adjustments, guidance on healthcare and repatriation arrangements, and assistance with contingency planning for major disasters overseas (e.g. pandemics, earthquakes, and civil unrest). At an individual level, OH input should focus on pre-travel preparation, support while overseas, and support on return home.

Pre-travel preparation

The objectives of pre-travel preparation are to assess the traveller's plans and determine potential health hazards; to educate the traveller and their families regarding the anticipated risks and preventive measures; to provide immunizations and medications for prophylaxis, self-treatment, or both; and to enable the traveller to manage their health while abroad. The key aspects are risk assessment, and health promotion with risk management (Box 17.1).

Box 17.1 Pre-travel preparation

Risk assessment
Traveller details

- Age.
- Medical conditions.
- Special conditions (e.g. pregnancy, recent surgery, disability, immunocompromise).
- Medications.
- Allergies.
- Immunization history.
- Prior travel.
- Risk tolerance.
- Risk-taking behaviour.

Trip details

- Itinerary (countries and regions, rural, urban, etc.).
- Timing (season, time to departure, duration).
- Reason for travel (e.g. tourism, business, visiting friends and relatives, volunteer, missionary, adventure, medical tourism).
- Travel style (e.g. independent travel, package tour).
- General hygiene standards.
- Transport and length of travel.
- Accommodation (e.g. luxury hotel, guest house, hostel or budget hotel, local home, tent).
- Planned activities.

Health promotion and risk management

- Personal behaviour, hygiene, safety, and security.
- Vaccination.
- Vector avoidance.
- Malaria prevention and chemoprophylaxis.
- Travellers' diarrhoea prevention and self-treatment.
- Sexual contact.
- Environmental hazards (altitude, heat, cold, animals, DVT prevention, etc.).
- Chronic disease management.
- Travel insurance and medical care overseas.
- Reporting of illness.

Risk will vary according to the area to be visited, endemicity of diseases, nature of travel, accommodation, activities, and duration of travel. It will also vary according to the health status of the traveller. Risk assessment should therefore focus on individual, occupational, and destination-related factors. For those who are travelling for work, preparation should also include a medical assessment of an individual's fitness to work abroad, and a process for managing problems identified before travel or while abroad.

Deep vein thrombosis in long-distance travellers

The association between long-distance travel and deep vein thrombosis (DVT) and venous thromboembolism (VTE) is well recognized.[12] Travelling for more than 4 hours doubles the risk of VTE compared with not travelling. The risk is highest in the first week following travel but persists for 2 months. The risk is similar whether travel is by car, bus, or train over a similar period. A number of factors can affect this risk (Table 17.1). The absolute risk of an individual developing a travel-related DVT remains low even if they are classed as being at relative moderate or high risk.

Fitness to travel and work abroad

OH departments have a role in ensuring that an individual is fit to work overseas without risk to themselves or others. There is little research that provides evidence-based guidance on pre-travel fitness assessments for overseas workers, but use can be made of a general traveller risk assessment and health questionnaires, telephone enquiry, face-to-face consultation, and, where appropriate, medical examination.

For certain occupations there may be industry fitness standards or best practice guidance, and where these exist, fitness assessment should be performed according to organizational policy.

Fitness assessment should be conducted by healthcare professionals who have an understanding of OH in an overseas context, and designed and performed in a way that allows identification of actual or potential health problems that may be problematic during the overseas assignment. The assessment should occur well in advance of the departure date so that there is sufficient time for identified health problems to be appropriately managed. Due to the different demands of overseas work, employees who are considered fit to work in the UK may not be fit to do the same work overseas.

While there should be no absolute health contraindication to work overseas, certain travellers are at higher risk of developing illness or injury while overseas; this includes those at the extremes of age, pregnant women, workers with pre-existing medical conditions, and those who are immunocompromised. Fitness decisions should be made on a case-by-case basis, with a thorough evaluation of the risks and tailored preparation and advice. Where pre-existing health concerns are identified, not only must the stability of the condition and any impact it has on functional ability be considered, but also the efficacy or advisability of preventive measures, the impact of travel, the overseas environment, the adequacy of local medical facilities, and the availability and adequate storage of medication and medical equipment. An easily managed illness in the UK can be a major challenge overseas[13] (Box 17.2).

Table 17.1 Deep vein thrombosis and venous thromboembolism in long-distance travellers

Risk	Risk criteria	Risk reduction advice for passengers
Low risk	◆ No history of DVT/VTE ◆ No recent surgery (in last 2 months) ◆ No other known risk factors	Keep mobile Choose an aisle seat when feasible Perform frequent calf muscle exercises Ensure hand luggage is not placed somewhere that it restricts movement of legs and feet Wear clothing that is comfortable and loose Avoid the use of tranquilisers, or sleeping tablets Maintain a normal fluid intake and avoid excessive alcohol consumption
Moderate risk	◆ History of DVT/VTE ◆ Surgery under general anaesthesia lasting >30 minutes within the last 4–8 weeks ◆ Known clotting tendency ◆ Pregnancy or postpartum ◆ Obesity (BMI >30 kg/m²) ◆ Clinically evident cardiac disease (e.g. recent myocardial infarction or uncontrolled heart failure) or other major acute illness (e.g. pneumonia) ◆ Combined oral contraceptives or hormone replacement therapy ◆ Varicose veins with phlebitis ◆ Family history of VTE in a first-degree relative ◆ Polycythaemia ◆ Lower-limb fracture in plaster	As for 'low risk' with the addition of graduated compression stockings proving 15–30 mm HG pressure at the ankle It is vital that compression stockings are measured and worn correctly Ill-fitting stockings could further increase the risk of DVT
High risk	◆ An active malignancy ◆ Undergone recent major surgery (within the previous 4 weeks) ◆ Had a previous unprovoked venous thromboembolism (VTE) ◆ Had a previous travel-related DVT with no associated temporary risk factor ◆ More than one risk factor for DVT	Recommend delaying or cancelling the trip if post surgery As for 'moderate risk' but seek specialist advice regarding use of low-molecular-weight heparin

Source: data from National Institute of Clinical Excellence (NICE). (2013) *DVT prevention for travellers*. London, UK: NICE. Copyright © 2013 NICE. Available at: https://cks.nice.org.uk/dvt-prevention-for-travellers#!scenario.

Therefore, for employees with pre-existing medical problems, preparation for an overseas assignment requires careful planning and informed decision-making, which may include liaison with treating doctors and, in some instances, doctors overseas.

Relevant disability or employment legislation must always be considered, but practicability and financial costs may preclude adjustments that would have been feasible in the

Box 17.2 Considerations for those with pre-existing health problems

- Pregnancy will limit immunizations and malaria chemoprophylaxis recommendations.[14]

- A worker with a previous history of DVT may require heparin prophylaxis during long-haul air travel.[13]

- Air travel is contraindicated for 7–10 days after an uncomplicated myocardial infarction and less than 10 days after abdominal surgery.[15]

- A type 1 diabetic may need to adjust their insulin for long-haul travel, and may find that their control is affected by hot climates.[16]

- An immunosuppressed traveller is more likely to become ill from travel-related infections compared to their healthy travel companions.[17]

- An expatriate with chronic liver disease may not be able to access specialist liver facilities in their host country.

UK.[18] The final decision on fitness for work overseas may also be influenced by country restrictions (e.g. entry restrictions for those infected with human immunodeficiency virus[19] or taking certain opiate analgesia), national travel advisories (e.g. for pregnant women travelling to countries affected by Zika virus),[20] or have to be balanced against organizational needs. An organization's working policy may require individuals with particular and unique skills to travel to areas where the risk to their health is higher than would ordinarily be accepted.

Psychological fitness

One of the most difficult areas to assess is psychological risk; travel may exacerbate or even precipitate a variety of psychological disorders, and while problems are multifactorial in origin, drug misuse, malaria chemoprophylaxis, and time zone changes have all been implicated.[4]

Data on business travellers show that frequent international travel is associated with increased insurance claims for psychological illness.[21] In this group, concerns regarding family disruption, isolation, health, and workload were the main stressors.[22]

Those on expatriate or long-term assignments appear to be at particular risk; expatriates have been shown to have a consistently higher incidence of affective and adjustment disorders, and mental health problems are one of the principal causes of premature departure and repatriation from overseas assignments.[11] Risk factors include a previous history of psychological problems, depressed mood, family history of mental ill health, home country anxieties, physical ill health, occupational anxiety, and work stressors. In the case of work stressors, over 40% of International Red Cross expatriates reported that their mission had been more stressful than expected, mostly due to the working environment.[10]

In British diplomats, the risk of ill health was significantly higher than that in their partners, suggesting that work demands could be a contributory factor to ill health overseas.[9]

Research in the 1960s suggested that overseas performance could be predicted if in-depth psychological assessment was carried out by experienced psychiatrists or interviewers familiar with the placement environment.[11] More recent research indicates that future mental health problems are associated with a number of identifiable risk factors such as a personal or close family history of psychosis, attempted suicide, personality disorder, attendance at a psychiatric outpatient department, consultation with a general practitioner for psychological reasons, or evidence of depressed mood at assessment.[23] Consequently, a more pragmatic approach for assessing psychological risk may involve screening questionnaires, with further medical assessment and onward referral to a psychiatrist where concerns are raised.

Occupational health hazards

Conventional OH hazards also need to be considered. These may pose a challenge as such exposures may be less well controlled overseas and opportunities for, and the quality of, health surveillance may be more limited. In some cases, hazards that are no longer routinely experienced in high-income countries (e.g. asbestos) may be prevalent.

Patterns of work on an overseas assignment—longer working hours, isolation, and leave arrangements—may create additional health risks or aggravate pre-existing ones. For certain occupational groups such as the armed forces, humanitarian aid workers, and healthcare workers, specific hazards (such as security, psychological trauma, and serious communicable disease) inherent to their work will require additional consideration. For some parts of the world, security represents one of the most challenging issues, as highlighted by high-profile events where foreign workers were targeted.[24,25] In these circumstances, robust and effective security systems are essential, and assistance may be required from the private sector.[26]

Assessment of dependants

In the case of expatriates there may also be a requirement to assess the fitness of partners and dependent children. Successful expatriate assignment often rests importantly on good family support, communication, and adjustment.[27] The problems that relocation may bring for the non-working partner must be considered, particularly if they abandon a career in their home country with no overseas job in prospect. However, the perception that partners are more susceptible to decreased well-being has not been confirmed in prospective expatriate studies.[28]

Children tend to adapt well to living overseas, but may have medical or developmental conditions or educational requirements that prove more difficult to manage overseas. In many countries, facilities for medical care of children are even less adequate than those for adults, and the threshold for seeking medical advice or repatriation may be correspondingly lower. Fitness considerations may pose a particular challenge both for children with pre-existing health problems and for healthy children who cannot access a suitable standard of medical care. In consequence, the organizational policy may occasionally preclude the overseas posting of children.

Travel health

In terms of travel health, much focus is given to vaccinations, despite vaccine-preventable diseases accounting for less than 5% of travel-associated morbidity.[29] Priority should be given to health problems that are common, preventable, treatable, and serious or potentially fatal. These include malaria, travellers' diarrhoea, sexually transmitted infections, and road accidents. Health hazards that are rare (e.g. Japanese encephalitis) should be put into perspective and discussed based on the individual traveller risk profile. Current best practice requires the health professional to balance the need for vaccination/prophylaxis against the realistic risk of infection, and the likelihood of adherence to preventive treatment. The latter will depend on many factors including perception of risk, concerns about side effects of preventive measures, and preferred risk management options. Travellers should be aware that no intervention is fully protective.

Provision of immunizations, malaria prophylaxis, and other preventive health advice should be started after an individual (and, if relevant, their family) is considered fit for their assignment. Employees should be encouraged to organize immunizations at least 4–6 weeks in advance of their departure date to allow for completion of courses, monitoring for adverse reactions, and time to mount an adequate immune response to vaccine-preventable diseases. For example, a full rabies course is given over 1 month (at 0, 7, and 21–28 days); it can take 2 weeks to develop protective immunity following typhoid vaccination; and the antimalarial mefloquine should be started 2–3 weeks prior to travel to ensure tolerance.

Detailed advice on immunizations, malaria prophylaxis, and other travel-related disease risks is beyond the scope of this chapter. Destination-specific requirements for travel health advice must be obtained from web-based resources from authoritative bodies. These bodies can provide the most up-to-date and valid information on the global distribution of infectious diseases and other health risks, the changing patterns of infection and antimicrobial resistance, advances in preventive measures, and the international health regulations. This information will help determine the additional immunizations needed, as a requirement of entry into a country (e.g. yellow fever vaccine), or recommended to counter endemic infections at the destination (e.g. hepatitis A vaccine). Similarly, it will help inform malaria prevention choices and advice on other protective measures.

These resources are also essential for highlighting disease outbreaks. Recent international outbreaks such as those caused by Ebola virus, Zika virus, and Middle East respiratory syndrome coronavirus, have highlighted the dynamic nature of travel health. While the risk of acquiring these infections is low for most travellers, certain occupations such as healthcare workers are at increased risk, and can play a role in international spread of disease.[30]

Support while overseas

The cost of healthcare overseas can be high, for example, at the time of writing, the cost of treating an individual with multiple leg fractures with an arterial tear in the USA and air ambulance repatriation to the UK was £500,000; and a hip fracture requiring treatment in a Spanish hospital and return flights to the UK cost about £15,000.[31] Additionally the medical (and dental) facilities in some parts of the world can be basic. It is vital, therefore, to ensure that adequate arrangements (including medical insurance cover) are in place to deal with medical and dental emergencies, which may extend to repatriation. Such arrangements must include the mechanism by which the costs of local care can be met, as in most countries medical care has to be purchased and, in many places payment, or guarantee of payment, is required before admission to hospital can be arranged or treatment commenced.

For expatriates or long-term assignees, arrangements should also include access to routine, non-urgent medical care, including cover for pre-existing medical conditions. Additional consideration needs to be given to the provision of OH support and employee assistance programmes for this group. If dependants accompany the employee, then their medical needs will also need to be addressed.

Importantly, employees must be familiar with medical cover arrangements and medical evacuation processes, regardless of whether they are travelling on a brief business trip or are on long-term assignment. The emergency evacuation of a sick employee is often a hazardous experience for the patient and an expensive, worrying, and time-consuming exercise for those organizing repatriation.

Return to the UK

The overseas worker should be advised of the possible need for follow-up after travel. In particular, all overseas workers should understand the importance of seeking expert medical advice immediately if fever develops after they return home.

The ill returned traveller

Prompt and effective treatment of travel-related illnesses reduces morbidity and mortality, and (for infectious diseases) reduces the risk of transmission to the community. OH departments do not generally manage acute illness, but are a point of contact for returned employees and can signpost them to sources of further medical care. Frequently the first port of call will be the individual's general practitioner although in some situations (e.g. febrile travellers returning from the tropics), may include referral to an infectious disease unit or tropical disease hospital.

Screening of asymptomatic travellers

The scientific literature on the cost-effectiveness of screening asymptomatic travellers is sparse. Screening may be valuable in certain groups; for example, as part of public health measures instituted for healthcare workers returning from Ebola-affected areas.[32] However, asymptomatic short-term travellers rarely need a post-travel medical examination, although in a cohort of UK travellers who had been in the tropics or subtropics for at least 3 months, it was found that potentially serious asymptomatic infection was common (e.g. schistosomiasis).[33] A careful itinerary-specific history with detailed questioning about potentially risky exposures, may help in identifying those who might benefit from screening, and should form the basis of the post-travel evaluation. This would, however, not generally be the role of an OH department.

Occupational health follow-up

OH follow-up may be required as part of a return-to-work plan for those who have significant illness, injury, or exposure (physical or psychological) while overseas. Additionally, certain groups such as long-term assignees and humanitarian aid workers require specific attention as, for some individuals, readjustment to home life can be difficult. On return home, up to 75% of aid workers reported difficulty in readjusting, 33% felt disorientated, and 73% felt inadequately supported on their return.[34] In one study, 46% of returned aid workers reported psychological difficulties, mainly depression, although 7% had chronic fatigue, and 4% post-traumatic stress disorder.[35]

Key points

- Travel-related health problems are common, but adequate preparation and support can reduce the risk of illness and injury in overseas workers.
- The most likely causes of mortality in travellers are accidental injury or a cardiovascular event, rather than an infectious disease.
- The key features of a pre-travel consultation are health risk assessment, and health promotion with risk management. Websites of authoritative national bodies should be consulted for comprehensive up-to-date information.
- Higher-risk groups of travellers include those with co-morbidities, pregnant travellers, and the very young or the elderly traveller.
- Medical preparation for overseas working is an essential precursor that should be completed well in advance of departure and, in the case of expatriates, should include every member of the family who is travelling.

Useful websites

Governmental travel medicine recommendations

Centers for Disease Control and Prevention (CDC). Travelers health (USA)	https://www.cdc.gov/travel
National Travel Health Network and Centre (NaTHNaC) (UK)	https://travelhealthpro.org.uk/
Public Health Agency of Canada (PHAC). Travel Health (Canada)	http://www.phac-aspc.gc.ca/tmp-pmv/index-eng.php
Travax (Scotland)	http://www.travax.nhs.uk/

World Health Organization (WHO). International travel and health — http://www.who.int/ith/en/

Travel warnings and consular information

UK Foreign and Commonwealth Office (FCO). Travel advice — https://www.gov.uk/foreign-travel-advice

Emerging diseases and outbreaks

CDC Health Alert Network — https://emergency.cdc.gov/han/index.asp

European Centre for Disease Prevention and Control. Outbreak reports and data — https://ecdc.europa.eu/en/threats-and-outbreaks/reports-and-data

NaTHNaC Outbreak Surveillance database — https://travelhealthpro.org.uk/outbreaks

PHAC Travel notices — hthttps://travel.gc.ca/travelling/health-safety/travel-health-notices

ProMed Mail — https://www.promedmail.org/

WHO Global Response and Alert Outbreak News — http://www.who.int/csr/don/en/

UK National Guidelines

Public Health England. Immunisation against infectious disease — https://www.gov.uk/government/collections/immunisation-against-infectious-disease-the-green-book#the-green-book

UK Advisory Committee on Malaria Prevention. Guidelines for malaria prevention in travellers from the UK (2017) — https://www.gov.uk/government/publications/malaria-prevention-guidelines-for-travellers-from-the-uk

References

1. **Office for National Statistics**. Travel trends 2016. Available at: https://www.ons.gov.uk/peoplepopulationandcommunity/leisureandtourism/articles/traveltrends/2016.
2. **Steffan R, Grieve S.** Epidemiology: morbidity and mortality in travellers. In: Keystone JS, Freedman DO, Kozarsky PE, Connor BA, Nothdurft HD (eds), *Travel Medicine*, 3rd ed, pp. 5–11. Philadelphia, PA: Saunders Elsevier, 2013.
3. **Harvey K, Esposito DH, Han P, et al.** Surveillance for travel-related disease – GeoSentinel Surveillance System, United States, 1997–2011. *MMWR Surveill Summ* 2013;**62**:1–23.
4. **Patel D.** Occupational travel. *Occup Med (Lond)* 2011;**61**:6–18.
5. **Richards C, Rundle AG.** Business travel and self-rated health, obesity, and cardiovascular disease risk factors. *J Occup Environ Med* 2011;**53**:358–63.
6. **Burkholder JD, Joines R, Cunningham-Hill M, Xu B.** Health and wellbeing factors associated with international business travel. *J Travel Med* 2010;**17**:329–33.
7. **Pierre CM, Lim PL, Hamer DH.** Expatriates: special considerations in pre-travel preparation. *Curr Infect Dis Rep* 2013;**15**:299–306.

8. **Chen LH, Wilson ME, Davis X, et al.** Illness in long-term travelers visiting GeoSentinel clinics. *Emerg Infect Dis* 2009;**15**:1773–82.

9. **Patel D, Easmon C, Seed P, et al.** Morbidity in expatriates – a prospective cohort study. *Occup Med* 2006;**56**:345–52.

10. **Dahlgren AL, Deroo L, Avril J, et al.** Health risks and risk-taking behaviors among International Committee of the Red Cross (ICRC) expatriates returning from humanitarian missions. *J Travel Med* 2009;**16**:382–90.

11. **Gamble K, Lankester T, Lovell Hawker D, Sharp E.** Expatriates and travel. In: Keystone JS, Freedman DO, Kozarsky PE, Connor BA, Nothdurft HD (eds), *Travel Medicine*, 3rd edn, pp. 305–16. Philadelphia, PA: Saunders Elsevier; 2012.

12. **Watson HG, Baglin TP.** Guidelines on travel-related venous thrombosis. *Br J Haematol* 2011;**152**:31–4.

13. **Wieten RW, Leenstra T, Goorhuis A, Van Vugt M, Grobusch MP.** Health risks of travelers with medical conditions-a retrospective analysis. *J Travel Med* 2012;**19**:104–10.

14. **Morof DF, Caroll D.** Pregnant travelers. In: **US Centres for Disease Control (CDC)** 'Yellow book': health information for international travel 2018. Available at: https://wwwnc.cdc.gov/travel/yellowbook/2018/advising-travelers-with-specific-needs/pregnant-travelers.

15. **Civil Aviation Authority. Assessing fitness to fly**. 2015. Available at: https://www.caa.co.uk/Passengers/Before-you-fly/Am-I-fit-to-fly/Guidance-for-health-professionals/Assessing-fitness-to-fly/.

16. **National Travel Health Network and Centre.** Diabetes. 2016. Available at: https://travelhealthpro.org.uk/factsheet/4/diabetes#undefined.

17. **Patel RR, Liang SY, Koolwal P, Kuhlmann FM.** Travel advice for the immunocompromised traveler: prophylaxis, vaccination, and other preventive measures. *Ther Clin Risk Manag* 2015;**11**:217–28.

18. *Cordell v. Foreign and Commonwealth office*. UKEAT/0016/11/SM.

19. **The Global Database on HIV Related Travel Restrictions. Homepage.** Available at: http://hivtravel.org/

20. **Public Health England.** ZIKV clinical and travel guidance. 2018. Available at: https://www.gov.uk/government/collections/zika-virus-zikv-clinical-and-travel-guidance.

21. **Liese B, Mundt KA, Dell LD, et al.** Medical insurance claims associated with international business travel. *Occup Environ Med* 1997;**54**:499–503.

22. **Striker J, Luippold RS, Nagy L, Liese B, Bigelow C, Mundt KA.** Risk factors for psychological stress among international business travellers. *Occup Environ Med* 1999;**56**:245–52.

23. **Foyle M, Beer M, Watson J.** Expatriate mental health. *Acta Psychiat Scand* 1998;**97**:278–83.

24. **Henderson B, Samuel H.** 'Briton killed' and '40 BP workers held hostage' in Algeria attack. *The Telegraph*, 16 January 2013. Available at: http://www.telegraph.co.uk/news/worldnews/africaandindianocean/algeria/9806305/Briton-killed-and-40-BP-workers-held-hostage-in-Algeria-attack.html.

25. **The Aid Worker Security Database. Homepage.** Available at: https://aidworkersecurity.org/.

26. **Foreign and Commonwealth Office.** Operating in high-risk environments: advice for business. 2014. Available at: https://www.gov.uk/guidance/operating-in-high-risk-environments-advice-for-business.

27. **Caliguri PM, Hyland MM, Joshi A, et al.** Testing a theoretical model for examining the relationship between family adjustment and expatriates' work adjustment. *J Appl Psychol* 1998;**83**:598–614.

28. **Anderzen I.** *The Internationalization of Work: Psychophysiological, Predictors of Adjustment to Foreign Assignment*. Stockholm: Karolinska Institute; 1998.

29. **Steffen R, Behrens RH, Hill RD, Greenaway C, Leder K.** Vaccine-preventable travel health risks: what is the evidence—what are the gaps? *J Travel Med* 2015;**22**:1–12.

30. **Cowling BJ, Park M, Fang VJ, Wu P, Leung GM, Wu JT.** Preliminary epidemiologic assessment of MERS-CoV outbreak in South Korea, May–June 2015. *Euro Surveill* 2015;**20**:21163.

31. **Foreign and Commonwealth Office.** Foreign travel insurance. 2017. Available at: https://www.gov.uk/guidance/foreign-travel-insurance.

32. **Public Health England.** Ebola: information for humanitarian aid and other workers intending to work in Ebola affected countries in West Africa. 2018. Available at: https://www.gov.uk/government/publications/ebola-virus-disease-information-for-humanitarian-aid-workers.

33. **Whitty CJM, Carroll B, Armstrong M, et al.** Utility of history, examination and laboratory tests in screening those returning to Europe from the tropics for parasitic infection. *Trop Med Int Health* 2000;5:818–23.

34. **Macnair R.** *Room for Improvement: The Engagement and Support of Relief and Development Workers.* London: Overseas Development Institute, 1995.

35. **Lovell DM.** *Psychological Adjustment Among Returned Overseas Aid Workers.* DClinPsy Thesis, University of Wales, 1997.

Chapter 18

Health effects of vibration

Ian Lawson and Roger Cooke

Introduction

There are two types of vibration that can have potential health effects: hand-transmitted vibration (HTV) leading to hand–arm vibration syndrome (HAVS) and whole-body vibration (WBV) affecting the lumbar spine. A survey in Great Britain for the Health and Safety Executive (HSE) estimated that approximately 4.9 million workers were exposed to HTV. Similar European surveys estimated that 350,000 and 6.7 million workers were exposed in Sweden and Germany, respectively.[1,2] There are many potential sources of HTV, the common feature being tools and equipment capable of transmitting an external source of vibrational energy to the hand–arm system. The main industries with exposure involve construction and heavy engineering, but significant exposures can arise in many trades, such as construction workers, metal-working and maintenance fitters, welders, miners, foresters, shipbuilders, foundry workers, utility service workers, and gardeners.[3,4] For WBV, exposure can arise in construction, agriculture, and transportation from driving heavy machinery, forklift trucks, tractors, and lorries with exposure estimated at 7.2 million men and 1.8 million women in Great Britain.[5] The prevalence of HAVS varies between occupational groups but two studies reported estimates of over 220,000 with the vascular component and 300,000 with the sensorineural component.[6,7] Despite this prevalence there have been no Cochrane systematic reviews or National Institute for Health and Care Excellence guidelines although the Faculty of Occupational Medicine (FOM) commissioned a systematic review in 2004. Advice on diagnosis, staging, and management has developed as a result of the latter along with consensus arising from international conferences, and medico-legal precedent setting.

Hand–arm vibration syndrome

HAVS comprises two main components resulting from exposure to HTV of sufficient intensity and duration:

- sensorineural (sensory)
- vascular (previously known as vibration white finger).

Musculoskeletal effects while common are less well explained. However, their effects can impact fitness for work decisions and should be considered in every case. The two main

---

Box 18.1 Diagnosis of HAVS

- A history of relevant exposure to HTV.
- The presence of symptoms compatible with such a diagnosis.
- Exclusion of other causes of such symptoms.

---

components usually develop concurrently but can occur in isolation. The prevalence of symptoms has been reported in one study as 48% sensory, 20% vascular, and 32% combined.[8]

Diagnosis is largely dependent upon history, supported by clinical examination findings (see Box 18.1). Other evidence includes validated photographs or witness accounts of finger blanching, or subjective sensory loss on sensorineural testing.

Relevant exposure

Although a detailed understanding of vibration assessment techniques is not required of the occupational health (OH) professional, a rudimentary knowledge of nomenclature and the interpretation of risk assessment is necessary. Vibration magnitude is measured in terms of its acceleration, averaged by the root-mean square method. Tool-mounted accelerometers measure frequency-weighted values (a_{hw}) in three axes relative to the tool handle. These are summated to produce the 'vibration total value' (defined in International Organization for Standardization (ISO) standard 5349-1, 2001).[9] Injury is assumed to relate to the total energy entering the hand, with a specific relation between time and vibration magnitude. The dose or 'daily vibration exposure' or '$A(8)$' is re-expressed in terms of the equivalent acceleration that would impart the same energy over an 8-hour reference period:

$$A(8) = a_{hw} \sqrt{(t / T_0)} (ms^{-2})$$

where:

$A(8)$ = the daily vibration exposure (8-hour energy-equivalent vibration total value or $a_{hw}(eq(8))$).

a_{hw} = the frequency-weighted vibration total value.

t = duration of exposure in a day to the vibration a_{hw}.

T_0 = 8 hours (in the same units as t).

There is no 'safe' level of HTV exposure, since there is considerable variation in individual susceptibility to exposure, although a daily $A(8)$ level of 1 ms^{-2} is regarded as posing negligible risk (ISO 5349, Annex C). In the UK, the HSE uses an $A(8)$ level of 2.5 ms^{-2} as an action level (exposure action value (EAV)), above which employers are required to introduce risk reduction measures, and introduce health surveillance.[10] This value is based on the ISO 5349 standard which refers to this magnitude of vibration producing symptoms of finger blanching in 10% of exposed people after a 10-year period. By contrast, the daily $A(8)$ which predicts the likelihood of onset of sensorineural symptoms of HAVS is uncertain.

It is generally accepted that lifetime cumulative HTV exposure is the major determinant of onset. Both occupational and non-occupational exposures contribute to lifetime exposure although non-occupational exposure is unlikely to contribute significantly to the total dose.

When taking a history of vibration exposure, the tool or equipment contact or 'trigger' time is important. It is notable that workers tend to overestimate this time (actual values typically 50–70% of estimate). For some tools, overestimation may be as high as 90%.[11]

Ideally, measurement of vibration magnitude should be undertaken by a qualified hygienist or safety engineer in accordance with ISO 5349. However, a lot of exposure information can be obtained from tool supplier data (equipment handbooks, suppliers' information sheets, European Union Good Practice Guides, and HSE Topic Inspection Packs). Partial doses from several tools can be summed to an equivalent daily dose. Tools may be conveniently grouped as 'high', 'medium', or 'low' risk but the same tools can vary in vibration magnitudes. HSE provides a ready-reckoner to estimate $A(8)$ from exposure time and vibration magnitude and an exposure calculator to facilitate the summation of doses from several tools (see 'Useful websites').

Clinical features of HAVS and differential diagnosis

Onset of symptoms

HAVS symptoms develop following the exposure, usually after a number of years. Sensory normally precede vascular symptoms. The interval between first exposure and symptom onset (latent interval), is primarily determined by magnitude and duration of exposure, but is also influenced by individual susceptibility. Latent interval can range from several months to 20 or more years (a rule of thumb for estimating latent interval in years for a given exposure is to divide 30 by the $A(8)$ value).

It is accepted that vascular symptoms may begin after cessation of exposure, although this may reflect a change in cold exposure rather than initial development of the condition. A workshop in Stockholm[12] and the HSE guidance, *Control of Vibration at Work Regulations 2005*, took a 1-year interval as an appropriate maximum for vascular symptoms, although a national scheme that compensated mineworkers in the UK accepted symptoms developing up to 2 years after exposure had ceased.[13]

Vascular symptoms

The vascular effect of hand–arm vibration is manifest as cold-induced Raynaud's phenomenon, which is episodic digital vasospasm. Although report of a classical triphasic history (whiteness, followed by blueness, followed by redness) varies, the diagnosis of Raynaud's phenomenon ideally requires certain features (see Box 18.2).

> ## Box 18.2 Features of Raynaud's phenomenon
>
> - Discrete episodes, typically 20–30 minutes (range 5–120 minutes).
> - Initial tingling or coldness followed by:
>   - numbness and clearly demarcated whiteness (blanching) uniform over affected area; normally extends around circumference of the finger
>   - whiteness that develops distally (at the finger tips) and spreads proximally.
> - The end of an attack is marked by return of normal colour beginning proximally. The affected area may take on a blue hue, resulting from the flow into the skin capillaries of deoxygenated blood, probably from the venules. This blueness is described by some individuals as the only noticeable feature.
> - Return of blood to the affected area, typically with tingling, pain, sensation of swelling ('hot aches'), and a bright red discolouration (reactive hyperaemia), precedes return of normal circulation and colour.

Attacks of vasospasm rarely occur at work unless there are cold conditions or the tool surfaces are cold. Raynaud's phenomenon also occurs naturally (primary Raynaud's phenomenon, Raynaud's syndrome, or Raynaud's disease). In the UK, about 5% of males and 15% of females are affected. It is important to differentiate a history of true vasospasm as described above from simple physiological vasoconstriction as occurs in 'normal' individuals following cold exposure. General cold sensitivity can occur for several months before the onset of finger blanching.

Where an underlying cause of the vasospasm is identified, it is known as secondary Raynaud's phenomenon. Vibration is one cause of secondary Raynaud's phenomenon. Others include connective tissue diseases (scleroderma, systemic lupus erythematosus, rheumatoid disease), trauma, frost bite, thoracic outlet syndrome, Buerger's disease and toxins, including medications (beta blockers and some cytotoxics) and chemicals at work. Secondary Raynaud's phenomenon associated with these other secondary causes is usually more severe and affects all four limbs. Primary Raynaud's phenomenon affects fingers only in approximately 50% of cases. Recent research concluded that vasospasm can also occur in the feet of those exposed to hand–arm vibration (albeit only when hands are affected), suggesting that this point of difference is not absolutely diagnostic.

The mechanism by which HTV produces Raynaud's phenomenon is not known, but it is thought to be multifactorial, with contributions from neural control, vascular wall changes, intravascular abnormalities, and vasoactive substances such as endothelins (see Box 18.3).[14]

There is increasing recognition that hypothenar hammer syndrome (damage to the ulnar artery as it courses round the hamate bone) may be associated with heavy manual work, and possibly with HTV. Thenar hammer syndrome (damage to the radial artery within

Box 18.3 Features suggesting that Raynaud's phenomenon may be due to HTV

- ◆ Onset and deterioration of symptoms after commencement of exposure to HTV and before 12 months after cessation of that exposure.
- ◆ The initial distribution of colour changes, typically, distributed over the hands and fingers most exposed to vibration.
- ◆ Stabilization or improvement of symptoms after cessation of exposure, if the condition is at an early stage.

the thenar eminence) and palmar arch damage may also be associated with manual work, but no link with HTV has yet been suggested. These conditions can be distinguished from HAVS by clinical assessment, including Allen's test and Doppler ultrasonography.[15] Investigation of severe symptoms by traditional or magnetic resonance angiography may assist in diagnosis, particularly when the symptoms are of acute onset and there is a view to possible surgical intervention.

Sensory symptoms

The neurological damage due to hand–arm vibration is thought to represent a combination of damage to mechanoreceptor nerve endings,[16] demyelinating neuropathy,[17] an increase in intra- and extra-neural connective tissue collagen, epineural oedema, and low myelinated nerve fibre density.[18] It may manifest as a peripheral digital neuropathy or a regional neuropathy (commonest affected is the median nerve). The separate roles of vibration, repetitive movements, grip and push forces, non-neutral postures, and other ergonomic stressors can be difficult to distinguish. Such disorders may be more appropriately identified as being caused by the work with vibrating tools than by exposure to HTV per se.

Sensorineural HAVS

The damage caused to neurological structures typically causes a 'diffuse neurosensory deficit in the fingers with numbness and/or tingling, loss of sensitivity, manual dexterity, and grip strength'.[19] The sensorineural component of HAVS develops through a number of phases (see Box 18.4)

It is generally accepted that pathological damage is present in phase 3, but prior to the development of pathological changes, the symptoms reflect a normal physiological response to vibration. It is widely thought that symptoms of tingling and numbness lasting 20 minutes or more after tool use mark the change from a normal physiological response to development of the pathological changes that are referred to as the sensorineural component of HAVS. However, this threshold is arbitrary and based on consensus, and legal decision in the UK, rather than scientific knowledge of the development of pathology.

Box 18.4 Phases of sensorineural HAVS

- Phase 1: exposure to HTV but no symptoms (the latent interval).
- Phase 2: exposure to HTV produces symptoms of tingling and/or numbness associated with vibration exposure and shortly thereafter.
- Phase 3: symptoms become more protracted and constitute the sensorineural component of HAVS.

The differential diagnosis includes systemic disease, medication, and neurotoxins, cervical spondylosis (50% report tingling and numbness of the fingers), thoracic outlet syndrome, and peripheral neuropathy due to alcohol or diabetes.

The 2005 HSE guidance[10] notes that 'numbness occurring separately from blanching is of prime interest as this may indicate the neurological component of HAVS'. The possibility of alternative causes will be raised by a history of dermatomal or peripheral nerve distribution of the neurological symptoms, and provocation by posture or pressure. Pain, tingling, or numbness associated with cold exposure, or an episode of Raynaud's phenomenon suggests those symptoms have a vascular basis. Pain per se is generally not a feature of sensorineural HAVS. There remains the diagnostic problem of those presenting with intermittent tingling or numbness, not associated with colour changes, and occurring in approximately 20% of presentations.

Carpal tunnel syndrome

Carpal tunnel syndrome (CTS) is the commonest of the nerve compression syndromes. It is usually regarded as arising from elevated pressure within the carpal tunnel, which has a direct effect and also interferes with capillary circulation to the median nerve leading to conduction block. If sustained, these effects may lead to demyelination and axonolysis. Additionally, it has been suggested that strain and relative stretching of the nerve causes a relatively diffuse nerve ischaemia. The pathological process in CTS associated with HTV is less well established but potential mechanisms have been suggested.

CTS is characterized by pain or paraesthesiae, or sensory loss in the median nerve distribution, and one or more of the following: Tinel's test positive, Phalen's test positive, nocturnal exacerbation of symptoms, motor loss with wasting of abductor pollicis brevis, and abnormal nerve conduction time.[20] Phalen's and Tinel's tests have significant false-positive and false-negative rates. Additional features that might support the diagnosis are absence of signs in the little finger and on the dorsum of the hand. However, caution needs to be exercised as it has been reported that symptoms in the little finger can occur in 39% of cases of clinical and neurophysiologically diagnosed CTS as a result of Martin–Gruber and other anastomoses between ulnar and median nerves.[21] Symptoms in the little finger in the absence of index finger symptoms point to an ulnar nerve problem in the Guyon or cubital tunnels although again anastomoses can produce atypical symptom

Table 18.1 CTS risk factors and causes

Risk factors	Causes
◆ Being a woman of menopausal age ◆ Obesity ◆ Diabetes or having a family history of diabetes ◆ Osteoarthritis of the carpometacarpal joint of the thumb ◆ Smoking ◆ Lifetime alcohol intake	◆ Tenosynovitis ◆ Over-use injuries ◆ Pregnancy (due to water retention) ◆ Old distal radius fractures ◆ Diabetes mellitus ◆ Hypothyroidism ◆ Acromegaly ◆ Amyloidosis ◆ Mycobacterial infections ◆ Tumours within the carpal tunnel space.

distributions in the latter. A history of successful surgery or steroid injection is strongly supportive of a diagnosis of CTS (Table 18.1). The Primary Care Rheumatology Society have developed useful criteria for clinical diagnosis of CTS.[22]

There are a number of reports of an association between primary Raynaud's phenomenon and idiopathic CTS, which may also lead to less clearly defined colour changes in the affected hands and digits.[23]

HTV exposure is associated with a neuropathy of the median nerve that may present in the same way as CTS, although it is thought that the pathological background may differ from that of classical CTS. An evidence-based review by the FOM supported a positive association with CTS and the use of vibrating tools, but the evidence was stronger for a combination of risk factors such as repetitive and forceful work, awkward postures and vibration combined.[19] Causation and attribution of CTS in vibration exposed remains contentious.[24-26] One meta-analysis controlled for non-occupational risk factors such as obesity reported an odds ratio of 5.4.[26] Yet a more recent publication supported the risk as only moderate[27] (Table 18.2).

Musculoskeletal effects and Dupuytren's contracture

Weakness of grip has been reported in workers with HAVS and is thought to be associated with dysfunction in the intrinsic muscles of the hands.[28-30] Although the pathological

Table 18.2 Symptom comparison matrix for vascular and sensory symptoms in HAVS

	Vascular	Sensorineural	CTS/median neuropathy
Numbness	Prior and during attack of RP	Yes	Yes
Tingling	Prior and after attack of RP	Yes	Yes
Hyperaesthesia	No	?	Yes
Pain	After attack of RP	No	Yes
Vascular symptoms	Yes	No	Yes

process and aetiology is unclear, a measure of grip strength should form part of the overall clinical assessment. Bone and joint disorders are recognized for state compensation in some countries, but it is difficult to differentiate these from the effects of heavy manual work. Similarly, studies on the association of HTV and Dupuytren's contracture have produced conflicting findings, with some in favour and others against an association.[31,32] At the time of writing, consideration is underway as to whether Dupuytren's should be added to the list of prescribed diseases following a command paper by the Industrial Injuries Advisory Council in 2014. As with CTS there are a number of non-occupational risk factors, none more so than genetic aspects and attribution to vibration is likely to remain conflicted for some time.

Clinical assessment and standardized tests

Following a detailed history to elicit the features described earlier, a clinical assessment primarily to assess other causes should be undertaken and should include the following:

◆ The overall condition, temperature, colour of hands, presence of scars, Dupuytren's nodules, fibrosis, and contracture (including Hueston's tabletop test).

◆ Bilateral measurement of blood pressure, radial and ulnar pulses, Allen's test, Adson's and/or Roos tests, and auscultation for subclavian bruits.

◆ An assessment of sensory perception using Semmes Weinstein or West monofilament fibres, and of tactile discrimination (moving two-point discrimination) and manipulative dexterity (Purdue pegboard). The distribution of abnormalities of sensation should be recorded.

◆ If appropriate, assessment of cervical spine, and vascular and neurological assessment of lower limbs.

◆ Phalen's and Tinel's tests for CTS.

◆ Tinel's test and fixed flexion test at the elbows if cubital tunnel syndrome is suspected.

It should be noted that many of these tests are of low discriminatory value for HAVS. Additional standardized tests and investigations may include the following:

◆ Thermal aesthesiometry and vibrotactile threshold assessment, which are likely to have particular value in determining severity.

◆ Doppler ultrasound, which may be useful in identifying thenar or hypothenar hammer syndrome or palmar arch damage.

◆ Nerve conduction studies of value in supporting a clinical diagnosis of CTS may also help to distinguish between receptor-level test results and those at wrist level. [33]

Good identifiable photographs of finger blanching are supportive evidence while cold provocation (rewarm) testing is no longer regarded as providing additional useful evidence (Figure 18.1).[10,34] A recent study found that finger systolic blood pressure had sensitivities and specificities greater than 90% in fingers reported to suffer blanching[35] and may have a role in distinguishing symptomatic from asymptomatic fingers when photography fails to capture blanching.

Grading

The vascular and neurological components are graded separately according to two scales that were developed by a workshop in Stockholm and published in 1987 (Table 18.3).[36,37]

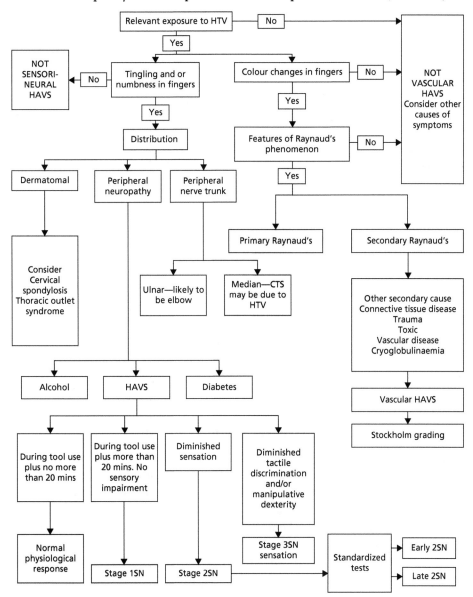

Figure 18.1 Diagnosis of HAVS.

Table 18.3 The Stockholm Workshop Scale for the classification of the hand–arm vibration syndrome

Vascular component stage	Grade	Description
0		No attacks
1V	Mild	Occasional attacks affecting only the tips of one or more fingers
2V	Moderate	Occasional attacks affecting distal and middle (rarely also proximal) phalanges of one or more fingers
3V	Severe	Frequent attacks affecting all phalanges of most fingers
4V	Very severe	As in stage 3, with trophic changes in the fingertips

Reprinted with permission from Gemne G et al., The Stockholm Workshop scale for the classification of cold induced Raynaud's phenomenon in the hand-arm vibration syndrome (revision of the Taylor Pelmear scale). *Scandinavian Journal of Work, Environment and Health* 13(4), 275–278. Copyright © 1987 Scandinavian Journal of Work, Environment & Health.

Sensorineural component stage	Description
0SN	Vibration-exposed but no symptoms
1SN	Intermittent numbness with or without tingling
2SN	Intermittent or persistent numbness, reduced sensory perception
3SN	Intermittent or persistent numbness, reduced tactile discrimination and/or manipulative dexterity

Note: the staging is made separately for each hand. The grade of the disorder is indicated by the stage and number of affected fingers on both hands, e.g. stage/hand/number of digits.

Reprinted from Brammer AJ et al., Sensorineural stages of the hand arm vibration syndrome. *Scandinavian Journal of Work, Environment and Health* 13(4): 279–83, Copyright © 1987 Scandinavian Journal of Work, Environment & Health.

These scales have international currency and have been modified in order to assist with the management of cases.[10]

Health surveillance and management of cases

Prior to giving any advice on health surveillance, it is imperative that the employer draws up a policy covering worker information on HTV hazards, identification and assessment of exposure, management of cases, and control measures. It is also advisable to include consultation with the company legal advisers and employee representatives. Those advising multinational enterprises should be aware of significant differences in regional legislation and approaches to health surveillance between global jurisdictions (Box 18.5).

In practice, the process begins with education and the encouragement of workers to report relevant symptoms to a responsible authority (doctor, nurse, line manager, or designated responsible person). In addition, for those exposed above the EAV, a screening

Box 18.5 Key elements of a health surveillance programme

- ◆ System of symptom reporting.
- ◆ Periodic health inquiry and examination.
- ◆ Formal clinical assessment of suspected cases.
- ◆ Management of affected individuals.
- ◆ Statutory record-keeping.

questionnaire is completed at regular intervals, at, say, the pre-placement stage and then annually (with a check during the first 6 months to identify early and unusual susceptibility). Direct inquiries are made about cold-induced finger blanching, sensorineural symptoms, problems of grip and dexterity, and sometimes other health effects.

The HSE suggests a tiered approach, as this is sparing of limited medical resources.[10] Evaluation by an appropriately trained and experienced clinician (having undergone a FOM-approved training programme) is needed for those with symptoms to confirm the nature, pattern, and history of complaints, to perform a clinical examination, and to consider differential diagnoses and the need for further tests and care.

At pre-placement assessment, consideration will be required of those who have pre-existing Raynaud's phenomenon. It would be appropriate to treat those with known HAVS in the same way as existing employees. Those who present at pre-placement with Raynaud's phenomenon due to another cause should be advised of a possible increased risk when exposed to HTV, but this should not be considered an automatic bar to employment. However, such workers should certainly be kept under more frequent surveillance as it will be impossible to determine whether any progression is due to the pre-existing disease or to the effects of HTV. Similar arguments may be applied to pre-existing peripheral neuropathy. With careful assessment, symptoms due to cervical spondylosis or thoracic outlet syndrome may be distinguishable from a peripheral neuropathy, and hence need not influence decisions regarding exposure to HTV.

Those with CTS in remission, whether through treatment or not, can use vibratory tools, although recurrence of symptoms will raise the question of whether that is due to vibration or the pre-existing condition. There is no evidence that HTV leads to exacerbation of pre-existing compressive CTS, although much work with vibratory tools also includes other risk factors for CTS; it is advisable to inform both employee and employer of the potential increased risks. This is true also of those returning to work after CTS surgery and each case should be considered individually.

Attacks of cold-induced blanching are a source of discomfort, and work and leisure-time interference, but do not appear to cause much loss of working time and have little effect on long-term function. Sensory impairment is a much more important cause of functional disability.

It is now accepted that vascular symptoms can improve on withdrawal from exposure, albeit slowly over several years. The likelihood of recovery is influenced by the age of the worker, severity of the disease, and duration of post-symptomatic exposure. In contrast, the neurological effects of HAVS do not seem to improve. The principle of management should be avoidance of progression to the more severe stage, which will increase the likelihood of improvement in symptoms as well as avoiding severe functional impairment which is likely to affect social and domestic activities as well as working ability. Because stage 2SN includes a wide range of severity of symptoms, it has become conventional to distinguish between early and late stage 2, with progression within stage 2 indicating the need to avoid further exposure to HTV. However, other factors will also need consideration, including the speed of development of the symptoms (which may reflect individual susceptibility) and the age of the employee. Hence, a 62-year-old worker with late-stage 2SN who has shown no progression for 10 years might continue work without restriction, while a 35-year-old worker who has progressed from asymptomatic to stage 2 in a few years should certainly be advised to avoid further HTV exposure.

In affected workers, HAVS tends to progress if the degree of exposure continues unchecked but the rate of progression varies between individuals and is not predictable. It depends on many factors, including vibration magnitude, operator technique, and (probably) personal susceptibility.

With regard to Dupuytren's contracture, there is no evidence to suggest that continuing vibration exposure has any deleterious effect. Fixed flexion contractures may, however, impact grip and health and safety considerations may come into play when handling vibrating tools.

Regardless of the decision on fitness for work, employers should receive a written record confirming that surveillance has taken place and of the outcome. This should be in accordance with General Medical Council and FOM guidance. These 'health records' need to be retained by the employer. Group anonymized results of the health surveillance should be offered to the employer with a review of control measures if required (Figure 18.2).

Distinction is needed between the likelihood of an individual developing worsening of symptoms and ability to do their job ('fitness for work'). Advice regarding either should always take account of age, equality, and biopsychosocial implications. Dupuytren's contracture increases with age and occupational attribution may be a consideration if developing at a young age, particularly in the absence of other risk factors. Older workers nearing retirement may acknowledge increased risks in HAVS but should be free to choose ongoing vibration exposure. CTS risks increase with a body mass index greater than 30 and workers should be supported to lose weight.

Industrial injuries benefit

In the UK, HAVS (A11) is prescribed for Industrial Injuries Disablement Benefit in employed earners for both vascular and sensorineural components if they have worked in a

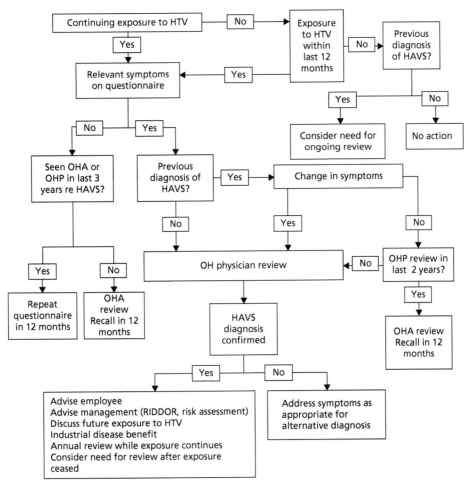

Figure 18.2 Occupational health management of cases. OHA, occupational health adviser; OHP, occupational health physician.

listed occupation (see 'Useful websites'). This state benefit may be claimed irrespective of fault and without a requirement for the individual to cease their job. Vibration-associated CTS (A12) is also prescribed. There are similar benefits in some European countries, some of which additionally compensate joint and bone disorders.

Reporting of Injuries, Diseases, and Dangerous Occurrences Regulations (RIDDOR)

Under separate legal provisions (RIDDOR), employers have a statutory duty to notify cases of HAVS to the appropriate enforcing authority (HSE or local authority), once they become aware that a diagnosis has been made by a medical practitioner, irrespective of the severity (grade) of the symptoms.

The OH professional may be called upon to give advice on primary prevention and control measures. The usual hierarchy of control should be used: avoidance (can the requirement be designed out?), substitution (of tool or material worked), interruption of the vibration transmission pathway (by isolation or vibration-damping), and safer systems of work.

Regular tool maintenance programmes are often offered by tool suppliers, routinely replacing worn-out tool parts. Training on tool usage, avoiding excessive grip and push forces, and the proper selection of tools for the tasks is also important. Sometimes tools and processes can be redesigned to avoid the need to come into contact with vibrating parts. Rest breaks and rotation of tasks that limit exposure time where practicable should be implemented. Although anti-vibration gloves are recommended in some countries, this is not presently the case in the UK.

Whole-body vibration

The health effects of WBV on the lumbar spine are supported by a significant body of research.[38] These include low back pain, sciatica, and intervertebral lumbar disc degeneration. Putative mechanisms have suggested increased compressive and shearing forces with cumulative exposure also likely to be a factor. An additional factor may be that of resonance, which varies in different organs or areas of the body, being about 4–5 Hz in the lower back and 3–5 Hz in the neck. It has been suggested that the voluntary and involuntary muscular contractions that may occur especially around the resonant frequency may be contributory to development of symptoms, but unsurprisingly, for such common conditions in the general population, the pathophysiology and dose–response relationship remains unclear. In addition, many vehicle driving roles include confounders such as prolonged sitting and manual handling. However, studies controlling for these have still reported increased risks. Other health effects including cervical spine, autonomic, and gastrointestinal symptoms are not supported by evidence. In a similar fashion to HTV, triaxial and frequency-weighted measurements are taken from seat-mounted accelerometers and used to express $A(8)$ values for WBV in accordance with ISO 2631-1.[39] The HSE recommends an $A(8)$ level of 0.5 ms^{-2} as an EAV and 1.15 ms^{-2} as an exposure limit value although these are likely to relate more to discomfort than any known level of risk to health (see 'Useful websites'). Health surveillance other than pre-placement screening for pre-existing low back pain is unlikely to be of any benefit. There should be training on risks and encouragement of early reporting of symptoms. Controlling the risk should follow standard hierarchy including elimination and avoidance where practicable.

Key points

- HAVS is one of the commonest occupational diseases comprising vascular and sensorineural components.

- The diagnosis of each component is dependent on history, relevant exposure, clinical examination supported by validated photographs of finger blanching, and where indicated, sensory nerve and receptor testing.
- The frequently reported association between work with vibrating tools and CTS should be considered in all clinical assessments.
- The Stockholm Workshop Scale or a modification should be used to grade clinical severity in HAVS but the management of cases should be based on individual factors.
- HAVS and CTS are both reportable and prescribed conditions.

Useful websites

Health and Safety Executive. Hand–arm vibration	http://www.hse.gov.uk/vibration/hav/source-vibration-magnitude-app3.pdf
Health and Safety Executive. Exposure points system and ready-reckoner	http://www.hse.gov.uk/vibration/hav/readyreckoner.htm
Health and Safety Executive. Exposure calculator	http://www.hse.gov.uk/vibration/hav/hav.xls
Health and Safety Executive. Industrial injuries benefit	http://iiac.independent.gov.uk/pdf/command_papers/Cm6098.pdf
Health and Safety Executive. Whole-body vibration	www.hse.gov.uk/vibration/wbv/index.htm
Industrial Injuries Advisory Council. Industrial injuries benefit	http://iiac.independent.gov.uk/pdf/command_papers/Cm6098.pdf

References

1. **Health and Safety Executive.** *Regulatory Impact Assessment of the Draft Control of Vibration at Work Regulations 2005 as they Relate to Hand-Arm Vibration.* Sudbury: HSE Books; 2004.
2. **Bovenzi M, Peretti A, Nataletti P, et al.** (eds). Workshop: 'Application of 2002/44/EC Directive in Europe'. In: *Proceedings of the 11th International Conference on Hand–Arm Vibration*, Bologna, Italy; 2007.
3. **Griffin MJ.** *Handbook of Human Vibration.* London: Academic Press; 1990.
4. **Palmer KT, Griffin MJ, Syddall H, et al.** Risk of hand-arm vibration syndrome according to occupation and sources of exposure to hand-transmitted vibration: a national survey. *Am J Ind Med* 2001;39:389–96.
5. **Palmer KT, Griffin MJ, Bendall H, et al.** Prevalence and pattern of occupational exposure to whole body vibration in Great Britain: findings of a national postal survey. *Occup Environ Med* 2000;57:229–36.
6. **Palmer KT, Griffin MJ, Syddall H, et al.** Prevalence of Raynaud's phenomenon in Great Britain and its relation to hand transmitted vibration: a national postal survey. *Occup Environ Med* 2000;57:448–52.

7. **Palmer KT, Griffin MJ, Bendall H, et al.** Prevalence of sensorineural symptoms attributable to hand transmitted vibration: a national postal survey. *Am J Ind Med* 2000;**38**:99–107.

8. **Stromberg T, Dahlin LB, Lundborg G.** Hand problems in 100 vibration exposed symptomatic males workers. *J Hand Surg* 1996;**21B**:315–19.

9. **International Organization for Standardization (ISO).** *Mechanical Vibration – Measurement and Evaluation of Human Exposure to Hand-Transmitted Vibration. Part 1: General Requirements.* ISO 5349-1. Geneva: ISO; 2001.

10. **Health and Safety Executive.** *Hand–Arm Vibration. The Control of Vibration at Work Regulations 2005. Guidance on Regulations.* L140. Sudbury: HSE Books; 2005.

11. **Palmer KT, Haward B, Griffin MJ, et al.** Validity of self-reported occupational exposures to hand-transmitted and whole-body vibration. *Occup Environ Med* 2000;**57**:237–41.

12. **Gemne G, Brammer AJ, Hagberg M, et al.** (eds). *Hand-Arm Vibration Syndrome: Diagnostics and Quantitative Relationships to Exposure. Proceedings of the Stockholm Workshop 94.* Solna, Sweden: NIOH/Arbete Och Halsa; 1995.

13. **Lawson IJ, McGeoch KL.** HAVS assessment process for a large volume of medico-legal compensation cases. *Occup Med* 2003;**53**:302–8.

14. **Stoyneva Z, Lyapina M, Tzvetkov D, Vodenicharov E.** Current pathophysiological views on vibration-induced Raynaud's phenomenon. *Cardiovasc Res* 2003;**57**:615–24.

15. **Cooke R, Lawson I.** Use of Doppler in the diagnosis of hypothenar hammer syndrome. *Occup Med* 2009;**59**:185–90.

16. **Ekenvall L, Nilsson BY, Gustavsson P.** Temperature and vibration thresholds in vibration. *Br J Ind Med* 1986;**43**:825–9.

17. **Takeuchi T, Imanischi H.** Histopathological observations in finger biopsy from thirty patients with Raynaud's phenomenon of occupational origin. *J Kumanato Med Soc* 1984;**58**:56–70.

18. **Dahlin LB, Sandén H, Dahlin E, Zimmerman M, Thomsen N, Björkman A.** Low myelinated nerve-fibre density may lead to symptoms associated with nerve entrapment in vibration-induced neuropathy. *J Occup Med Toxicol* 2014;**9**:7.

19. **Mason H, Poole K.** *Clinical Testing and Management of Individuals Exposed to Hand-Transmitted Vibration: An Evidence Review.* London: Faculty of Occupational Medicine; 2004.

20. **Harrington JM, Carter JT, Birrell L, et al.** Surveillance case definitions for work related upper limb pain syndromes. *Occup Env Med* 1998;**55**:264–71.

21. **Clark D, Amirfeyz R, Leslie I, Bannister G.** Often atypical? The distribution of sensory disturbance in carpal tunnel syndrome. *Ann R Coll Surg Engl* 2011;**93**:470–3.

22. **Burton C, Chesterton L, Davenport G, et al.** *Developing Agreed Clinical Criteria for the Diagnosis of Carpal Tunnel Syndrome in Primary Care – A Clinical Consensus Exercise.* Presented at: Society of Academic Primary Care Annual Conference: Nottingham, 4 July 2013: 2E.2.

23. **Hartmann P, Mohokum M, Schlattmann P.** The association of Raynaud's syndrome with carpal tunnel syndrome. *Rheumatol Int* 2012;**32**:569–74.

24. **Lozano-Calderón S, Anthony S, Ring D.** The quality and strength of evidence for aetiology: example of carpal tunnel syndrome. *J Hand Surg* 2008;**33A**:525–38.

25. **Palmer KT, Harris EC, Coggon D.** Carpal tunnel syndrome and its relation to occupation: systematic literature review. *Occup Med (Lond)* 2007;**57**:57–66.

26. **Barcenilla A, March LM, Chen JS, Sambrook PN.** Carpal tunnel syndrome and its relationship to occupation: a meta-analysis. *Rheumatology (Oxford)* 2012;**51**:250–61.

27. **Kazak A, Schedlbauer G, Wirth T, Euler U, Westermann C, Nienhaus A.** Association between work-related biomechanical risk factors and the occurrence of carpal tunnel syndrome: an overview of systematic reviews and a meta-analysis of current research. *BMC Musculoskelet Disord* 2015;**16**:231.

28. **McGeoch KL, Gilmour WH.** Cross sectional study of a workforce exposed to hand-arm vibration: with objective tests and the Stockholm workshop scales. *Occup Environ Med* 2000;**57**:35–42.

29. **Necking LE, Lundstrom R, Lundborg G, et al.** Hand muscle pathology after long term vibration-exposure. *J Hand Surg* 2004;**29B**:431–7.

30. **Lawson IJ, Burke F, McGeoch KL, Nilsson T, Proud G.** Hand-arm vibration and muscle weakness. In: Baxter PJ, Aw T-C, Cockcroft A, Durrington P, Harrington JM (eds), *Hunter's Diseases of Occupations*, 10th edn, pp. 500–2. London: Hodder; 2010.

31. **Burke FD, Proud G, Lawson IJ, et al.** An assessment of the effects to vibration, smoking, alcohol and diabetes on the prevalence of Dupuytren's disease in 97,537 miners. *J Hand Surg* 2007;**32E**:400–6.

32. **Descatha A, Jauffret P, Chastang JF, et al.** Should we consider Dupuytren's contracture as work-related? A review and meta-analysis of an old debate. *BMC Musculoskelet Disord* 2011;**12**:96.

33. **Lawson IJ.** The Stockholm Workshop Scale 30 years on—is it still fit for purpose? *Occup Med* 2016;**66**:595–7.

34. **Proud G, Burke F, Lawson IJ, et al.** Cold provocation testing and hand-arm vibration syndrome-an audit of the results of the Department of Trade and Industry scheme for the evaluation of miners. *Br J Surg* 2003;**90**;1076–9.

35. **Ye Y, Griffin MJ.** Assessment of two alternative standardized tests for the vascular component of the hand-arm vibration (HAVS). *Occup Environ Med* 2016;**73**:701–8.

36. **Gemne G, Pyykkö I, Taylor W, et al.** The Stockholm Workshop scale for the classification of cold-induced Raynaud's phenomenon in the hand–arm vibration syndrome (revision of the Taylor Pelmear scale). *Scand J Work Environ Health* 1987;**13**:275–8.

37. **Brammer AJ, Taylor W, Lundborg G.** Sensorineural stages of the hand–arm vibration syndrome. *Scand J Work Environ Health* 1987;**13**:279–83.

38. **Bovenzi M, Palmer K.** Whole body vibration. In: Baxter PJ, Aw T-C, Cockcroft A, et al. (eds), *Hunter's Diseases of Occupations*, 10th edn, pp. 513–22. London: Hodder; 2010.

39. **International Organization for Standardization (ISO).** *Mechanical Vibration and Shock: Guide for the Evaluation of Human Exposure to Whole Body Vibration- Part 1: General Requirements.* ISO 2631-1. Geneva: ISO; 1997.

Chapter 19

Mental health and psychiatric disorders

Richard J.L. Heron and Neil Greenberg

Introduction

Mental health disorders significantly impact well-being and productivity in the working age population (see Figure 19.1). They affect around 17% of the population[1] and their economic cost has been estimated at £70 billion or 4.5% of gross domestic product in the UK.[2] Mental health conditions are a leading cause of sickness absence with 70 million working days lost per year.[3] Over half of disabled people who are out of work have a mental health and/or musculoskeletal disorder as their main health condition.[4]

Overall, 'good' work and paid employment are generally beneficial for mental well-being.[5] Work also brings less tangible advantages such as social status and recognition, contact, and social support. It provides a forum for establishing supportive social relationships, daily routines, and a sense of personal achievement[6]; most people who are unable to work believe that working leads to better health.[7] Conversely, long-term, involuntary, unemployment is associated with despair, mental illness, and, in some cases, suicide.[8] However, the relationship between work and mental health is complex. Some serious mental health disorders, such as schizophrenia, are associated with challenging work limitations. However, the picture is less clear for common mental health disorders such as anxiety and depression. While the harmful effects of worklessness are well known, it is increasingly recognized that poorly managed or 'bad work' can contribute to mental ill health.

Organizations, ideally advised by occupational health (OH) professionals, have moral, legal, and economic reasons to support the mental health of their workforce and to consider workplace adjustments to accommodate employees with mental ill health. This chapter considers how work and mental health interrelate, and how employers can ensure that their workforce mental health needs are managed, opportunities for productivity are maximized, and psychiatric morbidity is minimized.

Prevalence of common mental disorders

According to the adult psychiatric morbidity survey of mental health and well-being in England, one in six adults (17%) met the criteria for a common mental disorder (CMD).[9]

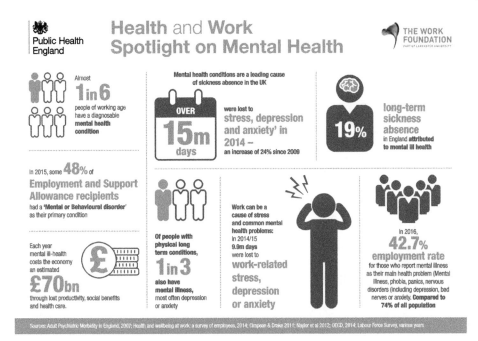

Figure 19.1 Spotlight on Mental Health.
Reproduced from Public Health England. (2014) *Health and work: infographics*. London, UK: Public Health England. © Crown Copyright 2014.

These include an increasing number of depression and anxiety-related disorders. The same study found that, in 2014, only one in three adults aged 16–74 (37%) with conditions such as anxiety or depression were receiving mental health treatment (although this is an increase from 25% in 2007). This is especially relevant given a longer-term, small, but steadily increasing prevalence of CMDs in women and a stable rate within the adult male population between 2000 and 2014. While not classified as a CMD in this study, around 1 in 20 (4.4%) also screened positive for post-traumatic stress disorder (PTSD) in the past month, with similar rates for men and women. This condition may be especially important when considering workers in trauma-prone roles (e.g. emergency ('blue-light') services, media, military, etc.).

During the same period (2007–2014), the proportion of people with more severe psychiatric disorders remained steady at around 0.4–0.7%[1] with no significant differences between men and women. At a population level, people with a severe mental illness are often more disabled than those with a CMD. However, at an individual level, the relationship between disability and diagnosis is not uniform. Some people with generalized anxiety disorders may be house-bound, and need significant support. Conversely, a person with a diagnosis of schizophrenia may be able to lead a relatively normal life in all respects other than the subjective experience of their symptoms.[10]

Employed adults were much less likely to have a CMD than those who were unemployed or economically inactive (see Table 19.1).

Table 19.1 Prevalence of CMD by employment status

Status	Prevalence of CMD (%)
Full-time work	14
Part-time work	16
Unemployed job seekers	28
Economically inactive	33

Source: data from McManus, S. et al. Adult Psychiatric Morbidity Survey: Survey of Mental Health and Wellbeing, England, 2014 [Internet]. NHS Digital. Copyright © 2014 NHS. Available from: http://digital.nhs.uk/catalogue/PUB21748.

The most frequently reported CMDs in all recipients of Employment and Support Allowance (ESA) were generalized anxiety disorder and depression.[1]

Employment rates for people with a mental health condition also vary according to the severity of the condition. People at the more severe end of the spectrum with, for example, psychotic disorders, have lower rates of employment and work in less secure jobs.[11] Among those receiving ESA, 41% were coded with a primary condition: 'mental or behavioural disorder'.[2] Approximately 14% of ESA claimants have psychosis compared to 0.1% in the working age population.

Patients with severe, enduring mental health problems account for 8% of long-term disabled people of working age. Of these, only 18% are in some form of employment, even though 30–40% are thought capable of working, compared with 52% of non-mentally long-term disabled people.[10]

People with less severe mental disorders (often referred to as neuroses) are still four to five times more likely to be permanently unemployed compared with the rest of the population: 61% of males and 58% of females with a single neurotic disorder are in work compared with 75% and 65% respectively in the general population.[12] Co-morbidities further reduce employment prospects. In patients with two concomitant neurotic disorders, the proportions in work fell further to 46% of males and 33% of females. Patients with phobic disorders had the bleakest employment record: only 43% of males and 30% of females were working. At the same time, up to 90% of patients state they would like to return to work.[12]

The economic burden of mental illness

Improving sustainable access to work for people with mental health conditions provides income and an improved standard of living to the employee, and reduces the financial burden on employers and the state. In 2016, mental health issues, including stress, depression, anxiety, and more serious conditions such as manic depression and schizophrenia, resulted in 15.8 million working days lost.[13]

On average, approximately 3000 people in the UK per week move onto incapacity benefit and mental health disorders are the second commonest reason accounting for

20%. In a recent review, the commonest reason for issuing a fit note (31%) in England between 2014 and 2017 was for a mental health or behavioural condition. During the same period, the number of fit notes written for anxiety and stress-related conditions by general practitioners increased by 14%.[14]

The direct costs of mental illness have been variably estimated at £70–105 billion/year of which 15% was due to lost economic output, sickness absence, and unemployment costs.[3,15]

Work as a health outcome

Irrespective of psychiatric diagnosis, successful return to paid work is perhaps one of the most meaningful yet least used measures of health outcome and an important positive prognostic indicator. Too many patients with mental health problems make a good clinical and functional recovery only to find themselves in an impoverished parallel world of social exclusion, becoming aimless, under-occupied, and unfulfilled. This existence potentially undermines an already fragile self-esteem and is itself a harbinger of further mental health problems. There is considerable opportunity for improving social inclusion, which has not been adequately addressed at a statutory or policy level. Moreover, traditional mental health services are focused on symptomatic improvement and pay too little attention to occupational outcome.

Common psychiatric disorders

Psychiatric disorders are ordinarily classified according to one of two classification manuals, the International Classification of Disease, tenth revision (World Health Organization (WHO)), and the *Diagnostic and Statistical Manual of Mental Disorders*, fifth edition (American Psychiatric Association). Not all healthcare professionals use either classification manual rigidly and examples of ill thought-out diagnostic labelling can often be found. This may be more common in primary care than secondary care settings. However, since most psychiatric disorders cannot be diagnosed using 'hard' tests, even mental health specialists may disagree about the nature of a psychiatric disorder. Another problem with classifying psychiatric disorders is that many diagnostic labels can also be found in lay use within everyday language. For instance, diagnostically, depression requires at least a 2-week history of the relevant symptoms, however the term depression is often used by lay people to describe unhappiness and some confusion may arise between the diagnostic and lay use of the term.

Wrongful use of a diagnostic label may mislead and OH psychiatric reports should always include a clear description of the symptoms and signs in any particular case. The following sections form a brief overview of some of the more common or important mental health conditions which OH professionals might encounter.

Adjustment disorders

Adjustment disorders are 'extreme' short- and medium-term reactions to stressful events. They occur more commonly in people with other mental health vulnerabilities and usually resolve within months of the stressor ceasing, but can persist when the stressful occurrence or its consequences continue. Individuals typically feel overwhelmed or unable to cope. They may experience marked symptoms of anxiety or depression and exhibit a range of unhelpful behaviours including, uncommonly, illegal acts. Symptoms may include a variety of somatic complaints including headaches, dizziness, abdominal pain, chest pain, and palpitations. People with an adjustment disorder may misuse alcohol or illicit substances as an (adverse) coping strategy. While most of these reactions are self-limiting, the severity of emotions and behaviours may be extreme. Damage to social and occupational relationships can be severe and enduring. Medication, including antidepressants and anxiolytics, may alleviate severe symptoms. However, providing temporary respite from stressful circumstances (potentially including the workplace) may also be appropriate. If the workplace is a major stressor, it is often helpful to maintain working in alternative roles in preference to sickness absence. Clinicians should ensure that those with an adjustment disorder do not cause themselves longer-term harm as a consequence of their behaviour. A graded return to normal functioning is itself generally therapeutic. The expectation should be one of full recovery. Adjustment disorders may evolve into more chronic illnesses such as major depression and other anxiety states. However, the absence of past psychiatric history and the presence of a 'robust' pre-morbid personality generally predict a good outcome.

Depression

Clinical depression is a potentially disabling but often eminently treatable CMD. Depression is often categorized as mild, moderate, or severe. People experiencing mild depression can usually continue with their usual pattern of life without substantial impairment. Moderate depression impairs but usually does not completely prevent an individual's usual routine. Severe depression is often associated with major functional impairment. The three key presenting features of depression are low mood, an inability to enjoy life (anhedonia), and pervasive feelings of tiredness/fatigue. Associated features include disturbances of sleep, appetite, and concentration, negative views of the future, lowered self-esteem, feelings of worthlessness, and thoughts of self-harm. Because some people with depression may find it difficult, or embarrassing, to discuss their emotions, patients commonly present with various physical complaints such as fatigue, pain, or with related psychological problems including anxiety. Depression may also be triggered by physical disorders where it may pass undetected but present a major obstacle to recovery. OH professionals should rely on sensitive direct questioning to identify depression such as 'What have your energy levels been like lately?' or 'What was the last thing you remembering enjoying?' Symptoms may develop insidiously and it may only be with hindsight that depression is identified as a cause of underperformance. Standard questionnaires to estimate symptoms have limited evidence of validity in OH settings for diagnostic purposes, and responses may be affected by work-context factors such as management disputes, and unresolved legal processes (see 'Fit for work? Assessment for employment'). Predictors of long-term outcome include pre-morbid personality, the presence of ongoing stressors, and the presence of co-morbid disorders, particularly substance misuse. There are a number of effective treatments for depression including antidepressant medications and psychotherapies such as cognitive behavioural therapy (CBT), interpersonal therapy, or behavioural activation. Non-specific interventions to reduce the impact of stressors such as lifestyle adjustments and exercise may also prove helpful.[16] The prospect of work can be intimidating for many depressed patients who may lack confidence and motivation; moreover, many perceive their employment (rightly or wrongly) as contributory to their disorder. However, a successful (most likely graded) return-to-work package can assist recovery through bolstering self-esteem and improving social contacts.

Post-traumatic disorders including PTSD

Most people who experience traumatic events do well and recover without the need for any formal healthcare assistance even if they experience short-term distress. However, a minority will develop more persistent disorders including PTSD, depression, other anxiety disorders, or substance misuse. PTSD is a persistent psychiatric condition that occurs in people who have been directly involved in, or witnessed, a traumatic event. Features include re-experiencing symptoms, avoidance symptoms, arousal symptoms, and changes in the way those affected think and feel about themselves and the world.

A diagnosis of PTSD should not be made unless functionally impairing symptoms have been present for at least 1 month. Most people who develop PTSD will do so within 6 months of the traumatic event, although their presentation to healthcare is often delayed. The correct management of post-traumatic disorders (including PTSD) should be of particular interest to employers of personnel in trauma-prone roles, not least because ill-considered psychological support post trauma may lead to litigation. Historically, the use of single-session critical incident stress debriefing, or psychological debriefing, was popular. However, randomized controlled trials have failed to demonstrate benefit from single-session psychologically focused debriefings,[17,18] which have actually been found to cause harm in some cases. Recently, less psychologically focused organization peer support interventions delivered by appropriately trained non-mental health professionals, such as the trauma risk management (TRiM) programme developed in the UK armed forces, have shown promise. TRiM is now routinely used in civilian settings including the emergency services, train operators, media companies, and similar settings.[19] Peer support programmes such as TRiM appear to mobilize informal social support post incident and help ensure access for the minority who need professional interventions. Post-incident education is commonly provided through briefings or leaflets. There is limited evidence of a modest benefit.[20] Formal post-incident mental health screening programmes, which are costly and administratively burdensome, have not been found to be effective[21] and may cause harm,[22] usually by incorrectly labelling normal reactions as pathological.

At times, the treatment of post-traumatic disorders can be complicated by litigation. It is noteworthy that lengthy legal proceedings and repeated examinations for legal reports are often unhelpful and can impede recovery. PTSD symptoms typically fluctuate and may deteriorate on anniversaries or following reminders of traumatic events. From an

OH perspective, it is important to encourage timely return to a supportive workplace, to ensure provision of evidence-based treatments, and avoid providing potentially harmful interventions such as single-session debriefings. Treatment for PTSD includes the use of trauma-focused CBT and eye movement desensitization and reprocessing as well as some antidepressants as a second-line approach or when treating co-morbid depression. It is important to note that the use of sedative medications such as benzodiazepines is contraindicated for PTSD.

Chronic mixed anxiety and depression

Low mood, sadness, worrying, and demotivation are features of normal life, experienced by most of the population at some time, and care should be taken not to over-medicalize such symptoms. Sometimes symptoms are severe enough to modestly, temporarily, impair normal daily activities but are insufficient to meet diagnostic criteria for either a depressive episode or other anxiety disorders. Some, but by no means all, warrant a specific diagnosis such as a depressive adjustment disorder or dysthymia, a persistent mood disorder characterized by longstanding feelings of being sad, 'blue', low, 'down in the dumps', and with little interest or pleasure in usual activities, or mixed anxiety and depression. Some people, who experience low-grade mood symptoms, including adjustment disorders or mild depression, might be considered as grumpy or persistent complainers and their presence in a workplace may negatively affect the well-being of colleagues. Medication is of uncertain value in more minor disorders and if used should be started as a trial and continued only if benefit is clear. Supportive counselling may be useful in the absence of adequate social networks but people with less serious mood problems benefit from retaining responsibility for their own recovery. Brief cognitive approaches that challenge unfounded worries or negative assumptions, problem-solving approaches, and relaxation techniques may also be useful. A variety of computerized CBT packages such as 'Living Life to the Full' and 'Beating the Blues' may also be helpful (see 'Useful websites'). Motivation, from the individual and their employers, and the willingness to accept responsibility is probably one of the best predictors of a successful outcome.

Bipolar (affective) disorder (also known as manic depression)

This disorder, along with schizophrenia, is often termed a serious mental illness (SMI). Bipolar affective disorder is characterized by episodes of depression, mania, or an admixture of both. Mixed affective states are common and mood and symptoms (see Box 19.1) may fluctuate and vary independently of each other.

Patients may manifest with predominantly depressive or manic symptoms (depressive presentations are more common with age) and presentations may change over time. Although full recovery from major mood swings is the norm, many patients display lesser degrees of emotional instability requiring treatment between episodes.

Factors to be considered in assessing the employability of bipolar patients include insight, relapse frequency, functional capacity during remissions, and adherence to any long-term treatment plan including compliance with mood stabilizing medication.

Box 19.1 Features of mixed affective states

- Fluctuating mood.
- Disordered thought including flight of ideas (the topic of conversation jumps in a non-predictable way).
- Altered motor behaviour (over- or underactivity).
- Arousal (irritability or withdrawal).
- Perceptual abnormalities including mood-congruous delusions (bizarre beliefs out of keeping with the facts behind the belief) or hallucinations (perceptions in the absence of a stimulus).
- Behavioural disturbances (retardation or disinhibition).

Patient insight and prompt withdrawal from work at the early stage of a relapse and before the florid symptoms can ease workplace re-entry after recovery. Co-morbid substance misuse during episodes is generally a poor prognostic sign. Disturbed sleep and sleep deprivation are important triggers for episodes of mania and shift work or work involving long-distance air travel may be ill-advised. While, when well, there may be a wide range of roles available for well-controlled individuals who suffer with this condition, suitability for safety-critical roles should be considered very carefully.

Schizophrenia

Schizophrenia is also a chronic SMI that is characterized by a range of symptoms. These include hallucinations, delusions and muddled thoughts based on the hallucinations, or delusions with associated (usually negative) changes in behaviour. Schizophrenia is a psychotic illness; individuals may often not be able to distinguish their own thoughts and ideas from reality. The exact cause of schizophrenia is unknown, but it probably results from a combination of genetic and environmental factors.

Schizophrenia is one of the most common SMIs, although the population prevalence is less than 1%. Men and women are equally affected. In men, onset is usually between the ages of 15 and 30 with a tendency to later onset in women (25–30 years). The risk of violence from someone who suffers with schizophrenia is small; violent crime is more likely to be linked to alcohol or other substance misuse. A person with schizophrenia is far more likely to be the victim of violent crime than the instigator.

From an occupational viewpoint, a third of people may recover completely, but those chronically affected are likely to find highly demanding work especially challenging. Stress may cause well-controlled schizophrenia to relapse. However, with good support, an understanding employer, and good liaison between OH professionals and specialists, people with schizophrenia can be highly effective employees when they are in remission. Specialists may be able to help employers understand the 'relapse signature' for the condition, which is often unique to that individual. For instance, before relapsing, someone with schizophrenia may become less socially integrated, spend more time mumbling to themselves, and perhaps wear strange combinations of clothes at work. An enlightened employer, aware of the implications of the changes in behaviour, would be enabled to assist the relapsing employee to seek early help.

Acute psychotic disorders

While all psychotic disorders are SMIs, not all are enduring. Although a first episode of a psychotic condition may eventually become chronic schizophrenia or bipolar affective disorder, some psychoses are transient and can occur as a result of extreme stress or be brought about by illicit drug use. While acutely psychotic, people are highly unlikely to be fit for work. Active psychosis may lead to unpredictable behaviour and while the exact nature of the psychosis is being determined a watch-and-wait approach in respect of work is often best.

Personality disorders

Personality disorders are maladaptive patterns of behaviour which manifest in late adolescence or early adult life, endure, cause difficulties for the person themselves and/or those around them, and represent the extreme ends of the normal spectrum of personality. Estimates vary from as low as 10% in the general population to 40% (or more) in prison settings. While there are many varieties of personality disorder, the term should not be used loosely. Diagnosis should only follow a high-quality assessment by an appropriately experienced mental health professional who has been provided with sufficient collateral historical information. It is notable that while personality is thought to be a static characteristic, there is evidence that some personality disorders (e.g. emotionally unstable personality disorder) may improve over time as a result of life experiences, maturation, and possibly therapeutic input. Also, personality may be altered by extreme experiences (e.g. repeated or severe trauma) or the impact of severe illness to the point that an acquired personality disorder may be diagnosed.

In broad terms, personality disorders fall into three clusters (see 'Useful websites'): cluster A is characterized by odd/eccentric behaviour including paranoid, schizotypal, and schizoid. People within this cluster can present as suspicious, unforgiving, bizarre, and cold. Many find it difficult to maintain relationships and indeed may have little interest in relationships at all.

Cluster B disorders include people with emotionally unstable (borderline), dissocial, or histrionic disorders. Individuals in this cluster may be hard to predict and likely to break rules. Individuals presenting with a borderline/emotionally unstable personality disorder often find emotional control difficult and may be at particular risk of self-harm.

People within Cluster C are often anxious and fearful and include those with obsessive compulsive—or anankastic—personality disorder. This is not the same as obsessive–compulsive disorder which is a distinct mental health condition. Often such people tend to be very rigid, highly judgemental, and are perfectionists. Those suffering anxious/

avoidant personality disorder tend to be anxious, tense, and worrisome and may react badly to perceived criticism. Those with dependent personalities tend to be passive, reliant on others, and very easily perceive abandonment.

The impact of personality disorder within the workplace also varies and extreme personality traits may be highly adaptive in some environments but less so in others (e.g. obsessional individuals may be effective quality assurers but less able to deal with significant organizational change). From an OH perspective, employees who suffer from a personality disorder are likely to be highly susceptible to pressure within the workplace or from other sources and their enduring personality traits may cause considerable difficulty among those who have to work with them. Treatment of these disorders is possible in some cases, usually through a psychotherapeutic process, but is often lengthy. Within the workplace they are likely to benefit from a patient and sensitive line manager more than most. While personality disorders may well be considered to fall under the Equality Act 2010, it may be difficult for employers to make reasonable adjustments to accommodate the behavioural manifestations of some personality disorders (e.g. aggressive outbursts as a result of a dissocial personality disorder).

Eating disorders

Eating disorders affect women up to ten times more commonly than men. While it is not entirely clear what causes these disorders, factors which are thought to be important include a desire or need to be in control, long-standing unhappiness, family attitudes towards food, low self-esteem, social pressures, and genetics. Eating difficulties may also form part of other disorder such as depression or bipolar disorder. There are three main types of eating disorders: anorexia nervosa, bulimia nervosa, and binge eating disorder.

Anorexic patients worry about their weight and body image; they restrict their food intake and often exercise excessively. They are often well below a safe weight and have body mass index (BMI) below 18.5. Women may experience irregular, or no, periods and in men sexual interest may be absent and testicles may shrink. The condition often begins in the teenage years although it can start at any time. Anorexia can be a dangerous condition which can lead to serious ill health and even death, especially in persons with lower BMIs.

Patients with bulimia also worry about their weight and body image but tend to binge eat and make themselves vomit and/or use laxatives as well as use exercise. They may have normal weight but experience guilt about this. This condition also often starts in the mid-teenage years although there may be a considerable delay to seeking help. Repeated vomiting brings a wealth of risks including cardiac problems secondary to potassium disturbance and dental problems because of regurgitation of stomach acid.

People with a binge eating disorder repeatedly diet and binge eat, but do not vomit. While distressing, it is not as harmful as bulimia. People with this condition are at risk of becoming overweight.

Within the workplace, these disorders may be problematic as poor nutrition may affect cognition and cause physical health problems. People with eating disorders may also be more vulnerable to other mental health conditions such as depression or adjustment disorders. There may be an element of social avoidance because of fears about having to eat or to hide weight reduction behaviours (e.g. purging).

There is good evidence that, if someone is motivated, talking therapies can be effective in helping people with eating disorders recover or at least minimize the health impacts of the conditions. Treatment is usually slow and progressive and, in more severe cases, specialist input, and very rarely hospitalization, is required. Informed managers and colleagues can be very helpful in supporting people with these conditions to recover.

Factitious disorders

Factitious disorder is a diagnostic term referring to patients who deceive others by feigning illness or injury. Symptoms can range from mild with slight exaggeration of symptoms to severe sometimes referred to as Munchausen syndrome. Individuals may also tamper with medical tests to convince others that treatment, such as high-risk surgery, is needed. Factitious disorder can also be imposed on another person (sometimes referred to as Munchausen syndrome by proxy), often taking the form of a parent or caregiver feigning the symptoms of those they care for (e.g. children). In some cases, the factitious disorder patient may actually harm those they care for.

A key feature of a factitious disorder is that it is not malingering. The 'gain' from feigning medical problems is not practical benefit (e.g. avoiding work or getting an insurance pay out). Instead there is an unconscious gain often in the form of recognition, attention, or sympathy. People who suffer with this disorder know they are causing their symptoms but will not consciously understand why they do so and may not recognize that they have a mental health problem.

Factitious disorders can be challenging to identify and hard to treat as those who have the disorder can go to great lengths to hide their deception. Often it is not easy for their colleagues, family, or healthcare professionals to understand why those affected feign symptoms or harm themselves, or others. People with the disorder do not simply cease their deception when presented with objective evidence that does not support their assertions.

Primary, secondary, and tertiary prevention in the workplace

Management of mental health disorders in an occupational environment can be considered in terms of primary, secondary, and tertiary prevention.

Primary prevention refers to an employer or line manager's accountability for addressing risks associated with the way work is organized, and the worker's responsibility to live a reasonably mentally healthy lifestyle.

Secondary prevention refers to the early identification of warning signs that indicate mental ill health. This allows for early workplace or health interventions to prevent progression or facilitate earlier improvement in health and occupational effectiveness. A mentally well-educated worker may improve stability using self-help techniques or seeking informal support.

Tertiary prevention refers to treatment and recovery, which aim to prevent longer-term disability. While line management support for tertiary prevention is beneficial, the responsibility for delivering the interventions is likely to rest with health professionals and the individual themselves to comply with treatment. OH and human resources professionals have a key role integrating evidence-based practices into organizational policies, raising awareness about them, and auditing implementation.

Primary prevention of work-related mental health disorders

Primary prevention is mainly non-medical and should focus on the preventive actions by employers to reduce workplace risk factors. Actions are usefully divided into:

- effective leadership, management, and organizational factors such as control of work delivery (methods and timing)
- the support of management and co-workers
- individual awareness, life-skills, and resilience in workplace settings.

Organizational factors

A wealth of evidence demonstrates that people working in well-led, mutually supportive companies can endure substantially higher levels of psychological pressure than personnel in less well-led and less cohesive groupings.[23] One important aspect of leadership is raising awareness about the nature, and impact, of mental health conditions, and encouraging their team's psychological resilience. Doing so includes challenging unhelpful intuitive beliefs, for example, that discretionary time away from work and work colleagues will be beneficial after a period of high-pressure working. Evidence, primarily from military samples, has shown repeatedly that maintaining work provides access to social support, minimizes guilt that can arise from a perception of letting colleagues or the organization down, and assists recovery.

A well-accepted model of occupational stress is known as the demand–control model.[24] This proposes that stress is an adverse reaction to excessive quantitative or qualitative demands[25] when unable to exert control over the work and when feeling unsupported. This model is incorporated within the UK Health and Safety Executive (HSE) stress management standards, which provide a framework for assessing six stressor areas: demands, control, support, relationships, role, and change.[25] Therefore, training to prepare personnel to carry out their role at work should provide employees with the ability to perform well and also support their well-being.

Another important model of stress at work is the effort–reward imbalance model,[26] which proposes that stress-related problems occur where there is an imbalance between high efforts and low rewards. Furthermore, the model suggests that highly committed individuals may be at especially increased risk of poor health outcomes. Timely recognition of employee effort, both informally and during organizational appraisal, can be seen as a mental health support tool. While other benefits such as financial bonuses or extra leave entitlement may be considered as rewards for good service, the evidence suggests that positive feedback also supports the mental well-being of employees.

Individual factors

An individual's psychological resilience is also a product of individual factors such as education, upbringing, family circumstances, and stressful life events. Therefore, primary prevention includes the provision of knowledge and skills to enhance coping and by enhancing resilience.

Evidence of the spread and popularity of mental health training can be found on many respectable health-related websites including the WHO, the National Institute for Health and Care Excellence (NICE), the UK Psychological Trauma Society, the Institute of Psychiatry, the National Center for PTSD, and the Uniformed Services University of the Health Sciences. Business in the Community in partnership with Public Health England has published mental health toolkits for employers. See 'Useful websites' for research evidence and toolkits. Training interested co-workers to recognize and support individuals with mental health problems has become increasingly popular. There is limited evidence that stigma may be reduced, together with self-reported increases in trainees' confidence to provide support to beneficiaries.[27] However, there is little evidence to suggest altered outcomes in those with mental health problems.

Few studies have established sustained or long-term protective effects from training. A systematic review of workplace resilience training was unable to identify the most effective format for resilience training, but did show evidence of improved personal resilience, psychosocial functioning, and performance after training.[28] Some military studies have shown mildly positive short-term effects in the prevention of psychological ill health after exposure to potentially traumatic situations.[29, 30] Cognitive behavioural training has been shown to reduce worry about work (affective work-related rumination) and chronic fatigue in workers attending a half-day work shop for up to 6 months.[31] Much attention has been paid to mindfulness interventions at work. While the overall impact of this intervention appears to be positive, the evidence is inconsistent and generally of poor quality.[32] Importantly, there are no randomized controlled trials, so firm views on its role in primary prevention should be reserved.

Although evaluation of stress management training has shown short-term individual benefits, their more important role may be to increase understanding of the management principles to reduce stress, improve coping,[33] and reduce the stigma associated with mental health conditions.[34] Stigma describes the set of beliefs which prevent people who may benefit from accessing support; these include a fear of what colleagues or bosses will think of the individual and the impact on career prospects. There is good evidence that stigma is a societal issue rather than limited to any specific occupational group.[35] Organizational policies and programmes that aim to reduce the stigma associated with mental health conditions have the potential to increase health and well-being of employees by encouraging them to seek collegial support and avoiding the need for professional support or medical treatment.

Reported stigma in the military has significantly decreased, although not disappeared, over the last 15 years. Within the wider UK community, many organizations have signed up to 'Time to Change', an anti-stigma campaign, which has been shown to have a significant impact on stigma and discrimination in the population.[36] The impact of Time to Change appears to have been especially evident as a result of lived experience, when people who have experienced mental health problems speak out about their journey back to health. However, it is important to note that stigma is not the only barrier to seeking help. Many people either fail to recognize their mental health difficulties or feel that they are not serious enough to warrant seeking healthcare. Overall, high-quality studies carried out in the UK suggest that only around one in three people who have a mental health disorder seek appropriate help for it.

Secondary prevention of mental health disorder

Secondary prevention refers to the early detection of at-risk employees to allow organizational-level interventions, including but not limited to temporary changes in duties and increased provision of informal social support. Where simple interventions are not successful, referral for professional assessment and management is generally recommended.

One challenge with providing secondary prevention at an organizational level is that most systems of early detection rely on individual 'case' identification. This usually defaults to a healthcare professional consultation, periodic medical examination, or specific screening programme. Substantial limitations of screening are discussed below. However, research suggests that many employees do not routinely seek help about work-related problems. This may be because they themselves lack insight that their difficulties result from mental health problems, their mental health problems go unnoticed by co-workers, or other perceived barriers to care, including but not limited to stigma.[37] Furthermore, many people prefer to use informal support mechanisms than seek professional help, especially for problems that they consider as being as minor. Indeed, initially avoiding medical help is not necessarily detrimental for most people who have good available support and who will, in any case, recover. However, even those who will go on to recover fully and rapidly may be temporarily unable to carry out some or all of their duties. The impact of so-called presenteeism has been well described as accounting for more loss of productivity than absenteeism.

How best to detect and manage persisting low grade symptoms, or more severe symptoms which do not come to the attention of health professionals, remains a substantial challenge. One popular mechanism is peer support programmes,[38] the rationale for which includes meeting the legal and moral duty to care for employees, and addressing multiple barriers to standard care (including stigma, lack of time, poor access to providers, lack of trust, and fear of job repercussions). Their format ranges from training non-professionals to deliver basic counselling interventions in the workplace, to more formalized early detection and management processes that are designed to support personnel who have been exposed to trauma.[39] Although evidence for their effectiveness is limited, peer support programmes are well accepted and may improve occupational function especially after traumatic events.[40]

Mental health screening has been proposed for early detection of latent mental health problems. However, there is currently no evidence of effectiveness either by questionnaire or face-to-face interview. Those identified using screening techniques differ from patients seen in routine clinical care in terms of severity, their interest in accessing health services, commitment to treatment, and their motivation to act on the results.[22] The low sensitivity of screening tools can generate false-positive diagnoses, resulting in inappropriate negative self-perceptions and inappropriate health service referrals and can potentially impact on employment outcomes. The first randomized controlled trial of psychological health screening in an organizational context failed to identify any evidence of a positive impact.[41]

An individual's friends and family may be the first to notice changes in character or symptoms of distress. They too are unlikely to let employers know of their concerns, unless they know how to and are confident that disclosure will not have an adverse work outcome. Family/employer liaison may therefore be a helpful mechanism to facilitate secondary prevention.

The secondary prevention stage is also critical from an employment law perspective. Once an employee is known to the employer to have a mental ill health condition, or even predisposing conditions, the issue of foreseeability of potential harm arises. By law, an employer may have to make reasonable adjustments for, and cannot unreasonably discriminate against, the employee (see Chapter 3).[42]

Reasonable adjustments including changes in working hours, responsibilities, or even work location and team may be required under the Equality Act 2010.[43] This is a two-way responsibility. Reasonable adjustments can only be made if the condition is known to the employer.[44]

Tertiary prevention

Tertiary prevention refers to the provision of rapid and effective treatment for those with mental health disorders. Identifying when medical intervention is indicated may be less of a problem for SMIs such as schizophrenia and bipolar disorder than is the case for CMDs. However, any behaviour that employers suspect as causing difficulty at work should be investigated. Prodromal individuals may resign or see contracts of employment terminated. This social drift (progressive loss of status, finances, and lifestyle) often precedes the onset of a serious mental health problem.

Ideally, effective treatment is instigated before social drift has occurred or before its progression is advanced. Although, the National Health Service (NHS) provides a wide range of treatment for mental health conditions, most specialist provision is targeted towards serious disorders. Poor access is an important issue for the much more prevalent CMDs. Average waiting times for mental health treatment can differ as much as 12 weeks across England.[4] NICE has issued a variety of guidelines for managing mental health conditions including depression, obsessive–compulsive disorder, PTSD, and recently CMDs (see 'Useful websites').

Specialist mental healthcare delivery is often consultant led and multidisciplinary. Initial assessments are 'holistic' to consider the presenting complaint and the wider psychosocial factors. In some cases, physical health complaints may directly cause mental health disorders (e.g. acute confusional state from hypoxia during a severe chest infection) but often causation is multifactorial. Importantly, where workplace relationships between colleagues or line managers are relevant, failure to resolve problems may prevent or delay return to work.

Mental healthcare, especially for CMDs, is likely to involve some psychotherapy or 'talking' treatments. 'Classic' (or Freudian) psychotherapy may take many months or years. However, most modern healthcare utilizes short-term psychological interventions often involving variants of CBT, which has considerable evidence of effectiveness in a wide range of conditions. Other time-limited, evidence-based therapies include interpersonal therapy and behavioural activation for depression or eye movement desensitization and reprocessing for PTSD. At the initial assessment, the most suitable therapeutic approach can be agreed with each patient. Establishing a 'therapeutic alliance' is important to almost all psychotherapeutic interventions. If a patient cannot trust, confide in, and work with their therapist after a few sessions, it is usually best to seek an alternative therapist. Non-complex disorders usually require 6–12, weekly, 1-hour sessions. However, complex cases may need considerably more sessions. An independent mental health specialist may periodically monitor therapeutic progress, since the therapist may find it difficult to make impartial occupational recommendations while balancing a sustained therapeutic alliance with the patient. The clear role of OH in advising about fitness for work can importantly protect the practitioner–patient relationship.

Over recent years, since the *Hatton* v. *Sutherland* ruling[45] supported their use, employee assistance programmes (EAPs) have grown in popularity. They provide confidential counselling services to employees (and in some case their families). Most EAPs provide only a limited number of sessions and evidence suggests that most access EAPs with non-work issues. There is a lack of evidence that EAPs improve the mental health or well-being of employees or improve organization effectiveness. However, it is possible that some are more effective than others.

In general, OH professionals should recommend evidence-based therapies such as those recommended by NICE. However, provided justification is clear and on the advice of a suitably experienced mental health consultant, other therapeutic techniques may be deemed appropriate. Ineffective therapy can waste scarce resources, render patients feeling untreatable, or deter them from seeking effective care.

How might mental health problems interfere with work?

Diagnostic labels do little alone to assist OH professionals in making fitness for work decisions. The mentally unwell, like all people, have individual strengths and weaknesses, so a thorough appraisal of abilities, deficits, and functional capacity should be integral to any occupational assessment. Excluding an individual on the basis of diagnostic labels is discriminatory and excludes potential talent from the workplace. Nevertheless, a diagnosis may focus a management plan and help clinicians make firm prognostic statements relevant to longer-term occupational fitness or eligibility for a disability pension.

An 'illness' model can be highly useful within acute psychiatric environments and in planning mental health service provision. But in the occupational environment, a 'disability' model, focusing on enduring problems, strengths, and weaknesses, is more appropriate. This approach informs the adjustments to enable early return to work, rather than simply waiting to 'get better'.

The social model of disability is consonant with government policy, and helps establish a joint understanding of problems that an individual with impaired mental health might experience. The model facilitates a consistent approach from the individual, their line manager, and medical advisers. This is important because the Equality Act 2010[43] focuses on preventing the discrimination and social exclusion that many mental health service users perceive to exist. Keeping the mentally unwell working will provide both the best opportunity for them to recover a social role and status and ensure that organizations meet their moral and legal obligations.

Psychiatric disorders may impair one or more domains of psychological or social functioning and it is important to assess these inclusively.

Impaired concentration and attention

Mental illnesses may significantly impair concentration and attention as a result of distractibility and preoccupying worries or rumination. More serious conditions such as hypomania and severe depression can alter thought processes. Malnourishment associated with eating disorders can also affective cognitive function. Many psychotropic drugs used in the treatment of these disorders are associated with marked behavioural effects (e.g. reduced concentration and attention span). Simple clinical tests of concentration and attention such as 'serial sevens' are crude indicators of actual performance and concentration. Some work roles require careful attention to cognitive function, and attentional deficits are best assessed using '*in vivo*' tasks that resemble those required in the workplace. This is especially important for people who work in safety-critical tasks such as professional drivers, those working at heights, or many healthcare professionals.

Impaired motor skills

Abnormal involuntary movements as well as a paucity of movement may hamper work performance. Psychomotor slowing is seen in many depressive disorders and the tremor associated with anxiety may impair skilled motor tasks, or increase self-consciousness especially in social situations such as meetings. Movement disorders can be a feature of conditions such as schizophrenia. These are both disfiguring and disturbing to others, making individuals more isolated and less integrated into their working environment.

Antipsychotic drugs including many of the newer atypical agents may produce marked extrapyramidal symptoms, which themselves may become a cause of significant disability.

Impaired communication and social skills

The ability to communicate effectively and form positive relationships with colleagues is one of the most important predictors of success at work. Many people with severe and enduring mental health problems work in isolated or low-paid manual roles, where relationships with co-workers are less impactful. Poor communication may be due to the illness itself, for example, the lack of self-confidence associated with depression, or paranoid thinking with schizophrenia, other psychoses, and personality disorders. Conversely, many of those who are mentally ill may simply lack practice and the opportunity to maintain and refine normal social skills and can do surprisingly well if they are gradually challenged.

Risk to self and others

A risk assessment is now an integral and explicit part of any psychiatric examination and a written statement regarding risk should form the outcome of all such examinations. Often the severity of the risks to self and others is couched in rather vague terms (low, moderate, or high), which may not enable employers to effectively manage risks. While the risk of self-harm and suicide is increased in those who are clinically depressed, many episodes of self-harm and/or violence do not result from formal mental health disorders. Alcohol misuse and impulsive personality traits also increase the risks of such behaviours. There is no substantive evidence supporting the use of suicide risk assessment tools in predicting who might go on to die by suicide.[46]

Higher risks of suicide are seen in certain occupations such as veterinary medicine and farming due in part to the ready availability of lethal means and knowledge as well as isolated, yet demanding and stressful working environments.

However, the risk to others associated with mental illness is overstated and grossly exaggerated by the media. The mentally ill are far more likely to harm themselves than others. The risk of a homicide conviction in mental health patients is largely related to coexisting substance misuse.[47] Nevertheless, OH professionals have a duty to reassure employers and expect a clear and unequivocal assessment of risk from the psychiatric team.

The effects of abnormal illness behaviour

Motivation, commitment, and willingness to work are perhaps the best predictors of success or otherwise in the workplace, irrespective of any psychiatric diagnosis. Many individuals with significant psychopathology are punctual, reliable, and hardworking employees, fit for their work, and show no signs of the underlying significant disorder. Indeed, some mental health conditions may actually be associated with especially high levels of conscientiousness and people with highly obsessional personalities may be well-suited to tasks that require attention to detail. Conversely, others with a similar disorder but with a lesser degree of symptomatology may be profoundly handicapped and incapable of work. It may be difficult at times for OH professionals to decide what proportion of poor working practice is attributable to illness and what relates to poor motivation or commitment. In the main, most mental health conditions should not be regarded as providing an excuse for poor behaviour but neither should their effects upon motivation and aptitude be ignored.

Fit for work? Assessment for employment

As well as a robust clinical assessment, a comprehensive occupational assessment has three key ingredients: an appreciation of the individual and their strengths and weaknesses; the nature of the workplace and demands of the job; and the desired outcome for both individual and employer. Individual factors to be considered include past employment history, skills, and work performance, and individual factors including motivation, confidence, and personal aspirations. Finally, the workplace itself should be considered in terms of the expectations of peers and managers, opportunities for supervision, training, and development and links to other employee development programmes.

Assessment requires skill and experience and can be an important intervention in its own right. The dichotomy between illness and disability models has already been described. In practice, this means that psychiatric reports alone are often unhelpful to OH professionals and fail to provide the necessary information to determine employability in a given work environment. Limitations in their content may also reflect efforts to protect patient confidentiality and maintain a strong therapeutic relationship.

Tests of intelligence, temperament, or aptitude have very poor predictive validity. Personal objectives, motivation, and confidence, however, are better predictors. Past behaviour is often the best predictor of future performance and detailed work histories combined with a secure understanding of job requirements give a good indication of an individual's employability. Getting a job can in itself be a powerful motivating factor, particularly for individuals who have been repeatedly unsuccessful, so it is important not to exclude apparently unmotivated individuals from employment opportunities.

While standardized psychological health measurement tools, such as the PHQ9 (patient health questionnaire) or GAD7 (generalized anxiety disorder assessment) may be used to aid clinical decision-making, they should not be relied upon to provide a diagnosis. Such scales are not validated diagnostic tools in the OH setting, and answers may be easily provided to achieve a patient's desired outcome either exaggerating or masking symptoms. Such scales may be useful in OH practice to measure change over time in patients receiving treatment for mental health problems.

Fitness for specific work

Notwithstanding an overall enabling approach, it should be acknowledged that there are circumstances in which caution in job placement should be exercised. For example, fitness assessment must consider the risk to the public, third parties, and personal safety in safety-critical jobs (e.g. airline pilots, train drivers, lorry drivers, fire fighters, electricians, and engineers employed by railway companies). In the NHS, the issue of pre-placement screening of nurses for psychiatric illness has been raised following patient deaths in spite of a lack of evidence that such an approach would improve patient outcomes. Where a pre-placement process is put in place, recent case law emphasizes the importance of specificity when defining pre-placement questions (see Chapter 2).

The General Medical Council (GMC) has similar concerns about mental illness and poor performance in doctors. Questions of fitness to practice should be asked in the early phases of treatment for florid psychoses, etc. and blanket judgements resisted, provided that no legal considerations apply. The GMC has also published guidance regarding mental ill health in medical students (see 'Useful websites'). Studies suggest that many medical students show signs of distress (often referred to as burnout) although it is not clear whether these symptoms are generically common among students on high-pressure university courses (e.g. law and veterinary science) or are more specific to medical students.[48]

An increasing focus on safeguarding children (up to 18 years) and vulnerable groups has highlighted the duty of OH professionals in assessing individuals with mental health problems. When the clients of OH services work in the area of safeguarding (e.g. the police services, health services, social care, and education) and OH professionals are called upon to assess fitness for work, their duty of care extends beyond the individual to children in their care. Specific guidance on their responsibilities and the limits of patient confidentiality has been produced by the Faculty of Occupational Medicine and the Royal College of Paediatrics and Child Health.[49]

Recovery and return to work

People who have had a period of (often lengthy) sick leave for mental health problems face a number of difficulties as they consider returning to work. An effective OH service can do much to maximize the likelihood of a successful outcome. Firstly, it should establish from the mental health team the likelihood and rate of return to pre-morbid functioning. Secondly, it should establish with local management the scope for flexibility in the duration and nature of work to rebuild confidence and reacclimatize the individual to a work routine. A detailed evaluation of the extent that the demands of the job itself may have contributed to the development of mental health problems is helpful, as is making a decision as to whether it is either safe or appropriate for the individual to return to their former job and working environment.

The Equality Act 2010[43] requires that 'reasonable adjustments' are made where an individual's health needs to be taken into consideration. When work-related stress underlies the absence, the HSE's 'Return to work' questionnaire can be used with the patient and the manager to establish relevant work stressors and opportunities for reasonable adjustment.[50] These may include phased return to work and modifications to the nature, duration, and complexity of tasks. The OH professional has an important role in advising on the monitoring of effectiveness of such recommendations clinically and operationally by manager and employee.

On occasions, employees may blame the organization, the system of working, or their manager for their health problem. This may be especially so for a stress-related absence, resulting in anxiety and/or depression. OH professionals may be able to help managers understand the benefits of discussing with the employee the reasons for absence and what will help ensure a successful return to work. On occasions, a different job or relocation may be a sensible solution.

Work schemes and sheltered employment

A variety of schemes are provided by both the statutory and voluntary sector to help re-introduce mental health service users to the workplace. However, there is little evidence of effectiveness. Statutory and voluntary sector employment schemes designed to return service users to the labour market will have limited effectiveness unless employers are more incentivized to recognize proactively the special needs of this group and do more to accommodate them within the workplace.

For those with more serious mental health problems or those never before employed, a variety of schemes exist that intend to ease the transition into the workplace. Sheltered employment and occupational rehabilitation are not new concepts. However, with the advent of community care, and the closure of large psychiatric or mental hospitals, the provision of employment schemes in community settings are increasingly provided by the voluntary sector. These may be haphazard and patchy, both geographically and in terms of quality and meeting local need. One of the few surveys conducted has shown a 40-fold variation in provision across health authority areas with the highest levels of provision generally found in the most affluent areas.[51] Across the UK, more than 130 different organizations offer some form of sheltered employment, including 77 providing open employment and with approximately 50 set up as 'social firms'.[52,53]

Models

A variety of models exist to facilitate a return to work. Sheltered workshops and employment support schemes (e.g. Remploy) offer work in a safe environment and occupations for those who would otherwise be unable to cope with the demands of open employment. Very few individuals in these schemes, however, move into the open employment market. These organizations often experience difficulty in maintaining profitability, putting their viability at risk. A more recent variant of sheltered employment is the 'social firm'. This is a commercial enterprise business with mental health service users employed throughout the organization. Social firms are not primarily engaged in rehabilitation and employees are paid the going rate for their work. Another variation, seen more commonly in Europe, is the 'social enterprise', a semi-commercial concern that also provides training and rehabilitation.

Pre-vocational training enables a period of preparatory training and a gradual reintro-duction to the workplace with the expectation of moving into the open employment market: 'train and place'. Tailored to individual need, this may include specific skills training, a period in a sheltered work environment, or in a job that is ring-fenced and sponsored by a rehabilitation agency.

'Supported employment' aims to place individuals directly into the workplace without lengthy preparation or training ('place and train'). Service users are expected to obtain work directly in the open employment market; they are hired competitively and employed on the same basis as other employees, with full company benefits, but with supervision and mentoring to maximize the likelihood of a successful outcome.[17] Assessment is on the job and support is continued as required. Perhaps this, more than any other model, most effectively bridges the gap between mental health services and the employment community. This approach is epitomized by the highly successful 'individual placement and support' for which there is excellent evidence of effectiveness.

Wellness recovery action planning

Wellness recovery action plans (WRAPs) are recovery-focused programmes which aim to improve the quality of life for people suffering with severe mental health conditions (e.g. psychotic illnesses).[54] Two randomized controlled trials of wellness recovery action planning, carried out in the US, found modestly positive impacts on quality of life and mental health symptoms in participants receiving WRAPs compared to either a neutral no active intervention. Developing a WRAP usually involves either a therapist or peers who have experienced mental health problems themselves. The plan, once developed, is owned by the patient and comprises self-help strategies to improve their ability to take responsibility for their own wellness and manage their symptoms.

Wellness recovery action planning is described as being 'values based' and is underpinned by five key concepts: hope, learning, self-advocacy, personal responsibility, and support networks. WRAPs are being used in some parts of the NHS as part of the recovery approach to mental healthcare. They may have some utility in helping people with more severe mental health difficulties stay at, or return to, work after experiencing an initial presentation or relapse of their mental health problems.

User employment programmes

Many NHS trusts now employ current or former (health) service users in jobs that demand a history of mental health problems as part of the personal specification for the post. Terms and conditions of service are identical to other employees and additional support is available as required. Many such posts involve patient advocacy and thus make use of the insight and personal experiences of former service users. Service users are increasingly employed in major service development roles such as National Service Framework Local Implementation Teams and increasingly serve as members of senior medical staff appointments advisory committees. Indeed, service user involvement has become a key performance indicator for all mental health trusts. This active participation of service users in high-profile positions of obvious importance within the NHS is of immense symbolic value, challenging stigma, prejudice, and the widely held poor expectations about the employability of mentally ill people in positions of responsibility in the workplace.[55]

Key points

- CMDs are among the most frequent ailments to affect employees and their performance at work.
- All employers should have plans in place to optimize the well-being of their employees and to manage mental health conditions as they arise.
- The OH professional has a significant role to play in primary, secondary, and tertiary interventions to prevent or minimize the impacts of mental health conditions in workplace settings:
  - Primary: have the risks to mental health from the context and content of work been assessed and addressed?
  - Secondary: are employees and their managers equipped to recognize the early signs of mental ill health at work, mentor them, and guide their employees in the direction of support?
  - Tertiary: are processes in place to accommodate those returning to the workplace after mental health problems, and are co-workers and managers equipped to receive them?
- Many mental health conditions are treatable and recovery is to be expected. While relapses may well occur at times of increased stress, early identification of signature patterns of symptoms may enable continued function within the workplace.

Useful websites

Business in the community (BITC)	https://wellbeing.bitc.org.uk/all-resources
Acas. 'Mental health in the workplace'	http://www.acas.org.uk/index.aspx?articleid=1900
MIND. 'Mental health at work'	https://www.mind.org.uk/workplace/mental-health-at-work/
Royal College of Psychiatrists (RCPsych). 'Work and mental health'	http://www.rcpsych.ac.uk/usefulresources/workandmentalhealth.aspx
RCPsych. Guide to personality disorders, 2011	http://www.rcpsych.ac.uk/healthadvice/problemsanddisorders/personalitydisorder.aspx
National Institute for Health and Care Excellence (NICE)	https://www.nice.org.uk/guidance/ph22/resources/mental-wellbeing-at-work-pdf-1996233648325

General Medical Council (GMC). Supporting medical students with mental health conditions	https://www.gmc-uk.org/education/undergraduate/23289.asp
Living Life to the Full	www.livinglifetothefull.com
Beating the Blues	http://www.beatingtheblues.co.uk/

References

1. **McManus S, Bebbington P, Jenkins R, Brugha T.** Adult Psychiatric Morbidity Survey: Survey of Mental Health and Wellbeing, England, 2014. NHS Digital; 2016. Available at: http://digital.nhs.uk/catalogue/PUB21748.
2. **OECD Publishing**. *Mental Health and Work: United Kingdom.* Paris: OECD; 2014. Available at: http://dx.doi.org/10.1787/9789264204997-en.
3. **Davies SC.** *Annual Report of the Chief Medical Officer 2013, Public Mental Health Priorities: Investing in the Evidence.* London: Department of Health; 2014. Available at: https://www.gov.uk/government/organisations/department-of-health.
4. **Department for Work and Pensions, Department of Health**. Work, Health and Disability Green Paper Data Pack. 2017. Available at: https://www.gov.uk/government/consultations/work-health-and-disability-improving-lives/work-health-and-disability-green-paper-improving-lives#fn:10.
5. **Waddell G, Burton AK.** *Is Work Good for Your Health and Well-Being?* London: The Stationery Office; 2006.
6. **Warr P.** *Work, Unemployment, and Mental Health.* Oxford: Oxford University Press; 1987.
7. **McManus S, Mowlam A, Stansfield S, Clark C, Brown V, Al E.** *Mental Health in Context: The National Study of Work-Search and Wellbeing.* London: Department for Work and Pensions; 2012.
8. **Bartley M.** Unemployment and ill health: understanding the relationship. *J Epidemiol Community Health* 1994;**48**:333–7.
9. **McManus S, Bebbington P, Jenkins R, Brugha T.** *Mental Health and Wellbeing in England: Adult Psychiatric Morbidity Study 2014.* Leeds: NHS Digital; 2016.
10. **Lelliott P, Tulloch S, Boardman J, Harvey S, Henderson M, Knapp M.** *Mental Health and Work.* London: Royal College of Psychiatrists; 2008.
11. **Marwaha S, Johnson S, Bebbington P, et al.** Rates and correlates of employment in people with schizophrenia in the UK, France and Germany. *Br J Psychiatry* 2007;**191**:30–7.
12. **Meltzer H, Singleton N, Lee A, Bebbington P, Brugha T, Jenkins R.** *The Social and Economic Circumstances of Adults with Mental Disorders.* London: Department of Health; 2002.
13. **Office of National Statistics.** Sickness absence in the UK labour market 2016. 2017. Available at: https://www.ons.gov.uk/employmentandlabourmarket/peopleinwork/labourproductivity/articles/sicknessabsenceinthelabourmarket/2016.
14. **Primary Care Domain, NHS Digital.** Fit notes issued by GP Practices. 2017. Available at: https://app.powerbi.com/view?r=eyJrIjoiYTRmMWViOWMtN2VjMC00ZTc5LWEzZmYtZGVjMzNjYzQ2NjEwIiwidCI6IjgwN2YzMwLWNhOGMtNDE5Zi1hMTc5LTVjNGZjN2E0YmY2YiIsImMiOjN9.
15. **Centre for Mental Health.** The economic and social costs of mental health problems in 2009/10. 2010. Available at: http://www.centreformentalhealth.org.uk/economic-and-social-costs-2009.
16. **Chu AHY, Koh D, Moy FM, Müller-Riemenschneider F.** Do workplace physical activity interventions improve mental health outcomes? *Occup Med* 2014;**64**:235–45.
17. **Becker D, Drake R.** Individual placement and support: a community mental health center approach to vocational rehabilitation. *Community Ment Health J* 1994;**30**:207–12.

18. **National Institute for Health and Care Excellence (NICE).** *Post-Traumatic Stress Disorder (PTSD): The Treatment of PTSD in Adults and Children.* Clinical guideline [CG26] London: NICE; 2005.

19. **Greenberg N, Langston V, Everitt B, et al.** A cluster randomized controlled trial to determine the efficacy of trauma risk management (TRiM) in a military population. *J Trauma Stress* 2010;**23**:430–6.

20. **Mulligan K, Fear NT, Jones N, Wessely S, Greenberg N.** Psycho-educational interventions designed to prevent deployment-related psychological ill-health in Armed Forces personnel: a review. *Psychol Med* 2011;**41**:673–86.

21. **Rona RJ, Hooper R, Jones M, et al.** Mental health screening in armed forces before the Iraq war and prevention of subsequent psychological morbidity: follow-up study. *Br Med J* 2006;**333**:991–4.

22. **Raffle A, Muir Gray J.** *Screening: Evidence and Practice.* Oxford: Oxford University Press; 2007.

23. **Jones N, Seddon R, Fear N, McAllister P, Wesseley S, Greenberg N.** Leadership, cohesion, morale, and the mental health of UK Armed Forces in Afghanistan. *Psychiatry* 2012;**75**:49–59.

24. **Mausner-Dorsch H, Eaton WW.** Psychosocial work environment and depression: epidemiologic assessment of the demand-control model. *Am J Public Health* 2000;**90**:1765–70.

25. **Health and Safety Executive.** Working together to reduce stress at work. A guide for employees. 2008. Available at: http://www.hse.gov.uk/pubns/indg424.pdf.

26. **Kouvonen A, Kivimäki M, Virtanen M, et al.** Effort-reward imbalance at work and the co-occurrence of lifestyle risk factors: cross-sectional survey in a sample of 36,127 public sector employees. *BMC Public Health* 2006;**6**:24.

27. **Mehta N, Clement S, Marcus E, et al.** Evidence for effective interventions to reduce mental health-related stigma and discrimination in the medium and long term: systematic review. *Br J Psychiatry* 2015;**207**:377–84.

28. **Robertson IT, Cooper CL, Sarkar M, Curran T.** Resilience training in the workplace from 2003 to 2014: a systematic review. *J Occup Organ Psychol* 2015;**88**:533–62.

29. **Iversen AC, Fear NT, Ehlers A, et al.** Risk factors for post-traumatic stress disorder among UK Armed Forces personnel. *Psychol Med* 2008;**38**:511–22.

30. **Mulligan K, Jones N, Woodhead C, Davies M, Wessely S, Greenberg N.** Mental health of UK military personnel while on deployment in Iraq. *Br J Psychiatry* 2010;**197**:405–10.

31. **Querstret D, Cropley M, Kruger P, Heron R.** Assessing the effect of a cognitive behaviour therapy (CBT)-based workshop on work-related rumination, fatigue, and sleep. *Eur J Work Organ Psychol* 2016;**25**:50–67.

32. **Wongtongkam N, Krivokapic-Skoko B, Duncan R, Bellio M.** The influence of a mindfulness-based intervention on job satisfaction and work-related stress and anxiety. *Int J Ment Health* 2017;**19**:134–43.

33. **Heron RJL, McKeown S, Tomenson JA, Teasdale EL.** Study to evaluate the effectiveness of stress management workshops on response to general and occupational measures of stress. *Occup Med* 1999;**49**:451–7.

34. **Osório C, Jones N, Fertout M, Greenberg N.** Changes in Stigma and barriers to care over time in U.K. Armed forces deployed to Afghanistan and Iraq between 2008 and 2011. *Mil Med* 2013;**178**:846–53.

35. **Woodhead C, Rona R, Iversen AC, et al.** Mental health and health service use among post-national service veterans: results from the 2007 Adult Psychiatric Morbidity Survey of England. *Psychol Med* 2010;**41**:363–72.

36. **Henderson C, Robinson E, Evans-Lacko S, et al.** Public knowledge, attitudes, social distance and reported contact regarding people with mental illness 2009–2015. *Acta Psychiatr Scand* 2016;**134**:23–33.

37. **Wang JL.** Perceived barriers to mental health service use among individuals with mental disorders in the Canadian general population. *Med Care* 2006;**44**:192–5.

38. **Levenson R, Dwyer L.** Peer support in law enforcement: past, present, and future. *Int J Emerg Ment Health* 2003;**5**:147–52.

39. **Greenberg N.** Managing traumatic stress at work. An organisational approach to the management of potentially traumatic events. *Occup Health Work* 2011;**7**:22–6.

40. **Greenberg N, Langston V, Iversen AC, Wessely S.** The acceptability of 'trauma risk management' within the UK armed forces. *Occup Med* 2011;**61**:184–9.

41. **Rona RJ, Burdett H, Khondoker M, et al.** Post-deployment screening for mental disorders and tailored advice about help-seeking in the UK military: a cluster randomised controlled trial. *Lancet* 2018;**389**:1410–23.

42. *Dickins v. O2 Plc* [2008]. EWCA Civ 1144 CA.

43. *Equality Act 2010.* Available at: http://www.legislation.gov.uk/ukpga/2010/15/contents.

44. *Wilcox v. Birmingham CAB Services Ltd.* [2011]. UKEAT 0293/10/2306.

45. *Hatton v. Sutherland* [2002]. EWCA Civ 76.

46. **Bolton JM, Gunnell D, Turecki G.** Suicide risk assessment and intervention in people with mental illness. *BMJ* 2015;**351**:h4978.

47. **Appleby L, Kapur N, Shaw J, et al.** *National Confidential Inquiry into Suicide and Homicide.* Manchester: University of Manchester; 2017. Available at: http://research.bmh.manchester.ac.uk/cmhs/centreforsuicideprevention/nci/reports/NCIAnnualReport2013V2.pdf.

48. **Dyrbye L, Shanafelt T.** A narrative review on burnout experienced by medical students and residents. *Med Educ* 2016;**50**:132–49.

49. **Smedley J, Steele A.** *Safeguarding Children: Guidelines for Occupational Health Professionals.* London: Faculty of Occupational Medicine; 2014. Available at: http://www.fom.ac.uk/wp-content/uploads/FOM-RCPCH-Safeguarding-Children-Guidelines-for-OHPs.pdf.

50. **Health and Safety Executive.** Return to work questionnaire. Available at: http://www.hse.gov.uk/stress/assets/docs/returntowork.pdf.

51. **Crowther RE, Marshall M.** Employment rehabilitation schemes for people with mental health problems in the North West region: service characteristics and utilisation. *J Ment Health* 2001;**10**:373–81.

52. **Grove B, Drurie S.** *Social Firms: An Instrument for Economic Improvement and Inclusion.* Red Hill: Social Firms UK; 1999.

53. **Crowther RE, Marshall M, Bond G, Huxley P.** Helping people with severe mental illness to obtain work: systematic review. *BMJ* 2001;**322**:204–8.

54. **Ashman M, Halliday V, Cunnane JG.** Qualitative investigation of the wellness recovery action plan in a UK NHS crisis care setting. *Issues Ment Health Nurs* 2017;**38**:570–7.

55. **Perkins R, Buckfield R, Choy D.** Access to employment: a supported employment project to enable mental health service users to obtain jobs within mental health teams. *J Ment Health* 1997;**6**:307–18.

Chapter 20

Musculoskeletal conditions, part 1: rheumatological disorders

Syed Nasir and Karen Walker-Bone

Introduction

Musculoskeletal pain affects up to 50% of the population at any one time. Consequently, low back pain, neck pain, and upper limb disorders are important causes of sickness absence. This chapter will focus on the common systemic rheumatological disorders, including osteoarthritis (OA), inflammatory arthritis, connective tissue disorders, and widespread pain syndromes. Spinal disorders, including back pain, are covered in detail in Chapter 21. Musculoskeletal disorders that affect specific anatomical sites (including upper limb disorders, both specific and non-specific) are covered in Chapter 22.

Many rheumatological conditions are long-term conditions and potentially disabling but there have been recent developments in medical therapies, especially in the inflammatory rheumatic conditions, which offer the prospect of controlling disease activity, reducing disability, improving quality of life, and enabling work.

Osteoarthritis

OA is the commonest form of arthritis, affecting at least 8 million people in the UK according to Arthritis Research UK (see 'Useful websites'). When the prevalence of OA is measured using radiological changes, one estimate has suggested that 80% of the population have OA after the age of 55 years.

The main affected joints are the knees, hips, hands, spine, and, less often, the feet. OA is a metabolically active, dynamic process involving all joint tissues (cartilage, bone, synovium, capsule, and ligaments/muscles), responding to injury which causes focal failure of articular cartilage. Damage of the articular cartilage triggers remodelling of adjacent bone and a hypertrophic reaction at joint margins, recognized radiographically as osteophytes. This remodelling and repair is efficient but slow and while it takes place, secondary synovial inflammation and crystal deposition can occur. Clinically, the patient experiences pain and stiffness in affected joint(s) with acute episodes of heat, redness, and swelling during secondary inflammatory phases. Longer term, the joint develops permanent structural change leading to functional limitation and disability.

Risk factors for osteoarthritis

OA affects women more than men and is more common with older age, although it is not uncommon in people of working age. Genetic factors are important, as is obesity. Weight bearing predisposes to hip and knee OA. Joint injury, recreational or occupational usage, joint laxity, reduced muscle strength, and joint malalignment are all established risk factors. There are also several medical conditions which predispose to secondary OA including congenital/developmental diseases, inflammatory joint diseases (e.g. rheumatoid arthritis (RA)), endocrinopathies (e.g. acromegaly), metabolic disorders (e.g. ochronosis), neuropathic disorders (e.g. diabetes), and disorders of bone (e.g. Paget's disease).

Occupational risk factors for osteoarthritis

Occupations which entail repetitive use of particular joints over long periods of time have been associated with the development of site-specific OA.[1] Thus, dockers and shipyard labourers have an excess of hand and knee OA; miners have an excess of knee and lumbar spine disease; cotton and mill workers develop an excess of hand OA at particular finger joints; workers using pneumatic drills have an excess of elbow and wrist OA; floor and carpet layers are more affected by knee OA; and farmers have more hip OA. The important exposures for lower limb OA are kneeling posture, jumping, climbing flights of stairs, and heavy lifting.[2]

Assessment of osteoarthritis

The course of OA varies considerably depending upon cause and the distribution of joints affected. Since OA is essentially a process of repair and regeneration, it can ultimately limit the damage and symptoms in most cases, but rates of progression and symptom severity vary by site (e.g. hand OA generally has a good prognosis except in the first carpometacarpal joints). Once knee OA has started, structural changes rarely reverse, but pain and disability can improve markedly. It has been estimated that, over time, one-third of knee OA patients will improve, one-third will stay the same, and one-third will worsen. The prognosis of hip OA has been less well studied but there is evidence that it generally progresses more than knee OA and that over 5 years, a significant proportion of patients require hip surgery.

Most patients with OA consult because of pain but the correlation between pain, disability, and structural changes can be poor, especially early in the disease course. The correlation improves with increasing severity of the structural changes. Within individuals there is an influence of personality, mood, occupation, psychosocial environment, and expectations, both on pain and response to treatment. The National Institute for Health and Care Excellence (NICE) guidance for managing OA recommends that the initial assessment should encompass a holistic approach[3]:

◆ *The patient's thoughts*: what are their concerns and expectations? What do they know about OA?

- *The patient's support network*: is the patient isolated or do they have a carer? If there is a carer, how are they coping and what are their concerns and expectations?
- *The patient's mood*: screen for depression and stresses
- *The patient's attitude to exercise.*
- *The impact of OA on*: occupation, activities of daily living, family responsibilities, hobbies, lifestyle, and sleep.
- *Pain assessment*: what self-help strategies are they using? Are they taking medicines? At what doses, how often, any side effects?
- *Other musculoskeletal pain*: could this be a chronic pain syndrome? Are there other treatable sources of pain (e.g. bursitis, trigger digit, or ganglion)?
- *Co-morbidities*: are there other medical problems? What impact might co-morbidities have on treatment options?

Management of osteoarthritis

Given the variable rate of disease progression, it is always appropriate to take a positive approach at presentation. The patient should be disabused of any view that OA universally worsens over time. Initial approaches focus on education, exercise, and self-management (Figure 20.1).[3] Exercise has two main aims: local muscle strengthening and general aerobic fitness. Patients should be advised about the importance of weight loss, which has been shown to reverse large joint progression. Education, given in one-to-one and group contacts, written or IT delivered, is an important treatment modality. The emphasis should be on a positive approach, exercise, simple measures such as shock absorbing footwear, heat and ice packs, and the importance of weight reduction. Although popular, there is no convincing evidence that glucosamine or chondroitin products are beneficial in OA and the NICE guidance for OA recommends that they should not be prescribed.[3]

Treatment approaches should commence at the centre of Figure 20.1 with education and exercise approaches and move outwards as required and appropriate when symptom control is poor.

Management of osteoarthritis in the workplace

Not only do occupational factors contribute to the causation of OA, but people with OA may experience difficulties performing work,[2] decreased productivity, sickness absence, work disability, and early retirement. The Department for Work and Pensions has estimated that around 36 million working days are lost annually because of OA at a cost of £3.2 billion in lost productivity.[4] As working lives are prolonged and the population prevalence of obesity increases, the costs of OA to employers seem set to grow. Measures to reduce the impact of OA on employees are urgently needed but there is little evidence on exactly what is required.[2] OA features frequently in long-term disability statistics but research rarely considers workplace outcomes, longitudinal data are not available, and

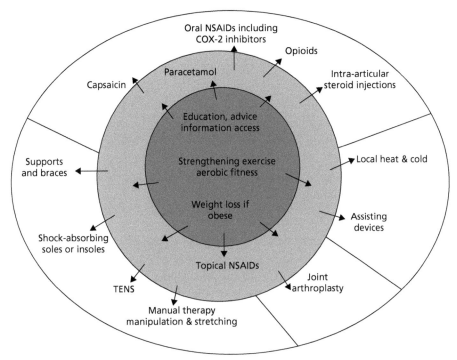

Figure 20.1 An algorithm for targeting treatment of osteoarthritis.

Reproduced from National Institute for Health and Care Excellence (NICE). (2014) *Osteoarthritis: care and management*, Clinical guideline [CG177]. London, UK: NICE. Copyright © 2014 NICE. Available fromnice.org.uk/guidance/cg177. Information accurate at time of publication, for up-to-date information please visit http://www.nice.org.uk.

few studies inform strategies to prevent sickness absence and early retirement.[2] This is a field where major research is needed.

Pragmatically, work that facilitates movement and encourages flexibility of the affected joints, thus avoiding stiffness, is likely to be of benefit—provided the tasks are not too physically onerous. An ergonomic workplace assessment may help in assessing postural strains and giving appropriate guidance. Where hand joints are affected, the provision of writing aids, the use of dictation or voice recognition software, or grasping aids may be helpful. Where knee joint symptoms are prominent, mobility will be restricted and standing should be reduced, together with work activities requiring climbing, walking over rough ground, kneeling, or crouching.

Inflammatory arthritis

There are many different inflammatory arthritides. These share in common an auto-immune basis in which the immune system triggers systemic inflammation of joints. In the absence of a clear understanding of pathophysiology, most of these conditions are distinguished by their clinical features and/or serological abnormalities. However, as understanding develops, new classification criteria are evolving.

Rheumatoid arthritis

RA is the commonest inflammatory arthritis, with a prevalence of 1–2%. It is a symmetrical polyarthritis, particularly involving the hands, wrists, and feet but can involve any joint. Some of its most disabling features are produced by systemic pro-inflammatory cytokines which cause fatigue, malaise, and low energy levels, which many patients report as debilitating, if not more debilitating than the pain. When joints are actively inflamed, they are hot, red, and exquisitely tender. Morning stiffness is a prominent feature, lasting anything from half an hour up until most of the day.

Risk factors for rheumatoid arthritis

RA affects women more than men and has a peak age at onset of 25–50 years, although it can present at any age. Possible independent risk factors for RA include obesity,[5] smoking, and genetic constitution, with the last of these contributing to disease susceptibility and/or severity. The higher rate in women has led to the suspicion that female hormonal factors are important in pathogenesis. In keeping with this, many women experience relative disease remission during pregnancy, but with greater risk of postpartum onset or flareup; nulliparity and breastfeeding seem to be risk factors; and oral contraceptives may be protective.

Occupational risk factors for rheumatoid arthritis

Several occupational exposures have potentially been implicated in the aetiology of RA, including vibration, exposure to mineral dusts, including silica, during mining,[5–7] farming, and exposure to pesticides.[8,9]

Diagnosis of rheumatoid arthritis

Recently, the diagnostic criteria for RA have been reviewed in light of the emergence of new effective treatments, which need to be started as early as possible after diagnosis to control disease activity and prevent joint damage.[10] A scoring algorithm is applied among patients who have at least one joint with definite clinical synovitis (swelling) that cannot be better explained by another disease (Table 20.1). A score of greater than 6 is required to classify the arthritis as RA.

Management of rheumatoid arthritis

Various treatments are available to manage RA, including medication, physiotherapy, occupational therapy, and surgery. Guidance from NICE, updated in 2017, emphasized the importance of rapid referral for early assessment in patients suspected of having inflammatory arthritis.[11] Once diagnosed, patients should be commenced on a combination of disease-modifying antirheumatic drugs (DMARDs), including methotrexate and at least one other DMARD, plus short-term glucocorticoids. The aim is to obtain control of disease activity, as measured by the Disease Activity Score (DAS28). It is well established

Table 20.1 Summary of the 2010 American College of Rheumatology/
European League Against Rheumatism (ACR-EULAR) classification criteria
for rheumatoid arthritis

	Score
A. Joint involvement	
1 large joint	0
2–10 large joints	1
1–3 small joints (with or without large joints)	2
4–10 small joints (with or without large joints)	3
>10 joints (at least 1 small joint)	5
B. Serology (at least 1 test is required)	
Negative RF *and* negative anti-CCP antibodies	0
Low-positive RF *or* low-positive anti-CCP antibodies	2
High-positive RF *or* high-positive anti-CCP antibodies	3
C. Acute-phase reactants (at least 1 test is needed)	
Normal CRP *and* normal ESR	0
Abnormal CRP *or* abnormal ESR	1
D. Duration of symptoms	
<6 weeks	0
≥6 weeks	1

Small joint is finger or thumb joint or wrists
Large joint is elbow, shoulder, hip, knee, ankle

CCP, cyclic citrullinated peptide; CRP, C-reactive protein; ESR, erythrocyte sedimentation
rate; RF, rheumatoid factor.

Adapted from Aletaha D et al., 2010 Rheumatoid arthritis classification criteria:
An American College of Rheumatology/European League Against Rheumatism
collaborative initiative, *Arthritis & Rheumatism*, Vol. 62, No. 9 September 2010,
pp. 2569–81 Copyright © 2010, American College of Rheumatology with permission
from John Wiley & Sons.

that adequate control of disease activity leads to markedly improved outcomes in terms
of joint destruction, function, and disability. Regular monitoring is required until stable
control is achieved, and therapy should be escalated as necessary to achieve this aim.
After at least two DMARDs have been tried (at therapeutic doses and including methotrexate), and in the presence of ongoing active disease (DAS28 score >5.1 on two occasions at least 1 month apart) and the absence of contraindications, patients become
eligible for biological treatment. First-line NICE-approved biologics are the tumour
necrosis factor (TNF)-alpha inhibitors, which are administered by subcutaneous injection weekly (etanercept), fortnightly (adalimumab or certolizumab pegol or abatacept),
monthly (golimumab), or can be given by intravenous infusion (infliximab, abatacept,

tocilizumab). These therapies are usually co-administered with methotrexate and act by lowering levels of circulating pro-inflammatory cytokines which are important to host defences.[12] Treated patients are therefore effectively immunosuppressed. The risk-to-benefit ratio heavily favours use of these therapies, but the occupational health (OH) team should be aware that these patients are at increased risk of infection, particularly upper respiratory tract infection (or reinfection in the case of tuberculosis), and should receive an annual influenza vaccination plus pneumococcal vaccination. In the absence of any specific safety or risk data among workers who are being treated with biological therapies, it is recommended that OH professionals perform a risk assessment based upon their knowledge of an individual's specific job requirements. Importantly, these patients may require antibiotic treatment at a lower threshold than other patients.

Beyond pharmacotherapy, the management of RA is multifaceted and is considerably enhanced by the involvement of a multidisciplinary team including occupational therapists and physiotherapists, podiatric services, and, as appropriate, counsellors, social workers, and pharmacists. NICE emphasizes the role of the specialist nurse in rheumatology in patient advocacy and coordinating case management.[11]

Management of rheumatoid arthritis in the workplace

Work disability is a serious and common outcome for people with RA.[13] Age, disease-related factors, and job characteristics have consistently been risk factors for work disability from RA. However, changes over the past two decades, such as improved pharmaceutical treatment,[14] a possibly milder disease course, increased workforce participation of older workers, and decreased physical demands of jobs may have somewhat reduced work disability. Certainly, more recent studies have suggested changing patterns in the prevalence of work disability.[15] Although rates have so far remained high, at about 35% after 10 years of disease, there are signs of improvement compared with the 50% reported in earlier studies. In one study, work disability was predicted by older age (odds ratio (OR) 1.2; 95% confidence interval (CI) 1.1–1.4) and lower income (OR 1.7; 95% CI 1.0–2.7), was worse among those with greater functional limitation and RA disease activity, but was not significantly associated with occupational hand use or overall job physical demands.[16]

Traditionally, outcomes in RA have been assessed by monitoring radiographic erosions and by functional measures such as the Health Assessment Questionnaire (HAQ). However, more recently, occupational outcomes have been evaluated using the RA Work Instability Score (WIS), a tool with some validity.[17] Using this instrument, intensive occupational therapy intervention has been shown to improve work-related outcomes among employed RA patients at risk of work disability.[18]

With early diagnosis and modern therapy according to NICE guidance,[11] OH professionals should remain positive in their approach to work participation among people with a new diagnosis of RA. There may be short-term work instability while the correct treatment regimen is established but the overall prognosis should be regarded as positive for long-term active working. The OH team should proactively support the employee, working closely with their rheumatologist and other team members, especially occupational therapists. A detailed assessment of permissible work activities, the ergonomic environment, and work station are advisable and may need to be repeated as the disease develops. Significant mechanical strain from force, repetition, or adverse postures may need to be avoided. Indoor work requiring skill, rather than strength, is likely to be better for the individual. Ergonomic adjustments or the provision of handling aids may be helpful. In extreme cases, relocation or retraining for less physically arduous tasks may help an individual to remain at work. Expert advice can be obtained from Access to Work, local disability employment officers, or NHS occupational therapy department on writing aids, electrically operated devices, or specialized hand-held tools.

Patients rate support from their managers and colleagues as important facilitators of continued working, as well as self-acceptance, self-efficacy, and professional advice on coping at work.[19] When considering the recruitment of an individual with established RA, a detailed history of symptoms and physical limitations, and a careful functional assessment are essential. Although employers may be unwilling to recruit an individual with aggressive disease, significant functional limitations, and an uncertain future, they must consider each case in the light of the requirements of the Equality Act 2010. Similarly, the Act is likely to require proactive attempts at reasonable adjustments if disease develops during employment.

Ankylosing spondylitis

The archetypal inflammatory spondyloarthropathy, ankylosing spondylitis, causes inflammatory low back pain frequently presenting in young men; 95% of those affected will carry the human leucocyte antigen (HLA) B27 genotype. The occupational management of this condition is described in Chapter 21. Best practice for its management is available from NICE.[20]

Seronegative arthritides

The seronegative arthritides are a group of clinical conditions which share in common seronegativity for rheumatoid factor and certain clinical, epidemiological, and genetic features—for example, asymmetrical joint involvement, sacroiliac joint involvement, risk of anterior uveitis, variable association with HLA B27, skin involvement (prominent in psoriatic arthritis), mucosal involvement (urethritis, conjunctivitis), enthesitis, and a variable association with bacteria or bacterial products.

Reactive arthritis

In most cases, reactive arthritis is an acute event, triggered by infection with a causative organism. Although patients may present feeling extremely unwell and with several hot, red, inflamed joints, providing the diagnosis is made promptly and appropriate treatment initiated for the causative organism, most cases settle within 6 weeks and the vast majority within 6 months. The prognosis is good and long-term disease-modifying therapy is not required. During the acute phase, the patient may require hospital admission or intensive outpatient management coupled with rest but in the long term, full functional restoration and return to work fitness can be expected.

Psoriatic arthritis

Psoriatic arthritis is a complex clinical entity. Psoriasis is a relatively common skin condition, affecting 2% of the population (see Chapter 28), and among sufferers of skin psoriasis, it has been estimated that between 1% and 42% develop inflammatory arthritis. (The wide variation in these figures is explained by different methodological approaches to estimation in settings that also differ.)

Psoriatic arthritis is equally common in men and women. It can occur at any age but peaks at age 45–54 years. HLA B27 is seen much less frequently among patients with psoriatic arthritis than ankylosing spondylitis, but more commonly than among the general population. HLA B27 tends to differentiate between those who suffer axial as compared with peripheral involvement. Ethnicity, geography, and workplace factors have an uncertain role but there is some evidence for a viral trigger, and patients with HIV and hepatitis C have an increased prevalence of psoriatic arthritis.

The management strategy for psoriatic arthropathy is modelled on that for RA, ankylosing spondylitis, and skin psoriasis. Assessment of disease activity must include assessment of the skin as well as joint involvement and patient-centred outcomes such as joint pain, disability, and function. Only recently have workplace outcomes been evaluated in a few studies of limited methodology.[21] Tillett and colleagues found 'intermediate-quality' evidence that rates of unemployment ranged between 20% and 50% and rates of work disability between 16% and 39% in psoriatic arthritis. Unemployment and work disability were associated with longer disease duration, worse physical function, high joint count, low educational level, female sex, erosive disease, and manual work.[22] There was sparse, low-quality evidence that workplace outcomes were worse in psoriatic arthritis than in psoriasis alone.

Among a young cohort (age 18–45 years) with psoriatic arthritis, Wallenius and colleagues found that 33% of women and 17% of men were receiving a permanent work disability pension.[23] Predictors of work disability were low educational attainment, long duration of disease, age, radiographic erosions, disability, and female sex. In a cohort of patients with psoriatic arthritis randomized to intravenous infusions of the anti-TNF-alpha infliximab or placebo, those receiving infliximab achieved greater productivity, with a trend towards increased employment and reduced sickness absence.[24] In the UK, prior to treatment with biological therapies, 39% of patients with psoriatic arthritis were work disabled (vs 49% of RA patients and 41% of ankylosing spondylitis patients). Prospectively, work disability over 6 months of follow-up was more likely among those with manual jobs and high disability scores.[25]

However, it should be borne in mind that the existing evidence is based upon people diagnosed and managed in the pre-biologic era. The treatment of severe inflammatory spondyloarthropathy and seronegative inflammatory arthritis including psoriatic arthritis is currently evolving as clinical trials demonstrate the effectiveness of the biologics developed for RA in these other diseases.[21] In consequence, functional impairment can be markedly slowed and it is to be expected that better workplace outcomes will soon be measureable. For this reason, OH professionals should take a more positive approach to the long-term work future of people recently diagnosed with these conditions. The biologic therapies are expensive and therefore NICE has restricted their use to all but the most severe cases but patients struggling to work should be advised to inform their rheumatologist as work instability would be an important consideration in recommending these drugs to individuals and requesting funding. As with RA, there may be some work instability while finding the ideal therapy for an individual, but the employer should be advised that the long-term is likely to be positive if they allow their employee to attend all their appointments and monitoring until the best solution is identified. For people with established disease, however, it is difficult for new therapies to 'reverse' functional loss and the needs/capabilities of the worker need to be assessed in relation to their work demands and support arranged as for RA patients.

Connective tissue diseases

There are a number of heterogeneous multisystem 'connective tissue' diseases that share in common systemic inflammation coupled with immune dysregulation. In most cases, the aetiology is poorly understood and therefore they are classified on the basis of clusters of clinical and/or serological features. All of these conditions are relatively uncommon. Systemic lupus erythematosus (SLE), the commonest, has an estimated prevalence of 1/1000 population.

Systemic lupus erythematosus

SLE affects women nine times more often than men, the highest prevalence being in the West Indies and California. It is notable for its diversity of clinical features which may present in a wide spectrum at onset or over the course of the disease. The commonest features are fatigue, malaise, oral ulceration, skin involvement (particularly the characteristic malar butterfly rash), arthralgia or arthritis, pleurisy, and pericarditis. More serious manifestations may occur in the central or peripheral nervous system or in the kidney. Haematological and immunological disorders are frequently observed, anti-double stranded DNA antibodies being the most specific positive immunological abnormality; positive antinuclear antibodies are less specific but more commonly detectable.

Risk factors for SLE

Gender, ethnicity, and genetic factors are the most important risk factors, and twin studies demonstrate a very high rate of concordance among monozygotic as compared with dizygotic twins. Infectious agents have long been implicated in aetiology, especially the Epstein–Barr virus. However, to date, no firm documentation of a viral cause has been shown.

SLE in the workplace

Until recently, there were few data on work outcomes in patients with SLE. In 2009, Baker and Pope undertook a systematic review of the literature and found 26 studies involving over 9500 patients.[26] They estimated a rate of work disability of 20–40% with some 46% of patients in employment. Workplace disability was associated with psychosocial factors and disease factors including age, race, socioeconomic group, educational attainment, activity and duration of the disease, levels of pain, fatigue, anxiety, and neurocognitive function.[26] In a longitudinal study of 394 SLE patients, Yelin et al. found that 51% were in employment at baseline of whom 23% experienced work loss over 4 years of follow-up.[27] Risk factors for job loss included older age, poorer cognitive and physical function, and depression. Over the same 4 years, 20% of the cohort started new work. This was more likely among those with fewer lung manifestations, better physical function, and shorter time since last employment. In younger patients (<55 years), low rates of employment were due to lower rates of starting work rather than higher rates of work loss, but after 55 years, both work loss and lower work entry were important.

Management of SLE

Mild disease often requires simple analgesia, input from the multidisciplinary team, and re-assurance with observation. Moderate to severe disease may require hydroxychloroquine, immunosuppression, and glucocorticoids, sometimes over the long term. Renal and central nervous system involvement needs urgent and aggressive management, often involving intravenous cyclophosphamide, a therapy which can cause significant side effects. If antiphospholipid antibody syndrome is present, treatment with aspirin or anticoagulation with warfarin may be required. However, over recent years, targeted immune therapies have been developed. The anti-B cell therapy (used for lymphoma) rituximab and more recently, belimumab,[28] seems promising in patients with active SLE affecting important organs.

Management of SLE in the workplace

There is little evidence to guide the practitioner beyond general principles. Where the disease is mild, work modifications are unlikely to be required; but in more severe cases, the extreme fatigue may require a change to less onerous, more sedentary, and perhaps paced, work. Work disability is common in SLE. Where possible, attention should be paid to potentially reversible factors which seem to increase work disability, particularly depression. Here, good communication with the rheumatology team and support from nursing staff with knowledge and understanding of the disease is likely to be helpful. Among patients requiring immunosuppressive therapy, employment exposing the individual to infective risk (e.g. hospital work and primary school teaching) may be unsuitable.

Chronic widespread pain and fibromyalgia syndrome

Some 13% of the population will report musculoskeletal pain which is chronic (lasting >3 months) and widespread anatomically. Chronic widespread pain is one of the core features of fibromyalgia syndrome (FMS), a syndrome which causes high levels of morbidity and high attendant costs to healthcare services. It is characterized by widespread pain, tenderness, fatigue, and sleep disturbances, and may overlap with irritable bowel syndrome, tension headaches, and features of the chronic fatigue syndrome.

Since the early 1990s, in order to characterize its epidemiology, risk factors, and the effects of treatment, this widespread pain phenomenon has been called FMS and subject to defined diagnostic criteria.[29] Using these criteria, the prevalence of fibromyalgia has been estimated at between 0.5% and 2.0%.

Risk factors for fibromyalgia syndrome

FMS is more common among women and has a peak age at onset of 30–50 years. It is more common among those of lower educational attainment and its impact is greater in this group. Familial clustering of cases has been observed but it is unclear whether this represents shared environmental or genetic factors. In cross-sectional studies, psychological and psychosocial stressors have been found to be more common among patients with FMS, but it is difficult to distinguish cause from effect with this study design. In a prospective study, patients with high baseline scores for depression without evidence of chronic widespread pain were twice as likely to develop widespread pain at follow-up 7 years later than those without depression.[30] Some but not all studies suggest that patients with FMS are more likely than controls to have a history of childhood physical and sexual abuse. Physical trauma may be a predisposing factor but this has not been evaluated in controlled prospective studies.

Management of fibromyalgia syndrome

A key factor in managing FMS is to recognize and explain it to the patient. Frequently, patients have considerable fear that they may have a major organic illness and need time and careful counselling to be reassured. Practitioners need to take a positive supportive approach as medical interventions have a limited impact in this condition and self-efficacy is vital. Supervised aerobic exercise training,[31] simple analgesics, antidepressants, and pregabalin and gabapentin can, however, improve control of symptoms and physical function. Management should also focus on ameliorating co-morbid complaints such as irritable bowel syndrome. Multidisciplinary rehabilitation is held to be effective although a Cochrane review found only limited data of poor quality to confirm this.[32]

Management of fibromyalgia syndrome in the workplace

The pain and discomfort of FMS are widespread, and FMS patients have significantly poorer health-related quality of life and lower productivity.[33] In one study, FMS patients felt that work needed to be paced so that they could perform their job well and obtain satisfaction while maintaining some energy for their home lives.[34] Support from managers and colleagues was rated as very important. A meta-analysis of four large randomized controlled trials of pregabalin versus placebo in FMS found that effective pain management with pregabalin was associated with reduced sickness absence from 2 days to 0.6 days/week.[35]

Practically, assessment of a patient with FMS should include physical and psychosocial factors, and in particular identify treatable co-morbidities such as depression. Workplace assessment should include exploring the workplace demands and facilitating appropriate pacing and flexibility of work schedule. Questioning the veracity and existence of the syndrome is a counterproductive approach. A positive, empathic approach, with emphasis on what the patient *can* do, is likely to be more rewarding.

Key points

- Musculoskeletal conditions, like back and neck pain, are very common and not infrequently cause significant problems in the workplace. For the most part, symptoms will be benign and self-limiting and need only short-term support and simple workplace measures in the expectation that most work is possible.
- This chapter, however, has focused on the more serious spectrum of rheumatic diseases in which biological effects of disease can be greater and more problematic. For such chronic conditions, the approach needs to be more long term and take account of change.
- Management benefits considerably from good communication between the OH and rheumatology teams, the patient, the manager, and the general practitioner.
- Patients often do not realize that they can, and indeed should, discuss their difficulties at work with the rheumatology team and should be encouraged to do so.
- With recent advances in the treatment of inflammatory rheumatic disease, improved workplace outcomes can be anticipated going forwards but the OH team should remain aware that more aggressive immunosuppressive therapy may carry infective risks in certain working environments.

Useful websites

Arthritis Research UK   https://www.arthritisresearchuk.org/

References

1. Hochberg M. Osteoarthritis. In: Silman AJ, Hochberg M (eds), *Epidemiology of the Rheumatic Diseases*, pp. 205–29. Oxford: Oxford University Press; 2001.
2. Bieleman HJ, Bierma-Zeinstra SMA, Oosterveld FGJ, et al. The effect of osteoarthritis of the hip or knee on work participation. *J Rheumatol* 2011;38:1835–43.
3. National Institute for Health and Care Excellence. *Osteoarthritis: Care and Management.* NICE Clinical Guideline [CG177]. London: NICE; 2014.
4. Arthritis and Musculoskeletal Alliance. *Standards of Care for People with Osteoarthritis.* London: Arthritis and Musculoskeletal Alliance; 2004.

5. **Silman AJ.** Rheumatoid arthritis. In: Silman AJ, Hochberg M (eds), *Epidemiology of the Rheumatic Diseases*, pp. 31–71. Oxford: Oxford University Press; 2001.

6. **Olsson AR, Skogh T, Axelson O, et al.** Occupations and exposures in the work environment as determinants for rheumatoid arthritis. *Occup Environ Med* 2004;**61**:233–8.

7. **Oliver JE, Silman AJ.** Risk factors for the development of rheumatoid arthritis. *Scand J Rheumatol* 2006;**35**:169–74.

8. **Gold LS, Ward MH, Dosemeci M, et al.** Systemic autoimmune disease mortality and occupational exposures. *Arthritis Rheum* 2007;**56**:3189–201.

9. **Parks CG, Walitt BT, Pettinger M, et al.** Insecticide use and risk of rheumatoid arthritis and systemic lupus erythematosus in the Women's Health Initiative Observational Study. *Arthritis Care Res* 2011;**63**:184–94.

10. **Aletaha D, Neogi T, Silman AJ, et al.** 2010 Rheumatoid Arthritis Classification Criteria. An American College of Rheumatology/European League Against Rheumatism collaborative initiative. *Arthritis Rheum* 2010;**62**:2569–81.

11. **National Institute of Health and Care Excellence.** *Rheumatoid Arthritis: The Management of Rheumatoid Arthritis in Adults.* NICE Clinical Guideline [CG79]. London: NICE; 2009 (Updated Dec 2015).

12. **National Institute of Health and Care Excellence.** *Adalimumab, Etanercept, Infliximab, Rituximab and Abatacept for the Treatment of Rheumatoid Arthritis after the Failure of a TNF Inhibitor.* NICE Technology Appraisal [TA195]. London: NICE; 2010.

13. **Verstappen SM.** Rheumatoid arthritis and work: the impact of rheumatoid arthritis on absenteeism and presenteeism. *Best Pract Res Clin Rheumatol* 2015;**29**:495–511.

14. **Yelin E, Trupin L, Katz P, et al.** Association between etanercept use and employment outcomes among patients with rheumatoid arthritis. *Arthritis Rheum* 2003;**48**:3046–54.

15. **Wolfe F, Allaire S, Michaud K.** The prevalence and incidence of work disability in rheumatoid arthritis, and the effect of anti-tumor necrosis factor on work disability. *J Rheumatol* 2007;**34**:2211–17.

16. **Allaire S, Wolfe F, Niu J, et al.** Current risk factors for work disability associated with rheumatoid arthritis: recent data from a US National cohort. *Arthritis Rheum* 2009;**61**:321–8.

17. **Tang K, Beaton DE, Gignac MA, et al.** The Work instability Scale for rheumatoid arthritis predicts arthritis-related work transitions within 12 months. *Arthritis Care Res* 2010;**62**:1578–87.

18. **Macedo AM, Oakley SP, Panayi GS, et al.** Functional and work outcomes improve in patients with rheumatoid arthritis who receive targeted, comprehensive occupational therapy. *Arthritis Rheum* 2009;**61**:1522–30.

19. **Detaille SI, Haafkens JA, van Dijk FJ.** What employees with rheumatoid arthritis, diabetes mellitus and hearing loss need to cope at work. *Scand J Work Environ Health* 2003;**29**:134–42.

20. **National Institute for Health and Care Excellence.** *Spondyloarthritis in Over 16s: Diagnosis and Management.* NICE guideline [NG65]. London: NICE; 2017 (Updated June 2017).

21. **National Institute for Health and Care Excellence.** *Etanercept, Infliximab and Adalimumab for the Treatment of Psoriatic Arthritis.* Technology appraisal guidance [TA199]. London: NICE; 2010.

22. **Tillett W, de-Vries C, McHugh NJ.** Work disability in psoriatic arthritis—a systematic review. *Rheumatology* 2012;**51**:275–83.

23. **Wallenius M, Skomsvoll JF, Koldingsnes W, et al.** Work disability and health-related quality of life in males and females with psoriatic arthritis. *Ann Rheum Dis* 2009;**68**:685–9.

24. **Kavanaugh A, Antoni C, Mease P, et al.** Effect of infliximab therapy on employment, time lost from work, and productivity in patients with psoriatic arthritis. *J Rheumatol* 2006;**33**:2254–9.

25. **Verstappen SM, Watson KD, Lunt M, et al.** Working status in patients with rheumatoid arthritis, ankylosing spondylitis and psoriatic arthritis: results from the British Society for Rheumatology Biologics register. *Rheumatology* 2010;**49**:1570–7.

26. **Baker K, Pope J.** Employment and work disability in systemic lupus erythematosus: a systematic review. *Rheumatology* 2009;**48**:281–4.

27. **Yelin E, Tonner C, Trupin L, et al.** Work loss and work entry among persons with systemic lupus erythematosus: comparisons with a national matched sample. *Arthritis Rheum* 2009;**61**:247–58.

28. **National Institute for Health and Care Excellence.** *Belimumab for Treating Active Autoantibody-Positive Systemic Lupus Erythematosus.* Technology appraisal guidance [TA397]. London: NICE; 2016.

29. **Wolfe F, Smythe HA, Yunus MB, et al.** The American College of Rheumatology 1990 criteria for the classification of fibromyalgia: report of the Multicenter Criteria Committee. *Arthritis Rheum* 1990;**33**:160–72.

30. **Magni G, Moreschi C, Rigatti-Luchini S, et al.** Prospective study on the relationship between depressive symptoms and chronic musculoskeletal pain. *Pain* 1994;**56**:289–97.

31. **Busch AJ, Barber KAR, Overned TJ, et al.** Exercise for treating fibromyalgia syndrome. *Cochrane Database Syst Rev* 2007;**4**:CD003786.

32. **Karjalainen KA, Malmivaara A, van Tulder MW, et al.** Multidisciplinary rehabilitation for fibromyalgia and musculoskeletal pain in working age adults. *Cochrane Database Syst Rev* 2000;**2**:CD001984.

33. **McDonald M, DiBonaventura M, Ullman S.** Musculoskeletal pain in the workforce: the effects of back, arthritis and fibromyalgia pain on quality of life and work productivity. *J Occup Environ Med* 2011;**53**:765–70.

34. **Bossema ER, Kool MB, Cornet D, et al.** Characteristics of suitable work from the perspective of patients with fibromyalgia. *Rheumatology* 2011;**51**:311–18.

35. **Straube S, Moore RA, Paine J, et al.** Interference with work in fibromyalgia: effect of treatment with pregabalin and relation to pain response. *BMC Musculoskelet Disord* 2011;**12**:125.

Chapter 21

Musculoskeletal conditions, part 2: spinal disorders

Birender Balain and John Hobson

Introduction

Non-specific low back pain (LBP) is one of the commonest conditions afflicting adults of working age. It represents a leading cause of disability and a major cause of sickness absence. Neck pain and its associated disability are scarcely less common. Collectively, back and neck pain pose a major challenge to employers. Occupational health (OH) professionals should be competent when assessing workers with these conditions, and be aware of evidence-based advances in the management and rehabilitation of mechanical LBP. Adoption of consensus guidelines has led to better coping and faster recovery.

In this chapter, we review these initiatives and the problem of assessing fitness for work in those with spinal pain. Emphasis is given to simple, non-specific spinal pain as this is the commonest presentation. Only rarely does the clinician make a more specific diagnosis, but occasionally serious pathology underlies symptoms and different responses are needed. Therefore, this chapter also considers more specific spinal problems and interventions.

Non-specific low back pain

Prevalence and natural history

Non-specific LBP is common and often recurrent. There is considerable heterogeneity among the back pain literature regarding prevalence and incidence. The main epidemiological estimates are summarized in Table 21.1.

Radiating leg pain has a lifetime prevalence of 14–40%, although by the strictest clinical criteria only about 3–5% of adults have true sciatica.[1]

The prevalence of symptoms is already high in adolescents, and rises modestly with age, peaking at 40–69 years.[1,3] Many episodes of LBP are short-lived and go unobserved by health professionals. Previous community studies show that most people with back pain consult their general practitioner (GP) about symptoms.[4] Just over two-thirds represent fresh episodes, 20% are acute-on-chronic exacerbations, and 10% are a continuation of chronic background discomfort. Three months later, a quarter will have resolved

Table 21.1 Epidemiology of non-specific LBP

Measure	Estimate (%)	Country
Lifetime prevalence	60–80[1]	UK
	39[3]	Global
1-year prevalence	1–82 (mean 38)[2,3]	Global
Point prevalence	17–31[1]	UK
	1–58 (mean 18)[2,3]	Global
Incidence	6–15 (first ever episode)[3]	Global
	1–36 (any episode)[3]	

and another quarter will have improved, but in the remainder, symptoms are either static (30%) or worsened (14%).

The likelihood of further attacks is greatest among those with recent symptoms and falls off with time (Table 21.2).[5] It has been estimated that 20% of people with LBP will continue to have symptoms of some degree over much of their life, while 5–7% will report these as chronic illness.[1]

Disability and sickness absence

Among 291 conditions studied in the Global Burden of Disease 2010 study,[6] LBP ranked highest for disability (years lived with a disability), and sixth for overall burden (disability-adjusted life years). Disability-adjusted life years increased from 58 million in 1990 to 83 million in 2010. Prevalence and burden increased with age.[6]

The Labour Force Survey 2016/2017 showed that of the half a million workers who reported work-related musculoskeletal disorders (MSDs), approximately 40% were LBP (see the Health and Safety Executive (HSE) website in 'Useful websites'). Collectively, MSDs accounted for almost 9 million lost working days although the long-term trend is

Table 21.2 Likelihood of further back pain according to time from the last episode

Time since last episode	Likelihood of attack in the next year (%)
<1 week	76
1–4 weeks	63
1–12 months	52
1–5 years	43
>5 years	28

Source: data from Biering-Sorensen, F. A prospective study of low back pain in a general population, I—occurrence, recurrence and aetiology. *Scandinavian Journal of Rehabilitation Medicine*. 15(2), 71–80. Copyright © 1983 Foundation of Rehabilitation Information.

a reduction in the rate of reporting of new and long-standing MSDs (a fall of almost 25% during 2002–2016). In 2016/2017, approximately 1500 per 100,000 workers reported new or long-standing MSDs caused or made worse by work. Industries reporting the highest rates were construction, agriculture, forestry and fishing, transportation and storage, and human health and social care.

Economically, the impact of LBP is considerable: 3.7 million people (7% of the adult population) consult their GP about back pain; 1.6 million attend a hospital outpatient department; 100,000 are admitted to hospital; and 24,000 have spinal surgery.[1]

Figure 21.1 provides an estimate of the distribution of work loss among workers with back pain. Most sufferers take a little time off work, while a small minority take many days off. Thus, 67% of workers with LBP episodes return to work within a week, 75% within a fortnight, and 84% within a month; but 10% exceed 60 days and at 6 months about 4% are still absent.

The probability of returning to work is a function of time. The longer a person is off work, the lower their chance of an eventual return. At 6 months, this probability falls to 50% and is even less for those with recurrent episodes. Deconditioning (both physical and mental) as a result of long-term absence is undoubtedly a factor in those not returning to work, especially where physical activity is part of the work role. These factors provide a rationale for encouraging early return to work, with special effort directed towards those

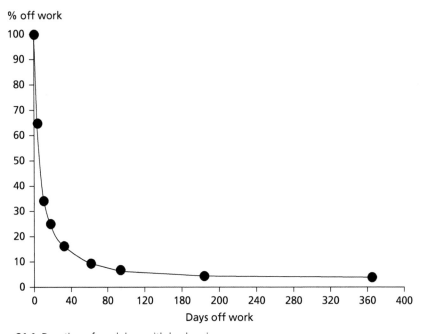

Figure 21.1 Duration of work loss with back pain.
Adapted from Clinical Standards Advisory Group. *Epidemiology review: the epidemiology and cost of back pain*, London, HMSO © Crown Copyright 1994.

in transition from the short-term to the long-term stages. Active intervention at 4–12 weeks is increasingly advocated.

Other factors

Between 1978 and 1992, inflation-adjusted expenditure on sickness and incapacity benefits for back pain rose by more than 200% compared to 55% for all incapacities and outpatient attendances for back pain increased fivefold.[1] These changes occurred at a time when the physical demands of work probably lessened. A comparison of two large population surveys a decade apart (1988–1998) found only a small rise in LBP overall with no corresponding rise in functional disability.[7] During 1997–2007, incapacity benefit awards for LBP declined and were overtaken by mental health disorders as the main reason for award, the change in trend beginning first in London and the South-East and only later spreading to other parts of Britain.[8]

These and other observations suggest that experience of disability may be influenced importantly by culture and prevailing societal beliefs and expectations about health. This idea, which is formalized in the biopsychosocial model of LBP,[9] has been incorporated into management strategies to rehabilitate the affected sufferer (see 'Active rehabilitation').

Risk factors

Many factors can contribute to the onset and severity of LBP, including age, gender, smoking habit, physical fitness, anthropometry, lumbar mobility, strength, psyche and mental well-being, other aspects of medical history, pre-existing spinal abnormalities, and physical demands of work. Evidence on these factors is not always consistent.[10,11]

Rates of back pain vary substantially by industry, occupation, and job title. In general, LBP is reported somewhat more often in people with heavy manual occupations, and workers in these jobs tend to lose significantly more time from work during back pain episodes.[12]

Certain physical exposures carry a consistently higher risk of reported back pain. These include lifting, forceful movements, exposure to whole-body vibration, and awkward working postures (Table 21.3).[11] The combination of adverse physical exposures, such as

Table 21.3 Evidence for a causal relationship between physical work factors and back pain

Risk factor	Strong evidence(+ + +)	Evidence (+ +)	Insufficient evidence (+/0)	Evidence of no effect (–)
Lifting/forceful movement	√			
Awkward posture		√		
Heavy physical work		√		
Whole-body vibration	√		.	
Static work posture			√	

Source: data from Von Korff, M. et al, Grading the severity of chronic pain. *Pain*. 50(2), 133–49. Copyright © 1992 International Association for the Study of Pain (IASP).

Table 21.4 Relative risk of lumbar disc prolapse according to posture and method of lifting

Lifting method	Relative risk	95% confidence interval
Avoids lifting with twisted body	1.0	Reference group
Lifts while twisting body, knees bent	2.7	0.9–7.9
Lifts while twisting body, knees straight	6.1	1.3–27.9

Source: data from Bernard, PB. (Ed) (2007) *Musculoskeletal disorders and workplace factors: a critical review of epidemiologic evidence for work-related musculoskeletal disorders of the neck, upper extremity, and low back.* Publication No. 97B141. London, UK: National Institute for Occupational Safety and Health (NIOSH). Copyright © 2007 NIOSH.

lifting and awkward posture, probably carries an even higher risk (Table 21.4).[13] However, back pain is also common in those with sedentary roles and some authorities consider that physical risk factors only account for a small proportion of the observed overall effect.

Psychosocial factors may be important. In a study conducted within The Boeing Company, psychological distress and dissatisfaction with work were the best predictors of new-onset LBP over follow-up.[14] They proved to be more important than any of the physical risk factors studied, although still not highly predictive. In the Manchester Back Pain Study, people free of back pain but more distressed at baseline were more likely to report a new episode over the next 12 months and more likely to see a doctor[15]; those who were dissatisfied with their work were also more likely to report a new episode. Psychological factors, including fear-avoidance beliefs and behaviours, have also been associated with delayed recovery among established cases[16]—these represent risk factors for chronicity and disability. Distress over somatic symptoms, in particular, has been associated with disabling and persistent regional pain, including back complaints.[17]

Assessing back pain and disability

Pain, by definition, is a subjective personal experience. Therefore, assessing its severity against objective benchmarks is an imprecise process. Several formalized clinical and research approaches have been employed, the simplest of which is use of a visual analogue scale.

Disability from back pain can be gauged clinically by its interference with activities of daily living—such as sitting, walking, sleeping, and dressing, together with more energetic activities. Well-recognized assessments, such as the Oswestry, and Rowland and Morris questionnaires, are quick, simple, and as robust as more complex approaches to assessing disabling pain.[18]

One *disadvantage* common to assessing LBP is the subjective reliance on the patient's own account.

When assessing LBP with or without sciatica, the National Institute for Health and Care Excellence (NICE) recommends using risk stratification, for example, the STarT Back risk assessment tool, at first point of contact with a healthcare professional. The Keele STarT Back Screening Tool (SBST) is a simple prognostic questionnaire that helps clinicians identify modifiable risk factors (biomedical, psychological, and social) for back pain disability (see 'Useful websites'). The resulting score stratifies patients into low-, medium-, or high-risk categories, with a matched treatment package for each category. This approach has been shown to reduce back pain-related disability and be cost-effective.

This allows simpler and less intensive support for people with LBP, with or without sciatica, likely to improve quickly and have a good outcome, including reassurance, advice to keep active, and guidance on self-management. This is very relevant in the OH setting.

More complex and intensive support is required for those at higher risk of a poor outcome, for example, exercise programmes with or without manual therapy or using a psychological approach.

Assessing the worker who presents with low back pain

As work limitation from LBP is frequent across all groups, most OH professionals will see patients with back-associated sickness absence and will need to assess their prognosis and fitness for work. There is only an approximate concordance between the severity of reported symptoms and disability, and likelihood of losing work time or seeking healthcare and the best predictor of future work loss is the past history of this behaviour (Box 21.1).[5]

Triage assessment and investigation

Back pain is a symptom and not a diagnosis. However, in an estimated 85% of presentations no underlying pathology can be identified and serious causes are rare. This has prompted a pragmatic approach to assessment, endorsed in a number of well-respected reports and based on the principles of triage. Cases of LBP should be classified on the basis of a few simple clinical criteria (Box 21.2)[9] into one of three groups:

1 Simple backache.
2 Nerve root compression or irritation.
3 Possible serious spinal pathology (<1% of all back pain).

The aim is to identify, among the many, the few requiring urgent investigation; and for the rest to follow a conservative approach bolstered, if recovery is stalled, by early active rehabilitation. This approach is advocated in the current NICE guidelines. Urgent specialist referral is required only in exceptional circumstances.

The role of investigation is limited. In the presence of so-called red flags (Box 21.2), screening blood tests for infection (such as erythrocyte sedimentation rate, C-reactive protein, and full blood count) and appropriate imaging, usually a magnetic resonance imaging (MRI) scan, would be indicated to rule out infection or suspected primary or metastatic lesions. In the absence of worrying features, investigation is rarely indicated. In particular, the use of computed tomography and MRI is unwarranted and inadvisable in most situations. NICE recommends that imaging should not be offered in a non-specialist setting; the health professional should explain to people that if they are being referred for specialist opinion, they may not necessarily need imaging. Both NICE and

Box 21.1 Questions that arise when assessing workers with LBP

- When will symptoms improve or resolve?
- Is this a short- or a long-term problem?
- Are any further investigations required to exclude serious pathology?
- Who (among the many with pain) should be referred for such an assessment?
- At what point should the OH professional intervene to hasten rehabilitation? And how?
- Has work contributed to symptom onset?
- Might work worsen or prolong symptoms?
- Is it appropriate to return the worker to the same job or does the work need to be modified?
- When is chronic spinal pain serious enough to declare a person permanently unfit for work?
- Could more be done to avoid or control the demands of work before that point is reached?
- Following spinal surgery, when will the patient be fit for work?
- Should special restrictions be considered and if so when?

At pre-placement

- Are there any specific inquiries (questions, examination findings, and investigations) predictive of future spinal pain leading to serious disability or sickness absence?
- How should these be utilized in assessing fitness for work?
- How should a past history of spinal pain be regarded?
- Are any characteristics sufficiently predictive to warrant restrictions?

In general

- What steps can be taken to promote fitness for work and to prevent spinal pain?
- What obligations exist under health and safety legislation and the Equality Act 2010?
- Do current policies on back pain promote well-being and avoid needless work restrictions?

Box 21.2 Diagnostic triage in patients presenting with LBP, with or without sciatica

Simple backache (90% recover within 6 weeks)

- Presents at age 20–55 years.
- Lumbosacral area, buttocks, and thighs.
- Mechanical in nature: varying with activity and with time.
- Patient well.

Nerve root pain (50% recover within 6 weeks)

- Unilateral leg pain greater than LBP.
- Dermatomal distribution.
- Sensory symptoms in same distribution.
- Straight leg raising reproduces the pain.
- Motor/sensory/reflex change only in one nerve root.

Red flags: possible serious spinal pathology

- Age at onset less than 20 or greater than 55 years.
- Violent trauma.
- Constant progressive pain.
- Thoracic pain.
- History of carcinoma, steroid use, drug abuse, or HIV.
- Unwell, weight loss.
- Widespread neurological features.
- Structural deformity.
- Features of CES (problems of micturition/faecal incontinence; saddle anaesthesia— anus, perineum, genitalia; progressive motor weakness; gait disturbance; sensory level).

Source: data from Waddell, G. (2004) *The back pain revolution*, 2nd Ed. Edinburgh, UK: Churchill Livingstone. Copyright © 2004 Elsevier.

the National Back Pain pathway state that imaging by a specialist (e.g. a musculoskeletal interface clinic or hospital) should only be considered if the result is likely to change management (see 'Useful websites'). In practice, imaging may be included in the clinical pathways within specialist services.

Box 21.3 Psychosocial ('yellow flag') risk factors

Factors that consistently predict poor outcomes:

- Belief that back pain is harmful or severely disabling.
- Fear-avoidance behaviour and reduced activities.
- Low mood and withdrawal from social interaction.
- Passive expectation of help (rather than a belief in self-participation).

Other issues in assessment

Psychosocial factors, 'yellow flags' (Box 21.3), should also be sought. Although imperfect indicators, these denote a higher risk of chronicity and disability, and so their presence may suggest the need for early active case management.[19]

Treatment of low back pain

There are very clear NICE guidelines on the treatment of LBP with or without sciatica and OH professionals should be aware of these and able to advise workers they see accordingly (Box 21.4).[20]

NICE recommendations on invasive treatment (NG59)[20] are that those with LBP should not be offered spinal injections, epidurals, spinal fusion, or disc replacement. In certain situations radiofrequency denervation and fusion can be considered, in chronic LBP for instance when other treatments have been unsuccessful or as part of a randomized controlled trial (RCT). In sciatica, epidurals and spinal decompression can be considered in certain circumstances.

Keeping active

A central component of all guidelines is advice to continue ordinary activities of daily living as normally as possible 'despite the pain'. Many trials indicate that this approach can give equivalent or faster symptomatic recovery from symptoms, and leads to shorter periods of work loss, fewer occurrences, and less sickness absence over the following year than advice to rest until completely pain free.

This advice is captured in a user-friendly way in 'Back Pain' from Arthritis Research UK which is a valuable handout for patients (see 'Useful websites').

Keeping active at work

Continuation of ordinary activities implies encouraging the worker to remain in their job, or to return to it promptly, *even if this still results in some LBP*. Direct evidence that this hastens rehabilitation is limited for the occupational setting (in contrast to primary care and community research), but the same general principles are thought to apply.

Most workers are able to follow this advice and remain at work or return to it within a few days or weeks. In some situations, a return to full normal duties may not be

Box 21.4 Non-invasive treatment in LBP with or without sciatica (NICE guidelines)

Recommended

- Self-management.
- Exercise.
- Psychological therapies using a cognitive behavioural approach but only as part of a treatment package including exercise.
- Return-to-work programmes.
- Consider oral non-steroidal anti-inflammatory drugs.
- Consider a combined physical and psychological programme, incorporating a cognitive behavioural therapy approach, preferably in a group context for people with persistent LBP or sciatica when they have significant psychosocial obstacles to recovery or when previous treatments have not been effective.

Not recommended

- Orthotics.
- Traction.
- Consider manual therapy (spinal manipulation, mobilization, or soft tissue techniques such as massage) but only as part of a treatment package including exercise.
- Acupuncture.
- Electrotherapies.
- Paracetamol alone, opioids routinely or in chronic LBP, antidepressants, or anticonvulsants.

possible—as when work requires exceptional levels of physical fitness (e.g. emergency rescue or military combat duties) or unavoidable manual handling of heavy loads, but such circumstances should be unusual. The Manual Handling Operations Regulations 1992 (as amended) require heavy physical tasks to be avoided or minimized, generally, by adaptation of the work and the provision of lifting aids. Guidance that accompanies the Regulations suggests ways in which lighter duties can be constructed.[21,22] The HSE has also developed risk assessment and other tools, to support job design and placement (see 'Useful websites').

Any prolonged period off work raises the chance that symptoms will become chronic. It is preferable to find or devise temporary restricted duties or an adapted pattern of work to encourage uninterrupted employment, and the earliest possible resumption of normal duties should be encouraged.

While doctors and managers commonly employ work restrictions in returning patients with LBP to the occupational environment, evidence for their effectiveness is limited. In 2003, Hiebert et al. reported a retrospective cohort study of patients who experienced absence from work because of LBP.[23] Forty-three per cent were provided with work restrictions. For a fifth of these workers restrictions were never lifted. Restricted duties did not reduce the incidence or duration of sickness absence and no significant reduction was observed in injury recurrence.

The advice given by health professionals is of critical importance. A recommendation to stay off work is often made on the basis of little or no evidence, but can seriously impair the prognosis.

Proper communication between the affected worker, the OH team, and line managers, and a shared understanding of the rehabilitation goal are fundamental for improvement in clinical and OH outcomes. An organizational culture that secures high stakeholder commitment may also reduce absenteeism and duration of work loss.

Managing the worker who still has problems after 1–3 months

A worker with LBP who is still having difficulty in returning to normal occupational duties at 1–3 months has a 10–40% risk of still being absent at 1 year. By the time 6 months has passed, the risk is higher still. Thus a need exists to identify workers off work with LBP before chronicity sets in. Intervention after 4 weeks is more effective than treatment received much later, and a system should be established to identify absence of this degree.

Active rehabilitation

A Cochrane systematic review and meta-analysis of multidisciplinary biopsychosocial rehabilitation for chronic LBP in 2015 found that multidisciplinary biopsychosocial rehabilitation interventions were more effective than usual care (moderate-quality evidence) and physical treatments (low-quality evidence) in decreasing pain and disability in people with chronic LBP. They concluded that for work outcomes, multidisciplinary rehabilitation seemed to be more effective than physical treatment but not more effective than usual care.[24]

The most recent NICE guidelines (NG59)[20] advocate the consideration of combined physical and psychological treatment programmes including elements of cognitive behavioural therapy. The NICE evidence review of multidisciplinary return-to-work programmes found sufficient evidence to support a general recommendation for encouraging return to normal daily activities and work. However, NICE did not find sufficient evidence to recommend specific work rehabilitation programmes.

Pre-placement assessment

A past history of symptoms should not be regarded as a reason for denying employment in most circumstances.

Caution should be exercised in placing individuals with a history of severely disabling LBP in physically demanding jobs, but the correct course of action involves a judgement.

Intuitively, it may seem obvious that individuals at higher recurrence risk should not be placed in jobs of high physical demand. Unfortunately, this logic has two problems—that of predicting future risk accurately enough, and that of distinguishing recurrence risk in a specific job from recurrence risk in any job (or no job). According to the HSE, the evidence base for matching individual susceptibility to a job-specific risk assessment is insufficient at present to achieve reliable health-base selection.

Investigations and clinical tests

Traditional clinical investigations do little to inform the decision of job placement. Future disability from LBP among job applicants is not predicted at all well by the following factors:

- Examination findings (e.g. height, weight, lumbar flexibility, and straight leg raising).
- General cardiorespiratory fitness.
- Isometric, isokinetic, or isoinertial measurements of back function.
- X-ray and MRI findings.

Symptom-free applicants with single psychosocial risk factors are at greater risk of incident LBP, but not to an extent that justifies exclusion.

Collectively these observations suggest a limited role for pre-placement health screening—perhaps just to avoid the very worst of mismatches between physical demands and back pain history.

Prevention and risk management

Success in preventing spinal disorders depends upon an informed assessment of risk, and a package of risk reduction measures, underpinned by suitable management systems for monitoring and enforcement. A similar approach can help the affected worker to return to work.

A number of preventive measures may have value:

1 Training, to ensure higher risk awareness and better working practices.
2 An induction period, to allow workers in unfamiliar roles to start out at a slower pace.
3 Job rotation and rest breaks, to avoid repetitive monotonous use of the same muscles, tendons, and joints.
4 A programme of phased reintroduction to normal work, with temporarily lighter duties or shortened working hours, after sickness absence.
5 Task optimization, for example, work reorganization to minimize the carrying load, improve the height from which loads are lifted, avoid awkward lifting and twisting, and replace manual handling by employing lifting aids instead.

Some excellent guidelines and case studies from the HSE illustrate this last approach (see 'Useful websites').

The case that such job modifications prevent back problems is intuitive and firmly rooted in ergonomic theory. It is also suggested by the research that identifies materials handling as a risk factor for LBP. But the evidence that well-designed workplace and job changes prevent LBP in practice is less clear cut. In part, this could reflect the difficulty of conducting well-controlled trials in the OH setting or of implementing change effectively. Another view is that the scope for preventing disability from LBP is limited, as it has other major non-physical explanations.

However, some well-conducted studies have shown a clear benefit. For example, Evanoff et al. examined injury and lost workday rates before and after the introduction of mech-anical lifts in acute care hospitals and long-term care facilities.[25] In the post-intervention period, rates of musculoskeletal injuries, mainly LBP, decreased by 28%, lost workday injuries by 44%, and total lost days due to injury by 58%.

In practice, ergonomic theory is likely to hold, at least to the extent that some tasks will aggravate pre-existing and current LBP and hinder the goal of remaining at work. Also in practice, there is a legal mandate to assess risks from manual handling and to min-imize unnecessary exposures within reasonable bounds. Simple ergonomic adjustments are likely to be construed as 'reasonable adjustments' within the scope of the Equality Act 2010 for workers with serious back problems.

Neck pain

Prevalence and natural history

Neck pain, like back pain, is common in the general population. Thus, for example, in a British population survey involving nearly 13,000 adults of working age, 34% re-counted neck pain in the past 12 months, 11% reported neck pain that had interfered with their normal activities over this period, and 20% had had symptoms in the past 7 days.[26]

Like back pain, neck pain is often persistent as some 14–19% of subjects report symp-toms lasting longer than 6 months in the previous year. Also like back pain, it is com-monly recurrent and a source of disability.

Occupational and personal risk factors

Occupational activities are sometimes blamed as a cause of neck pain. One systematic review concluded there was 'some evidence' for a relation with neck flexion, arm force, arm posture, duration of sitting, twisting or bending, hand–arm vibration, and work-place design.[27] A second review, by the US National Institute of Occupational Health, concluded that there was 'strong evidence' for an association with static loading of the neck–shoulder musculature, and 'suggestive evidence' of risks from continuous arm and hand movements and forceful work involving the same muscle groups.[11] A third review found reasonable evidence that repeated shoulder movements and neck flexion were as-sociated with neck pain with tenderness.[28]

Such evidence has tended to accrue from only a few occupations in industry. In com-munity samples, the findings have been less consistent. Thus, for example, in a Finnish population study there were no clear-cut differences in neck pain prevalence between blue-collar and white-collar workers[29] and in a UK population survey, no strong associations were found between occupational physical risk factors and neck pain.[26]

Psychosocial factors show a consistent relation to neck pain—in workplaces, in populations, and in outpatient clinics. Personal feelings of stress and tiredness, and psychosocial stressors such as high work pressures and low job control, are both relevant. The situation parallels that of LBP, especially when symptoms are non-specific and unrelated to trauma or serious local pathology.

Assessing and managing the patient with neck pain

Several clinical features predict sickness absence among workers consulting with neck pain. These include short duration, high pain intensity, report of continuous pain, and certain physical signs (pain in the upper limb during rotation of the head and pain in the shoulder during abduction of the arm).[30] Previous sickness absence attributed to neck pain is also predictive of future absence spells from this cause.[31]

Further investigations (e.g. radiology and MRI) are not indicated except in rare circumstances. Changes of osteoarthritis will often be found, but the correlation between symptoms and X-ray appearance is inconsistent, and the predictive performance of such tests for future incapacity is low.

Guidelines on managing neck pain are less developed than those on managing LBP. In principle, and by analogy, the optimal approach should be similar to that for LBP: initial assessment by triage, followed by advice to maintain activity and coping within the limits of pain for simple mechanical neck pain. A useful patient information leaflet is available from Arthritis Research UK (see 'Useful websites'). However, direct evidence on this is sparse.

Complex versions of such advice have been embedded in programmes of multidisciplinary biopsychosocial rehabilitation but there is little evidence at present to justify the effort. Specific exercise programmes, involving strength and endurance training, muscle training, stretching, and relaxation are also of uncertain benefit. Thus, strength and endurance training decreased pain and disability in women with chronic neck problems in one trial, where stretching did not.[32] In another randomized trial, dynamic muscle and relaxation training did not lead to better relief or recovery than continuation of ordinary activity.[33]

Perhaps the best that can be said at present is that most neck pain, like most LBP, does not have a serious underlying cause; that triage is a means of identifying the few cases needing further investigation; that such investigations will rarely aid fitness assessment in the work setting; and that symptomatic relief and advice to remain active is a sensible pragmatic approach, likely in most cases to be followed by an early return to work. Jobs that require workers to crane and twist their necks to an unusual degree (e.g. to inspect overhead electrical equipment in a confined space) and those that require full neck movements to ensure unrestricted field of view in safety-critical situations may justify a temporary fitness restriction. However, research evidence is currently lacking to support the view that workplace interventions will reduce the incidence of neck pain.[34]

Spinal surgery

Although back and neck pain episodes are frequent, few patients require surgery. Nonetheless, a small minority undergo such procedures. See also Chapter 11 for recommended return-to-work times following surgery.

Surgery for lumbar nerve root compression

The commonest indication for surgery in the lumbar spine is neurological compression, which has two main causes—prolapsed intervertebral disc (PID) and spinal stenosis.

The management of the patient with lumbar neurological compression starts with a clear definition of sciatica. Pain arising from the back, and radiating below the knee, is likely to be radicular in most cases, but not all. Non-specific LBP is defined as pain below the rib cage and above the buttock fold. Injecting hypertonic saline into the supraspinous ligaments demonstrates that distribution of pain referral patterns can exactly mimic dermatomal distribution. Pain felt in the lower limb can either be a radicular pain or be a referred pain pattern. The presence of sensory or motor symptoms helps to diagnose radicular pain. In the absence of sensory and motor changes, the distribution and characteristics of pain in the lower limbs along with its temporal association with back pain is important in differentiating referred pain from radicular pain. Asymptomatic disc prolapse can be found in some 20–30% of subjects of working age on MRI scans.[35] The unfortunate patient with a referred pain into the leg and a coincidental asymptomatic disc prolapse on an ill-advised MRI scan is at risk of unnecessary and ineffective surgical treatment.

Prolapsed lumbar intervertebral disc

The lifetime prevalence of sciatica is 40%, but the prevalence of sciatica due to disc herniation is only 1–3%. Only 1% of patients with acute LBP will have radicular pain from a disc herniation. Most cases occur between the ages of 30–50 years, with a higher proportion in males than females (2:1). Most of the cases are at L4/5 and L5/S1, with higher levels being more common with increasing age. The 1-year incidence of symptomatic PID lies between 0.1% and 0.5%.[36]

In most cases, the natural history of this condition is benign. Radiological evidence of disc herniation is far more common than the number of people presenting to medical professionals with sciatica. In 90% of cases, the pain substantially improves by 6 weeks, with most returning to activity in 4 weeks. Following a first episode of sciatica, 5–10% of patients will experience a recurrence. Following a second episode, recurrence rises to 20–30%, and 70% following three or more episodes.

In most patients, the history starts with acute lower back pain followed by a sharp and severe, burning/electric/stabbing type pain in the L5 and/or S1 dermatome distribution. This radicular pain is severe enough in the beginning to restrict the patient's ability to function normally, and they may have a varying amount of numbness/tingling, loss of sensation, and weakness associated with it. This weakness may restrict ability to get up on tiptoes (S1), or walk on the heels (L5).

The presence of nerve root tension signs is the hallmark of the physical examination. This includes the straight leg raising test, ankle dorsiflexion reinforcement test, Bowstring sign, or the slump test. The presence of any sensory loss and evaluation of muscle Medical Research Council (MRC) grade function in L4, L5, and S1 myotomes on both sides is important. Quick functional tests can be used to assess motor weakness, and these include the ability to walk on tiptoes and heels, and the ability to squat. L5 weakness may manifest as hip abductor function weakness as well.

Conservative management

Most patients can be safely treated conservatively. This includes bed rest for a short period, adequate analgesia using anti-inflammatories, opioids, and neuropathic pain medications according to symptom severity. It is also important for patients to avoid any posture, activity, or exercise that makes the leg pain worse. In the first few days or weeks, they may not be able to stand, sit, or lie down properly due to leg pain. As the pain settles down, they should be encouraged to be as active as they can be, but again avoid anything that makes the pain worse. As the pain settles, the resumption of normal activities is essential along with progressive maintenance exercises to promote muscle endurance and strength, where the help of a physiotherapist may be needed. Once the pain has settled, core stability exercises and advice about posture and 'back school' advice about lifting and bending should be given.

The acute effects of prolapse and the enforced rest can lead to significant muscular atrophy. Thus, it is important that normal activity is resumed as soon as pain allows and not left until the pain settles completely. As pain settles, in addition to resumption of normal activities patients should be advised to undertake progressive maintenance exercises to promote muscle endurance and strength.

Between 50% and 70% of conservatively treated cases of disc herniation will resolve completely, often with return to activity within 4 weeks.[37] The natural history of PID is favourable, irrespective of the size or location of the prolapse radiologically. Thus, conservative management is usually appropriate. Where necessary, epidural steroids or nerve root block can provide pain relief and reduce the need for surgery.[38]

Return to work

There is little evidence available concerning the return to work following conservative treatment of an acute disc prolapse. However, there is no evidence that resumption of work activities is harmful or capable of precipitating a relapse of symptoms, any more than other normal activities. Most patients who avoid activity do so because of pain, fear, and negative advice. The key messages, as with simple LBP in the absence of PID, are firstly that the more rapid the resumption of normal activities, the better the overall prognosis, and secondly that each incremental increase in activity may cause a temporary increase in discomfort. The patient can be reassured that this is not dangerous and advised of the difference between hurt and harm. If the patient has not had active management by 6 weeks, then involvement of a physiotherapist for advice, encouragement, and gentle mobilization may be helpful.

Surgical management

If the pain doesn't settle within 6 weeks or if the patient finds it difficult to bear the pain even before that, invasive interventions are an option. This includes the use of epidural injections and surgery in the form of discectomy (open, microscopic, or endoscopic).

The presence of progressive deterioration in neurology in the form of worsening sensory and/or motor loss (significant loss—usually assumed as distressing paraesthesia and/or MRC grade 3 or less weakness) is an indication for surgery. Some patients may have bilateral leg symptoms and symptoms and signs of perianal numbness, bladder and bowel disturbances, or loss of sexual function (cauda equina syndrome or CES) in which case emergency surgery is the best way to proceed. CES may present as a complete syndrome with retention (CESR), but can often present with incomplete sensory/motor loss of bladder/bowel function and is known as CES incomplete (CESI). Both CESR and CESI are indications for emergency surgery as every 12–24 hours delay in treatment can affect bladder and bowel function in the long term.

The role of surgery in the presence of established, but non-progressive neurological deficit is less clear. Evidence states that the number of patients that improve some muscle function is approximately two in three, whether they have surgery or not, implying that conservative management can also be easily advocated despite weakness, especially if the pain is settling or disappeared. If there is significant pain along with weakness, urgent surgery is definitely an option that needs to be discussed with the patient, although it is more predictable for pain relief rather than muscle function improvement.

Postoperative recovery is usually within 6-8 weeks, and use of gradual return to work and physiotherapy interventions may be necessary for people in occupations that involve repeated lifting and bending activities. Those with fear-avoidance behaviour and anxiety associated with the episode also benefit from physiotherapy input.

The risk of a recurrent disc herniation after surgery ranges from 6% to 9%, with the size of the annular defect being the biggest predictor. This is highest in the first year, but can happen after that as well. Most patients will be fearful of similar episodes happening again, but reassurance, posture advice, modifications in work-based environment, and use of regular core stability exercises is successful in most. For further episodes of recurrence, surgery is likely to be helpful.

Over the long term, there is approximately a 25% chance that those who have surgery will need another operation, and of those who have had conservative management, 25% will need one spine operation. A 10-year follow-up study of more than 500 patients found no difference in symptoms between those treated conservatively and surgically although the surgical patients were more likely to report that their LBP or leg pain had completely gone (56% vs 40%) and were more satisfied with the outcome (71% vs 56%). There was no difference in work and disability status.[39] Early surgery (within 8–12 weeks of symptom onset) results in faster recovery and earlier return to work in the short term, although there is no difference in outcomes at 1 year.[40]

Fear of recurrence led in the past to postoperative protocols that restricted activity. However, in a study in which patients were allowed to determine their own levels of activity postoperatively, or to return to full activity promptly,[41] the mean return-to-work time from surgery was 1.7 weeks and 25% of patients returned to work the following day; 97% of those working at the time of surgery returned to full duty by 8 weeks. At 2 years, no patient had changed employment because of back or leg pain. Recurrent disc prolapse occurred in 6% (three patients) of whom one required surgical intervention. Thus, when freed from restrictions imposed by healthcare professionals, patients returned to activities and work more rapidly and in apparent safety. Magnusson et al.[42] found no rational basis for lifting restrictions after lumbar spine surgery. By contrast, a Cochrane review found strong evidence that intensive exercise programmes commencing 4–6 weeks following surgery were more effective than mild exercise programmes in improving functional status and hastening return to work.[43] See Chapter 11 for recommended return-to-work times following surgery.

Lumbar spinal stenosis

This condition causes radicular pain most commonly after the age of 50 years. Younger patients can have stenosis if they have a congenitally narrow spinal canal or a lytic spondylolisthesis (most commonly seen at L5/S1 level). After the age of 50 years, either degenerative listhesis at L4/5 or facet degeneration-related hypertrophy and ligamentum flavum buckling can cause stenosis.

In the Framingham study, congenital lumbar spinal stenosis was observed in 4.7% of the population in relative terms (12 mm limit) and in 2.6% in absolute terms (10 mm limit). Acquired lumbar spinal stenosis was found in 22.5% in relative terms and in 7.3% in absolute terms.[44]

Neurogenic claudication causes symptoms of pain with or without numbness, heaviness, pins and needles, or paraesthesia in the legs. This pain comes on with standing and walking, and is relieved by bending or sitting down. This is thought to be related to the reduced dimensions of the spinal canal in extension, and the increased space available for the nerves in flexion. This claudication pattern has to be distinguished from vascular claudication. Neurogenic claudication varies from day to day, gets better with spinal flexion and not just standing still, starts from proximal to distal, and may be accompanied by abnormal neurological signs such as paraesthesia, loss of reflexes, and/or weakness. These patients can cycle for miles, but can only walk a small distance.

Lumbar spine stenosis gradually worsens with time, although the progress is slow in most patients. In a study of 49 patients with severe stenosis treated with conservative measures, nine had surgery and another five had deteriorated over an average of 33 months, and the rest had remained the same or improved.[45] Another study of 146 patients with moderate level lumbar stenotic symptoms not offered surgery over a median of 3.3 years revealed that only 7% patients revised their decision and proceeded to surgery, and 10–13% revealed worsening pain levels, favouring a non-operative course for moderate level symptoms. [46]

Injections don't work well in the medium or long term, but are of use for diagnostic and short-term pain relief in medically unsuitable patients. The mainstay of treatment is surgical decompression, usually with good results. Sometimes fusion is combined with a decompression, especially in the setting of degenerative listhesis causing significant back pain, or degenerative scoliosis, or a recurrent stenosis following previous decompression.

Recovery from a decompression-type procedure is quick, wound healing occurs in 2 weeks and the internal muscular/tendinous structures heal in 6–8 weeks. Most patients are back on their feet quickly, with improvements in their walking distance within the first 3 months, although they have to take precautions about lifting and bending for the first 6–8 weeks. [47] Most patients would be back to normal activities within 3 months, but the addition of a fusion would prolong recovery to 9–12 months. See Chapter 11 for recommended return-to-work times following surgery.

Surgery for low back pain

A number of procedures exist for the surgical management of LBP, of which the most common is spinal fusion. More recently there has been interest in total disc replacement.

Spinal fusion

Spinal fusion is the gold standard against which other surgical procedures for managing of LBP are judged. However, only a tiny fraction of patients presenting with LBP require surgery. Spinal fusion is a major operation, with success critically dependent on good patient selection. It may be appropriate in patients with chronic symptoms and significant disability, but the patient should already have undergone and failed a formal multidisciplinary intensive functional restoration programme, pain clinic interventions, and supervised physiotherapy programmes, before spinal fusion is considered according to NICE. Psychological distress and compensation claims are recognized predictors of poor outcome.

The efficacy of fusion surgery in appropriately selected patients has been supported by recent systematic reviews and a meta-analysis,[48,49] with benefits sustained over 5 years.

It is clear, therefore, that some chronic back pain patients in whom work restoration is unlikely with conservative treatment may be returned to work by fusion surgery and, moreover, that fusion surgery itself is not a contraindication to employment.

Most surgeons prefer to restrict vigorous activities until bony fusion has been achieved radiologically, a process taking 6–12 months. However, postoperative regimens vary considerably without apparent justification. See Chapter 11 for recommended return-to-work times following surgery.

There is evidence both in favour and against fusion for non-specific LBP. Fritzell et al. reported on a randomized controlled multicentre study of 294 patients with a 2-year follow-up by an independent observer.[50] The patients had suffered from LBP for a mean of 7.8 years for the surgical group and 8.5 years for the non-surgical group and been on sick leave due to back pain for a mean of 3.2 and 2.9 years, respectively. Back pain was significantly reduced in the surgical group by 33% compared with 7% in the non-surgical group. In the surgical group, 63% rated themselves as significantly 'much better' or 'better' compared with 29% in the non-surgical group. The 'net back-to-work rate' was significantly in favour of surgical treatment, or 36% versus 13%.

In a separate study of a fusion cohort of 3060 patients, derived from weighted averages of outcome scores from 26 articles after a systematic review, a 36.8/100 reduction in visual analogue scale score, Oswestry Disability Index (ODI) change of 22.2, and patient satisfaction of 71% were seen.[51] The body of literature, according to this study, supports fusion surgery as a viable treatment option for reducing pain and improving function in patients with chronic LBP refractory to non-surgical care when a diagnosis of disc degeneration can be made.

However, there have been studies that demonstrate that surgery is no better than cognitive behavioural therapy and an exercise-based approach. Mannion et al. presented a long-term clinical follow-up of three multicentre RCTs of surgery versus non-operative treatment (multidisciplinary cognitive behavioural, and exercise rehabilitation) in Norway and the UK.[52] Of 473 enrolled patients, 261 (55%) responded and after an average of 11 years' follow-up, the outcomes between fusion and multidisciplinary cognitive behavioural and exercise rehabilitation for chronic LBP were no different.

In a systematic review and meta-analysis of five RCTs, a total of 707 patients were divided into lumbar fusion and conservative management.[53] The pooled mean difference in the two groups was not significant. They concluded that either operative intervention by lumbar fusion or non-operative management and physical therapy remain two acceptable treatment methods for intractable LBP.

Total disc replacement

The indications for total disc replacement are similar to those for spinal fusion. Disc replacement has several advantages, including the avoidance of bone harvesting from donor sites, preservation of motion (which may reduce degeneration at adjacent levels), and immediate stability (which allows early mobilization). Return to work may thus be accelerated, although policies on postoperative rehabilitation vary and there is no consensus on optimum care. Potential disadvantages include displacement, long-term wear of the prosthesis, and the difficulties and complications of revision.

In a review of nine case series (564 disc replacements), de Kleuver et al. noted that 50% of patients had good results and 81% had excellent results.[54]

NICE guidelines from 2009 state that this procedure can be offered routinely as a treatment option in patients who have not improved after standard treatments or for whom standard treatments are unsuitable. The studies that NICE looked at mostly assessed patients for only a short time. NICE has encouraged further research into artificial disc replacement and encourages doctors to collect and publish longer-term results and include information about which patients were treated and whether further surgery was needed. A systematic review from 2013 concluded that in the short to medium term, the safety and effectiveness of lumbar artificial intervertebral disc replacement appears to be comparable to that of lumbar fusion.[55] However, a 2017 review has concluded that longer-term studies on safety and revision rates are needed prior to adopting this technique in treating patients.[56]

The cervical spine

Surgery to the cervical spine may be indicated for neurological compression or, more rarely, for cervical pain.

Cervical disc herniation will produce pain and neurological dysfunction in the distribution of the affected nerve root. Like sciatica, neurological compression may be differentiated from referred cervical pain by finding a specific nerve dysfunction. The natural history of cervical disc prolapse is reported as being less benign than for the lumbar region. Up to half of patients treated conservatively continue to experience radicular pain between 2 and 19 years of follow-up.[57] For those patients with insufficient relief from conservative measures, surgery may be considered. Common procedures (such as anterior discectomy with fusion and decompression with cervical disc replacement) generally give good functional results.

Return to work following cervical surgery, however, is influenced by length of prior sick leave, amount of postoperative pain, age, and claims for compensation.[58]

Postoperative management varies considerably between surgeons and there are no evidence-based reports to guide rehabilitation. However, no adverse effects have been found in patients returning to work within 6 weeks of surgery.[59]

Other spinal conditions

Ankylosing spondylitis

Ankylosing spondylitis (AS) classically presents with an inflammatory onset and involves the sacroiliac and costovertebral joints in the thorax and spinal column joints. Clinically, the pain is relieved by exercise and not relieved by rest, lumbar spine movement is limited, and chest expansion is decreased. Early morning stiffness taking some time to wear off is frequently observed. Of those presenting with LBP in general practice, 5% will have features of AS.

Management relies on analgesics, non-steroidal anti-inflammatory drugs, and disease-modifying antirheumatic drugs such as the tumour necrosis factor (TNF)-alpha inhibitors in those with uncontrolled disease. NICE have produced guidelines and clinical knowledge summaries last updated in 2013 (see 'Useful websites').

The National Ankylosing Spondylitis Society comments that 'most people with AS are motivated and reported to have less time off work than average, mostly remaining in full time employment' and evidence exists of this (see 'Useful websites'). Nonetheless, AS has an impact on functional work capacity. A study by Boonen et al.[60] found that work disability and incapacity increased steadily with duration of disease. Sick leave was found to vary from 12 to 46 days per year. Work disability increased from 3% at 5 years of disease duration up to 50% at 45 years' duration. After 5 years, 96% of patients retained employment, but at 45 years only 45% remained in work.

The difficulties are greater for manual workers. The same researchers found that among those with manual jobs there was a 2.3-fold higher risk of work-related job loss than in those with a non-manual job.[61]

Recently, the more effective pain relief afforded by TNF-alpha inhibitor therapy has improved the vocational prognosis for patients with AS. One RCT reported a significant improvement in work productivity and a reduction in AS-related absenteeism.[62] A caveat is that some TNF-alpha inhibitors are delivered by infusion in hospital outpatient settings, which may require time away from the workplace.

When at work, patients are advised to maintain a good posture, avoid needless forward bending, and to regularly change position. Prolonged car driving may increase pain and stiffness. Patients with rigid or stiff necks may be at greater risk in the event of driving accidents, and the car should be fitted with correctly adjusted head-restraints (and if necessary, additional mirrors to the windscreen or dashboard). Disease of mild severity will not preclude vocational driving, although this may not represent the best career choice in the longer term. Workers with a rigid neck or severe peripheral joint involvement may be unfit to drive vocationally and need to inform the Driver and Vehicle Licensing Agency of their functional limitations.

Patients with AS are at risk of fracture following surprisingly minor trauma. Persistent localized pain in a patient with AS following trauma should be investigated thoroughly. In the ankylosed spine, surgical fixation is frequently required to obtain satisfactory union.

About 6% of patients with AS require a hip replacement, which normally restores mobility and relieves pain. The work restrictions that ensue do not differ from those described elsewhere for hip replacement although patients tend to be younger than normal for this surgical procedure.

Rarely, in poorly managed and advanced cases of AS, extreme spinal curvature may occur, limiting normal mobility, posture, and vision. In rare cases, surgery is employed to straighten the spine. Other peripheral complications of AS sometimes arise, the most common being uveitis.

In most cases, the 'reasonable adjustments' required by the Equality Act 2010 (see Chapter 3) should enable AS sufferers to pursue gainful employment, although caution is indicated for occupations where there is an above-average risk of trauma (e.g. AS may preclude employment in military combat duties).

Scheuermann's disease

Scheuermann's disease is a kyphotic deformity developing in early adolescence. Estimates of its prevalence vary from 0.4% to 8%. The kyphosis, which is associated with a compensatory lumbar lordosis, is usually noticed clinically, but the diagnosis is radiological with the observation of end-plate irregularities, disc space narrowing, and wedging of a minimum of three adjacent vertebrae. Scheuermann's disease can produce a significant kyphosis, normally in the thoracic and thoracolumbar region of the spine.

In general, a history of Scheuermann's disease does not suggest the need for job restrictions or adapted work. In a long-term follow-up study, back pain was more common many years later and patients had taken up work with lower physical demands.[63] However, the number of days absent from work with back pain, the interference of pain with activities of daily living, social limitations, level of recreational activities, and use of medication for back pain were not dissimilar from the normal population. The magnitude of the spinal curvature was associated with pain but not with loss of time from work.

Treatment modalities, such as exercise, bracing, and surgery have little impact on work capacity.

Fractures

The thoracolumbar spine

Fractures in the thoracolumbar spine can be divided into three conceptual columns: anterior (anterior body wall and vertebral body), middle (essentially the posterior body wall), and posterior (the posterior elements). Fractures of the anterior column are principally wedge compression fractures and are generally stable. Fractures of both anterior and middle column are often referred to as burst fractures.

Most single-column injuries are treated conservatively. In general, the outcome is very satisfactory even in men still employed in heavy manual labour although job retention seems to be poorer in those claiming compensation.[64]

Burst fractures treated conservatively also have good results. The natural history of these fractures when they present without neurology is benign.[65] A follow-up by Weinstein et al.[66] found that 90% of patients could return to their pre-injury occupation.

Most other injuries (injuries of the posterior column) are treated with surgery by internal fixation. Patients with neurological deficit are more likely to undergo surgery, although a meta-analysis[67] concluded there is no evidence that decompression improves neurological outcome. Surgically and conservatively treated cases appear to have a similar long-term outcome, although immediate stabilization reduces immediate pain.[68]

Vertebral fractures occur in cancellous bone and may be expected to heal within 3–4 months. After this period more vigorous activities should be encouraged and work return considered. Surgically treated patients with bone grafting take longer to consolidate but return with restrictions on lifting may be contemplated earlier.

The cervical spine

The recovery from a cervical fracture is mainly influenced by concomitant spinal cord injury. If any significant cord deficit is present then the prognosis is that of the cord injury.

Atlantoaxial injuries are normally treated conservatively with a halo jacket or occasionally by surgical fixation and the results of management are good. The situation is similar for fractures in the subaxial region, although long-term symptoms are more prominent.

Fracture dislocations—a source of continuing pain—may be reduced by traction or surgically, to add stability and promote fusion of the injured motion segment.

Following fracture, mobilization may be vigorously commenced once bony union has been obtained, after 8–12 weeks. There is no general consensus on rehabilitation regimens.

Spinal cord injury

Injury to the spinal cord, including major injury to the cauda equina, is rare with an incidence of 20–30 per million per year in the UK. Tetraplegia and paraplegia are now equally common. The age of injured patients is increasing.

Employment rates following spinal cord injury vary from 21% to 67% according to one review.[68] Younger age and greater functional independence predict a positive outcome.

Functional independence is principally determined by the level of neurological injury and residual motor function. The other determinants of individual work capacity include the effects of cord injury on bladder and bowel function, the patient's vulnerability to pressure sores, physical limitations, and various practical barriers to employment (e.g. lack of suitable transportation, lack of work experience and training, physical barriers, and disability discrimination).[69] In general, the UK has a poor record of returning patients with spinal cord injuries to work. Just 14% are in employment, versus a European average of 38% and almost 50% in the US. This substantial underperformance is likely to be a combination of poor expectations among healthcare professionals and inadequate response from employers.

The Equality Act 2010 requires reasonable adjustments by employers to accommodate those with spinal cord injuries—including proper access to the place of work (e.g. ramps, widened doorways, a ground floor workstation or access to a lift, and special parking rights) and other reasonable assistance (e.g. choosing a job and work schedule to suit the worker's capability, reasonable time off for medical care, and adjustments to the workstation). Other than access, the most significant practical factor in returning to work is a toilet facility that has enough space and privacy for bladder and bowel management.

The Brain and Spine Injuries Foundation provides support to those with spinal cord injuries (see 'Useful websites'). Despite the provisions of the Equality Act 2010, spinal cord injury remains an area where patients in the UK are being significantly failed at present by the work rehabilitation process.

Key points

- Back pain is common, affecting 60–80% of the population at some point in their lives. It is an important cause of disability and work loss.
- Most back pain is non-specific, and 90% of this recovers within 6 weeks. A small proportion (<1%) have serious underlying pathology.

- Back pain is best managed according to a biopsychosocial model that acknowledges the impact of beliefs and behaviours on recovery. Early advice to remain active is an important aspect of back pain management.
- Early return to altered work is beneficial, and exclusion from work is only indicated for the very heaviest jobs.
- Even prolapsed discs are often now treated conservatively, but disc surgery and fusion are useful in selected patients. Recovery and return to work after fusion can take 6 months or more.

Useful websites

Health and Safety Executive (HSE)	http://www.hse.gov.uk
BackCare	http://www.backcare.org.uk/
The Keele STarT Back Screening Tool (SBST)	https://www.keele.ac.uk/sbst/startbacktool/
Health and Safety Executive. Manual handling charts	http://www.hse.gov.uk/msd/mac/index.htm
National Institute for Health and Care Excellence (NICE). 'Low back pain and sciatica in over 16s: assessment and management' (NG59)	https://www.nice.org.uk/guidance/NG59/chapter/Recommendations#assessment-of-low-back-pain-and-sciatica
Trauma Programme of Care: NHS England. 'National Low Back and Radicular Pain Pathway 2017' (including implementation of NICE NG59)	https://docs.wixstatic.com/ugd/dd7c8a_caf17c305a5f4321a6fca249dea75ebe.pdf
National Ankylosing Spondylitis Society	https://nass.co.uk/
The Brain and Spine Foundation	https://www.brainandspine.org.uk/spinal-injuries-units
Arthritis Research UK. Information for patients on back and neck pain	https://www.arthritisresearchuk.org/arthritis-information/conditions/back-pain.aspx https://www.arthritisresearchuk.org/arthritis-information/conditions/neck-pain.aspx

References

1. **Clinical Standards Advisory Group**. *Epidemiology Review: The Epidemiology and Cost of Back Pain.* London: HMSO; 1994.

2. **Hoy DG, Brooks P, Blyth F, Buchbinder R.** The epidemiology of low back pain. *Best Pract Res Clin Rheumatol* 2010;**24**:769–81.

3. **Hoy D, Bain C, Williams G, et al.** A systematic review of the global prevalence of low back pain. *Arthritis Rheum* 2012;**64**:2028–37.

4. **Croft P, Joseph S, Cosgrove S, et al.** *Low Back Pain in the Community and in Hospitals. A Report to the Clinical Standards Advisory Group of the Department of Health. Prepared by the Arthritis & Rheumatism Council.* Manchester: Epidemiology Unit; 1994.

5. **Biering-Sorensen F.** A prospective study of low back pain in a general population. I—occurrence, recurrence and aetiology. *Scand J Rehabil Med* 1983;**15**:71–80.

6. **Hoy D, March L, Brooks P, Blyth F, Woolf A, Bain C.** The global burden of low back pain: estimates from the Global Burden of Disease 2010 study. *Annals Rheum Dis* 2014;**73**:968–74.

7. **Palmer KT, Walsh K, Bendall H, et al.** Back pain in Britain: comparison of two prevalence surveys at an interval of 10 years. *BMJ* 2000;**320**:1577–8.

8. **Cattrell A, Harris EC, Palmer KT, et al.** Regional trends in awards of incapacity benefit by cause. *Occup Med* 2011;**61**:148–51.

9. **Waddell G.** *The Back Pain Revolution*, 2nd edn. Edinburgh: Churchill Livingstone; 2004.

10. **Riihimaki H, Viikari-Juntura E.** Back and limb disorders. In: McDonald C (ed), *Epidemiology of Work-Related Diseases*, 2nd edn, pp. 207–38. London: BMJ Books; 2000.

11. **Bernard BP** (ed). *Musculoskeletal Disorders and Workplace Factors. A Critical Review of Epidemiologic Evidence for Work-Related Musculoskeletal Disorders of the Neck, Upper Extremity, and Low Back* (Publication no. 97–141). Cincinnati, OH: US Department of Health and Human Sciences/NIOSH; 1997.

12. **Watson P, Main C, Waddell G, et al.** Medically certified work loss, recurrence and costs of wage compensation for back pain: a follow-up study of the working population of Jersey. *Br J Rheumatol* 1998;**37**:82–6.

13. **Kelsey JL, Golden A, Mundt D.** Low back pain/prolapsed lumbar intervertebral disc. *Rheumatic Dis Clin North Am* 1990;**16**:699–716.

14. **Bigos SJ, Battie MC, Spengler DM, et al.** A prospective study of work perceptions and psychological factors affecting the report of back injury. *Spine* 1991;**16**:1–6.

15. **Croft PR, Papageorgiou AC, Ferry S, et al.** Psychological distress and low back pain: evidence from a prospective study in the general population. *Spine* 1995;**20**:2731–7.

16. **Burton AK, Tillotson KM, Main CJ, et al.** Psychological predictors of outcome in acute and subacute low-back trouble. *Spine* 1995;**20**:722–8.

17. **Palmer KT, Calnan M, Wainwright D, et al.** Disabling musculoskeletal pain and its relation to somatization: a community-based postal survey. *Occup Med* 2005;**55**:612–17.

18. **Roland M, Morris R.** A study of the natural history of back pain. Part 1: development of a reliable and sensitive measure of disability in low back pain. *Spine* 1983;**8**:141–4.

19. **Kendall S, Burton AK, Main CJ, et al.** *Tackling Musculoskeletal Problems: A Guide for Clinic and Workplace – Identifying Obstacles Using the Psychosocial Flags Framework.* London: The Stationery Office; 2009.

20. **National Institute for Health and Care Excellence.** Low back pain and sciatica in over 16s: assessment and management. NICE guideline [NG59]. 2016. Available at: https://www.nice.org.uk/guidance/ng59.

21. **Health and Safety Executive.** *Manual Handling: Solutions You Can Handle.* HSG115. Sudbury: HSE Books; 1994.

22. **Health and Safety Executive.** *Guidance on Regulations*, 3rd edn. L23. Sudbury: HSE Books; 2004.

23. **Hiebert FR, Skovron ML, Nordin M.** Work restrictions and outcome of non-specific low back pain. *Spine* 2003;**28**:722–8.

24. **Kamper SJ, Apeldoorn AT, Chiarotto A, et al.** Multidisciplinary biopsychosocial rehabilitation for chronic low back pain: Cochrane systematic review and meta-analysis. *BMJ* 2015;**350**:h444.

25. **Evanoff B, Wolf L, Aton E, et al.** Reduction in injury rates in nursing personnel through introduction of mechanical lifts in the workplace. *Am J Med* 2003;**44**:451–7.

26. **Palmer KT, Walker-Bone K, Griffin MJ, et al.** Prevalence and associations of neck pain in the British population. *Scand J Work Environ Health* 2001;**27**:49–56.

27. **Ariens GAM, van Mechelen WV, Bongers PM, et al.** Physical risk factors for neck pain. *Scand J Work Environ Health* 2000; **26**:7–19.

28. **Palmer KT, Smedley J.** The work-relatedness of chronic neck pain with physical findings: a systematic review. *Scand J Work Environ Health* 2007;**33**:165–91.

29. **Takala J, Sievers K, Klaukka T.** Rheumatic symptoms in the middle-aged population in southwestern Finland. *Scand J Rheumatol* 1982;**47**:15–29.

30. **Viikari-Juntura E, Takala E, Riihimaki H, et al.** Predictive validity of symptoms and signs in the neck and shoulders. *J Clin Epidemiol* 2000;**53**:800–8.

31. **Smedley J, Inskip H, Trevelyan F, et al.** Risk factors for incident neck and shoulder pain in hospital nurses. *Occup Environ Med* 2003;**60**:864–9.

32. **Ylinen J, Takala EP, Nykanen M, et al.** Active neck muscle training in the treatment of chronic neck pain in women: a randomized controlled trial. *JAMA* 2003;**289**:2509–16.

33. **Viljanen M, Malmivaara A, Uitti J, et al.** Effectiveness of dynamic muscle training, relaxation training, or ordinary activity for chronic neck pain: randomised controlled trial. *BMJ* 2003;**327**:475.

34. **Aas RW, Tuntland H, Holte KA, et al.** Workplace interventions for neck pain in workers. *Cochrane Database Syst Rev* 2011;4:CD008160.

35. **Jensen MC, Brant-Zawadzki MN, Obuchowski N, et al.** Magnetic resonance imaging of the lumbar spine in people without back pain. *N Engl J Med* 1994;**331**:69–73.

36. **Kelsey J, White A.** Epidemiology and impact of low back pain. *Spine* 1980;**5**:133–42.

37. **Weber H.** The natural course of disc herniation. *Acta Orthop Scand Suppl* 1993;**251**:19–20.

38. **Datta S, Everett CR, Trescot AM, et al.** An updated systematic review of the diagnostic utility of selective nerve root blocks. *Pain Physician* 2007;**10**:113–28.

39. **Atlas SJ, Keller RB, Wu YA, Deyo RA, Singer DE.** Long-term outcomes of surgical and nonsurgical management of sciatica secondary to a lumbar disc herniation: 10 year results from the Maine lumbar spine study. *Spine* 2005;**30**:927–35

40. **Peul WC, van den Hout WB, Brand R, et al.** Prolonged conservative care versus early surgery in patients with sciatica caused by lumbar disc herniation: two year results of a randomised controlled trial. *BMJ* 2008;**336**:1355–8.

41. **Carragee EJ, Han MY, Yang B, et al.** Activity restrictions after posterior lumbar discectomy: a prospective study of outcomes in 152 cases with no postoperative restrictions. *Spine* 1999;**24**:2346–51.

42. **Magnusson ML, Pope MH, Wilder DG, et al.** Is there a rational basis for post-surgical lifting restrictions? 1. Current understanding. *Eur Spine J* 1999;**8**:170–8.

43. **Ostelo RWJG, de Vet HCW, Waddell G, et al.** Rehabilitation after lumbar disc surgery. *Cochrane Database Syst Rev* 2002;**2**:CD003007.

44. **Kalichman L, Cole R, Kim DH, et al.** Spinal stenosis prevalence and association with symptoms: the Framingham Study. *Spine* 2009;**9**:545–50.

45. **Simotas AC, Dorey FJ, Hansraj KK, Cammisa F Jr.** Nonoperative treatment for lumbar spinal stenosis. Clinical and outcome results and a 3-year survivorship analysis. *Spine* 2000;**25**:197–203.

46. **Wessberg P, Frennered K.** Central lumbar spinal stenosis: natural history of non-surgical patients. *Eur Spine J* 2017;**26**:2536–42.

47. **Budithi S, Dhawan R, Cattell A, Balain B, Jaffray D.** Only walking matters-assessment following lumbar stenosis decompression. *Eur Spine J* 2017;**26**:481–7.

48. **Mirza SK, Deyo RA.** Systematic review of randomized trials comparing lumbar fusion surgery to nonoperative care for treatment of chronic back pain. *Spine* 2007;**32**:816–23.

49. **Ibrahim T, Tleyjeh IM, Gabbar O.** Surgical versus non-surgical treatment of chronic low back pain: a meta-analysis of randomised trials. *Int Orthop* 2008;**32**:107–13. [Correction: *Int Orthop* 2008;**33**:589.]

50. **Fritzell P, Hägg O, Wessberg P, Nordwall A.** Lumbar fusion versus nonsurgical treatment for chronic low back pain: a multicenter randomized controlled trial from the Swedish Lumbar Spine Study Group. *Spine* 2001;**26**:2521–32.

51. **Phillips FM, Slosar PJ, Youssef JA, Andersson G, Papatheofanis F.** Lumbar spine fusion for chronic low back pain due to degenerative disc disease: a systematic review. *Spine* 2013;**38**:E409–22.

52. **Mannion AF, Brox JI, Fairbank JC.** Comparison of spinal fusion and nonoperative treatment in patients with chronic low back pain: long-term follow-up of three randomized controlled trials. *Spine* 2013;**13**:1438–48.

53. **Bydon M, De la Garza-Ramos R, Macki M, et al.** Lumbar fusion versus nonoperative management for treatment of discogenic low back pain: a systematic review and meta-analysis of randomized controlled trials. *J Spinal Disord Tech* 2014;**27**:297–304.

54. **De Kleuver M, Oner F, Jacobs W.** Total disc replacement for chronic low back pain: background and a systematic review of the literature. *Eur Spine J* 2003;**12**:108–16.

55. **Jacobs WC, van der Gaag NA, Kruyt MC, et al.** Total disc replacement for chronic discogenic low back pain: a Cochrane review. *Spine* 2013;**38**:24–36.

56. **Formica M, Divano S, Cavagnaro L, et al.** Lumbar total disc arthroplasty: outdated surgery or here to stay procedure? A systematic review of current literature. *J Orthop Traumatol* 2017;**18**:197–215

57. **Gore DR, Sepic SB, Gardner GM, et al.** Neck pain: a long term follow-up of 205 patients. *Spine* 1987;**12**:1–5.

58. **Bhandari M, Louw D, Reddy K.** Predictors of return to work after anterior cervical discectomy. *J Spinal Disord* 1999;**12**:94–8.

59. **Riew KD, Sasso RC, Anderson PA.** *Does Early Return to Work Following Arthroplasty and ACDF Result in Adverse Outcomes?* Presented at the Annual Meeting of the American Academy of Orthopaedic Surgeons, New Orleans 2010. Paper #539.

60. **Boonen A, De-Vet H, van-der-Heijde D, et al.** Work status and its determinants amongst patients with ankylosing spondylitis. A systemic literature review. *J Rheumatol* 2001;**28**:1056–62.

61. **Boonen A, Chorus AM, Miedema HS, et al.** Withdrawal from labour force due to work disability in patients with ankylosing spondylitis. *Ann Rheum Dis* 2001;**60**:1033–9.

62. **van der Heijde D, Han C, DeVlam K, et al.** Infliximab improves productivity and reduces workday loss in patients with ankylosing spondylitis: Results from a randomized, placebo-controlled trial. *Arthritis Rheum* 2006;**55**:569–74.

63. **Murray PM, Weinstein SL, Spratt KF.** The natural history and long-term follow-up of Scheuermann's kyphosis. *J Bone Joint Surg* 1993;**75A**:236–48.

64. **Aglietti P, Di-Muria GV, Taylor TKF, et al.** Conservative treatment of thoracic and lumbar vertebral fractures. *Ital J Orthop Traumatol* 1984;**9**(Suppl):83–105.

65. **Jaffray DC, Eisenstein SM, Balain B, Trivedi JM, Newton Ede M.** Early mobilisation of thoracolumbar burst fractures without neurology: a natural history observation. *Bone Joint J* 2016;**98B**:97–101.

66. **Weinstein JN, Collalto P, Lehmann ER.** Thoracolumbar burst fractures treated conservatively, a long-term follow-up. *Spine* 1988;**13**:33–8.

67. **McLain RF.** Functional outcomes after surgery for spinal fractures: return to work and activity. *Spine* 2004;**29**:470–7.

68. **Lidal IB, Huynh TK, Biering-Sørensen F.** Return to work following spinal cord injury: a review. *Disability and Rehabilitation* 2007;**29**:1341–75.

69. **Krause JS.** Employment after spinal cord injury. *Arch Phys Med Rehabil* 1992;**73**:163–9.

Chapter 22

Musculoskeletal conditions, part 3: disorders of upper and lower limbs

Sam Valanejad, Julia Blackburn,
and Karen Walker-Bone

Introduction

Musculoskeletal disorders (MSDs) are one of the major causes of disability and sickness absence in the working population. Two related chapters on musculoskeletal conditions have covered systemic rheumatological conditions (see Chapter 20) and spinal disorders including back pain (see Chapter 21) respectively. This chapter discusses the main conditions that affect the musculoskeletal system in the upper and lower limbs, classified by site and including both inflammatory conditions and trauma. Advice on return to work after orthopaedic surgery on the upper or lower limb is covered in detail in Chapter 11.

In assessing fitness for work in MSDs, two aspects should be borne carefully in mind. First, the rehabilitation aspects that would pertain irrespective of the cause of the condition—based primarily on function and capacity as well as the workplace conditions and demands of work. A second aspect arises when the musculoskeletal condition is caused or made worse by work (work related). Some musculoskeletal conditions have a strong association with certain types of work (e.g. repetitive work or awkward working posture), so adjustments to work manage the risk of recurrence alongside the impact of residual symptoms or dysfunction.

Biopsychosocial model

The general importance of the biopsychosocial model in work rehabilitation has been discussed elsewhere (see Chapter 10). This model is particularly relevant in advising about return to work in the context of work-related musculoskeletal conditions, both specific and non-specific. Fear of re-injury is important, but particularly if the injury was perceived as work related. Perceived level of control, social isolation, dissatisfaction in the workplace, and multiple co-morbidities are factors associated with sickness absence. Occupational health (OH) professionals should assess the individual's level of distress and perception of the workplace and address any barriers that perpetuate sickness absence. A 'biopsychosocial' model addressing all contributory elements to absence is recommended.

Work-related musculoskeletal disorders

The following sections cover musculoskeletal conditions of the upper and lower limbs that are associated with well-recognized causal risk factors in the workplace.

Work-related upper limb disorders

The term 'work-related upper limb disorders' (WRULDs) is used for a spectrum of different medical conditions affecting muscles, tendons, ligaments, bony structures, circulatory system, and nervous system, from fingers to shoulder with extension to the neck. Other older terms used for WRULD include repetitive strain injury or occupational overuse syndrome.

The prevalence of WRULDs in the UK in 2015/2016 was 690 cases per 100,000 employees, resulting in the loss of more than 3 million working days.[1] WRULDs were significantly more prevalent in female workers aged over 45 years, followed by male workers in the same age category.[1]

WRULDs are associated with repetitive work over a prolonged period, sustaining awkward or uncomfortable postures or prolonged excessive loads, extreme range of movement of the joints, poor working environment, psychological factors, and stress related-factors. The most recent epidemic of disabling arm pain occurred in Australia where it is generally thought that beliefs about a change in a keyboard, perceptions of harm and disability, and availability of compensation fuelled a rapid increase in the number of cases in a group of desk-based workers. WRULDs have been reported commonly among assembly line workers, meat and poultry processors, cleaning and domestic staff, construction workers, pottery workers, hairdressers, secretaries, and call centre workers. It should be noted that almost all of these disorders can have non-occupational causes, but progress of their symptoms can be exacerbated by repetitive work.

Common symptoms are pain, swelling, stiffness, weakness, tingling, and numbness. Diagnosis is based on general and occupational history and clinical examination supported by medical investigations in certain conditions.

The management of WRULD includes preventative measures in the workplace to reduce the risk of occurrence, and treatment for the condition. Preventative measures should be based on a thorough risk assessment. The Health and Safety Executive's (HSE's) Assessment of Repetitive Tasks (ART tool) and Manual Handling Assessment Charts (MAC tool) are useful means for quantifying and analysing the risk at different workplaces (see 'Useful websites'). Consideration should be given to the employee's pre-existing musculoskeletal problems during the risk assessment and implementation of adjustments. The adjustments may include improvement of the workplace and equipment ergonomics and lay out, job rotation, adequate rest breaks, training and clear instructions, and redeployment.

Medical treatment depends on the type of WRULD, and consists of pain-modifying medication and non-steroidal anti-inflammatory drugs (NSAIDs), local corticosteroid injection, local heat or ultrasound therapy, physiotherapy, immobilization or splinting of the affected area, and surgical interventions.

It is also extremely important that psychological, stress-related factors and the employee's satisfaction at the workplace be considered and appropriately assessed to achieve a more sustainable attendance at work and a successful return to work after sickness due to WRULDs.

Under the HSE's Reporting of Injuries, Diseases and Dangerous Occurrences Regulations 2013 (RIDDOR), some WRULDs occurring with certain work activities must be reported. These are carpal tunnel syndrome (CTS) where the person's work involves regular use of percussive or vibrating tools, cramp of the hand and forearm, hand–arm vibration syndrome (HAVS), and tendonitis or tenosynovitis. Elbow bursitis and forearm/hand tenosynovitis in manual labourers with repetitive movements, and also CTS and severe HAVS are covered by Industrial Injuries Disablement Benefit (IIDB).

The most common WRULDs as recognized by the HSE, with the exception of HAVS (see Chapter 18), are discussed in the following subsections.

Rotator cuff tendonitis and tear

Progressive degeneration of rotator cuff tendons can result in tears that are a common ageing-related pathology without a history of trauma. In the occupational setting, inflammation or degeneration of rotator cuff tendons is associated with repetitive shoulder flexion and abduction. Full tearing is asymptomatic in nearly a third of 65-year-olds that may predate a reported injury, although the injury may have caused an extension to a pre-existing degenerative tear. Improvements from physiotherapy can be anticipated over 12–16 weeks. A steroid injection may improve symptoms initially, facilitating earlier physiotherapy.

Full-thickness rotator cuff tears can be repaired either arthroscopically or by open surgery. Full benefit from repair may not be reached for 6–12 months after surgery. Failure and re-tear occurs in 20% of cases due to inadequate strength of the initial repair, inappropriate postoperative rehabilitation, and biological failure to heal despite strong initial fixation.[2] A French study demonstrated that return to full-time work took between 3 and 16 months after surgery, and most of the patients aged under 50 years returned to work, although age was not related to the length of sickness absence.[3] In this study, the type of work did not affect return to work but was directly associated with the time away from work, with heavy manual workers having longer sickness absences. The patient's operated limb will usually be in a sling for 4–6 weeks postoperatively, before physiotherapy and more dynamic range of motion exercises start. See Chapter 11 for recommended return-to-work times.

Bicipital tendonitis

Inflammation of the long head of the biceps tendon results in anterior shoulder pain that can be aggravated by lifting the arm. The condition occurs with repetitive overhead motion and heavy lifting, although it can coexist with rotator cuff tendinopathies. The conservative treatment consists of analgesics, NSAIDs, rest, ice packs, steroid injection, and physiotherapy. Consideration for surgical intervention should be given if the conservative treatment has failed after 3 months or when the tendon is severely damaged.[4]

Frozen shoulder (adhesive capsulitis)

Treatments initially target pain reduction. Surgical treatments for frozen shoulder are indicated once the pain has settled if shoulder movement remains very restricted. Treatments to improve motion include hydro-dilatation, manipulation under anaesthetic, and arthroscopic capsular release. The time course for improvement is unpredictable. The pain generally lessens over 3–6 months. Most symptoms improve over 18–24 months but improvement may extend over 2–5 years. Around a fifth will have residual symptoms, usually not sufficiently intrusive to restrict activities, although some manual tasks at work—especially those involving an extended range of shoulder movement and overhead work—will remain a problem and adjustments may be required.

The UK FROST trial is ongoing until 2019 to compare the effectiveness of physiotherapy and steroid injection, with manipulation under anaesthesia and arthroscopic capsular release.

Epicondylitis

This degenerative tendinopathy affects the common extensor origins (extensor carpi radialis and brevis in lateral epicondylitis or tennis elbow) or flexor origins (carpi radialis/pronator teres in medial epicondylitis or golfer's elbow) of the forearm muscles. Epicondylitis is considered an overload injury. Lateral epicondylitis is more common than medial epicondylitis affecting 1% of working age adults at any point in time.[5] Repetitive elbow flexion and extension for more than 1 hour per day is associated with both conditions.[5] Psychological distress and being a manual worker are other risk factors for lateral epicondylitis.[5] Pain during lifting and gripping initially localizes to the muscle origin at the elbow, later radiating into the forearm. There is local tenderness, maximal 2–3 cm distal to the bony attachment, with pain reproduced on resisted activation of the respective muscle groups. Resisted wrist or finger extension particularly provokes lateral epicondylar pain.

Medial epicondylitis is associated with ulnar nerve irritation; lateral epicondylitis is occasionally associated with radial tunnel syndrome. Forceful activities, high repetition, or awkward posture (particularly gripping) are associated with epicondylitis.

Symptoms are usually self-limiting and resolve in 80% of cases by 12 months. Activity modifications form the mainstay of long-term management. Braces around the muscle origins, with pads placed over tender points, can reduce symptoms during activities. Physiotherapy should involve deep friction, stretches of the affected muscles, and eccentric contraction strengthening exercises.

A single targeted steroid injection may have a short-term effect, confirm the diagnosis, and allow symptom relief until activity modifications are implemented, but physiotherapy or topical NSAIDs are more effective in the long term.[6] Other injection techniques (e.g. dry needling) have limited evidence of efficacy. Surgery to debride or release the tendon and degenerative tissues can help in resistant cases, good outcomes are reported in 75–80%; forceful gripping and lifting is restricted for 4–6 months. During surgery for medial epicondylitis many surgeons also decompress the ulnar nerve.

Useful adjustments at work may include reducing load and frequency, gripping require-ments, lifting with the palm up, and providing larger-diameter handles to tools. A vertical mouse may reduce pronation for desk workers. Consideration should be given to psycho-social factors in the workplace.

Elbow (olecranon) bursitis

The aseptic or inflammatory form of elbow bursitis is more commonly seen in occu-pations with a risk of regular elbow trauma or pressure on the bursa such as gardeners, carpet layers, mechanics, plumbers, roofers, truck drivers, and people with regular writing activities.[7] Common symptoms and signs are swelling, erythema, and local ten-derness with full range of movement usually preserved. Pain is not frequent in the aseptic form. The conservative treatment for inflammatory bursitis includes NSAIDs, rest or ac-tivity modification, compression, ice, well-padded splinting, possibly physiotherapy, and needle aspiration.[7] Surgery is rarely required and may increase the healing time. Failure of conservative treatment is an indication for surgical intervention, particularly when there is functional impairment. Open bursectomy is the procedure of choice, although arthroscopic bursectomy has shown the same success rate with less postoperative wound healing complications.[7]

De Quervain's disease and tenosynovitis of other forearm extensor and flexor compartments

De Quervain's disease is tendinosis of the abductor pollicis longus and the extensor pollicis brevis in the first dorsal extensor compartment of the wrist. It is found in approxi-mately 1% of the working population.[8] It is more prevalent in females aged 30–50 years, especially during pregnancy or lactation. Forceful grip with wrist pulling and twisting movements aggravate it, but the role of occupation in its aetiology is unclear. However, a study on a cohort of French workers showed an association between the disease and repeated or sustained wrist bending in extreme postures and using a screw driver more than 2 hours per day.[8]

Initial management through activity modification and splinting improves mild symp-toms. A steroid injection helps around 60% of patients. Physiotherapy aims to stretch the musculotendinous unit and reduce irritation. If symptoms persist, surgery to re-lease the tendon from its tunnel has been reported as effective in up to 90% of patients. Complications include tendon instability (a snapping sensation with forearm rotation) and scar tenderness due to irritation of the superficial radial nerve. Return-to-work times after surgery are given in Chapter 11.

De Quervain's is more common than other extensors tenosynovitis associated with work. Similar clinical and pathophysiological conditions are believed to affect the flexor carpi ulnaris and flexor carpi radialis tendons at the wrist and in particular in women between 50 and 70 years old.[9] They usually respond to activity modification and wrist splinting but are associated with systemic polyarthropathies, hence, systemic steroids may improve symptoms. Steroids, however, can precipitate tendon rupture. Therefore, the patient should avoid heavy (resisted) loading and a surgical opinion should be sought if there is concern about this or if swelling persists despite treatment.

Stenosing tenosynovitis (trigger finger/thumb)

This degenerative condition is caused by hypertrophy of the annular pulley (A1) of the fingers' fibro-osseous flexor sheaths over the metacarpophalangeal joints. It results in painful catching of the tendon and finger snapping particularly with extension of a flexed finger (the thumb may lock in extension). Many cases are idiopathic, some are secondary to other medical conditions such as diabetes, rheumatoid arthritis, and amyloidosis, and some are occupational. Forceful and/or repetitive gripping activities are occupational risk factors for trigger finger seen more commonly in construction and manual labour, assembly line occupations, and administrative work involving repetitive typing and mouse clicking duties.

Treatment includes activity modification, NSAIDs, hand therapy, and splinting. Corticosteroid injections are a safe and effective short-term treatment, but are associated with recurrent symptoms at 6 months. A single corticosteroid injection may be offered as a first-line treatment, but percutaneous release is a safe alternative. Surgical division should be considered if injection fails, symptoms recur, or the patient chooses it.[10] See Chapter 11 for recommended return-to-work times.

Dupuytren's contracture

This affects the fascia in the palm, with nodules and cords forming, causing contracture of the digits. Most of the epidemiological studies in recent years have confirmed the association between manual work and use of hand-held vibrating tools with Dupuytren's contracture[11] (see also Chapter 18). Nodule tenderness usually resolves over 9–12 months but progressive contractures require surgical intervention to divide or excise the cords. Percutaneous needle fasciotomy and fasciectomy are the common methods. In the former, a fine needle is used to cut the contracted cord. It can improve contracture but is associated with a higher rate of recurrence than fasciectomy. Injections of collagenase enzymes to break up the cords are also available but have even higher rates of recurrence than needle fasciotomy. The Dupuytren's Interventions: Surgery versus Collagenase (DISC) trial is ongoing to evaluate the effectiveness of collagenase injections compared to surgery.

In fasciectomy, the cords are surgically removed. It has a lower rate of recurrence and improves contractures more effectively in severe disease as shown by a Cochrane review.[12] Many surgeons use splints postoperatively to help maintain contracture correction, but evidence suggests it may not help.[12] Guidance published by the National Institute for Health and Care Excellence (NICE) in 2016 advises that in selected cases, radiotherapy can be used to prevent or postpone disease progression and potentially reduce the need for surgical intervention (see 'Useful websites' for NICE Interventional Procedures Guidance IPG573). Recurrence is common, requiring revision in 25–30% within 8–10 years. See Chapter 11 for recommended return-to-work times.

Non-specific forearm, wrist, and hand pain

The diagnosis of these conditions is established in the absence of other discrete disorders. They frequently occur in settings of physically demanding manual jobs or prolonged work on keyboards. They rarely last more than 2 months, and if they do, diagnostic tests should be considered for other underlying conditions such as cervical spine pathologies. Consideration should be also given to psychological issues and work-related stress in prolonged cases. Modification of job activities and ergonomic adjustments should be considered for affected workers.

Nerve compression (entrapment) syndromes

Nerve compression is often idiopathic but may arise due to structural anomalies, tenosynovitis, fluid redistribution (e.g. obesity, pregnancy), or systemic conditions (e.g. diabetes, rheumatoid arthritis, hypothyroidism, and alcoholism). It can arise at multiple sites. Assessment of nerve irritation should explore the different potential sites of compression. The neck must be screened in patients with upper limb neurological symptoms; shoulder posture protraction may indicate thoracic outlet plexus irritation.

It is important to remember the potential for nerve entrapment at multiple sites, termed the 'double crush' phenomenon. This can cause symptoms that are out of proportion to the electrophysiology changes. Treatment usually addresses distal compression sites first, as any surgery is usually less hazardous.

There is considerable overlap between median nerve and ulnar nerve compression symptoms. Asking patients to specify if the little finger or thumb is involved may help differentiate. The presence or absence of resting and nocturnal symptoms distinguishes between fixed structural and dynamic (functional) compression. The former occurs when a nerve is compressed by an abnormal or sizable fixed anatomical structure (e.g. an osteophyte or inflamed surrounding tissues), and the latter is the result of nerve compression by moving adjacent structures (e.g. group of muscles or tendons).

Nerve conduction studies help diagnosis, but with dynamic compressions, if no permanent nerve changes exist, the results may be normal. With brachial plexus lesions, normal electromyograms of muscle groups that are not clinically implicated help localize the lesion to the plexus as opposed to a peripheral nerve.

In the absence of objective neurological loss (clear weakness, muscle wasting, sensory loss, altered sensory threshold), initial treatment involves modifying activities (e.g. care with posture and pacing) (Table 22.1). Splinting also has a role. By placing the wrist in a neutral position, the volume of the carpal tunnel is maximized. Any objective neurological loss should prompt referral as delay may impair recovery, even following technically successful surgery.

Carpal tunnel syndrome

CTS is the most common peripheral compressive neuropathy. Symptoms are due to compression of the median nerve within the carpal tunnel and start gradually in the thumb, index, and middle fingers with tingling, numbness, or burning. With progression of the

Table 22.1 Management of upper limb nerve entrapments

Syndrome (nerve and site involved)	Typical pain site(s)	Characteristic clinical features	Investigation	Initial treatment(s)	Workplace modifications
Carpal tunnel (median nerve at wrist)	Hand and radial-sided digits (spares little finger)	Phalen's and Tinel's tests positive	NCS if doubt	Activity modification Wrist: neutral splintage Carpal tunnel injection	Reduce force/ vibration/repetitive flexion; pacing advice
Pronator (median nerve around elbow)	As for CTS, but more volar forearm pain and no night symptoms	Reproduced by resisted muscle activation (depends on site)	EMG (but may be normal)	Activity modification	As above
Anterior interosseous (AIN branch of median nerve in forearm)	Forearm; may be motor loss only	Cannot oppose tips of thumb and index	EMG	Observation	
Cubital tunnel (ulnar nerve at elbow)	Medial elbow; ulnar forearm and hand	Elbow flexion test	NCS	Provocation avoidance	Reduce elbow flexion and direct elbow pressure
Ulnar tunnel (ulnar nerve at wrist—Guyon's canal)	Ulnar-side digits	Normal sensation in dorsum of hand and negative elbow flexion test	NCS; imaging to look for cause (space-occupying lesion; hamate hook non-union)	Rest/splintage if no underlying structural cause Surgery (to address cause)	
Wartenberg's (superficial radial nerve compression in forearm)	Dorsoradial hand	Tinel's test provocation with forced wrist flexion, pronation, and ulnar deviation	Diagnostic anaesthetic injection	Wrist-neutral splintage (avoiding direct nerve pressure)	Avoid provoking activities
Posterior interosseous (PIN) (radial nerve at elbow, including radial tunnel)	PIN palsy: motor loss only Radial tunnel–proximal forearm	PIN palsy: wrist drop Radial tunnel– resisted wrist/middle finger extension, tender 3–5 cm distal to lateral epicondyle	PIN palsy: imaging to exclude space-occupying lesion, diagnostic anaesthetic injection	PIN palsy: surgical if mass lesion Radial tunnel–activity modification; wrist-neutral splintage	Pacing advice

(continued)

Table 22.1 Continued

Syndrome (nerve and site involved)	Typical pain site(s)	Characteristic clinical features	Investigation	Initial treatment(s)	Workplace modifications
Saturday night palsy (radial nerve in arm)	Motor and sensory (dorsum hand) loss	Wrist drop	NCS	Observation; wrist splint; maintain passive motion	
Thoracic outlet syndrome (neurogenic or vascular)	Arm symptoms	Adson's test Roo's test	Imaging (for cervical rib; arterial assessment if vascular symptoms; chest X-ray to exclude Pancoast tumour)	Shoulder posture and proprioception; surgical if vascular lesions	Ergonomics and pacing advice
Parsonage–Turner (neuritis of the brachial plexus)	Initial marked shoulder pains	Severe muscle weakness and numbness around shoulder	EMG	Shoulder posture	

EMG, electromyography; NCS, nerve conduction studies.

disease, grip power can reduce and performing manual tasks will become problematic. There are many known risk factors for CTS including occupation. Use of hand-held vibrating and percussive tools along with forceful and repetitive gripping have an established association with CTS (see Chapter 18).

Predominantly nocturnal symptoms may be relieved by a wrist-neutral splint. NSAIDs and diuretics do not improve symptoms. A steroid injection (with or without local anaesthetic) into the carpal tunnel (avoiding intraneural or intratendinous injection) temporarily alleviates symptoms in up to 80% of cases, with sustained improvement in 20%. Injections are useful if there is a clear reversible cause (e.g. pregnancy), early in the course of the syndrome, or if there is diagnostic doubt. A transient response indicates that surgical treatment may be helpful.

Surgery is usually effective. It may be open or endoscopic; endoscopic release allows slightly earlier return to work but has a higher rate of permanent nerve damage than open release. It usually takes about 3 months to regain full strength and a fully comfortable scar following carpal tunnel decompression surgery. The determinants for earlier return to full work are type of job (earlier for desk-based workers), younger age, altered work role, employees' motivation, and lack of anxiety and catastrophic thinking in response to pain.[13] Optimal safe return-to-work times are currently being researched in the REACTS trial but see Chapter 11 for the currently recommended return-to-work times.

Pronator syndrome

Pronator syndrome refers to compression of the median nerve around the elbow by either the pronator teres, flexor digitorum superficialis (FDS), or biceps. Nocturnal symptoms are rare (unlike CTS). Provocation clinical testing of the three muscles individually against resistance helps identify the compression site: elbow flexion with forearm supinated (biceps), forearm pronation with elbow extended (pronator), or middle finger proximal interphalangeal joint flexion (FDS). Conservative treatments should be tried—modifying activities, using a splint, and NSAIDs—as surgical treatment is extensive (requiring release of the nerve at all the above-mentioned sites) and the reported outcomes are variable. Half of cases managed conservatively resolve within 4 months. Up to 90% of those undergoing median nerve decompression surgery report good to excellent results.[14]

Cubital tunnel syndrome

Ulnar nerve compression most commonly occurs at the elbow, where it passes through the cubital tunnel into the forearm through the flexor carpi ulnaris. If the nerve is unstable, it subluxes anteriorly over the medial epicondyle with flexion (generally with a palpable snap at around 100 degrees of elbow flexion) and is more likely to require transposition surgery to move it anteriorly. In the absence of nerve instability or permanent neurology, initial conservative management includes reducing elbow flexion during activities (e.g. using a headset for telephone use), nocturnal elbow extension splints, and avoiding pressure from a desk or arm rest on the back of the elbow. Surgery decompresses the nerve; transposition is controversial, and reserved for cases where there is demonstrable nerve instability, an unhealthy nerve bed or in revision surgery. Endoscopic surgery is equivalent to open *in situ* decompression in terms of patient-reported outcome.[15]

Other upper limb conditions

The conditions covered earlier in this chapter are common upper limb disorders with strong or well-known occupational activities as risk factors. This section addresses some of the other upper limb conditions that may have less epidemiological association with work but either themselves or certain aspects of them can have a significant impact on fitness for work. Return-to-work advice following orthopaedic surgery to the upper limb is covered in Chapter 11.

Shoulder

Shoulder pain is common in adults. It may arise from the acromioclavicular (ACJ) or glenohumeral joint (GHJ), or the rotator cuff, and mixed disorders are common. Limitations in range of abduction indicate subacromial pathology and limitations in external rotation range indicate glenohumeral pathology. In the absence of 'red flag' signs that require urgent investigation and referral (Table 22.2), conservative treatment is recommended, including analgesia, physiotherapy, and workplace or activity modification.

The mainstay in the workplace is adaptation of tasks to minimize repetitive forceful shoulder motion, overhead reaching, vibration, and postures that provoke symptoms. Shoulder rehabilitation may take 12–16 weeks of treatment and exercises. Following surgery, rehabilitation generally involves a period of 4–6 weeks in a sling; see Chapter 11 for recommended return-to-work times. One-third of patients still have problems 6 months after treatment, particularly those with rotator cuff problems.

Table 22.3 lists some common causes of shoulder pain, their diagnosis, clinical management, and recommended workplace adjustments. A clinician's diagnostic flowchart and patient information booklet section can be found at the British Elbow and Shoulder Society website (see 'Useful websites').

Table 22.2 'Red flag' signs in the upper limb

Clinical feature	Possible pathology	Non-sinister causes
Night pain	Tumour; infection; acute rotator cuff tear	Frozen shoulder; arthritis of the ACJ
Significant trauma	Fracture; dislocation; acute cuff tear	
Redness/fever/systemic symptoms	Infection	
Recent convulsion followed by reduced rotation	Unreduced GHJ dislocation (posterior)	
Mass or swelling	Tumour; dislocation or fracture	Ganglion from ACJ

ACJ, acromioclavicular joint; GHJ, glenohumeral joint.

Table 22.3 Management of shoulder pain

Condition	Typical pain site(s)	Characteristic clinical features	Investigation(s)	Initial treatment	Workplace modifications
Subacromial impingement (also called rotator cuff syndrome or rotator cuff tendinopathy) Usual age: 30–50 years	Deltoid muscle and insertion	Painful abduction arc in mid-to-high zone	Ultrasound MRI	Analgesia Scapular- posture and control physiotherapy Subacromial bursal injection	Reduce: overhead activities Ergonomics to improve shoulder posture, reduce abduction/protraction
Rotator cuff tear Usual age: 50+ years (unless significant trauma)	As above plus resting/ night pains	As above plus possible abduction weakness	Ultrasound MRI	<60 years—consider referral; otherwise as per impingement	Reduce: overhead activities Ergonomics to improve shoulder posture, reduce abduction/protraction
ACJ arthritis Usual age: 50+ years	ACJ	High arc pain; pain on crossing body	X-ray	Analgesia ACJ injection	Reduce: overhead activities Ergonomics to improve shoulder posture, reduce abduction/protraction
GHJ arthritis Usual age: 60+ years	Deep in shoulder	Global restriction of active and passive motion	X-ray	Analgesia; consider GHJ injection	As above and reduce rotation
Recurrent GHJ anterior dislocation	Anterior with provoking motions	Apprehension on provocation testing	MR arthrogram	Proprioceptive retraining and cuff strengthening physiotherapy, surgical stabilization	Avoid contact/provoking activities, e.g. pulling/lifting
Frozen shoulder	Deep in shoulder (sometimes precipitant trauma) Nerve-pattern arm pains, night pain, commoner in diabetics	Global restriction of active and passive motion	X-ray	Ample analgesia (use neurogenic painkillers if radiating pain); GHJ injection; mobilization exercises *after* pain subsides	Avoid pain-provoking activities during painful phase

ACJ, acromioclavicular joint; GHJ, glenohumeral joint; MR, magnetic resonance; MRI, magnetic resonance imaging.

The mainstay of initial treatment is physiotherapy to improve the position of the shoulder blade. Strengthening of the rotator cuff (such as with resistance bands) should commence only *after* scapular posture has been addressed, for fear of worsening symptoms.

In the absence of a full-thickness cuff tear, the GHJ, subacromial bursa, and ACJ represent separate cavities. A response to local anaesthetic injections into one of these sites helps to confirm the diagnosis. Injection into the subacromial bursa reduces impingement pain in the short term while shoulder posture can be improved by physiotherapy. Steroid injections into the bursa are probably no more effective than alternative treatments (physiotherapy and NSAIDs).[6] Steroids can cause atrophy to tendons and joint cartilage, so generally a maximum of three injections is recommended. If no alternative treatments exist (e.g. arthritic joints), surgery may be justified to accelerate symptom relief. Injections of autologous blood or platelet-rich plasma have not been shown to be effective.

ACJ pain

Pain from an irritable ACJ can improve significantly by improving shoulder posture. Injection into the joint can provide short-lived relief. Surgery to remove the lateral end of the clavicle can be undertaken, generally with a successful return to full activities including work. See Chapter 11 for recommended return-to-work times.

GHJ arthritis and joint replacement

According to the National Joint Registry, 5221 primary shoulder replacements took place in England, Wales, and Northern Ireland in 2015, 57% of which were due to GHJ arthritis. Following surgery, the discomfort subsides over 6–8 weeks but physiotherapy for scapular posture is essential to avoid impingement. Over 90% of patients experience improvement in pain and range of movement. Loosening of the socket is seen after total shoulder replacement. Heavy activity can contribute to earlier implant failure. See Chapter 11 for recommended return-to-work times.

Subacromial decompression

Arthroscopic subacromial decompression surgery improves symptoms in 80% of patients with impingement, particularly if individuals have seen improvement from a steroid injection. Postoperative physiotherapy is essential (as for steroid injections).

GHJ stabilization

The risk of recurrent dislocation of the GHJ is greatest in males under 25 years of age. In these cases, investigation with magnetic resonance imaging (MRI) is recommended and arthroscopic anatomical stabilization may be required. Patients over 40 years old have around a 40% risk of associated rotator cuff tear so should also have specialist imaging as recommended by the British Elbow and Shoulder Society's guidelines.

The surgery may be either arthroscopic (which reduces the time in a sling to around 3 weeks) or an open procedure. Rehabilitation may involve no active movements of the shoulder joint for the first 6 weeks, then exercises to increase range of movement and adequate scapular control until 5 months, followed by exercises to increase strength. Ongoing improvements may be seen up to 1 year. See Chapter 11 for recommended return-to-work times.

Elbow

Elbow pain may arise from the joint, mainly due to arthritis, and the surrounding soft tissue attachments (lateral and medial epicondylitis and cubital tunnel syndrome, addressed earlier in this chapter).

Elbow osteoarthritis (OA) is usually a consequence of previous trauma or inflammatory arthritis. Patients may complain of pain, stiffness (loss of extension affects reach, loss of flexion affects getting the hand to the face), and intermittent catching or locking (from a loose body or inflamed synovium). There may be hand pain, numbness, and weakness from secondary ulnar nerve entrapment. Restricted forearm rotation limits the ability to place the palm facing upwards, producing difficulties with tasks that require cupping of the hands. Compensatory shoulder abduction may cause shoulder impingement when pronation is restricted.

Intra-articular steroids can reduce synovitic pain and locking due to synovitis. Physiotherapy may help overcome early stiffness. Appliances and adjustments to the workstation and work environment can help to overcome problems with reach. Surgery has a limited role. Arthroscopic removal of loose bodies and a synovectomy relieves intermittent catching or locking. Arthrolysis surgery may improve the range of motion (100 degrees of flexion–extension and forearm rotation enable 90% of tasks of daily living).

In the workplace, modifications should accommodate the restricted range of motion, and minimize lifting (where this precipitates pain). Following arthrolysis or ulnar nerve decompression, gentle activities can be resumed as symptoms allow. Significant lifting is restricted for 6–8 weeks after arthrolysis, and longer (up to 12 weeks) if the triceps tendon has been divided (see Chapter 11). Procedures vary between patients so liaison with the surgeon about rehabilitation is important.

Elbow arthroplasty

Most elbow replacement surgery is done for inflammatory disease such as rheumatoid arthritis. Elbow replacement can improve pain in patients with OA, but the ability to fully extend the elbow may not be restored.[16] Elbow replacement may not be suitable for younger patients with higher functional demand, as patients should never lift more than 2.5 kg after surgery to prevent early implant failure.

Wrist

Wrist pain

Pains felt around the wrist may arise from the joint (bones and ligaments) or adjacent nerves and tendons. CTS and Wartenberg's syndrome may present with wrist pain. Pains from the joints are described as 'deep' or as a 'band'; pain from nerves and tendons are described as 'longitudinal'; and nerve pain has associated paraesthesia. Tenosynovitis is associated with swelling along the tendons. Ganglion cysts are rarely the source of pain.

Wrist and hand problems affect grip strength that may affect the individual's safety to drive, climb ladders, use cutting tools, or work at heights. In this situation, decisions on fitness to work will depend on the scope for job modification (see Table 22.4) and the safety-critical aspect of the work.

Table 22.4 Management of wrist pain

Condition	Typical pain site(s)	Characteristic clinical features	Investigation	Initial treatment(s)	Workplace modifications
Arthritis: thumb-base	Thumb base	Worse on thumb ray compression	X-ray	Splint; analgesics; intra-articular steroid injection	Appliances to aid/avoid grip (e.g. ball type mouse)
Arthritis: wrist	Deep in wrist	Painful restriction range of motion			Reduce flexion/extension
Tenosynovitis: de Quervain	Radial aspect wrist and forearm	Worse on thumb traction (Finkelstein's test)	Ultrasound	Activity modification; splint; analgesics; tendon sheath steroid injection	Reduce grip and wrist twisting Ball type mouse
Tenosynovitis: flexor	Palmar aspect forearm	Tenderness along affected tendons			Reduce wrist flexion
Tenosynovitis: extensor	Dorsal aspect wrist and forearm				Reduce wrist extension
Ulnocarpal abutment	Runs down ulnar side of wrist or forearm	Worse on ulnar deviation of wrist or forearm rotation	Neutral rotation wrist X-ray	Radiocarpal intra-articular steroid injection	Split keyboard; vertical mouse
Scaphoid non-union	Radial sided	Local tenderness	Scaphoid plain X-rays	Surgical opinion	
Scapholunate ligament insufficiency	Dorsoradial	Watson's pivot shift test	MR arthrogram	Wrist flexor and extensor strengthening and proprioception exercises	

MR, magnetic resonance.

Ulnocarpal abutment

Some individuals have a relatively long ulna that predisposes to soft tissue and joint surface damage. Soft tissue damage can be debrided arthroscopically, following which manual tasks should be avoided pending wound healing. More significant lesions may require an ulnar-shortening osteotomy, following which delayed union and non-union of the osteotomy may occur, particularly in smokers. Heavy manual tasks should be avoided pending union (see Chapter 11). Alternatively, excision of the distal ulnar head (a wafer procedure) offers quicker rehabilitation.

Scaphoid non-union

An un-united scaphoid fracture can cause symptoms years later, as arthritis develops. Scaphoid reconstruction with bone grafting and fixation is recommended to reduce the long-term risk of arthritis. Delayed surgery is less likely to be successful. Postoperatively, splinting will be required for up to 12 weeks, and gripping may need to be avoided for a similar period, depending on the surgical findings (see Chapter 11). Wrist motion is likely to be reduced in the long term, and discomfort may persist.

Scapholunate insufficiency

After a fall onto the wrist, pain, weakness, a 'clunking', or giving way may be due to scapholunate ligament insufficiency. Ongoing symptoms, despite physiotherapy, may require ligament reconstruction and/or capsulodesis with a cast or splint for 6–8 weeks, during which time manual tasks must be avoided (see Chapter 11).

Wrist and thumb OA

Widening of the scapholunate space can occur in primary arthritic degeneration, hence this sign does not necessarily imply a traumatic origin, as it may predate any injury.

If conservative measures are insufficient, surgical options for the wrist may improve pain. Motion-preserving options include denervation (to reduce background aching pains), removal of the radial styloid process (for mechanical impingement pains), excision arthroplasty (to alleviate arthritic pain), and partial wrist fusion (fusing either the radiocarpal or the mid-carpal joint. Options for joint replacement exist, but are beset by problems of prosthetic loosening. NICE guidance is that wrist replacement surgery should only be used in selected patients by surgeons with special expertise (see 'Useful websites' for NICE guidance (IPG271)). The most durable solution to wrist arthritis is total wrist fusion, which requires lengthy rehabilitation of 3–4 months. Approximately 70% of individuals can then return to manual duties postoperatively.

Arthritis of the thumb base (carpometacarpal joint) may present with variable degrees of pain, reduction of thumb mobility, and joint deformity. Worsening OA at the thumb base can be reliably addressed by trapeziectomy as a form of excision arthroplasty. The long-term outcomes of trapeziectomy are good but pain may take 3 months to settle.

Following trapeziectomy, healing must occur before manual jobs can be considered (usually at 6 weeks). Fusion of the thumb base improves pain and allows young, higher-demand patients to return to heavy manual labour. After fusion surgery, manual tasks can only be undertaken after union (around 8 weeks). Total joint replacement surgery and interposition arthroplasty with a spacer device are also available, but are not widely used. The Norwegian Arthroplasty Register identified 479 total joint replacements over a 17-year period and found 90% implant survival at 10 years.[17]

Hand

The common hand conditions in relation to work have been addressed earlier in this chapter. General management of these conditions at the workplace depends on the type of the job, diagnosis, psychosocial factors, and available resources. For example, keyboard shortcuts can reduce mouse use and reprogrammed 'hot keys' and 'sticky keys' act as multiple keys simultaneously. Input device designs are manifold, including vertical mice (which reduce forearm pronation), ball or bar roller devices, graphics pens and pads, joysticks, and finger-held trackerballs. Voice-activated software helps if hand symptoms affect typing (it can be used in open plan offices but requires careful proof-reading). The charity AbilityNet advises disabled computer users (see 'Useful websites'). Electric staplers and hole-punchers reduce forceful wrist use. Larger-handled tools generally improve grip comfort for those with arthritic hands.

Digital arthritis

Small joint arthritis affecting the digits causes pain and stiffness. Multiple joints are commonly involved, often symmetrically. Initial treatments involve analgesia, physiotherapy, and advice from occupational therapists on the use of appliances. Fusion should improve pain and function but will prevent range of motion. Manual work is possible after 8 weeks. Metacarpophalangeal joint and interphalangeal joint replacements, typically made of a silicone-based material or newer ceramics, are available for end-stage arthritis. They have been shown to improve pain but may not improve range of movement (see 'Useful websites' for NICE guidance (IPG110)). Hand therapy can commence once the wounds have healed at approximately 2 weeks after surgery (see Chapter 11).

Hypothenar hammer syndrome

Thrombosis of the ulnar artery at the wrist is thought to be due to using the heel of the hand as a blunt instrument. It gives rise to pain, cold intolerance, and sometimes ulceration (in particular affecting the ring finger). Vascular reconstruction may be required.

Work-related lower limb disorders

Work-related lower limb disorders (WRLLDs) can be aetiologically classified into two major groups: those which result from acute injuries and those associated with overuse or cumulative injuries. The former occur when the affected structure in the lower limb fails as a result of exposure to a sudden and heavy load. Fractures, dislocations, meniscal tears, and acute ligament sprain or rupture are common examples. Overuse injuries are associated with exposure to less severe loads that over time exceed the tolerance of the affected structure. Examples include bursitis, OA, meniscal degenerative lesions, stress fractures, and Achilles tendinitis.

The general prevalence of WRLLDs has been reported by different studies as between 10% and 60% of all the work-related MSDs, depending on the specific worker popula- tions and type of study, with the knee being the most affected structure.[18] The prevalence of reported WRLLDs in 2015/2016 in the UK was 320 per 100,000 employees, totalling 103,000 cases.[1]

General workplace adaptations for lower limb problems

Lower limb problems may significantly limit work attendance. Maintaining work is im- portant, however, as employees who cease working while waiting for operative procedures are less likely to return. In one study of patients awaiting hip or knee surgery, 30% were off work because of their joint problems. The additional workplace flexibility afforded by larger employers may improve the patient's ability to keep working.[19]

Support for employees may include altered hours to avoid rush hour travel, provision of a parking space, temporary office relocation, and alteration of duties to reduce the distances walked or the time spent standing. Access to fire escapes, toilets, and dining fa- cilities must be considered. Individuals with a chronic disability may approach Access to Work to pay for taxis into work and specialist workplace adaptations. Arrangements for home working may help an individual awaiting surgery or convalescing. An individual with foot problems may struggle to wear safety footwear but a trainer-type safety shoe is sometimes suitable. Work using ladders or at heights may not be safe if there is concern about coordination, strength, or weakness of the lower limb.

Simple equipment (e.g. a trolley or chair) may significantly improve an individual's comfort or safety. If there is hip stiffness, a higher stool may be more comfortable than a low chair. A footstool can help if foot or ankle swelling is a problem. All equipment (including crutches) requires sufficient space to manoeuvre safely. Under the Equality Act 2010, employers have a duty to make reasonable access adaptations for the less mobile employee and for those with chronic health conditions.

Some of the common WRLLDs are discussed here. Return-to-work advice following orthopaedic surgery to the lower limb is covered in Chapter 11.

Knee

Bursitis

Bursitis is inflammation of the bursal sac accompanied by a fluctuant swelling arising over hours or days. Pain is felt on flexion of the knee as the bursa is compressed. Bursitis may be related to acute trauma from a fall, inflammatory conditions such as gout or rheumatoid arthritis, or repeated minor trauma related to occupation. An increased rate of recurrent bursitis has been shown in occupations involving prolonged practice of the following:

◆ Kneeling (e.g. suprapatellar bursitis, 'housemaid's knee', in cleaners, roofers, and plumbers).

◆ Leaning against the knee (e.g. fishermen resting against a boat side using their knees).

◆ Crawling (e.g. 'miners' knee').

In the carpet- and floor-laying industry, rates of up to 20% have been noted, particularly if 'knee kickers' (tools to smooth the carpet into the wall) are used.

The pain of bursitis usually settles within a few weeks with rest, ice, NSAIDs, and analgesia. In work, adaptation of the role or the use of cushioning knee pads may help, although the design of these must be appropriate. There is no evidence of the effectiveness of aspiration as a treatment for bursitis, and corticosteroid injection is not recommended routinely for the treatment of bursitis (see NICE Clinical Knowledge Summaries (CKS) in 'Useful websites'). If the bursitis becomes infected, antibiotics may be required. Recurrence is common. Incision and drainage or excision of the bursa is not advised acutely, but may improve chronic symptomatic bursitis.

Meniscal injuries

The menisci function as shock absorbers and allow a gliding action of the joint. They are at risk if the knee is twisted suddenly in a flexed position (e.g. playing rugby, football, and skiing). This often results in concurrent injury to the anterior cruciate ligament (ACL). Degenerative tears on minimal impact (e.g. getting up from a chair) occur in older individuals. Industries recognized as having higher rates of meniscal disorders include mining and carpet-laying.

Acute knee pain follows the injury but this may settle initially. Subsequent symptoms include pain, particularly on straightening the leg, stiffness and swelling, the sensation of giving way, and loss of range of motion. Patients may report a sudden painful 'catch' from the joint. A free fragment or a bucket handle tear can cause locking. Initial management includes rest, ice, compression, and elevation. Small peripheral tears occasionally heal spontaneously but tears that cause mechanical symptoms such as locking or giving way may be amenable to arthroscopic surgical repair or debridement. Arthroscopic debridement is not recommended for degenerative meniscal tears as it has been shown to be no better than exercise therapy.[20]

Knee arthroscopy

Arthroscopy is a low-risk procedure with a complication rate of 1% (infection, thrombosis, compartment syndrome, and haemarthrosis being the more severe problems). The patient returns home weight bearing but on crutches. For arthroscopy alone, without surgical repair, most people return to work within 1–2 weeks but remain off strenuous activities for 3–6 weeks (see Chapter 11).

Meniscectomy

Surgery is indicated for acute meniscal tears with persistent mechanical symptoms. Because loss of meniscal surface increases the progression rate of OA, surgery removes only the torn elements. If the knee is permanently locked, meniscal surgery should be undertaken promptly. Outcomes are very good and 85–90% of patients return to full function. Degenerative tears are generally managed conservatively with an exercise programme. Patients should avoid long journeys for the first 2 weeks to reduce the risk of deep vein thrombosis. See Chapter 11 for advice on recommended return-to-work times.

Meniscal repair

Young people with recent injuries and peripheral tears of the meniscus are most suitable for repair. Postoperatively they are more cautiously managed than after meniscectomy, but rehabilitation protocols differ between surgeons with little evidence to support any particular approach. In a young person with no significant arthritis, a meniscal transplant might be considered but the value in preventing long-term OA is uncertain.

After meniscal repair, rehabilitation takes about 3 months depending on the surgical technique. Early range of motion and immediate postoperative weight bearing have been shown to have no adverse effect on the success of meniscal repair, but rehabilitation protocols vary greatly.[21] Patients initially may require a brace, crutches, and physiotherapy. Leg elevation may be more comfortable and help reduce swelling. Many surgeons advise avoidance of deep squats for 3 months.

Anterior cruciate ligament injury

The ACL controls forward movement and rotation of the knee joint, which are essential for side stepping, pivoting, and landing from a jump. It is commonly injured in sports or traffic accidents and farming. Degenerative tears occur from more minor injuries. Half of ACL injuries involve other injuries, particularly to menisci and chondral surfaces.

Acute management includes rest, ice, and elevation. The acute swelling settles over 4–6 weeks and walking is possible. Injury is graded 1–3, where 3 (the majority) represents a complete tear and poor joint stability. Patients usually notice weakness or instability. Episodes of instability result in injury to the cartilages and joint surfaces that eventually lead to OA.

In degenerative knees in less-active individuals, conservative management is possible using bracing, joint stabilizing exercises, and pain relief. However, the patient may continue to experience symptoms of instability and need to restrict their subsequent activities.

Following complete rupture of the ACL, in an unstable knee, surgical reconstruction is recommended in younger patients who are active in pivoting sports.[22] Preoperative joint stability exercises are considered useful, and surgical reconstruction is not recommended until knee function has been optimized.[6] Reconstructive surgery usually involves arthroscopic grafting using autologous grafts such as a bone–patella–tendon or hamstring tendon graft. A satisfactory outcome with return to stability occurs in 90%. Graft failure occurs in approximately 2%, but rates are higher in younger patients. Other complications are rare but include deep vein thrombosis and sepsis.

Immediately after ACL reconstruction, weight bearing is encouraged. The majority of patients undergo day-case surgery with immediate intensive physiotherapy for at least 6 weeks. The majority can walk safely without crutches by 2 weeks postoperatively. Return to physical activity (e.g. gentle jogging) may not occur until at least 12 weeks postoperatively.

Postoperatively, 90% of patients regain near-normal knee function. Playing sport noncompetitively is possible at 4–6 months if adequate rehabilitation of the thigh musculature has occurred. See Chapter 11 for advice on return-to-work times.

Foot and ankle

Achilles tendinopathy (tendinosis and tendinitis)

This condition is related to degenerative change and excessive tendon loading. It is commoner in athletes and men aged in their 30s–40s. It is associated with obesity, biomechanical foot problems, fluoroquinolone use, increasing age, ankylosing spondylitis, and psoriatic arthritis.

Symptoms include pain, stiffness, and swelling that can be aggravated with exertion. Tendon rupture results in more acute and usually severe pain, with usually a positive squeezing (Simmond's) test.

Initial treatment should be conservative, including rest, weight loss, correction of excess pronation, and improved footwear. Eccentric exercises two to three times daily for 3 months reduce pain by 60%. NSAIDs and ice may help initially. Steroid injections can precipitate Achilles tendon rupture and are not recommended. NICE guidance for treatments in secondary care include low-level laser therapy and extracorporeal shock-wave therapy (ESWT), although it should be explained that the efficacy of ESWT is uncertain (for management of Achilles tendinopathy see NICE CKS in 'Useful websites'). Approximately 75% of cases settle with conservative management (footwear and exercises) over 6–12 months. The prognosis is worse if exacerbating factors are not addressed early on. In the acute phase, 'high-impact' activities (e.g. jumping and running) should be limited. Surgical management for the most recalcitrant cases usually involves debridement, with or without tendon transfer. Minimally invasive techniques, radiofrequency ablation, and laser ablation have similar results to conventional surgery. Most patients wear a splint after surgery with modified weight bearing for 4–6 weeks. The short-term outcome following surgery is satisfactory in about 60–85% of cases. See Chapter 11 for return-to-work advice.

Plantar fasciitis

Up to 10% of the population experience posterior heel pain, with 80% of cases associated with plantar fasciitis. The aetiology is multifactorial but intrinsic risk factors include age, obesity, and pronated foot posture. Extrinsic factors may include prolonged occupational weight bearing and inappropriate footwear.

Pain starts gradually around the medial or plantar aspect of the calcaneus. It is intense on first walking after a period of inactivity, easing initially then increasing again with activity and exacerbated by prolonged standing. Reproduction of the pain by extending the first metatarsophalangeal (MTP) joint is suggestive of the diagnosis. Ultrasonography and MRI may show a thickened plantar fascia (>4.0 mm) and fluid collection, X-rays may show a subcalcaneal spur.

Conservative interventions concentrate on reduction of biomechanical stressors, for example, weight loss, rest, specific stretching exercises, and arch-supporting footwear and shock-absorbing heel inserts. Over-the-counter shoe inserts, to prevent excess pronation, and custom-made night splints may be beneficial. A steroid injection may reduce pain but there is a risk of plantar fascia rupture and heel pad atrophy with repeated injections.

ESWT has limited evidence and NICE advises that injection of autologous blood should only be considered for patients with refractory symptoms (see 'Useful websites' for NICE guidance (IPG437)).

Surgical plantar fascia release helps a small subset of patients with persistent, severe symptoms refractory to non-surgical intervention. Surgical options include endoscopic release but success rates are variable.

Over 90% of patients recover with non-operative treatment over 6–12 months. Individuals require appropriate orthotics, supportive footwear, and physiotherapy to establish an exercise regimen. Some require a move to more sedentary duties for several months as symptoms dictate.

Tibialis posterior tendon dysfunction

This tendon supports the mid-foot arch and can become torn or inflamed by impact activities (e.g. court sports). Eventually this causes arch collapse or acquired adult flatfoot deformity. It is commoner in obese people, women over 40, and those with systemic inflammatory conditions. On walking and standing, the patient experiences pain along the medial border of the foot (or lateral pain if the foot collapses into valgus). There may be tenderness over the tendon, 'too many toes' seen from behind while standing, and difficulty rising onto tiptoe on one leg. Treatment includes activity modification, immobilization in a walker boot or cast, physiotherapy, appropriate analgesia, and arch support orthotics.

For patients without degenerative changes in the surrounding hindfoot joints, reconstruction of the failed posterior tibialis tendon with a tendon transfer is recommended. Surgical reconstructions require 6–8 weeks in plaster, mobilizing but non-weight bearing. It may take more than 1 year to detect maximal benefit from tendon reconstruction. Image-guided injections may be used for symptomatic degenerative changes in the hindfoot joints, then a 'triple fusion' of the subtalar, calcaneocuboid, and talonavicular joints is required. Postoperatively, patients are non-weight bearing for at least 6 weeks and recovery takes 6–10 months. The functional outcomes of triple fusion are not as good as reconstruction and maximal recovery may take more than 2 years. See Chapter 11 for return-to-work advice.

Bunions/hallux valgus

A bunion is a prominent medial bone and inflamed bursal sac over the first metatarsal head, usually associated with hallux valgus deformity of the first MTP joint; pain is from rubbing and pressure from the shoe. Bunions are commoner in women possibly due to ill-fitting footwear. Early severe pain arises from ligaments despite minimal deformity. Differentiation from hallux rigidus is essential, as degenerative disease in the MTP joint requires different treatment. Increasing deviation of the great toe causes subluxation of the first MTP joint, a 'hammer toe' deformity of the second MTP joint, and callosities. Patients complain principally of pain in the second toe. Increased use of the lateral foot area causes generalized metatarsalgia.

Initial conservative management includes use of comfortable footwear, a wide toe box, padding, toe splinting, and reducing the number of hours spent standing. High heels should be avoided. There is no evidence that night splints or orthoses improve mobility or slow progression, but they may improve pain after 6 months (see NICE CKS in 'Useful websites'). Surgery is indicated if conservative measures fail or if deformity causes a mechanical forefoot problem. Surgery is successful with around 85% satisfied with the results but 10% may have complications that can be severe (e.g. infection, joint stiffness, and ongoing pain). Long-term satisfaction rates drop to 60–70%.

Osteotomy is the mainstay of surgery but there is no evidence for the superiority of one operation over another. Minimal access techniques should only be undertaken as part of a research project (see 'Useful websites' for NICE guidance (IPG332)). Patients require 2–6 weeks of only heel weight bearing in a postoperative shoe or occasionally a plaster/rigid splint using crutches. Recurrence of deformity occurs in 8–15% of patients. Postoperatively, the individual should elevate the foot periodically and may need crutches. Older sedentary patients may undergo a bunionectomy with or without Keller's osteotomy (excision of the bony prominence). Recovery usually takes 2–3 weeks. See Chapter 11 for advice on return to work and driving.

Hallux rigidus

Hallux rigidus, often confused with bunions, is arthritis in the first MTP joint. Usually seen at 30–60 years of age, there may be a family history or a history of injury. Occupation is not thought to be causative but it often presents in farmers, sportsmen, and ballerinas. Symptoms include increasing joint pain and stiffness making walking difficult. Shoes that press on the joint or open-backed shoes requiring toe flexion cause discomfort. Examination shows joint swelling and reduced range of movement. X-rays show degenerative joint change and osteophytes.

Conservative management includes wearing flat shoes with a wide toe box. Rigid-soled footwear with a rocker bottom or a stiff orthotic brace ('shank') under the hallux also improves symptoms. These are available in the high street. Steroid injections, with or without manipulation, may offer temporary relief.

Cheilectomy for mild cases involves excision of obstructive osteophytes, thus allowing extension but preserving the joint. Recuperation involves 2–4 weeks in a rigid-soled shoe (see Chapter 11 for advice on return to work). Fifteen per cent of cases later require further surgery such as fusion or arthroplasty.

Metatarsophalangeal fusion

Fusion is appropriate in moderate to severe hallux rigidus. It usually controls pain but may limit footwear. Convalescence includes immediate weight bearing in postoperative shoes. Non-union of fusion for hallux rigidus occurs in up to 10% of cases. Some patients require a rocker bottom shoe long term and experience difficulty in squatting.

Morton's neuroma

Morton's neuroma, a common cause of metatarsalgia, is a perineural fibrosis of the plantar digital nerve as it passes between the metatarsal heads. Commoner in women, it may be related to footwear. Characteristic symptoms include pain, burning, or numbness in the affected metatarsal space or a 'pebble' feeling under the metatarsus. The third metatarsal space is most commonly involved, less often, the second or occasionally the fourth space.

Conservative management includes using rest, anti-inflammatory medications, wide toe box shoes, flat soles, and an insole with the metatarsal dome. There is little evidence for the use of supinatory insoles. Ultrasound-guided injections are highly successful and have made surgery virtually obsolete.

Radiofrequency ablation is a percutaneous treatment performed under local anaesthetic and image guidance causing thermal ablation of the nerve. Patients are advised to limit their walking for 1–2 days, and the procedure can be repeated if necessary after a few weeks (see 'Useful websites' for NICE guidance (IPG539)). It is effective at improving pain and avoiding the need for surgery.

Surgical treatment involves removal of the nerve. Success rates of 50–80% have been reported in non-randomized trials. Minor complications are common with recurrence rates of 4–8% and occasional severe refractory neuralgia. After surgery, patients return to full weight bearing over 2–6 weeks.

Osteoarthritis

Generalized OA is covered in Chapter 20.

Knee osteoarthritis and work

Systematic reviews have shown an increased risk of developing knee OA in workers who kneel or squat in their occupations with a dose–response correlation of kneeling or squatting more than 5000 lifetime hours.[23] Increased body mass index (BMI) accentuates the impact of repetitive kneeling and squatting.[24] Heavy lifting and climbing can also contribute.[23,24] The relevant industries include mining, forestry, farming, carpet and floor layers, and construction. Knee OA in underground coal miners with at least 10 years working in this industry, is a prescribed disease in the UK and covered by IIDB.

Employees may struggle with squatting, kneeling, climbing stairs, and walking on uneven ground. This may limit work participation in manual occupations more than sedentary ones, although moderate exercise is thought to have a role in clinical management and therefore is not contraindicated within the limits of pain. Adjustments and modifications of the activities at work in terms of job design or ergonomic interventions may help the affected employees to maintain an acceptable level of attendance and performance at work. Some evidence exists that symptomatic knee OA is less common in workplaces with the flexibility to allow job switching.[25] Severe cases awaiting surgery may well be covered by the provisions of the Equality Act 2010, requiring consideration of reasonable workplace accommodations.

Symptoms of OA include knee and anterior tibia pain on movement (e.g. going up or down stairs), difficulty kneeling, stiffness after rest that eases with movement ('gelling'), and night pain (late severe OA). Symptoms may worsen in damp weather and periods of low atmospheric pressure. Physical signs include crepitus, effusions, cysts, quadriceps wasting, stiffness, and valgus or varus deformity.

Initial management includes pain control, avoiding exacerbating activities, and maintaining function through activity (providing it is not painful), knee strengthening (particularly quadriceps) exercises, cycling or swimming, and weight loss. Paracetamol should be used initially in sufficient doses.[26] Assistive aids and management of sleep disturbance and mood are important. Knee taping may ease symptoms. There is insufficient evidence that heel wedges, knee braces, acupuncture, and hyaluronic acid are helpful.

Arthroscopy is indicated if there is a clear history of mechanical locking (suggesting a loose body). Newer techniques (e.g. microfracture, autologous chondrocyte implantation, and osteochondral grafting) may preserve articular cartilage in younger patients but longer-term studies are required. A realigning high tibial osteotomy may be used for single compartment arthritis in younger active patients, delaying the need for joint replacement for up to 10 years. Pain relief is comparable to that of joint replacement. These procedures require lengthy rehabilitation that varies considerably between surgeons. See Chapter 11 for recommended return-to-work times.

Knee arthroplasty is the definitive treatment for severe and progressively disabling OA. Referral for joint replacement should occur before prolonged established functional limitation and severe pain, refractory to non-surgical treatment, occurs. According to the National Joint Registry for the UK (excluding Scotland), nearly one-third of the total knee arthroplasties (TKAs) are carried out for patients under 65 years of age.[27] The majority of these prostheses survive more than 10–15 years. Partial or unicompartmental knee arthroplasty selectively replaces the damaged compartment, but is less commonly performed and has higher revision rates than a TKA (Box 22.1).

Hip osteoarthritis and work
Along with the aforementioned general risk factors for OA and within the occupational setting, heavy physical work and lifting, and prolonged standing have been associated with the development of hip OA.[31] Farming, construction, and other heavy labour industries are associated with the condition. Divers and compressed air workers have an increased risk secondary to aseptic osteonecrosis. In the UK, farmers with hip OA and a minimum of 10 years' work history are entitled to IIDB.

Pain is typically felt around the groin, the greater trochanter, and thigh, or referred to the back or knee and is characteristically worse after exercise. Stiffness worsens after resting. Painful internal rotation with reduction in the range of movement may be an early sign. Conservative management consists of pain relief, avoiding exacerbating activities, reducing biomechanical stressors (e.g. weight), use of walking aids, and cushioning footwear. Work-related activity that produces or maintains pain should be avoided. Deterioration to hip replacement often occurs over 1–5 years[26] with increasing functional limitation and absence from work.

Patients with advanced hip OA, who are limited by pain on weight bearing and walking, may struggle to undertake work in which these elements are prominent. More sedentary roles with opportunities for sitting may be considered as appropriate adjustments while the employee is waiting for a joint replacement (Box 22.2).

Box 22.1 Work implications: knee arthroplasty

Several studies have investigated the factors that predict the return to work after primary TKA, although their results have not been consistent in certain areas. A British-based study showed that age was the most important predicting factor for return to work as all the patients under 50 years who were working preoperatively returned to work, whereas less than a quarter of those aged over 60 years did so.[28] However, a Dutch study did not find any significant impact of age on return to work after TKA, while female sex, preoperative sick leave of more than 2 weeks, high BMI, and physically demanding jobs were associated with failed return to work.[29] Qualitative research has shown that delays in surgical intervention, inconsistent advice from healthcare professionals, and lack of rehabilitation from a patient's perspective influence the process of return to work.[30] The Royal College of Surgeons of England recommends that patients can expect to need to take analgesia for up to 12 weeks after their operation. Most individuals return to sedentary roles by 6–8 weeks (see Chapter 11). When sick leave exceeds 6 months, the prognosis for return to work is poorer. Postoperative stiffness is common. Stair climbing is affected if the knee does not flex beyond 90 degrees (and may need manipulation under anaesthesia). Patients report more difficulty with stairs, heavy domestic duties, and squatting than controls. Many forms of light manual and non-manual work are compatible with having a TKA and 80–100% of patients manage to return to their original work. It is possible to kneel after TKA, but it may be uncomfortable or unpleasant due to numbness around the scar. Very heavy work may not be appropriate after TKA. Similarly, high-impact activities that threaten joint loosening (e.g. jogging, contact sports, and military combat) are not recommended, although direct evidence on how the type of work affects prosthesis survival and functional outcome over the long term is lacking. Consideration of reasonable workplace accommodations should be considered in accordance with the Equality Act 2010.

Ankle osteoarthritis

Most ankle OA is post-traumatic from fractures (particularly malleolar and tibial plafond). Patients are younger than those with hip or knee OA. Symptoms include pain, swelling, stiffness, loss of range of movement, and valgus or varus deformity (end stage). Disability related to ankle OA can affect a person's quality of life profoundly.

Activity modification, use of a walking stick, ankle bracing, weight loss, analgesia, immobilization with lace-up boots, or ankle–foot orthoses, and physiotherapy to strengthen the ankle all offer benefit. British Orthopaedic Foot and Ankle Society (BOFAS) Commissioning Guidance (see 'Useful websites') states that there is no good evidence to support the use of phonophoresis (use of ultrasound to increase delivery of topical medications), prolotherapy (injection of dextrose), platelet-rich plasma injection, cryotherapy, or acupuncture and viscosupplementation is no more effective than

Box 22.2 Work implications: hip arthroplasty

Total hip arthroplasty or resurfacing significantly reduces pain and increases mobility. The majority of patients are expected to return to adjusted or regular work on average 12 weeks after their operation, with most of them carrying out their normal duties 12 months postoperatively[32,33] (see Chapter 11 for recommended return-to-work times). Standard postoperative movement restrictions include avoiding hip flexion beyond 90 degrees, hip adduction beyond neutral, and excessive hip rotation for 6–8 weeks to reduce dislocation risk. Most dislocations occur within 3 months of surgery. Patients are also advised not to lean forward while sitting in a chair, cross their legs, or turn their legs to reach their foot while sitting. It is also recommended that people sleep on their back for 6 weeks, as well as putting a pillow between their legs to avoid adduction.

Employees may need regular stretch breaks. A raised chair may help initially (chairs with wheels may be too unstable). Kneeling is usually possible. Flying is not recommended for 6–12 weeks postoperatively because of the risk of deep vein thrombosis. Patients may try to drive from 6 weeks (see guidance from the Driver and Vehicle Licensing Agency); most drive by 12 weeks. Many patients use ladders successfully but there is a risk of dislocation if the patient falls or lands heavily. There is concern that higher levels of physical activity after total hip replacement may increase the risk of implant failure by loosening, but evidence is limited.

physical therapy alone. Intra-articular steroid injections are a reasonable short-term measure (see 'Useful websites').

Bony spurs that cause impingement can be arthroscopically debrided to provide short-term pain relief. Distraction arthroplasty using an external fixator to allow movement has promising short-term results as an alternative to fusion in young patients. The external fixator aims to create 5 mm of distraction at the ankle joint that decreases the mechanical stress on the cartilage and improves pain. Postoperatively, patients are allowed to mobilize with full weight bearing by 2 weeks, and the external fixator removed at 3 months (see Chapter 11 for return-to-work times).

Both ankle joint fusion (arthrodesis) and ankle joint replacement are options for end-stage OA. Arthrodesis can be performed arthroscopically or as an open surgery. It controls pain in 90% of cases but can lead to arthritis in adjacent joints. The risk of non-union is almost three times higher in smokers (see BOFAS commissioning guidance in 'Useful websites'). Although outcomes are generally good there may be associated pain with limited functional improvement.

Total ankle joint replacement is less suitable for younger active patients because of the increased need for revision. Approximately 80–90% of ankle replacements last 10 years. However, up to 10% of patients report ongoing ankle pain that is not easily explained.

Patients may be in a plaster cast or walking boot and require crutches or a frame for up to 6 weeks after the operation. Range of movement is usually improved postoperatively and patients should be able to return to long walks, hiking, cycling, and certain sports such as golf (BOFAS patient information leaflet). More vigorous sports are not recommended as they may lead to earlier implant failure.

Trauma

Different biopsychosocial factors determine the success or failure of return to work following orthopaedic trauma sustained within or outside work. Poor outcomes are associated with older age, lower educational status, work-related injury, severity of injury, pre-existing medical or mental morbidities, compensations schemes, litigation, and an individual's pain perception.[34]

Fractures

With fractures, the associated soft tissue injuries are often more important in determining the long-term outcome. The clinician must consider whether the fracture needs reduction (perfect reductions are necessary when joint surfaces are involved, to reduce arthritis risk), whether the limb can be mobilized or needs protection, and the rate of rehabilitation. Bony union usually takes 6–8 weeks in the upper limb (and twice this in the lower limb). Loading is generally restricted until then. The bone then remodels over many months. Fractured bones can be stabilized with plaster casts, wires, external frames, internal plates, and screws or intra-medullary nails, and these allow earlier motion and loading.

For return to work, the ability to accommodate any splint, loading restrictions, and the required exercise programme needs consideration, bearing in mind safety in the workplace and the potential for reduction in employee performance. The need to elevate the injured limb (to reduce swelling, particularly if wound healing is not mature) and to restrict limb loading pending union of fractures, may delay return to work.

Removing metal works

Metalwork can be removed once fracture healing is assured, generally at least 9–12 months after injury. Implant removal may reduce local pressure problems (ulnar and ankle plates), improve range of movement (syndesmosis screws for ankle fracture), and allay concerns about infection and facilitate future reconstructions (e.g. if joint replacements are needed). Because there is a re-fracture risk, and often a higher complication rate with implant removal (than insertion), most implants will not be removed; however, employees may require 2 weeks off with initial restriction of high-impact activities on return.

Avascular necrosis

Fractures involving or adjacent to joints may disrupt the blood supply to articular bone giving rise to problems with union or avascular necrosis (AVN). Fractures of the scaphoid, talus, or anatomical neck of the humerus or femur carry a risk of this complication. AVN frequently leads to symptomatic OA. There are other potential risk factors for AVN such as HIV infection, sickle cell disease, alcoholism, chemotherapy, steroid use, and decompression episodes.

Pathological fractures

Pathological fractures occur following lower levels of energy transfer through areas of abnormal bone (e.g. tumour and osteoporosis), or repeated micro-trauma (i.e. a 'stress fracture'). The underlying condition influences the management. Stress fractures follow acute changes to loading patterns—either heavier loading with low repetitions/higher repetition of loading, or changing the way in which a bone is loaded. Increasing, persistent, task-related, and, later, resting pain after a recent change in activities raises the possibility of a stress fracture. Areas most often affected include the femoral neck, the tibial shaft, metatarsals, and the pars interarticularis of the lumbar vertebrae. The diagnosis is confirmed by isotope bone scan or MRI. Incomplete fractures may respond to rest. Persistent incomplete fractures or complete fractures require immobilization (potentially for months) or surgery, potentially with bone grafting. At work, risk assessment should address the provoking tasks and how to avoid recurrent stress fractures.

Dislocations

After joint dislocation, the duration of splinting depends on the subsequent stability of the joint—limited or none if the joint is stable, but longer if the joint remains unstable.

Interphalangeal joint dislocations without associated fractures can frequently be mobilized immediately with buddy-taping to the adjacent longer digit for a few weeks and attending hand therapy to help restore range of movement.

Patellofemoral dislocations may require immobilization for up to 6 weeks for a first dislocation (with or without surgical repairs or reconstructions) before mobilization.

Elbow dislocations tend to stiffen, so early mobilization is important (surgery to repair bone/ligamentous damage may be required). There is low-quality evidence that surgical management may reduce the recurrence rate, but no difference in function scores compared to non-surgical management.[35]

Anterior shoulder dislocations in younger individuals often cause significant soft tissue damage to the labrum and ligaments. The shoulder must be immobilized in a sling for a few weeks to reduce the risk of subsequent instability that is common in patients under 30 years. However, after any subsequent dislocations, early mobilization is permitted because the damage to the soft tissues has already occurred from the first injury. Older individuals have less risk of recurrent instability, so earlier mobilization is allowed.

Ligament injuries

After joint dislocation, significant ligamentous damage causes medium- to long-term problems unless recognized and treated promptly (e.g. tears of the knee ACL, the thumb metacarpophalangeal joint ulnar collateral ligament, or the wrist scapholunate ligament).

Ankle sprain

This common ligament injury is particularly related to sports activities, slips, trips, or previous strains. Lateral sprains (usually the anterior talofibular ligament), caused by foot inversion, account for over 90% of instances. They are graded depending on severity, from 1 (mild tenderness and swelling), to 3 (complete ligament tear with joint instability).

Ankle sprains should be managed initially with 'PRICE': protection, rest, ice, compression, and elevation for 48 hours with judicious anti-inflammatory medication. A semi-rigid support (e.g. a lace-up boot) and appropriate exercise is preferable to complete immobilization. Physiotherapy (but not ultrasound) may have positive short-term effects. Exercise therapy including wobble boards (focusing on restoring proprioception) may reduce recurrence rates and hence chronic ankle instability (which occurs in 10–20% of acute sprains depending on the injury severity). If significant ligament laxity is present, surgical intervention may be considered.

Most ankle injuries settle by 2 weeks and many patients do not require significant time off work. Those still absent after 2 weeks warrant further investigation to exclude occult injuries. Orthopaedic referral should occur if symptoms persist beyond 6 weeks. Patients may benefit from a footstool initially and a change to more sedentary work. Ankle instability may threaten safety at heights and on ladders. Post-sprain exercise therapy may reduce instability rates.

Many patients develop synovitis that causes persistent symptoms. This responds to a steroid injection or arthroscopy. Eighty per cent of osteochondral lesions of the talus improve following arthroscopy and debridement. Lateral ligament repairs have a good outcome in 90% of patients. Patients wear splints for approximately 6 weeks then lightweight splints and physiotherapy for a further 6 weeks. Sedentary workers should be able to return to work by 6–8 weeks and manual workers by 10–12 weeks. Return to running requires 4 months.

Tendon injuries

Tendons heal if their ends are apposed, but the associated scarring can cause long-term stiffness. This is prevented by using controlled active mobilization regimens following repair to minimize adhesion formation. If less than 50% of the tendon has been divided, partial tendon injuries are treated by bevelling off any tendon flap that may catch. The surgeon may restrict heavy manual tasks during the initial 4–10-week period, depending on the operative findings. If more than 50% of a tendon has been divided, full repair is needed. Following repair to flexor tendons in the hand a patient requires a splint to restrict function for 8 weeks. During this time, no gripping is permitted. Similar rehabilitation is seen after uncomplicated extensor tendon repairs. Repair re-rupture rates are around 5%; re-repair is possible, but should be done promptly and compliance with rehabilitation is essential.

Achilles tendon rupture

Acute Achilles tendon rupture classically occurs in men aged 30–50 years undertaking sports activities that load the tendon (e.g. squash). Chronic ruptures are usually seen after the age of 65, particularly if there is a history of chronic tendinitis and steroid tendon injections. Conservative and operative management produce similar outcomes. Early active weight-bearing produces better results than immobilization. Most ruptures heal if protected in plaster and then a 'range of movement' boot. A meta-analysis showed non-operative management had similar re-rupture rates to surgical treatment while offering fewer complications.[36]

Patients need casts or braces for 6–8 weeks as well as crutches and protected weight bearing. Manual workers may require 3–6 months off work. Long-term outcome depends on the timing of diagnosis and treatment. Most patients regain good function (at least 90% of power) if ruptures are treated in the first few days. Delayed (>4 weeks) treatment of the rupture results in an 80% restoration of power, which may affect function. Almost all younger patients in whom rupture is initially missed will require surgical reconstruction.

Amputation

Amputations are the result of vascular conditions, trauma, neoplasm, severe deformity, or infection. The majority of traumatic amputations occur in men younger than 40 years, often from road traffic accidents or combat situations. Early prosthetic fitting, rehabilitation, and psychological support facilitate successful functional recovery.

Problems in postoperative rehabilitation arise in relation to weight bearing, contractures, choke syndrome (venous pooling at the stump), wound care, and stump dermatitis. Phantom limb pain occurs commonly initially, but generally improves with time (Box 22.3). Transtibial (below-knee) amputees begin returning to work after 9 months, but following other major amputations, return to work can take 2 years.[37]

Lower limb amputation

Lower limb amputees take roughly 6 months to be fully weight bearing and return to work takes approximately 14 months.[37] They have a reduced capacity for walking, stamping, turning, and standing. Most prostheses do not allow ankle dorsiflexion, which affects stair climbing. The remaining healthy limb also undertakes significantly more work than in non-amputees and tires easily. Supportive adaptations include easy access to the workplace, and job modification to reduce the need for walking, running, lifting, carrying, and negotiating uneven surfaces. Work at heights or on ladders is contraindicated. The functional outcome of a transtibial amputation is generally better than that of a transfemoral or through knee because most amputees can use their prosthesis for a significant time per day. A higher level of amputation is associated with greater energy expenditure (physiological cost index) and reduced walking speed, although the use of crutches can mitigate this.[38] Amputees require restroom facilities to remove their prostheses occasionally. However, there are a wide range of sedentary jobs they can still perform and the Equality Act 2010 requires consideration of reasonable adjustments.

Box 22.3 Work implications: amputation

Return to work depends on amputation level, number of amputations, age, co-morbidity, mobility level, and ongoing stump or prosthesis problems. Educational level, salary, and employer and social support are also important. Sixty per cent of amputees return to work, often to a more sedentary role, and the majority of these are under 45 years old. Return to work should be phased.

Broadly, lower limb amputation affects mobility and standing while upper limb amputation affects manual dexterity and handling tasks. Both affect driving and carrying. The more proximal the amputation, the more functional the impact it has. An individual's pain control, mood, and confidence are substantially modified by their psychological status.

Upper limb amputation

Upper limb amputations are likely to arise from trauma or malignancy. Working age males predominate, the commonest amputation site being the digits. Upper limb amputation of anything more than a finger significantly hinders undertaking manual work. Loss of the thumb or finger affects fine grip and typing; loss of the hand (particularly the dominant hand) affects grasp and writing. Retaining part of the forearm permits some load carrying which is lost as the amputation level rises. Cosmetic silicone prostheses are helpful if aesthetics are important. Voice-activated software has made returning to administrative work possible.

A study in Canada found 82% of workers who experienced occupational upper limb amputation returned to work at a mean of 6 months after injury and to similar job types.[39]

Nerve damage

This may be in form of the following:

◆ *Neurapraxia*: damage to the myelin sheathes surrounding the axons. This usually recovers well over 6–8 weeks.

◆ *Axonotmesis*: damage to the axons, with the nerve remaining in continuity. This requires axonal regrowth to the end organ, so recovery is slow depending on the distance from the site of injury and the skin/muscle innervated by the nerve; regrowth occurs at an empirical rate of around 1 mm of nerve growth per day.

◆ *Neurotmesis*: macroscopic disruption of the nerve itself. This requires surgical repair to appose the damaged nerve ends for any recovery to occur. It carries a worse outcome.

Following nerve injuries, important outcome determinants include the patient's age, smoking status, systemic conditions such as diabetes, the integrity of the nerve, the likelihood of axonal regeneration reaching the appropriate end organ, and the injury mechanism (traction and crushing injuries damage a greater length of nerve and the neural blood supply worsening the outcome). Sensory recovery to the level of protective

> ## Box 22.4 Work implications: nerve damage
>
> After return to work, insensate areas must be protected from inadvertent damage (cuts, abrasions pressure, or thermal injury). This has safety implications in certain work environments (e.g. workshops, manufacturing, and catering industries). After 3–4 years it is unlikely that normal sensation will be restored. This may affect an individual's long-term ability to undertake fine manipulative tasks. After digital nerve repair in an index finger, individuals tend to grip without including the digit because of this impaired sensation, even if motion is unaffected. Joints affected by paralysed muscle groups need splinting and passive mobilization until motor recovery occurs to avoid fixed contractures (particularly important with ulnar and radial nerve lesions).

sensation should occur with time. Motor recovery depends on the distance to be covered by the regenerating axons—hence, proximal lesions may not recover before the motor end-plates decay irreversibly (Box 22.4).

Obesity and musculoskeletal problems

According to the governmental statistics, 58% of women and 68% of men in England were overweight or obese in 2015, nearly twice as many as the same statistics in 1993.[40] The global trend for increasing BMI is likely to continue, resulting in increased prevalence of obesity-related disorders in different body systems including the musculoskeletal system. There is a good body of evidence confirming the role of raised BMI as a risk factor for knee OA, and to a lesser extent hip OA.[41,42] Adipose tissue produces a number of cytokines involved in inflammatory processes. Some of these chemicals are specific to the adipose tissue (adipocytokines), most notably adiponectin, leptin, and resistin. Some studies have suggested a possible relationship between pro-inflammatory and inflammatory effects of these adipocytokines and the joint cartilage destruction in OA and inflammatory arthropathies such as rheumatoid arthritis.[43]

Obesity has been shown to be associated with foot and ankle tendinitis, plantar fasciitis, chronic plantar heel pain, meralgia paraesthetica (compression of the lateral femoral cutaneous nerve causing pain and sensory disturbances in the lateral thigh), and chronic lower limb pain with impaired mobility.[43]

A large-scale study on the Dutch working population with varied physical workload, demonstrated a significant increase in prevalence of musculoskeletal symptoms in overweight and obese workers.[44] The same study also showed that lower limb symptoms among obese workers in both low and high physically demanding jobs were more common. In another study on a small cohort of Portuguese workers, obesity and overweight were more common among 'blue-collar workers', and were associated with pain in the shoulders and the wrist/hand.[45]

There are several publications from Public Health England and NICE on prevention and management of obesity. Certain aspects of this literature can be applied in workplaces as part of health promotion programmes.

Reduction of musculoskeletal problems and other health conditions associated with obesity in the working population require a coordinated response to include education, culture, and organizational commitment to creating a health-oriented working environment.

Ageing workers and musculoskeletal disorders

The Office for National Statistics in a 2017 publication estimated that nearly 25% of the UK population will be over the age of 65 by 2046.[46] The same report shows that the working age population (16–64 years old) has contracted since 2006 and this contraction is set to continue. This suggests that a significant proportion of the workforce will consist of people with age-related musculoskeletal conditions who are beyond what is currently considered conventional retirement age. This group of workers have a higher prevalence of OA, other chronic arthropathies, joint prostheses, and regional musculoskeletal pain. These conditions, particularly when other co-morbidities exist, have a detrimental impact on older employees' functional capability for manual and physically demanding jobs.[47]

HSE's 'Ageing and work-related musculoskeletal disorders' report outlines that 'older workers suffer more serious, but less frequent, workplace injuries than younger workers, and that musculoskeletal disorders are often the result of a failure to match the work-based requirements of a task to the functional capacity of workers'.[47] This report concludes that older workers' decreased functional capacity make them more prone to work-related MSDs.[48]

The type of MSD and its treatment, retirement and pension benefits (or lack of them), the nature of work and its demands, employees' attitude towards remaining at work, and support from the employer for the implementation of appropriate adjustments at the workplace are the determining factors for the employment prospects of the ageing workforce.

Key points

- Work-related upper and lower limb disorders are major causes of short- and long-term incapacity, disability, reduced productivity, and sickness absence with unfavourable temporary or permanent outcomes for both the employee and the employer.
- These disorders either result from work itself through traumatic incidents, heavy load manipulation, repetitive movements, incorrect ergonomic postures, or a combination of these factors or are organic musculoskeletal conditions that can be worsened by work.
- OH management of these conditions, as for other occupational disorders, demands a holistic biopsychosocial approach with engagement of OH professionals, musculoskeletal

specialists, rehabilitation and physical therapy experts, supportive employers, and compliant employees in order to achieve favourable work outcomes.

◆ An OH professional is expected to be aware of the aetiology, relevant psychological and social factors, evidence-based therapeutic interventions, and prognosis of these disorders to provide robust recommendations to the employers on appropriate and suitable adjustments that could facilitate the affected employees' stay or return to work, even when they are still symptomatic to some extent.

◆ The ageing working population and the current increasing trend for obesity are expected to be challenging areas for health in the workplace and particular in the context of MSDs.

Useful websites

Health and Safety Executive (HSE). WRULD risk assessment	http://www.hse.gov.uk
National Institute for Health and Care Excellence (NICE)	https://www.nice.org.uk/guidance
NICE. 'Clinical Knowledge Summaries'	https://cks.nice.org.uk
British Elbow and Shoulder Society. Shoulder pain assessment	http://www.bess.org.uk
AbilityNet. Technology aids for disability	www.abilitynet.org.uk
British Orthopaedic Foot and Ankle Society (BOFAS)	https://www.bofas.org.uk/
BOFAS. Hindfoot arthritis	https://www.boa.ac.uk/wp-content/uploads/2016/11/Hindfoot-commissioning-path.pdf

References

1. **Health and Safety Executive.** *Work-Related Musculoskeletal Disorders (WRMSDs) Statistics, Great Britain 2016*, pp. 13–15. London: Health and Safety Executive; 2016. Available at: http://www.hse.gov.uk/statistics/index.htm.
2. **Lädermann A, Denard P, Burkhart S.** Management of failed rotator cuff repair: a systematic review. *J ISAKOS* 2016;**1**:32–7.
3. **Nové-Josserand L, Liotard J, Godeneche A, et al.** Occupational outcome after surgery in patients with a rotator cuff tear due to a work-related injury or occupational disease. A series of 262 cases. *Orthop Traumatol Surg Res* 2011;**97**:361–6.
4. **Churgay C.** Diagnosis and treatment of biceps tendinitis and tendinosis. *Am Fam Physician* 2009;**80**:470–6.

5. **Walker-Bone K, Palmer K, Reading I, Coggon D, Cooper C.** Occupation and epicondylitis: a population-based study. *Rheumatology* 2011;**51**:305–10.

6. **Coombes BK, Bisset L, Vicenzo B.** Efficacy and safety of corticosteroid injections and other injections for management of tendinopathy: a systematic review of randomised controlled trials. *Lancet* 2010;**376**:1751–67.

7. **Reilly D, Kamineni S.** Olecranon bursitis. *J Shoulder Elbow Surg* 2016;**25**:158–67.

8. **Petit Le Manac'h A, Roquelaure Y, Ha C, et al.** Risk factors for de Quervain's disease in a French working population. *Scand J Work Environ Health* 2011;**37**:394–401.

9. **American College of Occupational and Environmental Medicine.** Hand, wrist and forearm disorders guideline. Reed Group Ltd; 2016. Available at: http://www.dir.ca.gov/dwc/MTUS/ACOEM-Guidelines/Hand-Wrist-and-Forearm-Disorders-Guideline.pdf.

10. **Amirfeyz R, McNinch R, Watts A, et al.** Evidence-based management of adult trigger digits. *J Hand Surg Eur Vol* 2017;**42**:473–80.

11. **Palmer K, D'Angelo S, Syddall H, Griffin M, Cooper C, Coggon D.** Dupuytren's contracture and occupational exposure to hand-transmitted vibration. *Occup Environ Med* 2014;**71**:241–5.

12. **Rodrigues JN, Becker GW, Ball C, et al.** Surgery for Dupuytren's contracture of the fingers. *Cochrane Database Syst Rev* 2015;**12**:CD010143.

13. **Cowan J, Makanji H, Mudgal C, Jupiter J, Ring D.** Determinants of return to work after carpal tunnel release. *J Hand Surg* 2012;**37**:18–27.

14. **Lee M.** Pronator syndrome and other nerve compressions that mimic carpal tunnel syndrome. *J Orthop Sports Phys Ther* 2004;**34**:601–9.

15. **Aldekhayel S, Govshievich A, Lee J, Tahiri Y, Luc M.** Endoscopic versus open cubital tunnel release. *Hand (N Y)* 2016;**11**:36–44.

16. **Schoch B, Werthel J, Sanchez-Sotelo J, Morrey B, Morrey M.** Total elbow arthroplasty for primary osteoarthritis. *J Shoulder Elbow Surg* 2017;**26**:1355–9.

17. **Krukhaug Y, Lie S, Havelin L, Furnes O, Hove L, Hallan G.** The results of 479 thumb carpometacarpal joint replacements reported in the Norwegian Arthroplasty Register. *J Hand Surg Eur Vol* 2014;**39**:819–25.

18. **Okunribido OO, Lewis D.** Work-related lower limb musculoskeletal disorders: a review of the literature. In: Bust P (ed), *Contemporary Ergonomics and Human Factors 2010*, pp. 333–41. Abingdon: Taylor & Francis; 2010.

19. **Palmer K, Milne P, Poole J, et al.** Employment characteristics and job loss in patients awaiting surgery on the hip or knee. *Occup Environ Med* 2005;**62**:54–7.

20. **Siemieniuk R, Harris I, Agoritsas T, et al.** Arthroscopic surgery for degenerative knee arthritis and meniscal tears: a clinical practice guideline. *BMJ* 2017;**357**:j1982.

21. **O'Donnell K, Freedman K, Tjoumakaris F.** Rehabilitation protocols after isolated meniscal repair: a systematic review. *Am J Sports Med* 2017;**45**:1687–97.

22. **Meuffels D, Poldervaart M, Diercks R, et al.** Guideline on anterior cruciate ligament injury. *Acta Orthop* 2012;**83**:379–86.

23. **Verbeek J, Mischke C, Robinson R, et al.** Occupational exposure to knee loading and the risk of osteoarthritis of the knee: a systematic review and a dose-response meta-analysis. *Saf Health Work* 2017;**8**:130–42.

24. **Palmer K.** Occupational activities and osteoarthritis of the knee. *Br Med Bull* 2012;**102**:147–70.

25. **Chen J, Linnan L, Callahan L, Yelin E, Renner J, Jordan J.** Workplace policies and prevalence of knee osteoarthritis: the Johnston County Osteoarthritis Project. *Occup Environ Med* 2007;**64**:798–805.

26. **National Collaborating Centre for Chronic Conditions.** *Osteoarthritis: National Clinical Guideline for Care and Management in Adults.* London: National Institute for Health and Clinical Excellence; 2008. Available at: https://www.ncbi.nlm.nih.gov/books/NBK48984/.

27. **The NJR Editorial Board.** 11th Annual Report. National Joint Registry for England, Wales and Northern Ireland; 2014. Available at: http://www.njrcentre.org.uk/njrcentre/Portals/0/Documents/England/Reports/11th_annual_report/NJR%2011th% 20Annual%20Report%202014.pdf.

28. **Scott C, Turnbull G, MacDonald D, Breusch S.** Activity levels and return to work following total knee arthroplasty in patients under 65 years of age. *Bone Joint J* 2017;**99-B**:1037–46.

29. **Kuijer P, Kievit A, Pahlplatz T, et al.** Which patients do not return to work after total knee arthroplasty? *Rheumatol Int* 2016;**36**:1249–54.

30. **Bardgett M, Lally J, Malviya A, Deehan D.** Return to work after knee replacement: a qualitative study of patient experiences. *BMJ Open* 2016;**6**:e007912.

31. **Sulsky S, Carlton L, Bochmann F, et al.** Epidemiological evidence for work load as a risk factor for osteoarthritis of the hip: a systematic review. *PLoS One* 2012;**7**:e31521.

32. **Tilbury C, Leichtenberg C, Tordoir R, et al.** Return to work after total hip and knee arthroplasty: results from a clinical study. *Rheumatol Int* 2015;**35**:2059–67.

33. **Leichtenberg C, Tilbury C, Kuijer P, et al.** Determinants of return to work 12 months after total hip and knee arthroplasty. *Ann R Coll Surg Engl* 2016;**98**:387–95.

34. **Quested R, Sommerville S, Lutz M.** Outcomes following non-life-threatening orthopaedic trauma: why are they considered to be so poor? *Trauma* 2017;**19**:133–8.

35. **Smith T, Donell S, Song F, Hing CB.** Surgical versus non-surgical interventions for treating patellar dislocation. *Cochrane Database Syst Rev* 20152:CD008106.

36. **Soroceanu A, Sidhwa F, Aarabi S, Kaufman A, Glazebrook M.** Surgical versus nonsurgical treatment of acute Achilles tendon rupture: a meta-analysis of randomized trials. *J Bone Joint Surg Am* 2012;**94**:2136–43.

37. **Burger H, Marinček Č.** Return to work after lower limb amputation. *Disabil Rehabil* 2007;**29**:1323–9.

38. **Vllasolli T, Zafirova B, Orovcanec N, Poposka A, Murtezani A, Krasniqi B.** Energy expenditure and walking speed in lower limb amputees: a cross sectional study. *Ortop Traumatol Rehabil* 2014;**16**:419–26.

39. **Craig M, Hill W, Englehart K, Adisesh A.** Return to work after occupational injury and upper limb amputation. *Occup Med* 2017;**67**:227–9.

40. **NHS Digital.** Statistics on Obesity, Physical Activity and Diet, England 2017. 2017. Available at: https://www.gov.uk/government/statistics/statistics-on-obesity-physical-activity-and-diet-england-2017#history.

41. **Allen K, Golightly Y.** Epidemiology of osteoarthritis: state of the evidence. *Curr Opin Rheumatol* 2015;**27**:273–86.

42. **Lohmander L, Gerhardsson de Verdier M, Rollof J, Nilsson P, Engstrom G.** Incidence of severe knee and hip osteoarthritis in relation to different measures of body mass: a population-based prospective cohort study. *Ann Rheum Dis* 2009;**68**:490–6.

43. **Anandacoomarasamy A, Fransen M, March L.** Obesity and the musculoskeletal system. *Curr Opin Rheumatol* 2009;**21**:71–7.

44. **Viester L, Verhagen E, Hengel K, Koppes L, van der Beek A, Bongers P.** The relation between body mass index and musculoskeletal symptoms in the working population. *BMC Musculoskelet Disord* 2013;**14**:238.

45. **Moreira-Silva I, Santos R, Abreu S, Mota J.** Associations between body mass index and musculoskeletal pain and related symptoms in different body regions among workers. *SAGE Open* 2013;**3**:1–6.

46. **Office for National Statistics**. Overview of the UK population: July 2017. 2017. Available at: https://www.ons.gov.uk/peoplepopulationandcommunity/populationandmigration/populationestimates/articles/overviewoftheukpopulation/july2017.

47. **Palmer K, Goodson N.** Ageing, musculoskeletal health and work. *Best Pract Res Clin Rheumatol* 2015;**29**:391–404.

48. **Okunribido O, Wynn T.** Ageing and work-related musculoskeletal disorders. A review of the recent literature. Health and Safety Laboratory; 2010. Available at: http://www.hse.gov.uk/research/rrpdf/rr799.pdf.

Chapter 23

Neurological disorders

Jon Poole and Richard Hardie

Introduction

This chapter deals mainly with common acute and chronic neurological problems, particularly as they affect employees and job applicants. The complications of occupational exposure to neurotoxins and putative neurotoxins will also be covered in so far as they relate to the fitness of an exposed employee to continue working.

In addition to a few well-known and common conditions, many uncommon but distinct neurological disorders may present at work or affect work capacity. Fitness for work in these disorders will be determined by the person's functional abilities, any co-morbid illness, the efficacy or side effects of the treatment, and psychological and social factors, rather than by the precise diagnosis. This will also need to be put into the context of the job in question, as the basic requirements for a manual labouring job may be completely different from something more intellectually demanding. Indeed, even an apparently precise diagnostic label such as multiple sclerosis (MS) can encompass a complete spectrum of disability, from someone who is entirely asymptomatic to another who is totally incapacitated.

Furthermore, reports by general practitioners, neurologists, or neurosurgeons may describe the symptoms, signs, and investigations in detail, but without analysing functional abilities. These colleagues may also fail to appreciate the workplace hazards, the responsibilities of the employer, or what scope exists for adaptations to the job or workplace.

Size of the problem

About 10 million of the UK population have a neurological condition that significantly impacts their lives, and it has been estimated that 35% of disability-adjusted life years are due to brain diseases. One-quarter of those aged between 16 and 64 with a chronic disability have a neurological condition.

With the exception of malignant brain tumours and motor neurone disease (MND), relatively long survival rates mean that prevalence and disability rates of neurological diseases tend to be greater than their incidence. Neurological conditions account for about 5% of sickness absence and migraine headaches alone have been estimated to cost employers in Western Europe about €585 per affected person per year.[1]

Occupational causes of neurological impairment

The occupational health (OH) professional is more often involved with job adaptation and rehabilitation of patients with neurological disabilities than with eliminating the few known occupational neurotoxins from the workplace. However potential occupational exposure to organic solvents, organophosphates, pesticides, lead, mercury, or manganese, as well as traumatic brain injury should be considered in a worker with a behavioural or neurological problem.

Clinical assessment

This should include an assessment of the person's alertness and mental functioning, as well as their posture, balance, muscle power, coordination, and gait. Neurobehavioural disorders following head injury, stroke, encephalitis, or exposure to a neurotoxin may range from mild and transient effects that can only be detected by psychometric tests to severe and permanent impairment. Some are affected by communication disabilities including dysarthria or dysphasia, a visual field defect, or more global cognitive problems of which they lack insight. Dysphasia can preclude employment that requires good verbal communication, and dyspraxia may preclude work that requires good dexterity. Disturbance of spatial relationships may prevent the worker from driving, and the efficient integration of all cognitive functions is important for those with intellectually demanding jobs.

Disturbances of posture, balance, coordination, or gait are relatively easy to establish with appropriate clinical testing. Complaints of dizziness, light headedness, unsteadiness, or spatial disequilibrium should be distinguished from vertigo, which is a sensation of movement of the surroundings or of the patient. Parkinson's disease (PD) is a classic example of a movement disorder. Anti-parkinsonian drug treatment may minimize most work problems, but jobs that involve rapid or coordinated hand movements, good mobility, or fluent speech may still be difficult. Similarly, muscle spasticity associated with upper motor neurone disorders may prevent manual work, or even the ability to stand for long periods.

The consequences of neurological dysfunction may be different for manual and non-manual workers. Manual jobs that involve repeated lifting and moving require good muscle power, good coordination, and peripheral sensation, but a degree of impairment in intellectual function might be tolerable. If there is a radiculopathy from a slipped disc, specific movements of the vertebral column may exacerbate symptoms or disability. By contrast, an employee with paraplegia or a hemiparesis may still be able to undertake a desk-based job, although commuting to work may be a bigger problem than performing the job.

The impact of prognosis and rehabilitation on work

The impact of neurological symptoms on work can be considered broadly in three stages. The first stage covers workers with no health or disability problems who develop a condition, whether or not it is work related, that has the potential to affect job performance in the future if their condition deteriorates. The second stage is reached when the condition affects job performance, for which adjustments can be made. At the third stage, performance and attendance at work are adversely affected, but no further reasonable adjustments can be made, so for those in a pension scheme, eligibility to ill health retirement will need to be considered.

Some slowly progressive neurological conditions may move predictably through the three stages, but in others the clinical course may be unpredictably episodic, transient, or static. Such prognostic considerations are important to employment considerations and the disability provisions of the Equality Act. For example, the prognosis of MS is difficult to evaluate at the outset. The disease may never cause more than a transient episode of blurred vision or it may progress rapidly and inexorably to tetraplegia. Similarly, cerebrovascular disorders may range from a transient ischaemic episode with full resolution to a catastrophic intracerebral bleed. Most stroke patients recover, at least partially, so it is important wherever possible to keep their original job open, albeit if necessary in a modified form. Such modifications may be temporary or permanent and will require periodic re-evaluation. Co-morbid obstacles to returning to work such as depression, unhelpful beliefs, or non-medical factors need to be identified and addressed (see Chapter 10). The OH professional should identify the obstacles and advise on appropriate rehabilitation interventions.

After an acute episode, a neurologically impaired employee should not expect, or be expected, to have made a full recovery before work is resumed. The rehabilitation process will be enhanced if the patient can return initially to a modified or part-time job. Help with transport may also facilitate a return to work. The process of going to work and performing a job is an important outcome in itself, and ongoing rehabilitation will allow problems to be identified at an early stage. Therapy at the place of work can be of benefit to both employees and employers, but rarely occurs.

Similarly, those in whom slowly progressive disability is anticipated deserve careful planning to review their needs at intervals appropriate to the underlying pathology. Continuing at work may be a source of psychological strength to someone recently diagnosed with an incurable neurological disease, but both patient and employer must also be protected from unreasonable risk to health, performance, or productivity.

Specialist vocational rehabilitation services are available and the UK's Rehabilitation Council has drawn up rehabilitation standards for service providers (see 'Useful websites'). Disability Employment Advisers at local Jobcentres and Access to Work teams have financial and practical resources to help disabled people back to work and to make adjustments to the workplace.

How neurological illnesses may influence work

The disability that a patient suffers is dependent on the symptoms and impairments that the disease produces and not the disease itself. Certain disorders, and particularly brain injuries caused by a variety of pathologies, can lead to loss of function anywhere in the nervous system. The following headings provide a checklist to ensure comprehensive consideration of the key potential clinical aspects of a given neurological disorder.

Higher cerebral functions

Many neurological diseases will affect cerebral functioning. There are no guidelines that can be used universally and each case will need to be judged on its own merits.

Cognitive function and psychometrics

Possibly the most important consideration is the likelihood of a person with cerebral pathology suffering cognitive impairment that may render them unreliable or unsafe at work. In one community-based occupational survey, frequent or very frequent cognitive failures (e.g. problems of memory, attention, or action) and minor injuries were reported by about 10% of workers, and work accidents requiring treatment by almost 6%.[2] The extent to which cognitive failures could be attributable to organic neurological disease is not known, but they are clearly relatively common.

Detailed and objective psychometric evaluation may be necessary in the presence of some neurological disorders affecting the brain, depending on the person's responsibilities. For example, a person may require careful assessment to protect themselves from the risk of making errors that could lead to injuries to others or disciplinary action being taken against them, but also to protect their employer from claims of negligence. A feature of some cerebral pathology, such as dementia, is a lack of insight into one's own limitations, so it is imperative not to rely wholly on the patient's self-report.

The patient may already have undergone cognitive assessments, in which case the relevant reports should be obtained. It will be necessary to distinguish between results of screening tests, often administered by occupational therapists, and more definitive standardized neuro-psychological tests such as the Minnesota Multiphasic Personality Inventory used by clinical psychologists. In recent years, symptom validity (effort) tests have been developed by neuropsychologists to evaluate the validity of reported psychological or cognitive symptoms, such as memory loss. Inappropriate or inconsistent answers to questions or scores worse than chance are suggestive of deception. The best test to use for this will depend on the type of impairment being assessed, but the most popular in the UK are the Test of Memory Malingering and the Word Memory Test.[3]

The term 'ecological validity' has been coined to refer to the relevance of performance under formal test conditions to the patient's behaviour in 'the real world', which may of course be better or worse than expected from the tests. For example, a patient may perform well on specific tests of verbal memory in quiet conditions in an outpatient setting, but be incapable of taking telephone messages reliably in a noisy, hectic office environment. It is often better, if practicable, to allow an employee the opportunity for a work trial under careful but unobtrusive observation and supervision. This will help to build confidence, promote insight, and lead to better acceptance of a negative decision, and precautionary safeguards can be formalized or dispensed with. Memory loss can seldom be improved pharmacologically, but it can arise or be made worse by drugs such as anticonvulsants or psychotropic medication, in which case a reduction in medication before returning to work may be beneficial.

Simple memory aids are universally used at home as well as in the workplace, from the basic written 'to do' list or note stuck in a prominent position, to sophisticated paper-based organizers, 'smart' phones, and computer software. The demands of many jobs require such powers of cognitive processing that they would be beyond most average people without such aids. Nevertheless, behavioural approaches can be beneficial for the cognitive rehabilitation of those with memory impairment.

Behaviour and impulse control

Even when rigorous neuropsychological testing reveals no abnormality, a cerebral pathology can still give rise to disturbances of normal behaviour and impulse control with serious implications for employability. Sometimes these are apparent to lay colleagues and managers, particularly if they knew the employee before a traumatic brain injury or the onset of a neurological condition. Lack of attention to personal hygiene, appearance, and presentation at work may be a clue to the onset of frontal lobe dementia. Occasionally, and especially in MS, a euphoric mood may limit an employee's work potential.

Other changes can be more subtle and unpredictable, with outbursts of offensive language, physical aggression, or sexually inappropriate behaviour towards colleagues or customers giving rise to serious concern and perhaps disciplinary action. Such neurobehavioural changes can be associated with secondary problems that may be mistaken for the primary cause (e.g. marital breakdown, substance misuse, or side effects of medication), unless the connection is made by gathering information from a variety of sources with the necessary consent.

Disturbances of arousal and consciousness

Fixed deficits of alertness and attention are usually obvious, but certain conditions such as epilepsy can give rise to variable deficits, particularly where sleep is disturbed. Here the key occupational considerations are the risk of lapses in attention or awareness occurring at work, and the possible adverse effects of medication.

Sleep

Sleep disturbance is not uncommon in neurological conditions affecting cerebral function or associated with chronic pain or immobility, effects that can be magnified by stimulants and anti-parkinsonian drugs. Accurate diagnosis of the causes of poor sleeping is seldom achieved and simple effective measures such as reducing caffeine and alcohol intake or avoiding daytime naps are often not tried first[4] (see also Chapter 27, disorders of sleep). Epilepsy is the only neurological condition for which there is a relative contraindication to working at night (see Chapter 24).

Pain disorders

Certain neurological conditions may be entirely benign and yet associated with intense paroxysms of pain. Trigeminal neuralgia, for example, is characterized by lancinating facial pain that is difficult to treat. Post-herpetic neuralgia and migraine are other common pain disorders. Chronic regional pain syndrome (reflex sympathetic dystrophy) is frequently overdiagnosed in the presence of unexplained pain, but should normally be restricted to patients with localized allodynia, changes in skin colour or sweating, and, if prolonged, with muscular wasting. The key occupational considerations are the risk of incapacitation occurring at work due to pain and the possible adverse effects of medication.

Speech, language, and communication

Speech disorders, whether dysphasia, dysphonia, or dysarthria, can be helped by speech therapy, but it is rare for major improvement to occur without recovery of the underlying condition. Those who earn their living by talking will be most affected. It is often more effective to reduce the importance of speech in the job and to provide aids such as a word processor with text-to-speech software. A microphone and speech amplifier can be used if the voice is very weak, as can occur in laryngeal dystonia or functional dysphonia. Dysphasia can be associated with other language problems such as dyslexia, dysgraphia, and dyscalculia, and so in such cases communication as a whole must be considered.

Emotional state

Changes in mood state may occur with neurological disease. It is not uncommon to develop secondary depression if a condition is incurable, and progressive disability tends to be very frustrating. This can be helped by psychological support or antidepressant medication, particularly those with stimulant rather than sedative properties, provided that unwanted effects on mental function can be avoided. Patients with PD are prone to depression and those with MS may exhibit euphoria and denial of their problems as part of a psychological defence mechanism; it may also be a sign of incipient cognitive failure with frontal lobe dysfunction. Extreme emotional reactions may also cause a dissociative disorder, such as weakness of a limb, or non-epileptic seizures.

Symptoms related to cranial nerves

Problems relating to the nerves of the eye and ear are considered in Chapter 30 and Chapter 31 respectively. Impaired olfaction from a neurological cause occurs most commonly after head injuries, although local rhinological conditions or heavy smoking and advancing age are more likely causes in the general working population. In occupations using noxious substances, an employee with impaired olfaction might be at greater risk of hazardous exposure. Few jobs specifically require a good sense of smell, but with anosmia there is usually a concomitant loss of taste. Cooks and professional tasters would therefore be handicapped by such impairment.

Lesions of the trigeminal nerve rarely influence work capacity, although the risk of corneal trauma should be considered when sensation is impaired. In contrast, the pain of trigeminal neuralgia, combined with the sedative effects of analgesia, can interfere with concentration at work.

Bell's palsy is a fairly common cause of acute, painless unilateral weakness that involves the orbicularis oculi, frontalis, and other facial muscles. There should be no sensory loss.

It usually improves with time, but is disfiguring and can be embarrassing if the work involves talking to and meeting the public. The only danger is to the eye, when the cornea is at risk from drying and abrasion due to problems with lid closure and the tear mechanism. Fortunately, eye closure nearly always recovers, even if the lower facial paralysis does not. Bell's palsy and other facial palsies should rarely be a cause of a long-term inability to work. Synkinesis and facial spasm, common features of partial recovery, can be effectively managed with botulinum toxin injections. Plastic surgery techniques such as weighting of the upper lid may improve eye closure and cosmesis too.

After either trigeminal or facial nerve deficits, corneal protection is important in employees working with machinery or in dusty atmospheres. They should be educated to report new findings such as eye pain, discharge, or change in vision. Wearing goggles or safety glasses with side guards helps exclude draughts and dust. Lubricating drops can be applied regularly by day and a simple ophthalmic gel used at night. Those occupations necessitating the wearing of face masks or breathing apparatus may require special assessment.

The lower cranial nerves principally control swallowing and articulation. The development of portable ventilators has enabled some people with high cervical cord injuries and paralysis of the respiratory muscles to return to work part-time.

Motor symptoms related to the trunk and limbs

Patients with problems related to their trunk and limbs often find it difficult to describe their symptoms. Often the word 'weakness' is used to describe incoordination and sensory symptoms and 'numbness' is used to express weakness when there is no sensory change.

Weakness can be due to many causes including lesions of the upper or lower motor neurones or neuromuscular junction, muscle disease (myopathy), or psychological mechanisms. These can usually be distinguished from one another clinically. The management of the different causes and their effects on work capability, however, are different.

Upper motor neurone lesions, extrapyramidal disorders, and hypertonia

In acute upper motor neurone lesions, for example, after a stroke, difficulties can often be helped by rehabilitation. Physiotherapy aims to retrain movement patterns, posture and trunk control as the central nervous system (CNS) adapts, and hence function can be improved. Pure muscle strengthening exercises are usually contraindicated. However functional improvement after a year is unusual. Hypertonia in a long-standing upper motor neurone lesion leads to poor posture and clumsiness of movement that often affects fine hand movements or gait. Spasticity is often present, and causes problems with pain, involuntary spasms, and contractures that may require specific treatment or workplace adjustments, such as with botulinum toxin, splinting, or a keyboard guard.

In PD and other parkinsonian syndromes, increased tone and rigidity is associated with bradykinesia. It is the slowness of movements that usually causes the greatest disability. For example, a patient may walk easily for long distances in the open but with great difficulty in a crowded workshop where frequent changes of direction may be needed. Impaired dexterity or a tremor may be particularly problematic in someone who needs a steady hand, for which workplace adjustments and drug treatment are indicated. Safety to drive should also be considered.

Ataxia and incoordination

The effects of ataxia and incoordination can be similar to those of peripheral sensory loss, but the disability is likely to be worse particularly if other sensory input, such as vision, cannot be used in compensation. Unless the cause of the ataxia can be corrected, no amount of retraining will help. Loss of joint position sense is also very disabling and will make coordinated movements difficult. In these circumstances, where practicable, the workplace or job should be adapted.

Lower motor neurone lesions

With lower motor neurone lesions the situation is different. Unless there is very severe weakness and joint instability, the main difficulty is loss of power rather than decreased tone. In contrast to upper motor neurone lesions, physiotherapy should aim to strengthen the appropriate muscles. If there is complete paralysis of a muscle, other muscles may be strengthened and trick movements learnt. The long-term prognosis depends on the pathology. For example, in acute Guillain–Barré syndrome, full recovery can occur, but recovery is unusual in a hereditary peripheral neuropathy. In progressive diseases where treatment cannot halt the decline, excessive physiotherapy can lead to exhaustion and worsen symptoms, but orthoses such as a wrist or foot drop splint may help localized sites of weakness.

Disorders affecting the neuromuscular junctions

Disorders affecting the neuromuscular junctions, such as myasthenia gravis, are much less common than other neurological diseases. They are characterized by fatigability. Exercise makes the weakness worse and so muscle-strengthening exercises are inappropriate. The pattern of weakness is typically proximal and may also affect eye muscles causing ptosis and diplopia. Sedentary workers may have little or no difficulty apart from stairs, low toilet seats, and reaching files from high shelves, but manual workers will have most difficulty and will need adjustments.

Somatosensory impairments

The effects of sensory loss in the limbs can be more disabling than motor lesions. Humans rarely exert their maximum muscle power, but all modalities of sensory input are often used to the full. It is difficult to compensate for even mild cutaneous sensory loss in the fingers caused by a neuropathy or cervical myelopathy, and no amount of therapy or retraining will restore normal function. Employees with sensory loss are likely to encounter difficulty with skilled movements of the hands or unsteadiness of gait, but may be helped by, for example, using a thicker pen, a word processor, or a walking stick.

Loss of spinothalamic pain and temperature sensation produces different problems. If light touch and position sense are preserved, the patient's skilled use of the hands and walking are unaffected, but the normal protective response of withdrawing from dangerous stimuli may be impaired. Those with loss of pain sensation, such as from syringomyelia, are at risk of thermal injury if they come into contact with particularly hot or cold materials at work and remain exposed without realizing. Similarly, ill-fitting footwear may not be appreciated, resulting in skin damage. These difficulties occur most frequently in diabetic patients or those with other chronic neuropathies.

In more severely disabled employees with paraplegia, loss of sensation in the buttocks and legs results in increased risk of pressure sores. Proper seating to prevent trauma, both in the wheelchair and at the workstation, is important. Occupational therapists specialize in prescribing posture aids, seating cushions, and appropriate chairs.

Loss of sphincter control

Poor sphincter control is a feature of many neurological diseases. A catheter with a drainage bag or intermittent self-catheterization may be necessary where there is urinary retention or incontinence, but some patients learn how to stimulate their bladder to empty by abdominal pressure or other means and thereby regain control of micturition. Neuropathic bowel dysfunction may result in extremes of faecal incontinence or chronic constipation, sometimes alternating unpredictably between the two. Laxatives help to overcome constipation but may be avoided because they are assumed to make incontinence more likely. One method is to use bulk softeners or suppositories and to aim for a regular bowel action at a conveniently planned time.

Fatigue

Fatigue is a vague and imprecise term, and a normal emotional and physiological consequence of work. Rather than weakness, which is the inability to activate muscle power, physical fatigue denotes the inability to sustain power output and so can theoretically be measured objectively. However, fatigue can also affect mental performance and be influenced by factors such as motivation, mood, and arousal. It is reported in about 20% of the working population and has been found to be associated with long working hours and shift work that includes night work. It is also a subjective symptom that can be pleasant, but is usually regarded as unpleasant tiredness, weariness, or even exhaustion. Chronic fatigue syndrome is discussed later in this chapter.

Fatigue affects many people with neurological disorders, simply because mental and physical performance may already be impaired physiologically. For example, people recovering from simple concussion, let alone severe traumatic brain injuries, commonly complain of mental fatigue that is made worse by any form of sustained concentration. Those with corticospinal motor impairment from myelopathy or after stroke suffer from inefficient contraction of agonist and antagonist muscles and spasticity. Consequently they are prone to fatigue. PD, other involuntary movement disorders and cerebellar ataxia are all associated with greater energy demands, and myasthenia is characterized by objective muscle fatigability. However, it is MS that is most commonly associated with complaints of disabling fatigue, even in the absence of severe physical disability, either due to inefficient neurotransmission in the presence of demyelination, particularly in hot weather, or to psychological factors.[5]

Simple measures may assist the worker who is struggling to cope at work because of excessive fatigue. They may benefit from extra assistance at home with personal care that may be unduly time-consuming, or with mobility aids and transport. Sometimes gentle persuasion to accept provision of a wheelchair or motorized scooter can help someone previously determined to remain ambulant at all costs. Cardiovascular fitness can sometimes be improved with an appropriate exercise programme, and relative immobility is not an exclusion criterion because paraplegics can work out using a hand bicycle, for example. Flexible work practices should be considered, with reduced hours and increased rest periods. Relaxation techniques, sleep hygiene, and psychological interventions may also be beneficial.

Drug management

Patients with neurological disease are sometimes overmedicated, which can limit their capacity for work. As a general rule, any drug acting on the CNS will interfere with arousal, awareness, and cognitive function to some degree, particularly when given in higher doses. Therefore, it is important to review any medication and liaise with medical colleagues responsible for the clinical management about stopping non-essential treatment. Not infrequently, drugs are initiated by specialists in an acute setting, but not tapered off when the patient is discharged.

The OH consultation prior to a return to work may be the ideal opportunity to rationalize medication. Analgesia requires particular care, as patients do not always appreciate the potential adverse effects as much as the benefits. The underlying cause of the pain must be treated, but skill is required in selecting the correct analgesia. Working while taking an opiate, such as morphine or tramadol, is common but the patient should not be experiencing side effects or drowsiness that might impact on ability to carry out safety-critical or business-critical activity. Certain types of neuropathic pain may respond to particular drugs, such as carbamazepine, gabapentin, or pregabalin, all of which have sedating side effects. Hypnotics can be particularly helpful when taken at night for a few weeks to improve sleep, which itself may ameliorate pain. Tranquillizers should be used with caution during the daytime as drowsiness can make driving or other safety-critical work dangerous and reduce efficiency at work. Because of their addictive potential, hypnotics and tranquillizers should not be taken for more than a month at a time.

Explicit advice must be given about dose frequency, because some patients tend to take too much, while others take inadequate pain relief. If the pain is continuous or regular then the therapy needs to be taken regularly. An employee who waits to take analgesia until breakthrough pain impedes their work has probably waited too long. On the other hand, medication overuse may be a significant factor perpetuating, for example, chronic headache, sedation, or poor concentration.

Antispasticity medication with baclofen or tizanidine can relieve painful and disabling muscle spasms. The dose may have to be carefully titrated against functionally relevant criteria, but not infrequently is increased simply because spasticity is still detectable on examination without taking into account possible adverse effects. These include increasing muscle weakness, which is actually the mechanism of action, and sedation that may interfere with work capacity.

Drug treatment is relatively straightforward in the early stages of PD, but special neurological expertise is required to manage longer-term complications of anti-parkinsonian medication, such as fluctuations in motor response, drug-induced dyskinesia, and impulse control disorder.

Although rare in absolute terms, immunosuppressive therapy is being used more frequently for neurological disorders such as MS, some acquired neuropathies, as well as inflammatory myopathies and autoimmune conditions such as myasthenia and vasculitis. The OH professional will need to be mindful of relevant potential side effects such as anaemia, leucopenia, skin changes, steroid-induced diabetes, myopathy, and osteoporosis in those who return to work on this treatment.

Driving

Decisions on fitness to drive can be extremely difficult for patients with neurological conditions.[6] The standards of medical fitness to drive and the role of the Driver and Vehicle Licensing Agency (DVLA) are discussed in Chapter 15 and the particular problems arising in relation to epilepsy are discussed in Chapter 24. With trauma or other pathology affecting the nervous system, the challenge is to determine whether the resulting neurological deficit itself or the future risk of an alteration to consciousness constitutes an unacceptable driving hazard.

The commonest conditions where licence holders should not drive include following any unprovoked seizure, unexplained blackout or vertigo, and immediately after a craniotomy, severe traumatic brain injury, or acute stroke. Those with a static, or progressive, or relapsing neurological disorder likely to affect vehicle control because of impairment of coordination and muscle power must inform the DVLA of their condition. Doctors have a professional duty to advise patients of their statutory obligation to notify the DVLA of any medical condition that may affect their ability to drive safely and if such advice is not heeded, to inform the DVLA directly.

Factors affecting neurological function

Temperature and humidity

Neurological disease may be adversely affected by extremes of temperature or humidity. At high ambient temperatures, the symptoms of MS worsen temporarily as core temperature rises because of slowing of nerve conduction through demyelinated plaques, but recover when the body is cooled. A similar adverse effect occurs with low ambient temperatures, which also slow peripheral nerve conduction and neuromuscular actions generally, posing a particular problem for those with neuropathic or myopathic disorders. Such patients should, wherever possible, avoid working where extremes of ambient temperature are likely to occur. Little has been written about any clinical consequences of disordered sweating in neurological patients. Excessive facial sweating can occur with cluster headache and after incomplete lesions of the spinal cord, but this is unlikely to present practical problems.

Light

Poor lighting at work is a particular problem for the visually impaired (see Chapter 30). Both poorly lit and dazzlingly bright workplaces may cause headaches. It is thus important that the employee has optimum illumination. Photosensitive epilepsy is considered in Chapter 24. Flashing lights can also precipitate migraine. Some patients with dyslexia report sensitivity to bright lights, or the shimmering of black print on a white background, for which the term scotopic sensitivity syndrome has been used and coloured overlays recommended.

Chemical factors

Naturally occurring or synthetic chemical agents in the environment, including the workplace, may sometimes cause changes in neurological structure or function. For example, parkinsonism can be a feature of poisoning by carbon disulphide, carbon monoxide, or manganese. Observational studies have shown an association between farming or living in parts of France with a high density of vineyards with PD. A longitudinal study of a large cohort of vineyard workers in France with long-term exposure to pesticides has shown a significant decline in their scores on neurobehavioural tests compared with controls (odds ratios of 1.35–5.60) in keeping with an evolution towards Alzheimer's disease.[7] A recent systematic review of the literature came to the conclusion that exposure to pesticides is associated with about a 50% increased risk of developing PD.[8]

Chronic mercury exposure is classically associated with tremor (hatters' shakes), ataxia, and peripheral neuropathy. Neuropsychological effects, such as impaired dexterity, can also be detected at lower levels of exposure. Exposures to high doses of manganese, such as when welding, may also be associated with parkinsonism and a psychological disturbance known as manganism due to deposition of the metal in the basal ganglia.[9]

The occupational evaluation of anyone exposed to a neurotoxin should include clinical examination, neuropsychological tests, and biological monitoring such as blood or urinary analysis.

Toxic neuropathies

Inorganic lead characteristically causes a motor peripheral neuropathy with wrist or foot drop. Arsenic and organic solvents such as *n*-hexane and methyl-*n*-butyl-ketone cause a mixed sensory and motor peripheral neuropathy, whereas mercury and polychlorinated biphenyls cause a predominantly sensory neuropathy. Investigation of suspected cases should include nerve conduction tests and biological monitoring. Regeneration usually follows slowly and uneventfully provided exposure is halted at an early stage. It would be inadvisable for any employee with a pre-existing neuropathy of any aetiology to be exposed knowingly to such an additional hazard, regardless of the standard safety precautions in the workplace.

Heavy metal toxicity and organic solvents

An acute encephalopathy associated with exposure to aluminium was first described in smelter workers. It was known as 'pot room palsy', and characterized by incoordination, poor memory, and impaired abstract reasoning. The finding of raised levels of aluminium in the brains of patients with dementia in 1973 led to a hypothesis that aluminium was a neurotoxic factor in the pathogenesis of Alzheimer's disease. Aluminium may cause dialysis encephalopathy in patients with treated chronic renal failure, which has been referred to as dialysis dementia. If identified early enough, aluminium intoxication can be treated with the chelating agent desferrioxamine. An accidental contamination of drinking water in Camelford, UK, with aluminium sulphate in 1988 led to many residents complaining of neuropsychological symptoms some of which were found to have an objective basis.[10] A longitudinal study of aluminium welders showed no adverse cognitive or neurological effects when compared with age and educationally matched controls.[11] There is, however, increasing evidence that inorganic lead impairs cognitive functioning, particularly in children, at blood levels of lead of less than 10 micrograms/dL[12] and in adults, damage to cognitive performance and peripheral nerve function has been observed in the 30–50 micrograms/dL range.[13]

Organic solvents are widely used in the manufacturing industry, dry-cleaning, degreasing, and paint production and application. The acute effects of organic solvents range from mild fatigue to frank psychosis. A review of mainly cross-sectional studies of the long-term effects of low-dose solvent exposure has shown impairments of memory and motor performance when compared with controls, but no effect size could be calculated due to the difficulty of obtaining reliable information about exposure, the absence of an exposure–response relationship, and the many confounding factors in addition to age and educational level.[14] Investigation by biological monitoring is essential for acute exposures but is unlikely to be helpful in chronic low-dose exposures.

Organophosphate pesticides

Well-established acute toxic effects of organophosphate pesticides from spraying or dipping arise from their capacity to inhibit acetyl cholinesterase in the CNS and autonomic nervous systems and at the neuromuscular junction. An acute cholinergic crisis, muscle weakness, or a polyneuropathy have been seen, most commonly in agricultural workers in developing countries, after excessive exposure that should not occur if the chemicals are used while the worker is in a protected machine or with appropriate personal protective equipment (PPE). A review and meta-analysis of 14 studies found a significant association between low-level exposure to organophosphates and impaired cognitive functioning to include psychomotor speed, executive functioning, visuospatial ability, and memory.[15]

Identification and prevention of occupational neurotoxicity

A detailed occupational and environmental history is advisable when assessing the potential for chemical exposures to cause or aggravate a neurological condition. This should cover the employee's tasks, use of PPE, and contact with specific chemicals. Risk assessments, safety data sheets, and the results of any environmental measurements should be inspected. A visit to the workplace to understand how the job is done and the controls that are in place is also important before making any judgements about exposure.

Questions about the use of specific natural remedies which may contain heavy metals, the use of recreational drugs which may be contaminated with methyl-4-phenyl-1,2,3,6-tetrahydropyridine (MPTP), and the source of residential water supply which in some parts of the world is contaminated with arsenic are also important.

Education and advice about work hazards and the provision of PPE may not always reduce exposures due to operational pressures. If PPE is poorly fitting, or uncomfortable to wear for long periods of time or in hot climates, then poor compliance may limit protection. Health surveillance should aim to provide evidence of exposure and to identify early adverse health effects or markers of biological effect.

Assistive technology

Computerized environmental control devices are available for home use under the NHS, but at work they may allow a disabled person to continue useful work. Such technology might include a lightweight electric wheelchair, a keyboard with large, easy-to-use keys, a key guard or sticky keys for a patient with a tremor, keyboard emulation such as a joystick or head pointer, and speech recognition software. A large computer screen, a speech synthesizer, or an electronic reading machine may also helpful. For those in work, specialist help from the UK government's Access to Work scheme can be sought when choosing and purchasing such technology.

Specific neurological disorders

The neurological diagnosis is also important in assessing prognosis and in guiding decisions about whether a person should be employed, the timing and nature of adjustment(s), or eligibility for medical retirement.

Headache

Daily in the UK more than 90,000 people are absent from school or work due to headache. Eighty per cent of the population have tension type headaches, 2–3% of adults have chronic tension type headaches (on >15 days per month), 10–15% have migraines, and 4% have chronic daily headaches, with 1 in 50 having medication overuse headaches. Organic disease is a very uncommon cause unless the headache is of recent origin, has changed its character, or it is associated with symptoms of raised intracranial pressure such as being aggravated by straining, lifting, sneezing, or bending, or associated with vomiting, visual loss, and papilloedema. In the older worker, temporal arteritis should also be considered.

Migraine may occur with or without aura, typically a visual disturbance although other transient focal neurological deficits may occur simultaneously or sequentially, such as dysphasia or sensory disturbance. It then progresses to a unilateral or generalized headache with nausea and/or vomiting. Migraine aura can occur without headache. The manifestations of the migraine can change with time, and migraine is only rarely symptomatic of an underlying localized pathology.

A high proportion of workers attribute headaches to stress, dissatisfaction with work, or worry about losing their jobs. Education about headaches, relaxation, and neck and shoulder exercises have been shown in community studies to be effective in reducing the prevalence of headaches.[16]

In spite of advances in medication and management guidelines, migraine and other forms of headache are underdiagnosed and undertreated. A variety of questionnaire instruments have emerged to help manage them better. History taking should pay particular attention to coexisting stress, depression, and anxiety. Thus, depression and stress are often features of morning headaches that prevent people getting to work. A stress-prone personality or an individual's perceived capacity to exercise self-control is a factor in the aetiology of headaches that can be improved with cognitive behavioural therapy. Chronic headaches can also result from medication overuse, including the triptans (5-hydroxytryptamine-1A agonists), which also needs to be considered.

Precipitating factors such as workplace chemicals (including perfume or deodorant), volatile organic compounds from building materials, extremes of temperature, humidity, or light, prolonged periods of close work, irregular meals, or altered sleep patterns (particularly sleeping in late) should be elicited in an occupational history. There are many modes of medication delivery including nasal sprays, injectable, sublingual formulations, and suppositories, and regular prophylaxis with beta blockers or amitriptyline such that effective treatment is available for the majority.

Employees with headaches are unlikely to fall under the disability provisions of the Equality Act 2010 as normal day-to-day activities are possible between attacks and for the majority during a headache as well. Workplace adaptation might require a change to ambient lighting, humidity, or temperature and a quiet, dark room when a sufferer needs to rest. Migraineurs may be precluded from safety-critical jobs that have a pre-set incapacitation rate set by their industry, as is the case for airline pilots, air traffic controllers, and aerial climbers (see Chapter 15). There are also additional published specific criteria for migraine and other neurological conditions set by the Civil Aviation Authority.

Disorders of awareness and sleep

Disturbances of awareness include blackouts, seizures, and fluctuations in wakefulness. A patient who has lost consciousness, unless it was a simple faint while standing, who is a group 1 or 2 licence holder must be advised not to drive and to inform the DVLA.

Daytime somnolence can be a normal physiological phenomenon, particularly after a heavy lunch. However, obstructive sleep apnoea is increasingly being recognized as a cause of excessive daytime somnolence (see Chapter 27).

The classical narcolepsy syndrome is very rare, comprising cataplexy, hypnogogic hallucinations, and sleep paralysis as well as an irresistible desire to sleep even while eating, talking, or driving. Cataplexy is the sudden decrease or loss of voluntary muscle tone following emotional events in which the patient collapses. It is potentially dangerous for the patient and others, but the frequency of attacks can be reduced by optimizing nocturnal sleep duration, and allowing planned daytime naps as well as appropriate medication such as modafinil, sodium oxybate, and amphetamines. In the UK, anyone with narcolepsy who holds a driving licence must report their illness to the DVLA.

Return to work following stroke and transient ischaemic attacks

The effects of an acute stroke are determined both by the extent and location of damaged brain tissue. This combination will also determine the rate of recovery and the occupational prognosis.

Cerebrovascular disease results in two different pathologies, ischaemia or haemorrhage, with infarction, gliosis, and atrophy as the end result of both. Typically haemorrhage is intracerebral, but it can be subarachnoid from either aneurysms or vascular malformations.

Transient ischaemic attacks (TIAs), by definition, cause focal neurological disturbance for less than 24 hours. TIAs have more limited occupational implications, such as for driving. However, it is not uncommon for incomplete neurological assessment or clinically silent cerebral infarction to occur in this context.

Risk of recurrence/incapacitation

It would be wrong to prevent a person returning to non-safety-critical work just because the employer is concerned that a further episode might occur. Each employee should have an assessment of prognosis and reasonable adjustments to work practices. The absolute risk of a first stroke following a single TIA, or of a second stroke following a first one, is statistically quite low. Nevertheless, the risk of recurrent TIAs is highest within the first 6 weeks of an initial event, and the lifetime risk of a second stroke is double compared with those who have never had a stroke (Box 23.1).[17]

Such analysis may have implications for those who work in isolation or in safety-critical roles. The DVLA's medical standard is no driving for 1 month after a single TIA for group 1 drivers, no driving for 3 months with notification of the DVLA after multiple TIAs, and no driving for 1 year with notification of the DVLA for group 2 drivers (see Chapter 15).

Medication

As with all employees, any potentially adverse effect of prescribed medication should be identified. For safety reasons, postural hypotension, sedation, and cognitive impairment are particularly important. There may be a need to assess those who are on anticoagulants

Box 23.1 Prognostic factors for stroke after a TIA

- ◆ Increasing age.
- ◆ Unilateral weakness with or without speech impairment.
- ◆ Duration of the deficit.
- ◆ The coexistence of hypertension.
- ◆ The coexistence of diabetes.

Source: data from Johnston, SC. Et al. Validation and refinement of scores to predict very early stroke risk after transient ischaemic attack. *Lancet*. 369(9558), 283–92. Copyright © 2007 Elsevier.

for risk of injury and subsequent haemorrhage. For example, members of the uniformed services might be restricted to administration and training, rather than frontline duties. Access to facilities for measurement of blood clotting time may also be relevant.

Functional deficits

The time to maximum recovery after a stroke varies widely, but can be a year or more. However, after about 4 months it is usually possible to give a reliable prognosis, as by then the functions that are recovering can clearly be discerned and any function that has not started to recover is unlikely to do so completely. Ideally, a final prognosis should not be given until the employee has received optimum rehabilitation.

Physical deficits such as a residual hemiparesis are usually apparent to everyone, including the employee, their managers, and work colleagues. Assessment should determine any reasonable adjustments to the workplace or job, for which advice may need to be sought from Access to Work or an occupational therapist. Subtle deficits of cognitive function may occur, particularly following non-dominant hemisphere strokes affecting frontal lobe executive functions and non-verbal abilities. Those who have had a dominant hemisphere lesion may not only have residual dysphasia with word-finding difficulties apparent in normal conversation, but also coexistent dysgraphia, dyslexia, and dyscalculia which should be sought where appropriate with the help of a neuropsychologist. Visual field deficits, whether absolute, or for simultaneous stimuli presented in opposite visual fields, may require careful assessment, together with other tests for visual agnosia or other perceptual difficulties. This is particularly important where driving or other safety-critical work is undertaken.

Cerebral tumours

Unlike tumours elsewhere in the body, primary cerebral and spinal cord tumours do not metastasize outside the CNS. Their histological grade can still vary from benign to rapidly malignant, but ultimately the anatomical site determines prognosis. Even the most benign tumour can be incurable if it is deeply inaccessible within the brain. Fortunately, most benign tumours can be treated successfully by surgery, some of the malignant ones can be halted by radiotherapy, and a few are sensitive to chemotherapy.

After treatment, an assessment of the employee's functional ability and information about the prognosis usually facilitates decisions about work. Return to work will be determined by:

- the natural improvement that will occur with rehabilitation and recovery after treatment such as surgical excision, not dissimilar to recovery from a stroke
- the natural history of the tumour, which has a worse long-term prognosis if malignant or likely to recur
- the liability to seizures from the tumour or as a consequence of craniotomy
- the nature of the job, with driving and other safety-critical work needing to be considered. The individual who hold a group 1 or group 2 driving licence should be told not to drive and to inform the DVLA unless the tumour is asymptomatic and an incidental finding not requiring treatment.

Parkinson's disease

PD is, after stroke, the second most common cause of acquired physical disability from a neurological condition in later life. Its incidence increases progressively with age, and it affects about 1% of the population above retirement age. Nevertheless, a significant minority of cases occur at younger ages, occasionally even under 40 years. The average life expectancy after diagnosis is between 7 and 14 years. The cardinal features of parkinsonism are the classical triad of slowness of movement or bradykinesia, resting tremor, and cogwheel rigidity, together with impairment of postural righting reflexes.

Before reaching a diagnosis of primary parkinsonism, that is, idiopathic PD characterized by Lewy body neuropathology, the physician must attempt to rule out other causes of parkinsonism (Box 23.2).

Environmental neurotoxicity hypotheses

Although the aetiology of idiopathic PD is unknown, one popular hypothesis concerns one or more hitherto unidentified environmental toxins, perhaps affecting only those exposed subjects with a genetic susceptibility. Epidemiological studies have suggested that drinking well water, exposure to industrial chemicals or living near industrial chemical plants, or exposure to pesticides or herbicides increases the risk of getting PD.[18] Of interest, MPTP, a selective dopaminergic neurotoxin, was industrially developed as a potential herbicide, but instead has been used to produce an animal model of PD. It may also be a contaminant of heroin, sufficient to cause severe PD. The herbicide rotenone has also been used to produce an animal model of PD.

The OH professional should consider any potential neurotoxic exposure in the employee's workplace. For example, long-term exposure to manganese dust may cause parkinsonism (manganism) and clinical progression continues even 10 years after cessation of exposure.[19] There was a tenfold increase in the prevalence of parkinsonism in

Box 23.2 Causes of parkinsonism

- Any acute cerebral pathology, for example, encephalitis, traumatic brain injury, anoxia, or ischaemia.
- Parkinsonism-plus syndromes such as progressive supranuclear palsy and multiple system atrophy which are associated with non-Lewy body neurodegenerative disease.
- Chronic exposure to prescribed medication that blocks dopamine receptors in the brain, for example, major tranquillizers, prochlorperazine, and metoclopramide.
- Environmental toxins such as manganese, carbon disulphide, pesticides, or MPTP.

a sample of male welders in Alabama compared with the general male working population[20] as well as a report of a group of heavily exposed welders with manganism.[21] Parkinsonism due to manganese exposure is a Prescribed Disease in the UK's Industrial Injuries Disablement Benefit (IIDB) scheme.

Occupational considerations

In the early stages, motor impairments may be completely corrected with dopamine replacement therapy, although problems with micrographia and a slow shuffling gait may gradually become more apparent. In those occupations dealing directly with members of the public, prominent tremor can be embarrassing, although patients are sometimes remarkably resourceful in disguising their disabilities using various trick manoeuvres. When speech is impaired through dysphonia, speech therapy and the use of a voice amplifier, for example, on the telephone, may be needed. A keyboard guard and adjustments to the 'stickiness' of the keys may also be helpful (Box 23.3).

Cognitive impairment is rarely a feature of PD, unless it has been present for a decade or more, but depression is remarkably common and may have a similar neurochemical

Box 23.3 The main fitness for work considerations in someone with PD

- The worker's functional capacity in relation to the degree of motor impairment and tremor; the need for workplace adjustments and advice to notify the DVLA if the worker is a vehicle licence holder.
- Concomitant cognitive and emotional factors.
- Ensuring optimal symptomatic control with medication while minimizing adverse side effects.
- Periodic reviews to monitor disease progression.

basis of catecholamine deficiency to the motor impairment. Antidepressant medication can improve quality of life.

As the underlying disease progresses slowly after the first few years, the requirement for medication may increase. A significant proportion of patients, particularly younger ones, also develop fluctuations in motor performance during the course of a day that often co-incide with cycles of drug absorption and metabolism, resulting in its extreme form in the 'on–off phenomenon'. This can result in spectacular oscillations between someone who is immobile and frozen one minute, and moving freely the next. Sometimes this latter phase is associated with drug-induced dyskinesia, with involuntary movements that can be embarrassing and disconcerting to colleagues. Titration of the timing of oral medication may be insufficient to control these fluctuations. Specialist neurological advice should be sought concerning other available strategies, such as the use of longer-acting dopa-mine receptor agonist drugs, modified-release levodopa formulations, the use of subcuta-neous apomorphine, either by intermittent injection or by infusion, and even deep brain stimulation.

Most anti-parkinsonian drugs, particularly with the larger doses required in the later years of the condition, have the potential to cause psychiatric side effects including im-paired attention, confusion, visual hallucinations, and overt delusional states. These can arise idiosyncratically with certain powerful dopamine receptor agonists, and may resolve completely following withdrawal of the drug.

Although disability in PD does steadily progress, normally it does so only slowly over the course of a decade or more. This may be sufficient for the employee to reach retire-ment age. The OH professional should be proactive in arranging to review the employee at appropriate intervals. Parkinson's UK takes a particular interest in providing advice and support for sufferers who are still in active employment, and its regional network can provide information and training for employers locally (see 'Useful websites'). In the case of those in professional practice, a notice in the waiting room that Mr X has PD but his condition is being regularly monitored, may help to avoid questions about health or fitness to be at work.

Essential tremor

Essential tremor is an idiopathic condition, often familial and dominantly inherited, that is ten times more common than PD, but not associated with bradykinesia or rigidity. It almost always affects both upper limbs symmetrically, and less commonly the head, lower limbs, tongue, and voice. Older textbooks refer to it as benign, but it is a lifelong disorder that gradually worsens. It can cause significant interference with handwriting, employment, and activities of daily living, and also with social functioning because of embarrassment.

Many patients with essential tremor require nothing more than an accurate diagnosis and reassurance that a more sinister disease is not present. The avoidance of stimulants such as caffeine and the judicious consumption of ethanol which may ameliorate the tremor are helpful to some patients. Approximately half benefit from either primidone or beta-adrenergic blockers such as propranolol. Response to one drug does not predict response to the other, but complete suppression of tremor is rare.

Dystonia

There are various forms of dystonia but, rather like essential tremor, they are probably underdiagnosed, usually idiopathic but with a significant genetic component, and poorly understood. Primary generalized dystonia normally starts in childhood and gives rise to severe motor dysfunction ('dystonia musculorum deformans') that is seldom compatible with work. Secondary causes are extremely rare except as a side effect of drugs such as major tranquillizers.

However, focal forms of adult-onset dystonia are probably more common than PD in those of working age, and are classified according to their anatomical involvement. They usually cause irregular involuntary muscle spasms such as dystonic torticollis, writer's cramp, dysphonia, or blepharospasm. They are usually persistent and remission is uncommon, but they do vary in severity and can be controlled to some extent by voluntary strategies such as trick movements. Rarely are they so severe as to prevent working. Formerly, they were classified erroneously as psychogenic conditions, but there is now good evidence that they are associated with basal ganglia dysfunction. Focal dystonias respond poorly to anticholinergic medication such as benzhexol, but the introduction of botulinum toxin treatment has revolutionized their management.

Traumatic head and brain injuries

The first step when assessing an employee's capacity to undertake their duties after head injury is to estimate the severity of the injury to the brain, which is the best indicator of prognosis. Most people use the term 'head injury' loosely to refer to any traumatic event, but the term 'traumatic brain injury' is preferred to underline this distinction. Various data can be used to estimate the severity, of which the Glasgow Coma Score, and the durations of coma and of post-traumatic amnesia are most useful prognostically, providing they are not prolonged by anaesthesia, sedative medication, or systemic factors. A poor prognosis is associated with an initial low Glasgow Coma Score less than 9, a coma lasting longer than 6 hours, post-traumatic amnesia for more than 24 hours, and recovery longer than 3 months in duration.[22]

However, there are many patients whose injuries are not obviously very severe yet have difficulty returning successfully to their previous work. There are two possible explanations for this: either the severity of the underlying brain injury has been underestimated, or there are associated non-organic factors that are contributing to a vicious cycle of ongoing cognitive difficulties, low mood, negative perceptions, muscular deconditioning, and medico-legal issues. The eventual outcome will be the result of interactions between injury severity, intrinsic recovery, and individual personal and environmental factors.

Even with concussive injuries involving little or no period of loss of consciousness, injuries to the brain can occur with focal contusions and disruption of cerebral connections secondary to diffuse axonal injury. However, the physical signs of organic disease can be minimal. Diagnostic pointers include other features of high kinetic energy impact (e.g. high-speed collisions, craniofacial fractures, spinal or proximal long bone limb fractures, visceral rupture). Magnetic resonance imaging (MRI) can usually demonstrate brain injuries objectively long after the event, provided that the correct sequences are requested and the films reported by an experienced neuroradiologist. Finally, formal neuropsychological assessment may help distinguish between focal cognitive impairments, general intellectual under-functioning compared with estimated pre-morbid ability, deficits more in keeping with anxiety and depression, or even deliberate exaggeration of difficulties (see symptom validity testing, discussed in 'Cognitive function and psychometrics').[23]

Approving return to work after concussion and minor brain injury

In certain occupations, for example, safety-critical jobs or sports professionals, even a minor head injury requires careful assessment before allowing the person to resume their usual activities. The potentially fatal risks of so-called second impact syndrome have been exaggerated, but clearly carry enormous medico-legal implications. The national governing bodies of certain sports in many countries now insist upon a medical examination as part of a 'return to play' protocol.[24] The basic requirement is that the person is fully recovered from whatever effects they may have suffered, but this is sometimes hard to confirm with certainty (Box 23.4).

After a minor head injury, there are three main areas for the physician to consider:

Symptoms
Seemingly, it should be easy to be satisfied that someone has returned to their pre-injury state—just ask the patient! However, those doctors who manage elite sports athletes know only too well that patients' accounts can sometimes be misleading. Incentives exist for the professional athlete to conceal the truth if the consequences of not competing are likely to affect their prize money or chances of being picked for the squad. Similar motives may influence other workers, especially those involved with litigation.

Box 23.4 Traumatic brain injury and the DVLA

Group 1 driving may resume after 3 months and the DVLA need not be informed provided

+ There is full clinical recovery with no visual field or cognitive defects likely to affect safe driving.
+ There are no seizures.
+ Post-traumatic amnesia did not last longer than 24 hours.
+ There was no intracranial haemorrhage or contusion on brain imaging.

Signs

Unfortunately, the neurological examination is not sensitive enough to identify people who are still symptomatic. Minor abnormal neurological signs are uncommon even after moderately severe traumatic brain injury, and after milder injury findings are more likely to reflect pre-existing conditions. Perhaps one of the most sensitive signs of impaired recovery is subtle impairment of coordination and balance. Although not usually part of the standard examination, stringent tests of high-level balance such as single-leg stance, and walking along a low beam, as well as standard heel-to-toe gait will be examined routinely by sports physicians. In practice, vocational tests in a protected training or simulator environment should be undertaken before allowing, for example, pilots to return to work or professional athletes to return to competition.

Cognitive functioning

Neuropsychological tests have long been thought to be the most sensitive and objective measure of recovery after minor head and brain injury. Simple tests of orientation, attention, and recall have been incorporated into standardized concussion assessment tools such as the Sport Concussion Assessment Tool (SCAT) by consensus groups, but they have not been scientifically evaluated. They can be used for contact sports on the sidelines during a match, or by the roadside after an accident and can be extended to evaluate satisfactory recovery.[24] More detailed pencil and paper tests can also be used to chart and confirm recovery, and do not necessarily require a trained clinical neuropsychologist. However, the selection of appropriate tests that can be administered repeatedly to the same subject while avoiding practice effects does require special expertise.

Computerized neuropsychological test batteries have also been developed that claim to minimize practise effects while remaining sensitive to significant slowing of information processing speed and other relevant impairments. By using such instruments in a comprehensive programme of pre-season baseline testing, governing bodies such as the English Rugby Football Union and the Jockey Club have established databases for participants in their respective sports that can be used to compare an individual's performance after a single head injury. They may also identify those with a trend of deteriorating performance that might provide evidence of cumulative harm from repetitive head injuries.[24]

Vocational rehabilitation after moderate–severe brain injury

Early liaison with relevant healthcare professionals and support organizations such as Headway is highly desirable (see 'Useful websites'). Psychometric testing will usually establish the extent of any organic impairment which may be integral to a person's rehabilitation back to work.[25] Participation in a brain injury education programme may be beneficial to increase insight into residual difficulties, anticipate areas of potential difficulty at work, and identify compensatory strategies. The information can usefully be communicated to colleagues and line managers to facilitate understanding and adjustment. Ideally, this should be an integral part of a formalized managed process of vocational rehabilitation. Employees should be advised to do as much as they can for themselves, take regular meals, go to bed at reasonable hours, and adjust their lifestyle. Alcohol should be avoided, both because of reduced tolerance to intoxication and increased adverse neurobehavioural effects.

As with other organic lesions of the brain, functional improvement does occur, but takes time and may be incomplete. Shift work is best avoided and medication that might impair concentration or cognition should be minimized. For many employees after prolonged absence, returning to work too abruptly can be counter-productive and a graduated return is preferable, taking on limited responsibilities at first and then adding to them. This is because of a combination of physical deconditioning, particularly if commuting involves long journeys, and mental fatigue induced by cognitive inefficiency and increased multitasking.

Meningitis and encephalitis

Most infections of the CNS begin acutely over the course of hours or a few days, and involve both the meninges and brain to some extent. Many different viral, bacterial, and even fungal pathogens can cause an identical acute neurological syndrome with intense headache, fever, malaise, and drowsiness that may progress to coma and seizures, depending on the extent of cerebral involvement. After the first few days and appropriate timely antimicrobial treatment, the course is mostly one of slowly progressive improvement over several days or weeks. The prognosis and influence on work capacity vary according to the organism and extent of underlying cerebral damage. Herpes simplex encephalitis, the most common cause of severe sporadic encephalitis in the Western world, can cause considerable memory impairment and these patients may never return to intellectually demanding occupations. Other less severe infections usually result in full recovery.

Better treatment for opportunistic infections and the development of highly active antiretroviral therapies has greatly reduced morbidity and mortality in those infected with HIV, and a marked decrease in the incidence of HIV-associated dementia. Nevertheless, because of their high prevalence, a high index of suspicion must be kept for neurological disorders in the HIV or AIDS patient (see Chapter 34).

Alzheimer's disease and other pre-senile dementias

Dementia usually develops insidiously, most often after retirement, but poses a diagnostic and management problem when it arises in someone of working age. If the employee has been in the same job for many years, cognitive failure may be less obvious. They can work relatively well in familiar surroundings at routine tasks, but new tasks are difficult. Colleagues may become aware of deterioration in memory or work performance.

Dementia from occupational neurotoxic exposure was discussed earlier in this chapter. Unfortunately, reversible causes of dementia (e.g. metabolic, normal-pressure hydrocephalus, and certain drugs including alcohol) are uncommon. Dementia may be inherited such as Huntington's disease, early-onset familial Alzheimer's disease, and frontotemporal dementia, but most are sporadic. Advice about continuing employment must be based objectively on competency and reasonable adjustments. Any safety-critical activities should be prohibited, and administrative safeguards instituted at diagnosis if medical retirement is not effected immediately. The individual, and sometimes a relative as well, must be told not to drive and to inform the DVLA of their illness. Such advice should be confirmed in writing.

Sporadic Creutzfeldt–Jakob disease (sCJD) generally presents after the age of 50 years with much more rapid progression over weeks or months (although cases aged below 40 years have been described), and 10% of cases are familial with autosomal dominant inheritance. A new variant of the disease (vCJD) due to an abnormal prion protein was first described in 1996 by the UK National CJD Surveillance Unit based in Edinburgh, which maintains a website with up-to-date research and advice.

Neurological disorders of childhood

Cerebral palsy includes a group of childhood syndromes (historically classified as either spastic or dystonic) resulting from genetic and acquired insults to the developing brain, causing abnormalities in tone, posture, and movement. It is important to appreciate that cerebral palsy includes a wide range of infectious, hypoxic–ischaemic, endocrine, and genetic conditions. Other developmental disorders of the posterior fossa and spinal cord, such as Chiari malformations and spina bifida, may cause similar disabilities, not least because of their association with hydrocephalus. Poliomyelitis and autism spectrum disorders should be viewed in a similar way.

At the start of employment, it is advisable to have a full medical and functional capability assessment so that work can be adjusted to allow the employee to use their skills most efficiency. A systematic approach to a prospective employee, often a young school leaver, allows accurate identification of the key occupational considerations and prognosis, and avoids the danger of stereotyping, as someone with severe physical disability may have no intellectual impairment at all.

Employment prospects are usually established during education and training, enabling a young person to develop their potential abilities and attain appropriate vocational qualifications. It is usually valuable to obtain previous statements of educational needs that document the subject's abilities systematically. Minor motor impairments rarely pose a problem except during highly skilled activities. Machinery, office equipment, and vehicles can usually be adapted.

Spinal cord injury and disease

The commonest neurological disease affecting the spinal cord itself is MS (described in the next section). Primary tumours arising within the spinal canal are rare and are usually benign, the commonest being a neurofibroma. However, the commonest cause of acute myelopathy is trauma, which tends to affect younger adults engaging in risk-taking activities and a significant proportion occur at work. Some patients return to work after spinal cord injury with the help of adaptive technology, particularly those who need to work and who are in sedentary jobs. The employee may require reasonable time and space to use a standing frame during the working day, or to self-catheterize intermittently. The occurrence of autonomic dysreflexia with postural hypotension or hypertensive storms also needs to be considered in those with high thoracic injuries.

Multiple sclerosis

MS is the commonest neurological disorder affecting young adults. The diagnosis traditionally requires two or more CNS lesions separated in time and space, not caused by other CNS disease. The manifestations vary enormously because lesions can occur anywhere in the CNS. Common presentations include a single episode, lasting only a few weeks, of visual impairment, ataxia, or focal motor or sensory disturbance.

MRI and cerebrospinal fluid analysis are abnormal in more than 95% of definite cases. MRI has also become essential to rule out conditions that could mimic MS. Updated diagnostic criteria use new MRI lesions to define separation in time and space.[26] The majority present with relapsing and remitting disease, but MS is progressive from onset (primary progressive MS) in about 10% of cases, particularly with later age of onset. More typically, there are three phases: initially relapses with full recovery, then relapses with persisting deficits, and later secondary progression. In the progressive phase, clinical remissions disappear, but constant low-grade immune activation continues or worsens.

The time course is extremely variable, as some patients may spend years or even decades in each phase, whereas about 10% rapidly become severely disabled. About 25% of patients have a benign form of MS that is not disabling. The prognosis is relatively good when sensory or visual symptoms predominate and there is complete recovery from individual relapses, a pattern commonest in young women. Negative prognostic predictors include cerebellar or pyramidal signs, frequent early attacks, development of secondary progression, or a primary progressive course, and age over 40 years at onset. Later-onset MS is more common in men and often primary progressive; even when it begins as relapsing–remitting disease, secondary progression occurs earlier.

After a single episode with full recovery, an employee should be able to return to normal work. If recurrent attacks are infrequent with full recovery, the amount of time off work over a period of years should be small. In more chronic cases, regular assessment will be required to decide about capability, adjustments, and medical retirement. Disease-modifying drugs such as interferon, glatiramer, and various biological agents such as natalizumab may be used, but their long-term value is uncertain.

The initiating event for the first attack is unknown, but genetics and environmental factors both interact. Epidemiological studies have found an association between MS and residential latitude in different parts of the world, but the significance of those factors remains unclear. Trauma and stress have been implicated anecdotally as causing MS or triggering exacerbations, but the occurrence of any specific exacerbation cannot yet be causally linked to any specific stressor. Fatigue is one of the most common complaints among patients with established and disabling MS, typically magnification of post-exertion fatigue with sensitivity to heat and humidity. Some studies have shown modest benefit from treatment with amantadine and from energy-conserving courses.[27] High temperatures are not well tolerated and some patients like to work in slightly colder environments than is usually desired by other employees as this reduces their symptoms. Poor sleep, worry, or depression, as well as cognitive deterioration also need to be considered by the OH professional. Euphoria can be an early sign of frontal lobe dysfunction, causing abnormal contentment with physical disability.

The factors relating to remaining in work are mainly disease related, such as balance and walking abilities, but the physical requirements of the job and the motivation of the employee to remain at work are also relevant. Financial and practical help with travel is available from the UK government's Access to Work scheme. To remain in work, people with MS need good healthcare management such as an orthotic support for foot drop, or an indwelling catheter for urinary incontinence, as well as workplace or job adjustments such as wheelchair access, or adjustments to their role. Flexible working hours, time off work for physiotherapy or medical appointments, and increased absence due to relapses of MS are also reasonable adjustments that will help patients remain in work. Regular occupational screening for visual field loss or cognitive decline may be necessary for employees in safety-critical jobs. An individual with MS that may affect vehicle control should be advised to inform the DVLA of their illness. It is not sufficient for patients to decide when they are fit to drive. They should also be encouraged to join self-management groups run by the MS Society (see 'Useful websites').

Multidimensional scales for objectively assessing impairment and disability of patients with MS have been developed, such as the Kurtzke Expanded Disability Status Scale (EDSS). The full scale is 0–10 but most people with MS who are in work will have a score of 5 or less. The functional systems that are scored are pyramidal, cerebellar, brainstem, sensory, bowel/bladder, visual, mental, and other. Alternative scales are the Multiple Sclerosis Functional Composite, and the Incapacity Status Scales, but they all have their limitations, such as the need for self-reported information and maximal effort by the patient, an overreliance on walking ability, and no assessment of energy levels or quality of life. Information such as the EDSS is usually contained within the neurological records, or it can be requested from the treating neurologist.

Miscellaneous genetic disorders

A small but significant proportion of neurological disease is caused by single-gene mutations, which can present at working age. Neurocutaneous genetic syndromes share a dominantly inherited predisposition to developing tumours of the nervous system. Such a diagnosis is compatible with working, but the risk of developing complications is unpredictable and may justify some form of regular occupational screening, such as for acoustic neuromas in type 2 neurofibromatosis or for visual acuity or field loss due to haemangioblastomas in von Hippel–Landau disease.

An employee with limb-girdle or facio-scapulo-humeral muscular dystrophy affecting the shoulder or pelvic girdle may need adjustments to their job or workplace if, for example, they have difficulty lifting their arms above their shoulders, climbing stairs, or rising from a squatting position. Someone with dystrophia myotonica will have difficulty releasing their grip in cold weather, so will need to be moved indoors and, because of their propensity to develop cataracts, regularly screened for deteriorating visual acuity.

Motor neurone diseases

The term MND describes a family of rare disorders resulting from selective loss of function of lower and/or upper motor neurones controlling the voluntary muscles of the limbs or bulbar region. Four main syndromes are recognized—amyotrophic lateral sclerosis, progressive muscular atrophy, bulbar palsy, and pseudo-bulbar palsy. Some forms progress rapidly, in which case medical retirement is appropriate, whereas others are more benign and compatible with work with the help of adaptive technology. Mental ability is unimpaired so the patient may be able to control their environment and, for example, operate a telephone or computer with assistive technology. Life expectancy is less than 3 years from the onset of symptoms for about 50% of cases. In a large longitudinal study of Danish utility workers exposed to low-frequency magnetic fields, a significant increase in dementia, MND, MS, and epilepsy was found in those with the highest estimated exposures.[28] However, in another longitudinal study of Central Electricity Generating Board workers in the UK there was no increased risk of mortality from dementia, MND, or PD.[29]

Peripheral neuropathy

Neuropathy is a common condition with a very broad differential diagnosis (Box 23.5). It is typically insidious in onset with glove and stocking sensory loss and produces gradually increasing disability. Progress is usually slow and many cases are asymptomatic or have little disability. The main exception is acute idiopathic inflammatory polyneuropathy or Guillain–Barré syndrome, in which symptoms develop rapidly over days and then resolve, usually completely, within weeks or months. Return to work is usually possible when the patient becomes fully ambulant, although occasionally residual muscle weakness may persist indefinitely so each case will need to be assessed for functional capacity (Box 23.5). Guillain–Barré syndrome has been associated with exposure to *Campylobacter jejuni* in poultry and swine farmers.[30]

About 15% of all patients with diabetes mellitus have a significant peripheral neuropathy (PN). Symmetrical sensory or autonomic neuropathy with postural hypotension, incontinence, and impotence, or isolated peripheral nerve lesions, or multifocal neuropathies may occur and mixed syndromes are common. Walking aids such as ankle–foot orthoses may be helpful when there is foot drop.

Hereditary neuropathies, such as Charcot–Marie–Tooth disease, usually affect both motor and sensory nerves and present during school years with foot deformities or difficulty in walking. A family history makes the diagnosis easier, but sporadic cases may arise by recessive inheritance or new mutations.

PN is a recognized complication of many toxic chemicals and therefore the onset of a PN should always alert the doctor to the possibility of toxic chemical exposure at

---

Box 23.5 Causes of peripheral neuropathy

Non-occupational

- Cryptogenic.
- Alcohol misuse.
- Metabolic and endocrine such as diabetes, uraemia, amyloid, and hypothyroidism.
- Inherited neuropathies.
- Nutritional deficiencies such as vitamins B1, B6, B12, and E and folate.
- Chronic inflammatory demyelination.
- Drugs such as cytotoxic agents, isoniazid, and amiodarone.
- Paraproteinaemias.
- Connective tissue disorders.
- Neoplastic and paraneoplastic disorders.
- Infections such as HIV, hepatitis B, Lyme disease, and shingles.

Occupational

- Hand–arm vibration syndrome.
- Toxins such as inorganic lead, mercury, arsenic, thallium, cobalt, acrylamide, diethylene glycol, carbon disulphide, methyl bromide, arsenic, the plasticizer tri-ortho-cresyl phosphate (TOCP), solvents such as *n*-hexane, 2,5-hexanedione and methyl *n*-butyl ketone (MBK) and pesticides such as the organophosphates, carbamates, and rotenone.

---

work. Symptoms of exposure might include weakness, paraesthesiae, or neuropathic pain in the limbs. The neuropathy may be subclinical and therefore only detected by electrodiagnostic investigation. Appropriate investigations would include motor and sensory nerve conduction tests with peak latency and sensory action potential wave amplitude measurements, as well as biological monitoring of blood or urine for the suspected toxin or a metabolite of the toxin. Some PNs are prescribed diseases under the UK's IIDB scheme.

Progression of PN is usually slow allowing most patients to be able to continue to work for several years. Care of the feet is vitally important in any sensory neuropathy, to prevent minor injuries being left untreated, the development of chronic ulceration, and possibly even amputation. There is guidance available from the Health and Safety Executive (L140) on when exposure to hand-transmitted vibration should cease, but in general the worker should be identified by health surveillance when sensory perception in the fingers is impaired, but before manual dexterity is lost (Box 23.6).

Box 23.6 Checklist for workers with peripheral neuropathy (or if suspected)

- Check gait, balance, foot drop, and grip strength with a dynamometer.
- Check sensory perception in hands and feet for light touch with cotton wool, pin prick with Neurotips™, monofilaments and vibration perception with a 64 Hz and a 128 Hz tuning fork, as well as proprioception in the great toe and little finger. Standardized thermal and vibration perception tests are available at Tier 5 health surveillance for sensorineural hand–arm vibration syndrome.
- Check that footwear is not overly restrictive.
- Advise adjustments to work so as to minimize amount of standing, walking, jumping, running, or climbing.
- Advise smoking cessation so as to optimize peripheral blood flow.

Neuromuscular junction disease

Neuromuscular junction diseases are rare. The most prevalent is myasthenia gravis, an autoimmune disorder in which antibodies interfere with normal neuromuscular transmission. Repeated or sustained exercise induces focal weakness, usually affecting limb girdle muscles, the extra-ocular muscles, or bulbar-innervated muscles, so an employee may first complain of proximal weakness when asked to do physical work, or of transient diplopia, or difficulty with chewing. If suspected, examination should be carried out before and after exercise, such as repeated abduction of the arm or walking, and positive serum acetylcholine receptor antibodies are diagnostic, but seronegative cases require more specialist investigation.

Provided the correct diagnosis is made, few cases become gravely ill nowadays because most respond well to treatment with the anticholinesterase drug pyridostigmine and immunosuppressants, including steroids. Most patients then enter remission, but may require treatment indefinitely and adverse drug effects need to be monitored. Certain classes of drug such as D-penicillamine and aminoglycosides aggravate myasthenic weakness so should be avoided, and muscle-strengthening exercises are inappropriate. A small proportion of cases require thymectomy, either because of an associated thymoma, or thymic hyperplasia in early-onset seropositive subjects. Unless the job is particularly physically demanding, the majority of employees with myasthenia should be able to continue working.

Muscle diseases

Muscle disease is less common than CNS disease. Some acquired myopathies are associated with drug treatment (e.g. corticosteroids or statins), or some other endocrine or malignant disease, on which its prognosis will depend. Polymyositis appears to be a syndrome of diverse causes that often occurs in association with systemic autoimmune diseases, viral infections, or connective tissue disorders such as lupus and rheumatoid arthritis. Chronic polymyositis can give rise to mainly proximal weakness with periodic flare-ups that may require increasing doses of steroids and other immunosuppressant therapy.

Persistent muscle weakness and fatigue may affect survivors of acute respiratory distress syndrome and other critical illnesses, who may encounter unexplained difficulties upon returning to work apparently fully recovered. The possibility of myopathy, polyneuropathy, or muscular deconditioning secondary to critical illness should be considered in anyone who has had a prolonged stay on an intensive care unit.

Entrapment neuropathies

The median nerve may be compressed in the carpal tunnel of the wrist causing nocturnal pain and paraesthesiae in the affected hand or forearm. Carpal tunnel syndrome is considered in Chapter 22. A cervical rib from the seventh cervical vertebra may produce a similar picture by compressing the C8 and T1 nerve trunks causing pain down the medial aspect of the forearm and weakness of abductor pollicis brevis.

The ulnar nerve is most commonly compressed in the cubital tunnel of the elbow, but may also be damaged in Guyon's canal between the pisiform and hammate bones in the wrist. The ulnar nerve divides into superficial and deep branches in the canal causing sensory loss in an ulnar nerve distribution or weakness of the intrinsic muscles of the hand when damaged. A ganglion in the wrist may produce similar symptoms.

The lateral cutaneous nerve of the thigh may be compressed as it passes under the inguinal ligament causing burning or numbness over the anterior thigh (meralgia paraesthetica), the common peroneal nerve may be compressed against the neck of the fibula causing foot drop, and the posterior tibial nerve may be compressed in the tarsal tunnel causing pain and numbness in the sole of the foot.

Chronic fatigue syndrome

A degree of limiting fatigue has been reported by 27% of working adults, but the prevalence of chronic fatigue syndrome is 0.1–2.6% depending on the criteria used for its definition. The underlying mechanisms remain poorly understood, but psychosocial factors and poor sleep are thought to be relevant. Chronic fatigue syndrome should be diagnosed when fatigue sufficient to interfere with normal physical and mental functioning has lasted for more than 6 months and no medical or psychiatric cause for the fatigue has been found. The only treatments that have been shown in clinical trials to work are cognitive behavioural therapy and graded exercise therapy.

Adjustments to work such as a phased return, the ability to pace work with regular breaks, a reduction in workload, the resolution of interpersonal difficulties, and additional support are helpful when rehabilitating someone with chronic fatigue back to work. As such patients are usually relatively young, medical retirement is rarely justified on the grounds of permanent incapacity until normal retirement age. Prognosis is highly variable but many patients improve spontaneously or sufficiently with treatment to return to work or normal functioning, although they may still report feelings of fatigue.[31] A sense of control over symptoms and not attributing illness to a physical cause are associated with a good outcome. Medical retirement should not be recommended until the patient has engaged with these adjustments and treatments.

The effects of ageing

It is generally accepted that the mature human CNS loses a large number of neurones each year naturally through a combination of apoptosis, degeneration, and various exogenous insults. Fortunately, there seems to be sufficient redundancy that most people can survive into retirement and old age with little clinical evidence except perhaps some mild cognitive impairment, motor slowing, weakness, and tremor. Indeed it has been suggested that if humans lived long enough they would all display features of dementia and parkinsonian as brain dopaminergic function naturally declines.

In those of normal working age, however, it is the effects of premature or accelerated ageing superimposed upon an underlying neurological condition that concern the OH professional. Some of the neurological conditions that are described in this chapter are degenerative in nature, and thus by definition they progress naturally with the passage of time. Motor neurone disease and young-onset dementia and parkinsonism are prime examples. By contrast, single-insult acquired disease such as traumatic or vascular injury to the brain or spinal cord typically remains static for many years once the acute phase and rehabilitation are complete. However, functional deterioration is more likely to occur 10–20 years after the event as the ability to compensate is exhausted. Furthermore, there may be long-term biomechanical complications from continuing to work with a chronic hemiparesis or paraplegia.

Key points

- Most neurological illnesses have implications for working, driving, flying, and serving in the armed forces.
- Migraine headaches have been estimated to cost employers €585 per affected person per year.
- Chronic exposure to pesticides has been found to be associated with a 50% increased risk of PD.
- Exposure to heavy metals, solvents, pesticides, or vibration may cause PN.
- The EDSS is a commonly used method for quantifying disability in MS.

Useful websites

Parkinson's UK	https://www.parkinsons.org.uk/
Headway (the brain injury association)	https://www.headway.org.uk/
MS Society UK	https://www.mssociety.org.uk/
United Kingdom Rehabilitation Council. 'Rehabilitation Standards'. 2009	http://rehabcouncil.org.uk/wp-content/uploads/2018/03/UKRC_Rehabilitation_Standards.pdf

References

1. **Stovner LJ, Andree C.** Impact of headache in Europe: a review for the Eurolight project. *J Headache Pain* 2008;**9**:139–46.
2. **Simpson SA, Wadsworth EJ, Moss SC, et al.** Minor injuries, cognitive failures and accidents at work: incidence and associated features. *Occup Med* 2005;**55**:99–108.
3. **Professional Practice Board.** *Assessment of Effort in Clinical Testing of Cognitive Functioning for Adults.* Leicester: British Psychological Society; 2009.
4. **Morgan K, Kucharczyk E, Gregory, P.** Insomnia: evidence-based approaches to assessment and management. *Clin Med* 2011;**11**:278–81.
5. **van Dijk FJH, Swaen GMH.** Fatigue at work. *Occup Environ Med* 2003;**60**(Suppl. 1):1–2.
6. **Drazkowski JF, Sirven JI.** Driving and neurologic disorders. *Neurology* 2011;**76**(Suppl. 2):S44–9.
7. **Baldi I, Gruber A, Rondeau V, et al.** Neurobehavioural effects of long-term exposure to pesticides: results from the 4-year follow-up of the PHYTONER study. *Occup Environ Med* 2011;**68**:108–15.
8. **Gunnarsson L-G, Bodin L.** Parkinson's disease and occupational exposures: a systematic literature review and meta-analyses. *Scand J Work, Environ Health* 2017;**43**:197–209.
9. **Furbee B.** Welding and parkinsonism. *Neurol Clinics* 2011;**29**:623–40.
10. **Altman P, Cunningham J, Dhanesha U, et al.** Disturbance of cerebral function in people exposed to drinking water contaminated with aluminium sulphate: retrospective study of the Camelford water incident. *BMJ* 1999;**319**:807.
11. **Schaper M, Buchta M, Schaller KH, et al.** Longitudinal study on potential neurotoxic effects of aluminium: assessment of exposure and neurobehavioural performance of Al welders in the automotive industry over 4 years. *Int Arch Occup Environ Health* 2009;**82**:1191–210.
12. **Lidsky TI, Schneider JS.** Lead neurotoxicity in children: basic mechanisms and clinical correlates. *Brain* 2003;**126**:5–19.
13. **Gidlow DA.** Lead toxicity. *Occup Med* 2015;**65**:348–56.
14. **Meyer-Baron M, Blaszkewicz M, Henke H, et al.** The impact of solvent mixtures on neurobehavioural performance – conclusions from epidemiological data. *Neurotoxicology* 2008;**29**:349–60.
15. **Ross SM, McManus IC, Harrison V, Mason O.** Neurobehavioural problems following low-level exposure to organophosphate pesticides: a systematic and meta-analytic review. *Clin Rev Toxicol* 2013;**43**:21–44.
16. **Mongini F, Evangelista A, Rota E, et al.** Further evidence of the positive effects of an educational and physical program on headache, neck and shoulder pain in a working community. *J Headache Pain* 2010;**11**:409–15.

17. **Johnston SC, Rothwell PM, Nquyen-Huynh MN, et al.** Validation and refinement of scores to predict very early stroke risk after transient ischaemic attack. *Lancet* 2007;**369**:283–92.

18. **Tanner CM, Ross GW, Jewell SA, et al.** Occupation and risk of parkinsonism: a multicenter case-control study. *Arch Neurol* 2009;**66**:1106–13.

19. **Huang CC, Chu NS, Lu CS, et al.** Long-term progression in chronic manganism: ten years of follow-up. *Neurology* 1998;**50**:698–700.

20. **Racette BA, Tabbal SD, Jennings D, et al.** Prevalence of parkinsonism and relationship to exposure in a large sample of Alabama welders. *Neurology* 2005;**64**:230–5.

21. **Bowler RM, Nakagawa S, Drezgic M, et al.** Sequelae of fume exposure in confined space welding: a neurological and neuropsychological case series. *Neurotoxicology* 2007;**28**:298–311.

22. **Sherer M, Struchen MA, Yablon SA, et al.** Comparison of indices of traumatic brain injury severity: Glasgow Coma Scale, length of coma and post-traumatic amnesia *J Neurol Neurosurg Psychiatr* 2008;**79**:678–85.

23. **McCauley SR, Boake C, Pedroza C, et al.** Correlates of persistent postconcussional disorders: DSM IV criteria versus ICD-10. *J Clin EXP Neuropsychol* 2011;**30**:360–79.

24. **McCrory P, Meeuwisse WH, Dvorak J, et al.** Consensus statement on concussion in sport: the 5th international conference on concussion in sport, Berlin, October 2016. *Br J Sports Med* 2017;**51**:838–47.

25. **British Society of Rehabilitation Medicine and Royal College of Physicians.** *Rehabilitation Following Acquired Brain Injury: National Clinical Guidelines.* London: Royal College of Physicians; 2003.

26. **Thompson AJ, Banwell BL, Barkhof F, et al.** Diagnosis of multiple sclerosis: 2017 revisions of the McDonald criteria. *Lancet Neurol* 2018;**17**:162–73.

27. **Lee D, Newell R, Ziegler L, et al.** Treatment of fatigue in multiple sclerosis: a systematic review of the literature. *Int J Nursing Practice* 2008;**14**:81–93.

28. **Pedersen C, Poulsen AH, Rod NH, et al.** Occupational exposure to extremely low-frequency magnetic fields and risk for central nervous system disease: an update of a Danish cohort study among utility workers. *Int Arch Occup Environ Health* 2017;**90**:619–28.

29. **Sorahan T, Mohammed N.** Neurodegenerative disease and magnetic field exposure in UK electricity workers. *Occup Med* 2014;**64**:454–60.

30. **Davis MF, Kamel F, Hoppin JA, et al.** Neurologic symptoms associated with raising poultry and swine among participants in the Agricultural Health Study. *J Occup Environ Med* 2011;**53**:190–5.

31. **Cairns R, Hotopf M.** A systematic review describing the prognosis of chronic fatigue syndrome. *Occup Med* 2005;**55**:20–31.

Chapter 24

Epilepsy

Ian Brown and Martin C. Prevett

Introduction

Epilepsy is a common condition that affects large numbers of working people. In about one-third, epilepsy is the only condition, and in others there are additional neurological, intellectual, or psychological problems. Uncontrolled epileptic seizures can lead to injury and may impact education and employment, but antiepileptic drug (AED) treatment is effective in approximately 70% of people with epilepsy.

Definitions

Epileptic seizures

Epileptic seizures are the clinical manifestation of an abnormal excessive discharge of cerebral neurons and may involve transient alteration of consciousness and motor or non-motor phenomena (sensory, autonomic, emotional, or cognitive). Epileptic seizures are caused by a wide variety of cerebral and systemic disorders, and may be *provoked* (acute symptomatic seizures) or *unprovoked*:

- Provoked or acute symptomatic seizures occur during an acute cerebral or systemic illness and do not constitute a diagnosis of epilepsy.
- Unprovoked seizures may be the late consequence of an antecedent cerebral disorder such as meningitis, head injury, and stroke, or be due to other structural, genetic, metabolic, and immune disorders. However, often there is no clear aetiology.

Epilepsy

Epilepsy is defined as a tendency to experience recurrent unprovoked epileptic seizures.

Classification of epilepsy

The international classification of epilepsies was updated in 2017 to reflect scientific advances since the last classification in 1989.[1] The updated classification is based on a diagnostic framework, which includes seizure types, epilepsy types, and epilepsy syndromes. It also incorporates aetiology and co-morbidities. The starting point of the updated classification is the classification of seizure type. In the classification of seizures proposed by the International League Against Epilepsy (ILAE) in 1981, seizures were divided into two main categories: partial and generalized.[2] Partial seizures were subdivided into simple partial, complex partial, and secondarily generalized seizures. Distinguishing between simple and complex partial seizures was sometimes difficult and the term 'secondarily generalized' was used inconsistently. In the updated 2017 ILAE classification, seizures are divided into focal onset, generalized onset, and unknown onset (Table 24.1).[3]

Focal onset seizures

In focal onset seizures, the abnormal neuronal discharge starts in a localized area of the brain. Clinical manifestations vary widely depending on anatomical localization and spread of the neuronal discharge. Focal onset seizures may occur with or without impairment of awareness and may evolve into a bilateral tonic–clonic seizure. Focal onset seizures can be further subdivided according to motor and non-motor features.

Generalized onset seizures

In generalized seizures, the abnormal neuronal discharge is widespread and involves both cerebral hemispheres from the onset. Generalized onset seizures are subdivided into motor and non-motor (absence) seizures. Tonic–clonic, typical absence, and myoclonic seizures are the commonest types of generalized seizure in people without other neurological or learning problems. Tonic, atonic, and clonic seizures tend to occur in people with diffuse cerebral disorders associated with learning disability. The updated 2017 classification introduces some new categories of generalized seizure including myoclonic absence, myoclonic–tonic–clonic, myoclonic–atonic, and epileptic spasms. In all generalized seizures there is an abrupt onset without any warning or aura.

Incidence and prevalence of epilepsy

A British study of treated epilepsy showed an incidence rate of 81 (95% confidence interval (CI) 77–85) per 100,000 per year.[4] Between the ages of 16 and 65 years, new cases

Table 24.1 ILAE 2017 classification of seizure type

Focal onset		Generalized onset	Unknown onset
Aware	Impaired Awareness	**Motor** Tonic–clonic Other motor **Non-motor (absence)**	**Motor** Tonic–clonic Other motor **Non-motor**
Motor onset **Non-motor onset**			**Unclassified**
Focal to bilateral tonic–clonic			

Source: data from Fisher, RS. Et al. Operational classification of seizure types by the International League Against Epilepsy: Position Paper of the ILAE Commission for Classification and Terminology. *Epilepsia*. 58(4): 522–30. Copyright © 2017 John Wiley & Sons, Inc.

of treated epilepsy occurred at a rate of approximately 75 per 100,000 per year. The lifetime risk of having a seizure is estimated to be 2–5%.

The prevalence of treated epilepsy in England and Wales in 1995 was estimated to be 5.15 cases per 1000.[4] The National General Practice Study of Epilepsy (NGPSE) found that 52% of patients had focal seizures and 39% had generalized seizures. Tonic–clonic seizures were the most common form of generalized seizure, other types being rare. Overall tonic–clonic seizures (either generalized or of focal onset) occurred in 62% of patients.[5] Seizure frequency varies enormously between individuals with about a third experiencing less than one seizure per year and about 20% more than one per week.

Causes of epilepsy

A cause can be established confidently only in a minority of new cases of epilepsy (20–40%). The most common causes of epileptic seizures in adults are listed in Table 24.2. The proportion of patients in whom a cause is identified depends on the extent of investigation, particularly neuroimaging (computed tomography or magnetic resonance imaging (MRI)). Advances in MRI technology have allowed identification of more subtle structural causes, such as disorders of cortical development. In a large series of patients with focal epilepsy, MRI revealed a structural cause for the epilepsy in 20%, but among patients with drug-resistant epilepsy, detailed MRI can detect a potential cause in up to 85%.[6] In addition to structural causes, the updated 2017 ILAE classification of the epilepsies lists five other aetiological categories: genetic, infectious, metabolic, immune, and unknown.[1]

The proportion of patients with epilepsy with an identifiable cause increases with age. Toxic causes of epilepsy are rare. Seizures may very occasionally occur as a result of lead encephalopathy, almost always in children. Seizures have occurred in employees overexposed

Table 24.2 Common causes of adult onset epileptic seizures

Cause	Proportion of identifiable cause (from the NGPSE[5])
Cerebrovascular disease	15% (49% in >60 years age group)
Cerebral tumour	6%
Head injury (and neurosurgery)	3%
Central nervous system infection (meningitis, encephalitis, cerebral abscess)	2%
Vascular malformation (cavernoma, arteriovenous malformation)	All other causes accounted for 7%
Disorders of cortical development	
Perinatal injury and hypoxia	
Genetic	
Immune disorders (e.g. anti-LGI1 encephalitis)	
Degenerative disorders (e.g. Alzheimer's disease)	

during the manufacture of chlorinated hydrocarbons, and ingestion of or gross overexposure to organochlorine insecticides has resulted in status epilepticus.[7] The organochlorine dichlorodiphenyltrichloroethane (DDT) is known to interfere with potassium, sodium, and calcium transport across the neuronal membrane, leading to repetitive discharges in neurons and tremors, seizures, and electrical activity triggered by tactile and auditory stimuli. Epileptiform abnormalities on electroencephalography (EEG) have also been recorded in asymptomatic individuals exposed to methylene chloride, methyl bromide, carbon disulphide, benzene, and styrene, although the significance of these observations is uncertain.

Recurrence of seizures

Estimates of recurrence rates after a first seizure have varied from 27% to 84%, the variation reflecting selection bias in the study population.[8] Aetiology has an important influence on the risk of recurrence. In the NGPSE, seizures associated with neurological deficits presumed to be present from birth had a 100% rate of relapse within the first 12 months, whereas seizures associated with a lesion acquired postnatally carried a risk of relapse of 75% by 12 months.[9] The presence of generalized spike and wave activity on EEG also appears to increase the risk of recurrence.

The risk of recurrence decreases as time elapses after the first seizure, a fact that is of importance in resolving concerns about safety at work. In the NGPSE (in which only 15% of patients with a first seizure received treatment), the 3-year risk of recurrence after a seizure-free period of 6 months was 44%, after 12 months of being seizure free the risk was 32%, and after 18 months of being seizure free the risk fell to 17% (Figure 24.1).

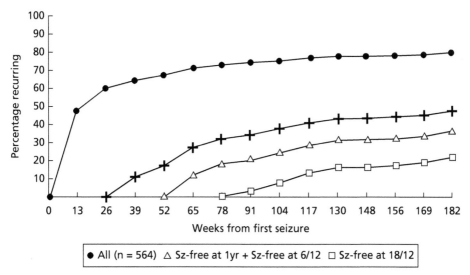

Figure 24.1 Actuarial percentage recurrence rates after a first seizure for those still free of recurrence at 6, 12, and 18 months, and for all patients.
Reproduced with permission from Hart, YM et al. National General Practice Study of Epilepsy: recurrence after a first seizure. *Lancet.* 336(8726), 1271–4. Copyright © 1990 Elsevier.

Randomized studies have shown that the risk of recurrence after a first seizure is reduced by AED treatment.[10,11] Patients started on treatment after a first seizure are, however, no more likely to achieve remission than patients in whom treatment is delayed until after two or more seizures. Bonnett et al. undertook a further analysis of the multicentre study of early epilepsy and single seizures and concluded that at 6 months after the index seizure (for those taking AEDs), the risk of recurrence in the next 12 months was 14% (95% CI 10–18%).[12] For patients who did not start AED treatment, the risk estimate was 18% (95% CI 13–23%). These data have resulted in a change to the driving restrictions after a first seizure (see 'Lifting of restrictions').

Chances of remission

Although there is a modest and measurable risk of recurrence after a first seizure, most people who develop epilepsy become seizure free. In the NGPSE, if patients with single or provoked seizures are excluded, 62% achieved a 5-year remission after 9 years of follow-up.[13] In another population-based study, the 5-year remission rates were 65% at 10 years and 76% at 15 years.[14] Most patients who enter remission do so within 2 years of diagnosis and, as time elapses without seizure control, the chances of subsequent remission decreases. Factors such as a previous neurological insult and seizure type may influence time to remission.[15] A syndromic classification can be useful prognostically. Benign epilepsy with centrotemporal spikes (benign rolandic epilepsy) develops in childhood and spontaneous remission occurs in 98–99% of cases by the age of 14 years. Juvenile myoclonic epilepsy, however, develops in adolescence and although responsive to treatment, is associated with a lifelong disposition to seizures and over 90% of patients will relapse if treatment is withdrawn.

Twenty to thirty per cent of patients continue to experience seizures despite drug treatment.[16] The introduction of more than ten new therapies since 1990 has had little impact on this figure. There is no evidence that the newer drugs are any more effective than standard treatment and a poor response to initial treatment with any drug appropriate to the type of epilepsy, whether standard or new, tends to predict a poor response to other drugs. A prospective study found that among previously untreated patients, 47% became seizure free with their first AED and 14% became seizure free during treatment with a second or third drug.[17]

Withdrawal of antiepileptic drug treatment

For those patients who go into remission and remain seizure free for 2 years or more, withdrawal of treatment is an option. The risk of relapse in this group is 30% (95% CI 25–30%) in the first 12 months after discontinuing treatment.[18] Given the implications of relapse for work and driving, most patients elect to continue treatment indefinitely.

Prevention of epilepsy in the workplace

Primary and secondary prevention

In the workplace, avoidance of head injuries through risk assessment and implementation of appropriate controls is the most important preventive measure. The use of seat belts and safety helmets is important. Where there is a risk of falling objects, netting can be rigged below the work area, warnings given for those in the vicinity, and the wearing of hard hats made compulsory. However, a safety helmet will not protect an individual from serious head injury if anything heavy is dropped from a height. The other main preventive measure is the avoidance of precipitating factors, some of which are described below.

Epilepsy does not follow a trivial head injury; but if the head injury is associated with a depressed fracture (especially if the dura is torn), an intracranial haematoma, or focal neurological signs, then there is a significant risk of later epilepsy.

A large community survey of a head-injured population[19] confirmed findings by previous workers that the risk of early seizures (within 7 days of injury) and late seizures (7 days or more days after injury) can be determined by assessing the severity of the brain injury. Severe head injuries (loss of consciousness, amnesia lasting more than 24 hours, subdural haematoma, and brain contusion) are accompanied by a substantially increased risk of epilepsy over the next decade (standardized incidence ratio 17.0, 95% CI 12.3–23.6). Because of this risk, patients who have suffered a serious head injury should be treated in a similar way to those who have already suffered a seizure, including a 6–12-month ban on driving. The use of antiepileptic medication does not affect the risk of developing post-traumatic epilepsy but it does reduce the frequency of early seizures.[20]

Shift work

Seizures are common just before and after waking, especially in idiopathic generalized epilepsy, so it might be supposed that the introduction of a shift system into the work routine of a person with well-controlled epilepsy would predispose them to an increased frequency of seizures. This has not been documented possibly because people with epilepsy elect to avoid shift work.[21] Many people with well-controlled epilepsy, however, can work on rotating shifts without problems.

Night work may be an exception. Patterns of sleep are disturbed by night work and to a lesser extent by other types of shift work. Night workers sleep for shorter periods during their working week and sleep longer on rest days to make up the deficit.[22] Sleep deprivation is an important precipitant of seizures for some individuals and is best avoided by those with idiopathic generalized epilepsy.

Stress

Stress is a frequently self-reported precipitant of seizures in patients with epilepsy. Changes in brain arousal lead to changes in excitability and this may affect neuronal discharges, particularly of those neurons that surround an epileptic focus. Many patients report that the frequency of their seizures increase when they are exposed to stress, but stress itself may also be associated with other seizure-provoking factors such as drinking alcohol and sleep disturbance, and there may be reporting bias as people search for an explanation for exacerbations of their condition. Stress mediators (corticosteroids, neurosteroids, etc.) probably contribute to this phenomenon.[23]

Paradoxically, inactivity and drowsiness may also be related to an increased seizure frequency. The possibility that stress and its associated factors may affect seizure control should be considered when employees with epilepsy are moved to different areas of responsibility.

Photosensitivity and visual display equipment

Photosensitivity epilepsy is a form of reflex epilepsy that is rare in adults and usually associated with idiopathic generalized epilepsy. It may need to be considered where a light source flickers. The overall prevalence is 1 in 10,000 and more common in women. Ninety per cent of patients have suffered their first convulsion due to photosensitivity before the age of 25 years.[24–26] Photosensitivity may be increased following deprivation of sleep and spontaneous seizures may also occur in photosensitive subjects.

The diagnosis of photosensitive epilepsy is supported by performing an EEG with photic stimulation and eliciting a photoparoxysmal response. This is usually a generalized discharge of spike wave activity elicited by the flickering stimulus and persisting after the stimulus has ceased. False-positive tests can also arise: some individuals have a paroxysmal EEG response to photic stimulation without evidence of having had a seizure.[24-26] The now obsolete electron gun televisions were a precipitant of photosensitive epilepsy, but modern light emitting diode and plasma screen televisions do not present the same risk. The use of display screen equipment (DSE) in employment constitutes a much smaller risk than viewing television. The probability of a first convulsion being induced by DSE is exceedingly small; seizures are unlikely even in an established photosensitive subject. Sufferers of epilepsy are therefore fit to work with DSE. Other precipitants include flickering sunlight (e.g. through the leaves of a tree or when swimming), faulty and flickering artificial lights, and helicopter rotor blades and aeroplane propellers. The Civil Aviation Authority has recognized the special risks that may be associated with flying, and these are covered in Chapter 15.

Other types of reflex epilepsy

Although reflex epilepsy may occasionally be induced by reading, concentrating, being suddenly startled, and auditory stimuli, this is extremely rare.

Alcohol and drugs

Alcohol misuse increases the risk of epileptic seizures. Seizures may be caused by alcohol withdrawal, a direct toxic effect of alcohol, or an associated metabolic disturbance (e.g. hypoglycaemia). Seizures may also occur with chronic alcohol misuse in the absence of withdrawal or other identifiable causes. Alcohol misuse may also complicate established epilepsy, increasing the risk of seizures and other complications.

A number of drugs lower seizure threshold, especially tricyclic antidepressants but also isoniazid, penicillin, lignocaine, and antipsychotics such as chlorpromazine and haloperidol. Some of the newer antipsychotic drugs, notably olanzapine, are associated with epileptiform abnormalities on EEG.

Box 24.1 What to do if a seizure occurs

If a seizure is likely to occur at work, supervisors and workplace colleagues should be warned and instructed in appropriate first-aid measures, with agreement. Convulsive seizures are almost always short-lived and do not require immediate medical treatment:

- The person should be made as comfortable as possible, preferably lying down (eased to the floor if seated).
- The head should be cushioned and any tight clothing or neckwear loosened.
- The patient should remain attended until recovery is complete.
- During the attack, the patient should not be moved, unless they are in a dangerous place, for example, in a road, by a fire or hot radiator, at the top of stairs, or by the edge of water.
- No attempt should be made to open the mouth or force anything between the teeth.
- After the seizure has subsided, the person should be rolled on to their side, making sure that the airways are cleared of any obstruction, such as dentures or vomit, and ensuring that there are no injuries that require medical attention.
- When the patient recovers consciousness there is often a short period of confusion and distress. They should be comforted, reassured, and allowed to rest.
- An ambulance or hospital treatment is not required unless there is a serious injury, the seizure has lasted more than 5 minutes,[27] the person has had a series of seizures without recovering consciousness between them, or the seizure has features which differ significantly from the patient's usual pattern.

Fluctuating serum levels of AEDs, which may arise from poor compliance with treatment or interactions with other drugs, increases the risk of seizures. Sudden withdrawal of AEDs, especially phenobarbital and benzodiazepines, may also result in seizures (see Box 24.1).

The Epilepsy Action website (see 'Useful websites') provides excellent practical advice for those with epilepsy on many aspects of employment. They also produce a card that provides details about an individual's epilepsy and advice about what to do if the person is found unconscious.

Responsibility of the occupational health professional in the workplace

The first task is to establish without doubt that a seizure has occurred. The employee should attend the occupational health (OH) department as soon as possible and remain off work in the interim. A detailed history of the event should be obtained and information sought from the patient and any reliable witness to try to establish the nature of the event. Interviewing work colleagues and relatives who witnessed the event can be extremely useful, as the subject usually remembers little beyond the first few seconds. It is unwise to rely solely on the patient's account, written reports from witnesses, or second-hand anecdotal information.

The past medical history may reveal risk factors for the development of epilepsy, such as febrile seizures in childhood, previous significant head injury, or stroke. Relevant points about the family history and consumption of drugs or alcohol should also be obtained. The patient should always be fully examined, as a seizure may occasionally be the first symptom of a serious systemic illness such as meningitis, or of a structural cerebral lesion—detailed medical assessment is therefore always necessary.

Permission to contact both the general practitioner (GP) and any hospital consultant should be obtained from the patient. It is often useful to contact these physicians infor-mally and discuss the situation that has arisen. This should be followed by a formal letter giving a concise account of events and the examination findings, and requesting any fur-ther relevant information (with informed consent).

Not all episodes of unconsciousness are epileptic seizures. The most common differen-tial diagnoses are syncope (vasovagal or cardiac) and dissociative seizures (non-epileptic) with an underlying psychological basis. Other possible diagnoses include transient is-chaemic attacks and migraine.

Prolonged cerebral anoxia due to syncope may produce some stiffening, twitching, and even incontinence, although a generalized tonic–clonic seizure (secondary anoxic seizure) is unusual. The circumstances of the event, prodromal symptoms, and rapidity of recovery will usually allow distinction between syncope and an epileptic seizure. Dissociative seizures can be very difficult to distinguish from epileptic seizures and spe-cialist advice is usually required.

Focal ischaemia of a transient ischaemic attack does not usually involve a loss of con-sciousness but often causes neurological deficits such as aphasia or paresis, and only rarely muscle jerking (clonus).

Once it has been established as far as possible that a single, unprovoked, seizure has occurred, the procedure listed in Box 24.2 should be adopted.

Consideration of potential new employees

The majority of jobs are suitable for those with epilepsy but job placement may require a detailed risk assessment. Epilepsy falls within the disability provisions of the Equality Act 2010 even if it is medically controlled. However, precedence is given to the Health and Safety at Work etc. Act 1974 (HASAWA) when safety issues arise. Sufficient thought must be given to the possibility of making 'reasonable adjustments to the workplace or the job'. With epilepsy, this is nearly always possible except where there is a statutory bar (e.g. the driving of large goods vehicles). Often a safe place of work can be found for an employee, unless the hazard and risk is an integral part of the job (e.g. working as a steeplejack or on an oil rig). Similarly, provided that driving is only a small component

---

Box 24.2 Procedure following a seizure

1. The medical notes must state clearly the course of events and that a seizure has taken place.

2. The management should be contacted and given clear and concise recommendations, in writing, regarding the employee's placement. Such written recommendations should be constructed with the agreement of the employee and should observe codes of medical confidentiality. If epilepsy has been confirmed (not just a single seizure), some employees prefer to inform their immediate supervisor. It is worth discussing the possibility of such disclosure with the patient.

3. The OH professional must become familiar with any AED prescribed and have a sound knowledge of potential side effects.

4. Consideration should be given to sensible employment restrictions. This should include advice to the individual on driving and their responsibility to inform the DVLA (see 'The driving licence regulations and their effects'). See also Chapter 15.

---

of the job (<15%), an employee should not be refused employment if they do not hold a driving licence. The training manual prepared by the International Bureau of Epilepsy[28] provides excellent practical advice, an assessment questionnaire, and some illustrative cases with vocational scenarios.

Sensible restrictions on the work of people with epilepsy

Proposed restrictions must be discussed with the employee and with management. Clear written instructions should be given to management regarding placement, responsibilities, and review. Confidentiality must not be breached. Restrictions should be no more than necessary on common-sense grounds, as would apply equally to any individual subject to sudden and unexpected lapses in consciousness or concentration, however infrequent.

The success rate in placing people with epilepsy is far greater if they have fewer than six seizures per year. In general, minor seizures are less disruptive than major ones, but periods of automatism (performance of acts without conscious will), may upset colleagues. Other disadvantageous characteristics are prolonged periods of postictal confusion and atonic and tonic seizures where the possibility of serious injury is increased. See Box 24.3 for sensible restrictions regarding avoidance of activity.

There are also certain jobs with special hazards where the risk of even one seizure may give rise to catastrophic consequences. These jobs fall into two groups:

1. Jobs in transport, including vocational drivers, train drivers, drivers of large container-terminal vehicles, crane operators, aircraft pilots, seamen, and commercial divers.

Box 24.3 Epilepsy restrictions

◆ Climbing and working unprotected at heights.

◆ Driving or operating motorized machinery.

◆ Working around unguarded machinery.

◆ Use of hand-held powered tools that can be left in the 'on' position.

◆ Working near fire or water.

◆ Working for long periods in isolation.

2. Jobs that involve work unprotected at heights (e.g. scaffolders, steeplejacks, and fire-fighters), work on mainline railways, with high-voltage electricity, hot metal, dangerous unguarded machinery, or near open tanks of water or chemical fluids.

The working environment and equipment to be used by the employee with epilepsy should always be inspected by the OH professional and the safety officer. The employee's immediate supervisor should also be involved in any decisions.

It is important to remind the employee that contravention of agreed restrictions may endanger not only their own safety, but also the safety of others. It may also be impossible to make a personal injury insurance claim for financial compensation should an accident occur as a result of evasion of the agreed restrictions.

Lifting of restrictions

A policy should be established for terminating any restriction on work practices. This should be made known to the affected employee and altered only in exceptional circumstances. There is little place for partial lifting of restrictions. If a work restriction is removed after a period of freedom from seizures, the employee should be instructed to report any further seizure to the OH staff or to a personnel officer or manager. If AED treatment is stopped or changed, consideration should be given to close monitoring at work for a period, or to the temporary reintroduction of restrictions.

It may be that, following the introduction of medication, control is poor with an unacceptable rate of seizure recurrence. Every effort should be made to improve control before the individual is rejected or restrictions imposed on employment or promotion. There may be specific and avoidable precipitating factors (e.g. alcohol or poor adherence to medication). It may be appropriate to consider whether the diagnosis is correct and the possibility of dissociative seizures (psychogenic seizures) has been eliminated. Also that an appropriate AED has been chosen, there is concordance with treatment, and adequate blood levels have been achieved (see 'Effect of antiepileptic drugs on work performance').

A planned date for a review of restrictions should be offered, as this will affirm that the employee is a valued member of the workforce. In this respect, it seems reasonable to follow, for employment purposes, guidelines issued by the Department of Transport for ordinary driving licences (see Driver and Vehicle Licensing Agency (DVLA) guidance listed in 'Useful websites'). An employee who is safe to drive a car should be safe to undertake most industrial, production, or commercial duties. (Jobs with special hazards are listed earlier.) After an initial seizure, the Department of Transport advises car driving is restricted for 6 months (unless there is a high risk of recurrence). If there is considered to be a 20% or greater risk of recurrence after a first seizure or there has been more than one seizure, a 1-year ban on driving is applied.

Effect of antiepileptic drugs and other common co-morbidities of epilepsy on work performance

Many additional factors should be considered once reasonable or complete seizure control has been achieved. All AEDs will alter brain function to some extent, and this will be discussed in greater detail later in this section. A number of other factors may impact work and employment. Approximately 20–30% of patients with epilepsy have psychiatric disturbances[29] (a 6–12-fold increase compared to the general population), with a prevalence of about 7–8% in patients with treatment-refractory temporal lobe epilepsy. The most common psychiatric conditions in epilepsy are depression, anxiety, and psychosis (Table 24.3).[30]

The problem may be simply the result of having to cope with a chronic disorder, as a result of the AEDs or a concomitant neuropsychological disorder. Neuropsychiatric prescription can affect seizure control adversely. Epilepsy may also have an effect on learning, memory, and cognition—a result of the seizure events or the AED prescribed. Cognitive impact is increasingly recognized, and may predate the diagnosis of epilepsy. There is a relationship between memory impairment and measures of anxiety and depression.[31] Memory impairment can be related to temporal lobe dysfunction, but it has been argued that memory complaints in epilepsy could partly reflect difficulties adjusting to the diagnosis (discussed in 'Epilepsy and epileptic seizures').[32]

AED treatment aims to control seizures without significant adverse effects, and in most patients this is achievable. For others, particularly those requiring combination therapy, a balance must be struck between seizure frequency and adverse effects.

Table 24.3 Prevalence rates of psychiatric disorders in patients with epilepsy and general population controls

Psychiatric disorder	Controls (%)	Patients with epilepsy (%)
Major depressive disorder	11	17
Anxiety disorder	11	23
Mood/anxiety disorder	20	34
Suicidal Ideation	13	25
Others	21	35

Acute adverse effects are usually rapidly reversible on drug withdrawal or dose reduction. The chronic adverse effects of AEDs are more difficult to control and can impact work performance. However, it is often difficult to separate the effects of AEDs from the effects of the underlying disorder and of the seizures themselves.[33]

In patients treated with a combination of AEDs, reducing drug intake improves cognitive function. It is generally considered that adverse cognitive effects are greater with phenobarbital than with phenytoin, carbamazepine, and valproate. There is evidence to suggest that some of the newer AEDs (e.g. lamotrigine and oxcarbazepine) are better tolerated. The wider range of AEDs now available increases the likelihood of achieving a treatment regimen without adverse effects.

The OH professional should work closely with the neurologist to determine whether the patient's drug regimen is appropriate for their epilepsy and explore the therapeutic options that match their specific employment requirements.

Special work problems

Disclosure of epilepsy to employers

Ideally, individuals with epilepsy would freely disclose how their seizures affect them, enabling the OH professional to better advise about employment which maximizes the employee's potential and minimizes any risk to themselves or others. However, people with epilepsy may feel they are at a competitive disadvantage and that their choice of vocation is limited. They may have concerns regarding their mobility and promotion within a company, whether they can join the pension fund, and may face suspicion and scrutiny from their fellow workers.

Therefore, the presence of epilepsy is often concealed from employers. A survey of people in London with epilepsy showed that over half of those who had had two or more full-time jobs after the onset of epilepsy had never disclosed their epilepsy to their employer, and only one in ten had always revealed it.[34] If seizures were infrequent, or usually nocturnal, such that the applicant considered that they had a good chance of successfully concealing it, then the employer was virtually never informed. Among those who declared their condition, two variables correlated with failure to gain employment: frequent seizures and lack of any special skills.

Educational programmes are important in addressing this situation as well as a clear definition of the jobs that can be undertaken as published by the International Bureau for Epilepsy.[35] This considers the vast majority of jobs to be suitable for people with epilepsy, especially where the person possesses the right qualifications and experience. Blanket prohibitions should be avoided and the organization of work practices should be reviewed to reduce potential risk to an acceptable level.

Accident and absence records of those with epilepsy

There is no evidence that people with epilepsy are more accident-prone or have worse attendance records than other workers although many studies are biased as workers with epilepsy tend to get placed in inherently less risky work. The most significant (old but landmark) study of work performance that attempted to eliminate this bias was conducted by the US Department of Labour.[36] A statistical comparison was made of ten groups with different disabilities, including people with epilepsy, with matched unimpaired controls in the same jobs. Within the epilepsy group, no differences were found in absenteeism and while their incidence of work injuries and accident rates was slightly higher, this was not statistically significant. The general conclusion was that people with epilepsy perform as well as matched unimpaired workers in the same jobs in manufacturing industries.

Another study demonstrated that discriminatory practices against the recruitment of people with epilepsy are unwarranted, if based on the belief that they have worse accident rates, attendance, or productivity.[37] These positive findings were reinforced by a recent study[38] which concluded that epilepsy did not contribute importantly to workplace injury in Britain. A study of epilepsy in the British Steel Corporation[21] generally supported these findings. There was no significant difference between epilepsy and control groups with regard to overall sickness absence, accident records, and five different aspects of job performance. Work performance, however, was significantly reduced in people with epilepsy who also had an associated personality disorder. However, any applicant with epilepsy must be assessed individually with regard to seizure control and other associated handicaps. Employers should have a receptive policy for recruitment and job security. This may encourage employees to admit the problem and allow industry an opportunity to appraise their abilities and place them appropriately. A major task for OH professionals is to challenge and change the often firmly held prejudices of employers.

Current employment practices

Employment practices are increasingly flexible, particularly since the Equality Act 2010. However, certain restrictions apply in situations determined by health and safety regulations.

Proven cases of epilepsy are not accepted for new entrance to the UK armed forces, and those who have suffered a single seizure less than 4 years before entry are also rejected. For serving personnel, a single seizure after entry necessitates full examination, restricted activities, and observation for 18 months. Full reinstatement is awarded only after assessment by a senior consultant. Air crew who have suffered a single seizure after entry are grounded permanently (see Chapter 15) and servicemen who suffer more than one seizure will be considered for discharge on grounds of disability. The policy for civilians employed in the armed forces is more flexible than for servicemen, allowing for work adaptations to accommodate their medical history.

Epilepsy is not an absolute contraindication for employment in the police force, although the police expect all their officers to be fit for all duties. All cases are individually assessed in the Metropolitan Police.[39] The Epilepsy Action website lists other employment where restrictions might be required but a number relate to driving licence restrictions (see DVLA website in 'Useful websites').

Employers should consider their obligations according to the Equality Act 2010 having given consideration to any safety-critical work. Epilepsy declared at the pre-placement stage is rarely an absolute bar and requires OH assessment. Epilepsy developing in service can often be accommodated if the employee is willing to be relocated, although this may involve some loss of earnings and status. In some occupations, retirement on the grounds of ill health may be considered if there is no alternative to terminating employment.

The Department for Education relies on the employer (usually the school) to make an assessment on fitness to teach and will engage an experienced occupational physician to make this assessment to ensure that the teacher can perform their duties safely at all times. The NHS has made considerable progress over the last decade but still has no national guidelines. Guidelines have been constructed by the Association of National Health Occupational Physicians, stating that all healthcare workers with epilepsy must be assessed, although emphasizing that the epilepsy should be well controlled and patient safety is paramount.

The Civil Service has a documented policy on the recruitment and employment of people with epilepsy. The health standard for appointment requires that a candidate's health does not disqualify him/her for the position sought, and that the person is likely to give regular and efficient service for at least 5 years or for the period of any shorter appointment. The Civil Service OH service stresses that epilepsy per se is not a bar to holding any established appointment apart from those posts with special hazards.

Getting employers to understand about epilepsy

Many people with epilepsy are unemployed. Epilepsy Action's survey found that 14% of respondents were unemployed, although actively seeking work. This is significantly higher than the International Labour Organization unemployment rate of 8.8% for disabled people. Even if employed, many workers with epilepsy are still frequently denied promotion. In a survey of employers in the US, it was found that few would employ people known to have had a generalized seizure within the previous year.[40] Employers gave the reason that people with epilepsy 'create safety problems for themselves and other workers'. Such misconceived reasoning has not varied for more than two decades. Encouragingly, this study provided evidence of a positive change in attitude and law in the US, probably attributable to the continued efforts of public and private agencies. A more recent study examining employers' attitudes in the UK[41] revealed that 21% thought that employing people with epilepsy would be a 'major issue' and 16% considered there were no suitable jobs in their company for a person with epilepsy. It is therefore unsurprising that concealment of the condition remains high.

Informal health education seminars at work could improve employers' understanding. A programme that involves the human resources department, OH team, and union representatives may prevent problems. Topics such as epilepsy, stress, and alcohol misuse should be discussed openly with the benefit of expert advice on hand. OH can play a major part in health education and changing attitudes. For such a common complaint (prevalence 5–10 per 1000 of the population), misconceptions among employers are surprising. Many employees, both on the shop floor and in management, consider that someone with epilepsy also has some degree of mental handicap combined with a lesser or greater physical infirmity. Certainly such problems may coexist but not in the majority. It is essential that health professionals dispel myths, bringing a sense of proportion.

Medical services and opportunities for sheltered work

A minority of people with epilepsy will only be able to work in a sheltered environment. Poorly controlled seizures, physical disability, learning disability, and poor social adaptive skills will pose additional problems. The following specialized facilities are available in the UK for people with epilepsy.

NHS medical services

All patients with a suspected first seizure should be seen as soon as possible by a specialist in the management of epilepsy.[42] Those patients entering remission will usually be referred back to primary care. The care of the 20–30% whose epilepsy proves difficult to control is usually shared between general practice and hospital clinics. Epilepsy nurse specialists attached to hospital services or based in primary care provide enormous support for people with epilepsy and are an integral part of the epilepsy care team. Epilepsy nurses are very specifically trained, often to degree level and run their own hospital clinics supporting the epileptology team. They also act as the first responders when problems crop up with medication, seizure frequency, or domestic difficulties. Some regional neuroscience centres also provide tertiary epilepsy services with facilities for specialist investigation and surgical treatment.

Residential care

Residential care is required for a small proportion of people with severe epilepsy and is usually provided by social services. In addition, there are epilepsy charities, residential centres, and special assessment centres that cater for the more complex needs of patients with epilepsy, as outlined in the following sections.

Epilepsy charities

The Epilepsy Society

The Epilepsy Society (formerly the National Society for Epilepsy), founded in 1892, is the UK's largest epilepsy charity. It provides residential care, medical services (in conjunction with the National Hospital for Neurology and Neurosurgery in London), information, support, and training. A wide range of written information is available including information for patients on epilepsy and work. The Epilepsy Society is also committed to campaigning for improved services for people with epilepsy.

Epilepsy Action (British Epilepsy Association)

Epilepsy Action aims to raise awareness and modify regressive attitudes towards epilepsy. It also provides a wealth of advice and information about the condition.

Residential centres and schools for people with epilepsy

In the UK, there are a number of special schools and centres for epilepsy, the largest of which are the Chalfont Centre for Epilepsy, the David Lewis Centre, and the National Centre for Young People with Epilepsy. These provide residential care for people with epilepsy, who are unable to live independently in the community. Some provide sheltered employment. Financial support is usually provided through the local authority, the health service, or private or charitable funds.

Special assessment centres

There are several special assessment centres in the UK providing short-term and social in-patient assessment for people with severe or complicated epilepsy. The largest is the Chalfont Centre for Epilepsy. Others include Boundary Brook House (formerly known as Park Hospital) in Oxford for children and the David Lewis Centre in Cheshire.

Relationship between the occupational health professional, neurologist, and general practitioner

Recommendations received from the neurologist may conflict with the OH professional's perceptions about the best interests of the patient in their particular working environment. The GP, who is likely to have closer knowledge of the patient and their family, can liaise with these two specialists. It is advantageous if all the medical professionals involved work together to avoid conflicting advice. In companies with an OH service, an employee with epilepsy should be encouraged to discuss problems with OH as they arise. The OH service has a special role in counselling and health education. Detailed confidential notes should be kept. Employees with epilepsy should be reviewed regularly by the OH service (at least annually).

Existing legislation and guidelines for employment

For a more detailed discussion of legal aspects, see Chapter 3 and also Carter.[43] The HASAWA makes no reference to disability and applies to all employees regardless of their health. People with epilepsy who do not disclose it to an employer may contravene section 7 of the HASAWA, if they knowingly accept a job that poses significant risks. The Equality Act 2010 imposes a legal duty on the employer to make reasonable adjustments or modifications to working arrangements to safely accommodate the disabled person.

Someone who suffers from epilepsy will be considered disabled even if their condition is controlled by medication. A common example might be an applicant for a job who is presently unable to hold a group 1 driving licence because of a seizure. The job applied for requires the applicant to hold a group 1 driving licence but the driving component of the job is only about 10% of the duties. Under these circumstances, it would probably be reasonable for the employer to provide an alternative means of transport for the employee. However, if the driving component were a substantial part of the job, then it would not be reasonable for the employer to provide an alternative means of transport. The disability advisor at Jobcentre Plus will be able to give additional advice in these circumstances and may be able to help with temporary transport needs using the Access to Work scheme.

For those in employment who develop epilepsy, the employer should also consider reasonable adjustments and reasonable in this context means that such adjustments must be achievable and practical without incurring excessive cost. Some employers are also under the misconception that an applicant with a history of epilepsy will not be accepted into the pension fund. While this is generally untrue, the pension scheme assessors may consider all cases on their merits, and very occasionally restrictions are placed on those with specific medical problems. Life cover or ill health retirement provision may be reduced if the risk is considered very significant, but this will only be in relation to an accident or disability that is directly related to the specific declared disability. In most cases, there is no restriction and occupational pension schemes are more liberal than independent life assurance schemes.

No special insurance arrangements are necessary for a worker with epilepsy. The employer's liability insurance covers everyone in the workplace, provided the employer has taken the disability into account when allocating the individual's work. Failure to disclose epilepsy will render the employer's insurance invalid, and should an accident occur as a direct result of the condition it is unlikely that a claim for compensation will be honoured by the insurance arrangements.

The driving licence regulations and their effects

Licensing for driving is one of the few areas in which there is legislation related to epilepsy (see also Chapter 15). Regulation is deemed necessary because seizures are a potential cause of road traffic accidents in drivers suffering from epilepsy. Although the overall incidence of road traffic accidents may not be higher in people with epilepsy, the risk of serious accidents and fatal accidents is increased.[44] Ideally, legislation should balance the excess risks of driving against the social and psychological disadvantage to the individual of prohibiting driving. In the UK, it is the licensing authority (DVLA), not the sufferer's personal medical advisers, who makes the decision on licensing. The regulations are based, where possible, on research into the risks of seizure recurrence in different clinical circumstances. Licensing is divided into two groups, with more stringent conditions applied to group 2 licences because more time is spent driving and the consequences of accidents are often more serious (Box 24.4). Reference should also be made to DVLA guidance.

Box 24.4 Group 1 and group 2 driving licences

◆ *Group 1 licences* (motorcars and motorcycles): an applicant for a licence who suffers from epilepsy shall satisfy the following conditions:

- He/she shall have been free of any epileptic attack during the period of 1 year immediately preceding the date when the licence is granted; or
- An applicant who has seizures only while asleep, and has never had a seizure while awake, shall have demonstrated a sleep-only pattern of seizures for one year or more. If the applicant has ever experienced a seizure while awake, they must have demonstrated a sleep-only pattern of seizures of 3 years or more.
- An applicant who has demonstrated, over the course of 1 year from the date of the first seizure, a pattern of seizures which neither affect awareness nor cause any functional impairment, and has never experienced any other type of unprovoked seizure.
- The person complies with advised treatment and check-ups for epilepsy, and the driving of a vehicle will not be likely to endanger the public.

◆ *Group 2 licences* (large goods vehicles and passenger-carrying vehicles, i.e. vehicles over 7.5 tonnes, or nine seats or more for hire or reward): an applicant for a licence shall satisfy the following conditions:

- No epileptic attacks shall have occurred in the preceding 10 years.
- The applicant shall have taken no AED treatment in the preceding 10 years.
- There will be no continuing liability to suffer epileptic seizures.

The purpose of the third condition is to exclude people from driving (whether or not epileptic seizures have actually occurred in the past) who have a potentially epileptogenic cerebral lesion, or who have had a craniotomy or complicated head injury, for example.

Following a first unprovoked seizure, the regulations require 6 months off driving for group 1 licence holders unless there are clinical features which indicate a high ($\geq$20% per year) risk of a further seizure. For group 2 licence holders, driving can be resumed after 5 years if recent assessment indicates that the risk of a further seizure is 2% or less per year and they have taken no antiepileptic medication throughout the 5-year period prior to the granting of a licence.

If a seizure is considered to be 'provoked' by an exceptional condition which will not recur, driving may be allowed once the provoking factor has been successfully treated or removed and provided that a 'continuing liability' to seizures is not also present. For group 1 licence holders, treatment status is not a legal consideration but it is recommended that driving be suspended from the commencement of drug reduction and for 6 months after drug withdrawal.

Van, crane, and minibus drivers will need to be found alternative employment, as with those whose job also involves driving. The safety of forklift truck drivers will depend on individual circumstances.

Key points

- Many people do not disclose a history of epileptic seizures when applying for a job or during a routine examination at the workplace.
- The disability provisions of the Equality Act 2010 confer some protection on those with epilepsy.
- Responsibility for the employment and placement of a person with epilepsy rests with the employer and they should take appropriate medical advice. Each case must be judged on its merits in light of the available information, which must include a sound and complete understanding of job requirements.
- A competent OH service, trusted by both shop floor and management, can be invaluable in educating both employer and employee, resolving conflicts, and giving advice. The development of good rapport and mutual trust will encourage disclosure.
- Employees with epilepsy should be reviewed regularly.

Useful websites

Epilepsy Action	http://www.epilepsy.org.uk
The Epilepsy Society	https://www.epilepsysociety.org.uk/
DVLA. Guidance on fitness to drive with epilepsy	https://www.gov.uk/guidance/assessing-fitness-to-drive-a-guide-for-medical-professionals
Access to Work. Help at work if you are disabled or have a health condition	https://www.gov.uk/access-to-work
Remploy. Employers guide to epilepsy	http://www.remploy.co.uk/info/20140/a_-_z_of_disabilities/36/epilepsy

References

1. Scheffer IE, Berkovic S, Capovilla G, et al. ILAE classification of the epilepsies: position paper of the ILAE Commission for Classification and Terminology. *Epilepsia* 2017;**58**:512–21.
2. Commission on Classification and Terminology of the International League Against Epilepsy. Proposal for revised clinical and electroencephalographic classification of epileptic seizures. *Epilepsia* 1981;**22**:489–501.
3. Fisher RS, Cross JH, French JA, et al. Operational classification of seizure types by the International League Against Epilepsy: Position Paper of the ILAE Commission for Classification and Terminology. *Epilepsia* 2017;**58**:522–30.

4. **Wallace H, Shorvon S, Tallis R.** Age-specific incidence and prevalence rates of treated epilepsy in an unselected population of 2 052 922 and age-specific fertility rates of women with epilepsy. *Lancet* 1998;**352**:1970–3.

5. **Sander JWAS, Hart YM, Johnson AL, et al.** National General Practice Study of Epilepsy: newly diagnosed epileptic seizures in a general population. *Lancet* 1990;**336**:1267–71.

6. **Craven IJ, Griffiths PD, Bhattacharyya D, et al.** 3.0T MRI of 2000 consecutive patients with localization-related epilepsy. *Br J Radiol* 2012;**85**:1236–42.

7. **Davies JE, Dedhia HV, Morgade C, et al.** Lindane poisonings. *Arch Dermatol* 1983;**119**:142–4.

8. **Chadwick D.** Epilepsy after first seizures: risks and implications. *J Neurol Neurosurg Psychiatry* 1991;**54**:385–7.

9. **Hart YM, Sander JW, Johnson AL, et al.** National general practice study of epilepsy: recurrence after a first seizure. *Lancet* 1990;**336**:1271–4.

10. **First Seizure Trial Group.** Randomized clinical trial on the efficacy of antiepileptic drugs in reducing the risk of relapse after a first unprovoked tonic-clonic seizure. *Neurology* 1993;**43**:478–83.

11. **Marson A, Jacoby A, Johnson A, et al.** Immediate versus deferred antiepileptic drug treatment for early epilepsy and single seizures: a randomised controlled trial. *Lancet* 2005;**365**:2007–13.

12. **Bonnett LJ, Tudur-Smith C, Williamson PR, et al.** Risk of recurrence after a first seizure and implications for driving: further analysis of the Multicentre Study of Early Epilepsy and Single Seizures. *BMJ* 2010;**341**:c6477.

13. **Cockerell OC, Johnson AL, Sander JW, et al.** Remission of epilepsy: results from the National General Practice Study of Epilepsy. *Lancet* 1995;**346**:140–4.

14. **Annegers JF, Hauser WA, Elveback LR.** Remission of seizures and relapse in patients with epilepsy. *Epilepsia* 1979;**20**:729–37.

15. **Bonnett LJ, Tudor Smith C, Smith D, et al.** Time to 12-month remission and treatment failure for generalized and unclassified epilepsy. *J Neurol Neurosurg Psychiatry* 2014;**85**:603–10.

16. **Sander JWAS.** Some aspects of prognosis in the epilepsies: a review. *Epilepsia* 1993;**34**:1007–16.

17. **Kwan P, Brodie MJ.** Early identification of refractory epilepsy. *N Engl J Med* 2000;**342**:314–19.

18. **Bonnett LJ, Shukralla A, Tudur-Smith C, et al.** Seizure recurrence after antiepileptic drug withdrawal and the implications for driving: further results from the MRC Antiepileptic Drug Withdrawal Study and a systematic review. *J Neurol Neurosurg Psychiatry* 2011;**82**:1328–33.

19. **Annegers JF, Hauser WA, Coan SP, et al.** A population based study of seizures after traumatic brain injuries. *N Engl J Med* 1998;**338**:20–4.

20. **Temkin NR, Dikmen SS, Wilensky AJ, et al.** A randomised double blind study of phenytoin for the prevention of post-traumatic seizures. *N Engl J Med* 1990;**323**:497–502.

21. **Dasgupta AK, Saunders M, Dick DJ.** Epilepsy in the British Steel Corporation: an evaluation of sickness, accident and work records. *Br J Ind Med* 1982;**39**:146–8.

22. **Wilkinson RT.** Hours of work and the 24 hour cycle of rest and activity. In: Warr PB (ed), *Psychology at Work*, pp. 31–54. Harmondsworth: Penguin; 1971.

23. **Joels M.** Stress, the hippocampus, and epilepsy. *Epilepsia* 2009;**50**:587–97.

24. **Kasteleijn-Nolst Trenité DGA.** Photosensitivity in epilepsy: electrophysiological and clinical correlates. *Acta Neurol Scand* 1989;**125**:3–149.

25. **Wolf P, Goosses R.** Relation of photosensitivity to epileptic syndromes. *J Neurol Neurosurg Psychiatry* 1986;**49**:1386–91.

26. **Jeavons PM, Harding GFA.** *Photosensitivity Epilepsy*. London: Heinemann; 1975.

27. **Lowenstein DH, Bleck T, Macdonald RL.** It's time to revise the definition of status epilepticus. *Epilepsia* 1999;**40**:120–2.

28. Troxell J, Thorbecke R. *Vocational Scenarios: A Training Manual on Epilepsy and Employment.* Second Employment Commission of the International Bureau for Epilepsy. Heemstede: International Bureau for Epilepsy; 1992.

29. Vuilleumier P, Jallon P. [Epilepsy and psychiatric disorders: epidemiological data]. *Rev Neurol (Paris)* 1998;**154**:305–17.

30. Tellez-Zenteno JF, Patten SB, Jetté N, Williams J, Wiebe S. Psychiatric comorbidity in epilepsy: a population-based analysis. *Epilepsia* 2007;**48**:2336–44.

31. Rayner G, Wrench JM, Wilson SJ. Differential contributions of objective memory and mood to subjective memory complaints in refractory focal epilepsy. *Epilepsy Behav* 2010;**19**:359–64.

32. Baxendale S. Epilepsy: cognition and memory in adults. In: Shorvon S, Guerrini R, Cook M, Lhatoo S (eds), *Oxford Textbook of Epilepsy and Seizures*, pp. 367–74. Oxford: Oxford University Press; 2012.

33. Kwan P, Brodie MJ. Neuropsychological effects of epilepsy and antiepileptic drugs. *Lancet* 2001;**357**:216–22.

34. Scambler G, Hopkins AP. Social class, epileptic activity and disadvantage at work. *J Epidemiol Community Health* 1980:**34**:129–33.

35. **Employment Commission of the International Bureau for Epilepsy**. Employing people with epilepsy. Principles for good practice. *Epilepsia* 1989;**30**:411–2.

36. **US Department of Labor**. *The Performance of Physically Impaired Workers in Manufacturing Industries*. US Department of Labor Bulletin No. 293. Washington, DC: US Government Printing Office; 1948.

37. Udell MM. The work performance of epileptics in industry. *Arch Environ Health* 1960;**6**:257–64.

38. Palmer KT, Stefania DA, Harris EC, Linaker C, Coggon D. Epilepsy, diabetes mellitus, and accidental injury at work. *Occup Med (Lond)* 2014;**64**:448–53

39. **Metropolitan Police**. The medical assessment for police officer, special constable, police community support officer and designated detention officer. Available at: http://www.metpolicecareers.co.uk/media/doc/medical_assessment_officers.doc.

40. Hicks RA, Hicks MJ. The attitudes of major companies towards the employment of epileptics: an assessment of 2 decades of change. *Am Correct Ther J* 1978;**32**:180–2.

41. Jacoby A, Gorry J, Baker GA. Employers' attitudes to employment of people with epilepsy: still the same old story? *Epilepsia* 2005;**46**:1978–87.

42. **National Institute for Health and Care Excellence (NICE)**. *Epilepsies: Diagnosis and Management.* Clinical Guideline [CG137]. London: NICE, 2012.

43. Carter T. Health and safety at work: implications of current legislation. In: Edwards F, Espir M, Oxley J (eds), *Epilepsy and Employment*, pp. 9–17. London: Royal Society of Medicine; 1986.

44. Taylor J, Chadwick D, Johnson T. Risk of accidents in drivers with epilepsy. *J Neurol Neurosurg Psychiatry* 1996;**60**:621–7.

Chapter 25

Diabetes mellitus and other endocrine disorders

Ali Hashtroudi and Mayank Patel

Introduction

Diabetes mellitus is a metabolic disease characterized by hyperglycaemia. More people of working age now live with diabetes. If glucose levels are well controlled through diet, lifestyle, and treatment adherence, the risk of hyperglycaemia affecting employment is reduced. Well-controlled diabetes can also reduce the risk of associated complications, which can affect the ability to work. Those with diabetes may require adjustments at work to facilitate their employment and help them control their diabetes better. They may also require precautionary measures such as monitoring glucose levels while undertaking safety-critical roles to reduce the risk of debilitating hypoglycaemia and minimize the risk of harm to them and others. Many people live with other endocrine diseases, which usually do not affect the ability to work but may need specific considerations in the workplace.

Diabetes

An appropriate level of functioning insulin secreted by the pancreas is essential to keep blood glucose levels (BGLs) stable. Insulin acts as a key to promote the cellular uptake of glucose, for use as an energy source. Insulin ensures that hepatic glucose output is controlled and not excessive, and has an anabolic role in promoting fat and protein synthesis.

Diabetes mellitus is a metabolic disease characterized by hyperglycaemia, resulting from inappropriate action of endogenous insulin. There are two common types. Type 1 diabetes mellitus (T1DM) results from autoimmune-mediated damage to the pancreas, which incapacitates insulin production. Type 2 diabetes mellitus (T2DM), the most common type worldwide, occurs when the body becomes resistant to the effects of insulin, often with associated impaired insulin secretion.

The American Diabetes Association has also defined type 3 diabetes as a result of other pathologies or situations in which insulin production is reduced or insulin resistance is increased, such as total pancreatectomy or haemochromatosis.[1] Other types include gestational diabetes mellitus (GDM) and monogenic diabetes (a familial form).

Epidemiology of diabetes

Diabetes UK estimates that 4 million people in the UK live with diabetes,[2] with the global prevalence of 415 million estimated to increase to 642 million in 2040.[3]

Aetiology and pathophysiology

Type 1 diabetes

Autoimmune-mediated islet cell destruction is a key precipitant of T1DM, but the precise trigger for this process remains unclear. Environmental factors, in particular viral infections, have been implicated in the aetiology. The resulting islet cell damage causes absolute insulin deficiency, necessitating lifelong insulin treatment. Over 370,000 adults in the UK currently live with T1DM.[4]

Type 2 diabetes

Insulin resistance is the hallmark of T2DM, although insulin deficiency is observed too. Obesity, sedentary lifestyle, and reduced physical activity are key risk factors, as are family history or ethnicity (particularly African or South Asian). Women who developed GDM, even if it is resolved after pregnancy, are also at increased risk. Abdominal obesity in particular is associated with release of fatty acids from stored visceral fat, which can worsen insulin resistance through increasing hepatic glucose output and reducing peripheral glucose uptake. It has been demonstrated that a waist size over 40 inches (102 cm) in men and 34.5 inches (88 cm) in women increases the risk of developing T2DM similar to those who are clinically obese.[5] More recently, the Leicester Practice risk score,[6] has been advocated by NICE and Diabetes UK for identifying those at risk of diabetes (calculated using age, sex, body mass index (BMI), ethnicity, family history of diabetes, and presence of treated hypertension).

Consequences of hyperglycaemia

Regardless of diabetes type, left unaddressed, the clinical hallmark is hyperglycaemia. It can cause short-term physical symptoms (lasting hours to days) (see 'Emergencies in diabetes'). Long-term (months to years) uncontrolled hyperglycaemia can contribute to premature occlusion of key blood vessels. The commonest manifestations of vascular damage from diabetes are blindness, kidney disease, foot disease, and premature heart disease. Vascular risk in diabetes is markedly increased in association with uncontrolled hypertension, hyperlipidaemia, and smoking. This vascular-mediated damage gives rise to the 'complications' of diabetes (Table 25.1).

Diagnosis of diabetes

For diagnosis, hyperglycaemia must be confirmed. Once the BGL is above a threshold at which concurrent insulin levels cannot promote its cellular uptake, hyperglycaemia

Table 25.1 Complications of diabetes

Macrovascular	Microvascular
Coronary heart disease	Retinopathy
Cerebrovascular disease	Neuropathy
Peripheral vascular disease	Nephropathy

will result. Glucose enters the urine, increasing diuresis. The body is then deprived of a key energy source. Uncontrolled acute hyperglycaemia is often associated with a short history of osmotic symptoms (polyuria, polydipsia, and nocturia), with or without unplanned weight loss, blurred vision, and fatigue, which have usually developed over a few weeks. Recurrent genitourinary or skin infections may also suggest hyperglycaemia.

An oral glucose tolerance test (OGTT) is not often used in clinical practice to diagnose diabetes. Its main use in the UK is in diagnosing GDM. The presence of glycosuria, though a key screening test for diabetes, is insufficient to confirm the diagnosis. Further blood-based glucose-level evaluation is needed.

Type 1 diabetes

A short history of osmotic symptoms, with a raised random BGL above 11.1 mmol/L is highly suggestive of T1DM. The presence of ketones in the blood or urine, ketonuria (above +2 on urine dip), or ketonaemia (above 1 mmol/L on blood ketone testing) implies that insulin deficiency has prompted preferential use of fat as an energy source, as appropriate glucose uptake cannot occur. This partly explains unplanned rapid weight loss.

Insulin autoantibodies (glutamate decarboxylase and islet cell antibodies) further support the diagnosis, although (because of varying sensitivity and specificity) these are not measured routinely if baseline investigations confirm T1DM.

Type 2 diabetes

T2DM can often be missed in asymptomatic individuals. As they continue to produce some insulin, symptomatic hyperglycaemia is variable. The presence of glycosuria detected during a routine screening may provide the first clue. Some people report several months of fatigue, or recurrent skin or urinary infections prior to formal diagnosis. Since 2011, the World Health Organization (WHO) has advocated the use of glycosylated haemoglobin (HbA1c) to diagnose T2DM.[7] Fasting is unnecessary and the HbA1c level reflects mean glycaemia for the preceding 2–3 months. An HbA1c value of 48 mmol/mol or above confirms the diagnosis.

Notably, HbA1c cannot reliably diagnose T2DM in certain situations, including pathologies affecting red cell turnover (anaemia, chronic kidney disease, and pregnancy), haemoglobinopathies, and acute pancreatic injury. Moreover, HbA1c cannot be used to diagnose T1DM, as the history could be too short to affect it. Steroid or antipsychotic

Table 25.2 WHO diagnostic criteria for diabetes (when HbA1c not reliable)

	BGL mmol/L (mg/dL)	
	Fasting	OGTT
Normal	<6 (108)	<7.8 (140.4)
Diabetes	>7 (126)	>11.1 (199.8)
Gestational diabetes	>5.6 (>100.8)	>7.8 (140.4)

drugs in recent weeks may also affect measured HbA1c by increasing insulin resistance. If in doubt, the HbA1c measurement should be repeated within a few weeks and use of a fasting BGL and OGTT can be considered (Table 25.2). Note that the diagnostic criteria summarized in Table 25.2 do not distinguish between diabetes types.

Gestational diabetes mellitus

This can only be diagnosed in pregnancy. Regardless of type, diabetes during pregnancy increases the risk to mother and fetus of miscarriage, pre-term labour, stillbirth, and congenital malformations. Women who have risk factors are screened for GDM at 24–28 weeks (Box 25.1).

Cautions in diagnosis

Longstanding observations that T1DM occurs only in children and younger adults, and T2DM only in older adults, no longer hold true. T1DM can be diagnosed in older adults, as well as in people of increased weight although T2DM in a lean individual should prompt consideration of alternative pancreatic pathology and reasons for weight loss (e.g. thyroid disease). In adults with T2DM, who do not respond to usual therapy, or have osmotic symptoms, insulin autoantibodies and ketones should be measured to exclude latent autoimmune diabetes of adults ('LADA') (a form of slow-developing T1DM).

Box 25.1 Risk factors for GDM

- BMI greater than 30 prior to pregnancy.
- Previous baby weighing more than 4.5 kg.
- Previous GDM.
- First-degree relative with diabetes.
- Family origins (South Asian, Chinese, African-Caribbean, or Middle-Eastern).

Treatment of diabetes

General management

Once diabetes is confirmed, appropriate treatment should be commenced promptly. Regardless of diabetes type, appropriate diet and lifestyle advice should be offered early. It should be clarified to patients that these are ongoing parts of diabetes management, alongside medical treatment. There is no 'diabetic diet' to advocate; the emphasis is on healthy food choices and portion awareness (Box 25.2).

Good vascular and general health must be promoted, such as ensuring blood pressure (BP) and cholesterol levels are controlled and smoking is discouraged. It has been observed that while improved glycaemic control favours reduction of microvascular complications, both lipid and BP lowering reduce risk of macrovascular problems particularly in T2DM.[8] Diabetes UK provides educational resources to support living well with diabetes.

Increased physical activity is encouraged with care. Overactivity without a sufficient intake of carbohydrate can increase the risk of hypoglycaemia, which can reduce confidence with exercise. Increased fitness can promote increased insulin sensitivity and weight loss, particularly in T2DM. It is essential to empower people to take an active interest in their diabetes where possible.

People with diabetes are encouraged to attend a structured education course as part of treatment, offering the chance to obtain essential skills about living well with diabetes.[9] Examples include DAFNE (Dose Adjustment For Normal Eating) for T1DM and DESMOND (Diabetes Education and Self-Management for Ongoing and Diagnosed) for T2DM in the UK. These courses typically require a few days' attendance, and those who adopt the learnings are likely to achieve better diabetic control. This helps maintain productivity (e.g. by reducing sickness absence and avoiding complications that reduce ability for particular tasks). Therefore, an economic case can be made for employers to permit time away from work to attend a diabetes course.

Box 25.2 Healthy eating in diabetes

- ◆ Eat:
  - Regular meals and minimize snacking.
  - Minimum of five portions of fruit and vegetable daily.
  - Starchy foods (slowly absorbed carbohydrate; e.g. rice, pasta, and potatoes) daily.
  - Protein-containing foods daily, with one or two portions of oily fish weekly.
  - Dairy (milk, cheese, and yoghurt).
- ◆ Keep daily salt intake below 1 teaspoon (6 g) per day.
- ◆ Foods high in fat and sugar should be considered as occasional treats.

Treatment of type 1 diabetes

The latest UK guidelines for T1DM[4] provide a framework for overall management. Several classes of insulin are available, classified by their duration of action (Table 25.3).

For T1DM, the favoured insulin regimen is 'basal-bolus' therapy, which seeks to mimic natural insulin physiology. A single or twice-daily intermediate or long-acting basal (background) dose is administered at a similar time daily, with bolus rapid or short-acting insulin administered with meals. Thus, persistent background insulin is available, and meal-related blood glucose spikes are addressed by the bolus dose. Carbohydrate counting is importantly taught on courses. This enables patients to calculate the bolus dose for particular meal choices, depending on the carbohydrate content. Making the carbohydrate content of food available in the workplace canteen is invaluable. It is also important to educate the individual to consider adjusting bolus insulin doses ahead of planned exercise, increased physical activity (e.g. at work), or at times of acute illness.

Table 25.3 Summary of insulins available for clinical use

Type	Examples	Duration of action (hours)	Notes
Rapid-acting bolus[a]	Novorapid® Humalog® Apidra®	3–5	Taken with meals
Short-acting bolus[a]	Actrapid® Humulin® S	6–8	Taken with meals
Intermediate-acting basal[a]	Insulatard® Humulin® I	12–18	Once or twice daily
Biphasic[a]	Humulin® M3 Novomix® 30 Humalog® Mix 25	12–14	Fixed combinations of short and intermediate acting, taken with breakfast and the evening meal
Long-acting basal[a]	Glargine® Detemir®	Approximately 24	Occasionally twice daily is needed
Ultra-long acting basal[a]	Tresiba® (U100)	Up to 42	Once daily or two to three times weekly
Biosimilar[a]	Abasaglar® (similar to Lantus®)	Approximately 24	
Concentrated (contains >100 units/mL of insulin)	Tresiba® (U200), Humalog® 200 (both 200 units/mL) Insulin Toujeo® (U300: 300 units/mL) Humulin® R (U500: 500 units/mL)		If high volume of insulin is needed, typically in severe insulin resistance

[a] All insulin vials or cartridges only contain 100 units of insulin/mL (U100).

Some people find administering several daily injections challenging. Twice-daily biphasic insulin is an option. However, this is less flexible than variable timed basal-bolus regimens, and biphasic insulin should be injected at a similar time daily: before breakfast and evening meals. Particular adjustments to the work pattern may be necessary to support this treatment.

Factors affecting insulin performance

'Physical' issues can influence how insulin acts. Insulin needles should only be used once; a needle size of 4–6 mm is appropriate for most people. Care must be taken with insulin storage. Unopened insulin should be stored in the fridge until needed. It can be stored at room temperature for up to 28 days while being used, although direct sunlight can cause damage. Employees who travel to places where a fridge is not available should have a cool bag for warm environments. Insulin should be allowed to reach room temperature prior to administration, with attention paid to injection timings, and ensuring that injection sites are rotated and 'lump free'. Lumpy sites (lipohypertrophy) can be associated with erratic insulin absorption.

Insulin equipment disposal

Consideration should be given to the disposal of the sharps (needles and lancets). Employers should be advised to either permit the individual to bring their safe disposal device or to provide alternative safe disposal (sharps bin).

Monitoring glucose and ketones

It is essential that insulin users undertake regular self-monitoring of BGL and are confident in adjusting doses to optimize control. For certain safety-critical roles, there might be a requirement to measure the BGL at certain intervals (e.g. every 2 hours), before a particular task (e.g. driving), or to provide a record of BGL monitoring over a period of time (to demonstrate that BGLs are controlled), especially from a hypoglycaemic perspective.

Employment in some safety-critical roles requires a diabetologist review at defined intervals to confirm good control. This may need to be funded by the employer if not indicated clinically.

In view of the risk of hypoglycaemia on insulin treatment, regular BGL monitoring should be performed, at least four and up to ten times daily. Prompts for glucose testing include before meals, recurrent hypoglycaemia, acute illness, and during periods of critical tasks (e.g. driving). The UK Driver and Vehicle Licensing Agency (DVLA) recommends a particular schedule of monitoring for insulin-treated drivers (Table 25.4) which can be also used for other safety-critical duties (see 'Useful websites'). The advice is to maintain BGL over 5 mmol/L and stop driving (or safety-critical activity) at levels below 4 mmol/L or if hypoglycaemic symptoms occur.

For bus and lorry drivers (group 2 licence), a glucose meter with memory functions is required to ensure 3 months of readings are available for assessment. This should also be considered for other vocational drivers so that BGL can be established in the event of altered consciousness while driving.

Table 25.4 Blood glucose monitoring for drivers

Car and motorcycle	Bus and lorry
◆ BGL testing no more than 2 hours before the start of the first journey ◆ Every 2 hours while driving ◆ More frequent self-monitoring may be required with any greater risk of hypoglycaemia (physical activity, altered meal routine)	◆ Regular BGL testing—at least twice daily including on days when not driving and ◆ No more than 2 hours before the start of the first journey and ◆ Every 2 hours while driving ◆ More frequent self-monitoring may be required with any greater risk of hypoglycaemia (physical activity, altered meal routine)

Anyone with T1DM should also have the equipment to measure their blood or urine ketones at times of acute illness, to warn of developing diabetic ketoacidosis (DKA). See 'Emergencies in diabetes'.

The role of personal insulin pumps

The use of continuous, subcutaneous insulin infusion-based therapy (insulin pumps) has increased in recent years. In the UK, it is suggested for people with T1DM who have recurrent disabling hypoglycaemia or sustained poor glycaemic control (HbA1c >69 mmol/mol) despite intensified use of subcutaneous insulin injections.[10] The pump is worn continuously, infusing only rapid-acting insulin at a very slow rate through an abdominal cannula. Insulin pump treatment requires initiation, training, and surveillance by a specialist diabetes team, and a high level of user motivation and engagement. Training is essential and should cover carbohydrate counting and action in case of emergencies. Their use is associated with improved BGL control, reduced hypoglycaemia, and potentially reduced cardiovascular mortality.[11]

From a safety perspective, the pump should be worn in an appropriate place for the activity/job being performed. A direct blow and extremes of temperature could damage the pump. It is important that the user keeps well hydrated, particularly in warm environments, to reduce the risk of dehydration and associated hyperglycaemia that could lead to ketone production and DKA. All pump users must also have a supply of rapid- and long-acting insulins to provide emergency cover in the event of pump malfunction.

Treatment of type 2 diabetes

Healthy diet and lifestyle choices play a major role in the management of T2DM, and therefore should be strongly promoted. Individuals should be reminded of the progressive nature of T2DM and that healthy lifestyle and weight loss may contribute to prolonging pancreatic function and insulin sensitivity.

An increasing number of pharmacological options are available (Table 25.5). The majority of cases are expected to be managed[12] in primary care (including choosing treatment, setting up therapeutic targets, and monitoring). Specialist referral is reserved for more complex cases.

Table 25.5 Pharmacological options in type 2 diabetes

	Drug class	Mode of action	Advisory notes
Older treatments	*Biguanides* (metformin)	Reduces hepatic glucose output and increases peripheral insulin sensitivity	◆ **No risk of hypoglycaemia** ◆ Weight neutral ◆ Risk of lactic acidosis with significant volume loss and poor tissue perfusion (e.g. diarrhoea and vomiting), hence suspend in acute illness ◆ Commencing at low dose and gradual dose titration can reduce gastrointestinal side effects ◆ Use has been recommended alongside insulin in T1DM, particularly if BMI >25
	Sulphonylureas (e.g. gliclazide, glipizide, glibenclamide)	Act on the pancreas to stimulate insulin release	◆ **Insulin released is at a level unrelated to the circulating BGL; hence a risk of hypoglycaemia** ◆ Anabolic function of insulin may cause weight gain ◆ With stage 4–5 chronic kidney disease, there is an increased risk of reduced sulphonylurea clearance, and associated increased risk of hypoglycaemia
	Glinides (e.g. repaglinide, nateglinide)	Similar to sulphonylureas, but shorter-acting	◆ Similar side effect profile to sulphonylureas ◆ **Hypoglycaemia may be less frequent**
	Alpha-glucosidase inhibitors (acarbose)	Inhibits the intestinal alpha-glucosidase, resulting in reduced carbohydrate absorption	◆ **Low risk of hypoglycaemia** ◆ Limited use due to flatulence and diarrhoea
	Thiazolidinediones (pioglitazone)	Increases insulin receptor sensitivity and augments the effects of endogenous insulin	◆ **Low risk of hypoglycaemia** ◆ Can cause fluid retention, weight gain, dilutional anaemia, osteopenia in postmenopausal women
Newer treatments	*GLP-1 agonists* (subcutaneous injection; exenatide, liraglutide, dulaglutide)		◆ **Low risk of hypoglycaemia** ◆ Help weight loss, therefore recommended when BMI >35 ◆ Reduced cardiovascular risk[14] ◆ Stop if HbA1c not improved or no weight loss after 6 months ◆ Bloating and nausea ◆ Abdominal pain should be investigated (reports of pancreatitis) ◆ Provision of safe needle disposal
	DPP-4 inhibitors (sitagliptin, linagliptin, saxagliptin)	Inhibition of the enzyme DPP-4, which partly metabolizes GLP-1	◆ Weight neutral ◆ **Low risk of hypoglycaemia** ◆ Abdominal pain should be investigated (reports of pancreatitis)

(continued)

Table 25.5 Continued

Drug class	Mode of action	Advisory notes
SGLT2 inhibitors (dapagliflozin, canagliflozin, empagliflozin)	Actively causing glycosuria by reducing glucose reabsorption in kidney	◆ **Risk of hypoglycaemia increases if used with insulin and sulphonylureas** ◆ Can help weight loss ◆ Risk of genital thrush and urinary tract infections ◆ Risk of DKA[15] ◆ Reduced risk of cardiovascular morbidity and mortality (empagliflozin)[16]

Newer treatments in type 2 diabetes

Incretins are naturally occurring gut hormones such as glucagon-like-peptide 1 (GLP-1), the levels of which are low in T2DM.[13] They stimulate pancreatic insulin production proportionately to blood glucose concentration, reduce pancreatic glucagon secretion, and delay gastric emptying. These actions collectively result in lower BGLs without hypoglycaemic risk.

Evidence suggests that sodium–glucose co-transporter (SGLT2) inhibitors can increase the risk of DKA. If a treated individual becomes unwell, ketone testing is required irrespective of BGL, with onward referral to exclude DKA if necessary (see 'Emergencies in diabetes'). They should be suspended in acute illness and other states that can be associated with hypovolaemia.

Insulin: using insulin in T2DM is increasing. When non-insulin-based therapies cannot maintain normoglycaemia in T2DM, insulin is the only option, usually starting with intermediate or once-daily long-acting insulin at night. The dose is up-titrated until the fasting BGL is satisfactory. Twice-daily biphasic (e.g. Humulin® M3), or basal-bolus regimens, similar to T1DM, may be indicated. Most other treatment agents are stopped when insulin is commenced. Metformin, dipeptidyl peptidase-4 inhibitors, GLP-1 agonists, and SGLT2 inhibitors can be used with insulin.

Monitoring blood glucose in type 2 diabetes

Regular BGL monitoring should be considered in T2DM in:

◆ insulin treatment

◆ other agents that can cause hypoglycaemia and working in safety-critical roles

◆ recurrent hypoglycaemia

◆ pregnancy or considering pregnancy.

Treatment of diabetes in pregnancy

Ideally any woman with existing diabetes who becomes pregnant should be under the joint care of an obstetrician and a diabetologist. They may need to regularly self-monitor their BGL and/or be regularly reviewed (every 1–2 weeks) throughout pregnancy. If medication is contraindicated in pregnancy and/or BGL is not well controlled, insulin may be needed. GDM increases the lifetime risk of developing T2DM, therefore a healthy diet and lifestyle should be reinforced.

Assessing glycaemic control in diabetes

There are several means to assess glycaemic control:

Urine dipstick monitoring detects glycosuria, but it is not quantitative so cannot inform overall glycaemic control. It is an initial screening method to decide if further tests for diabetes are required.

HbA1c is the most widely used marker to assess glycaemic control. The ideal range without risking hypoglycaemia, or in those with other significant co-morbidities, is between 48 and 58 mmol/mol (previously 6.5–7.5%). Key trials have informed the appropriate level of glucose control to reduce the risk of microvascular complications.[17,18] HbA1c reflects an average BGL over the preceding 2–3 months and takes no account of daily BGL fluctuations. Therefore, while an HbA1c within the range could be commended, caution is needed to avoid missing frequent hypoglycaemia, especially if asymptomatic. A rapid HbA1c rise (e.g. more than 8–16 mmol/mol over 3–6 months) should raise questions about treatment adherence or (less likely) concurrent endocrine problem, such as thyroid disease.

Morbidity and mortality increase in people aged over 55 years who have had T2DM for at least 10 years plus another cardiovascular risk factor.[19,20] Therefore with ageing, the focus should shift from tight glycaemic control, to controlling BP and lipid levels. Regardless of age, antihypertensive drugs and a statin are used regularly in T2DM to reduce cardiovascular risk. The BP target is less than 140/80 mmHg (<130/80 mmHg if renal complications). Atorvastatin 20 mg daily is advised if the estimated risk of cardiovascular disease is greater than 10%, using the QRISK®-2 risk assessment tool.[21]

Self-monitoring of BGL establishes real-time values and is most often used in those who administer insulin. The results should inform decisions, such as adjusting insulin doses or the ability to undertake a certain task, taking into account factors that may contribute to erratic readings. Meters must be validated regularly with glucose test solutions.

Glucose sensors measure interstitial subcutaneous fluid glucose levels in real time. The current UK DVLA guidance is based on plasma glucose therefore these sensors cannot be used to establish the fitness to drive. This is under review and further guidance is expected in the near future.

Continuous glucose monitoring is attached to the abdomen and measures interstitial glucose levels and can be connected wirelessly to an alarm that warns of critical glucose thresholds. This is most useful in hypoglycaemic unawareness, to reduce the risk of injury to self or others.

Diabetes health checks

In the UK, diabetes health checks are offered at least annually. Key metrics (Box 25.3) identify early evidence of vascular damage, review general health, and ensure treatment adherence.

Box 25.3 Metrics used at health checks

- BMI.
- BP.
- HbA1c.
- Cholesterol.
- Smoking status.
- Foot examination.
- Serum creatinine.
- Urine albumin/creatinine ratio.
- Retinal screening.

Emergencies in diabetes

Acute hyperglycaemia

Symptoms suggesting acute hyperglycaemia can develop over hours to days. They can include osmotic symptoms, blurred vision, fatigue, headache, and general malaise. Intermittent hyperglycaemia, that is, 1–2 high readings among otherwise normal glucose readings, may warrant reviewing the dose, adherence, and lifestyle (work pattern, meal choices). With more persistent or worsening hyperglycaemia (BGL >14 mmol/L for >3–4 successive hours), it is imperative to establish the cause (Table 25.6) and encourage increased hydration.

Diabetic ketoacidosis

This critical diagnosis should have a low threshold for exclusion. DKA most often occurs in T1DM and is usually related to insulin omission or intercurrent illness, such as infection. The importance of never stopping insulin in T1DM, even if not eating, must be remembered. DKA can be observed in T2DM treated with SGLT-2 inhibitors. DKA can be preceded by non-specific symptoms of hyperglycaemia. A relative deficiency of insulin impedes glucose uptake and instigates fat breakdown, of which ketoacids are a by-product.

Vomiting is a common presenting symptom, regardless of cause, and may be a consequence of acute ketosis with impending acidosis. This can occur over a matter of hours. If there are concerns that DKA could be developing, hospital referral is advisable (e.g. an unwell individual, with BGLs above 14 mmol/L, and a blood ketone level above 1.5 mmol/L, or more than +2 urine ketones). Confirmed DKA requires inpatient care for intravenous fluids and insulin. It is essential to identify and treat the precipitant. DKA morbidity and mortality is now very low and unless it is recurrent, there are no particular work implications.

Table 25.6 Causes of hyperglycaemia

Causes	Example
Physical	Erroneous reading Dirty hands (clean with alcohol-free agents and reassess) Faulty glucometer Missed medications
Acute catabolic state	DKA or HHS New diagnosis of diabetes Intercurrent illness (sepsis) Alternative pancreatic disease
Drugs	Steroids Antipsychotics Antiretrovirals Thiazides
Mechanical	Device failure (e.g. damaged insulin pen or pump) Problem with injection technique or site (oedematous, lipohypertrophy) Incorrect insulin type or dose Mixed insulin not agitated properly prior to use
Gastrointestinal	Overtreatment of hypoglycaemia Increased eating after a period of reduced intake Inappropriate snacking Use of high-sugar supplements Constipation
Endocrine	Menstruation Pregnancy Thyroid disease

People with T1DM should be aware of 'sick day rules', that is, to measure ketones, preferably blood, when unwell. They should be advised to:

◆ increase fluid intake

◆ consume food containing glucose

◆ administer additional bolus doses of rapid- or short-acting insulin

◆ seek medical advice if glucose and ketone levels continue rising despite the above, especially if vomiting.

Hyperglycaemic hyperosmolar state

A hyperglycaemic hyperosmolar state (HHS) usually occurs in older individuals with T2DM and is uncommon in workplace. It takes a few days to develop and may be precipitated by infection, dehydration, or high-dose steroids. People with HHS become severely dehydrated but usually not ketotic; typically with increasingly drowsiness and a very high BGL. Hospital treatment is essential for fluid replacement and to identify the cause. HHS has higher mortality than DKA, usually due to thrombotic complications from marked dehydration.

Table 25.7 Symptoms and signs of hypoglycaemia

Autonomic	Sweating
	Palpitations
	Hunger
Neuroglycopenic	Confusion
	Drowsiness
	Odd behaviour
	Speech difficulty
	Incoordination
	Seizures
	Coma
General	Malaise
	Headache
	Nausea

Acute hypoglycaemia

This can be defined as a BGL less than 4 mmol/L (Table 25.7).

Once hypoglycaemia is confirmed, it should be treated promptly. Usually the individual knows how to treat it, but if unable to self-manage, treat as per Box 25.4.[22]

It is essential to establish the cause (Table 25.8) and take steps to reduce the risk of recurrence, such as medication dose reduction. Extremely tight blood glucose control should be avoided in those at increased risk or who have recurrent hypoglycaemia. Relevant dietary knowledge should be reviewed, and ensure appropriate BGL monitoring. The stress of acute hypoglycaemia often induces rebound hyperglycaemia (partly by increasing the stress hormones adrenaline and cortisol). Hence, the next due insulin dose should not be omitted, although dose reduction (10–20%) should be considered.

Hypoglycaemia and work

Hypoglycaemia can cause transient cognitive impairment, which can present risks in the workplace. This is particularly important in safety-critical work, or when working in hazardous situations (e.g. driving or operating machinery). People prone to hypoglycaemia, especially those who lack awareness, may need adjustments, tight monitoring, or restriction depending on their job to ensure the safety of themselves and others.

After a hypoglycaemic event, including asymptomatic individuals found through monitoring, the resumption of work activity (especially if safety critical) must be delayed for at least 45 minutes. With guidance from the specialist and occupational health (OH) professional it is sensible to keep a hypoglycaemia kit in the workplace. This should include glucagon and rapid-acting carbohydrate (dextrose sweets, glucose gels). First aiders or a colleague should be trained in how to manage hypoglycaemia, but with an emphasis on summoning help.

Box 25.4 Treatment of acute hypoglycaemia

Conscious, able to swallow

1. 15 g of rapid-acting carbohydrate every 15 minutes, or one or two tubes of glucose-based gel squeezed into the mouth.

2. 1 mg of intramuscular glucagon if an appropriate oral treatment is not available—*use only once.*

3. Repeat step 1 up to twice more if needed. Consider calling an ambulance if there are clinical concerns.

4. When the BGL is greater than 4 mmol/L and the person has recovered, give them longer-acting carbohydrate (slice of bread or toast, 200–300 mL milk, or two biscuits).

   • A larger carbohydrate load is needed if glucagon was administered.

5. Monitor BGL closely up to minimum 2 hours post recovery, ensure there is no sign of recurrent hypoglycaemia, and perform regular BGL monitoring for 24–48 hours.

Unconscious person

1. Put them in the recovery position.

2. 1 mg of intramuscular glucagon promptly:

   • Do not administer oral treatment (unsafe).

   • Low threshold to call an ambulance.

3. For uncomplicated recovery after glucagon, follow steps 3 and 4 as for 'Conscious, able to swallow', if safe.

Hypoglycaemic unawareness

Most hypoglycaemic events are 'mild', self-recognized, and self-managed. 'Severe' episodes requiring third party assistance are rare, comprising less than 5% of hypoglycaemic events.[23]

A particular risk factor for severe hypoglycaemia is hypoglycaemic unawareness, where there is a lack of or significant reduction in symptoms of impending hypoglycaemia.[24] This can occur with long-term T1DM, autonomic neuropathy, and recurrent hypoglycaemia. It can be addressed partly by temporarily relaxing glucose control (to avoid hypoglycaemia) for several weeks, following which warning signs may reappear. Use of an insulin pump or continuous glucose monitoring are alternatives.

People with diabetes may become aware of their low BGL at different levels and the presentation varies. Therefore it is important to ascertain each individual's awareness of their symptoms. An important distinction is that not all cognitive functions are affected at the same rate and level. Complex tasks are more susceptible to hypoglycaemia than

Table 25.8 Causes of hypoglycaemia

Causes	Example
Medication	Injection site problem (lipohypertrophy)
	Reduction of steroid without reducing insulin
	Quinine
	Alcohol
	Sulphonylurea (typically 4–8 hours post dose)
	Polypharmacy (drug interaction)
Reduced glucose intake or absorption	Nausea
	Vomiting
	Gastroenteritis
	Reduced appetite, irregular, smaller, delayed, or missed meals
	Lack of usual snacking
	Inadequate treatment of previous hypoglycaemia
Relative insulin excess or increased insulin sensitivity	Rapid- or short-acting insulin without food
	Incorrect insulin (dose, type)
	Sulphonylurea with reduced or no food intake
	Exocrine pancreatic insufficiency and missed creon (less glucose absorption)
	Reduced renal function (reduced insulin clearance)
	Endocrine disease (thyroid, hypoadrenalism)

simple ones.[25] An individual may be capable of performing a simple task at a low BGL, but struggle with a complex task at the same level. Hypoglycaemia can reduce the speed of task completion, although the final outcome can be unchanged.[26] Therefore in assessing fitness to work in an individual at risk of hypoglycaemia, the complexity and speed of reaction should be taken into account.

Another aspect is whether hypoglycaemia can impair insight and risk perception. In two separate studies, subjects with BGLs of 2.6 mmol/L[27] and 4 mmol/L[28] considered themselves safe to drive. This reiterates the importance of assessing BGL, symptom awareness, and also education about hypoglycaemia.[29] The above-discussed intelligence should be balanced with the suggestion that hypoglycaemia in the workplace is uncommon.[30]

Complications of diabetes

Complications of diabetes are caused by impaired blood supply due to vascular changes subsequent to uncontrolled hyperglycaemia (Table 25.1). Advanced complications, such as visual impairment, limb loss, and dialysis interfere with life and work. Neuropathy can be debilitating. For example, autonomic neuropathy may cause postural hypotension (dizziness) and gastroparesis (vomiting and diarrhoea). Peripheral neuropathy may affect tasks that rely on good tactile perception.

Relatively few adults of working age develop such severe complications. When they occur, they can compromise the ability to undertake a specific task or entire role. An individual assessment of abilities is required to assess fitness for a particular role and also identify any modifications or restrictions to enable the individual to perform their tasks safely. Any physical symptoms should be evaluated carefully, as they may suggest the development of complications.

Cognitive decline

The long-term impact of recurrent hypoglycaemia on cognitive functioning is controversial.[31] While some studies have failed to show significant cognitive decline,[32] others indicate mild cognitive impairment in those over 60 years,[33] a lower IQ in young adults diagnosed 12 years earlier,[34] and slowness.[36] Microvascular changes in the brain and changes in the hippocampus neurons[35] are causally implicated.[36]

Cognitive decline identified in tests may not necessarily translate into significant functional limitation. Also in the older population, experience accumulated over years at work can offset mild cognitive decline. It is imperative that the OH professional carries out an individual assessment of cognitive capability in the context of job requirement.

Employment

Diabetes can affect employment in multiple ways including the risk of unemployment, reduced productivity, sickness absence, or the inability to undertake certain tasks because of complications. Certain work activities such as shift work can increase the risk of insulin resistance, which may result in the development of diabetes or hamper achieving good glucose control.

Impact of diabetes on employment metrics

Rate of employment

Previous evidence indicated that having diabetes did not decrease the rate of employment.[37] However, recent studies demonstrate variable and largely inferior rates of employment among those with diabetes (adjusted odds ratio (OR) 0.53 (95% confidence interval (CI) −0.28–1.00)[38] for people with diabetes compared to those without; rate of employment 0.81 and 0.57 in sample without and with diabetes respectively[39]). Several factors contribute to unemployment, including disease-related factors (complications or uncontrolled hypoglycaemia) that undermine capacity or safety. It may also indicate misplaced prejudice by prospective employers that someone with diabetes may not work safely or effectively. In countries with anti-discrimination legislation, prohibition of unjustified discriminatory exclusions have probably improved the employment rate of people with diabetes closer to general population levels.

Sickness absence

The majority of research shows a higher rate of absenteeism in people with diabetes.[40–42] While many of these studies tried to control for confounders, other factors including co-morbidities such as depression[43] can influence the findings.

Early retirement

The rate (OR 1.3; 95% CI 1.05–1.68[44]) and probability (hazard ratio 1.6; 95% CI 1.5–1.8[45]) of early retirement in those with diabetes are reported to be higher than those without, although not all confounders were adjusted for.

Impact of employment on diabetes

It is well documented that shift work can be associated with increased insulin resistance. A meta-analysis showed a higher risk of diabetes in people who had ever done shift work (OR 1.09; 95% CI 1.05–1.12) which was more prominent in men.[46] Long working hours have also been implicated in developing diabetes, but only in people from a low socioeconomic background.[47] Shift work can result in poorer glycaemic control in T1DM[48] or T2DM.[49] Notably, work-related stress did not appear to have an adverse impact on glycaemic control in working adults with diabetes.[50]

Diabetes prevention in the workplace

Given the shift from physically demanding professions to more sedentary roles coupled with lifestyle factors, health promotion initiatives such as encouraging physical activity and healthy eating will help reduce the risk of diabetes. The workplace provides an excellent opportunity for health promotion and employers should be encouraged to invest in health and well-being programmes for their staff. This is more relevant in industries that rely on shift work, where in addition to general health promotion, other measures including offering healthy dietary options day and night is highly recommended.

The value of direct screening (e.g. measuring random BGL) in the workplace is debatable. It may identify those with T2DM who otherwise would not have been screened. However, this should be balanced against confidentiality, logistics, relationship with the primary care physician, and cost. Health and well-being initiatives that utilize health risk assessment in the workplace along with health education and signposting is a reasonable approach.

Fitness assessment

Assessment of fitness to work considers the impact of the illness and its treatment on functional capability to perform a particular task safely.

Many individuals with good glycaemic control have no functional limitations and are capable of performing most work. Certain jobs, mainly those which are classed as safety critical, may require tight monitoring of BGLs to ensure an acceptably low risk of disabling hypoglycaemia. Safety-critical roles typically include some roles in transport, construction, and emergency services, and those requiring firearms use. However the decision about whether a particular role or a task is safety critical relies on a risk assessment to evaluate the impact of sudden incapacity (e.g. caused by severe hypoglycaemia) on safety. The DVLA guidance for vocational drivers (Table 25.6) recognizes up to a 2% risk of incapacity as an acceptable threshold to hold a group 2 licence and can be used as a benchmark for risk assessment, fitness assessment, and monitoring in other industries or roles where there is no industry-defined standard.

It is important to reiterate that although sudden incapacity due to hypoglycaemia is usually the main concern, the overall glucose control is important too because persistent or erratic high BGLs may result in more aggressive treatment by agents that may in turn cause hypoglycaemia. For example, the UK Civil Aviation Authority requires a medical review if the HbA1c level is between 69 and 86 mmol/mol (8.5% and 10%) and revoking of the licence if it is over 86 mmol/mol (10%).[51]

Diabetic complications and fitness to work

In the event of diabetic complications, the impact on function and fitness to work and the necessary adjustments and restrictions warrant an individual functional assessment. Some diabetic complications cause obvious loss of function (e.g. the impact of advanced retinopathy on visual acuity). However, other complications may cause subtle limitations (e.g. postural hypotension due to autonomic neuropathy). Therefore, OH and other health professionals who advise on fitness to work must assess individual signs and symptoms comprehensively to ensure that subtle changes are detected.

Shift work

Traditionally, there have been concerns about shift work in the context of insulin treatment. This was mainly on the basis of how to adjust the insulin dose given the disruption of sleeping and eating pattern by rapidly rotating shift patterns. Newer insulin preparations with predictable profiles offer different durations of action. Additionally, educating people with diabetes facilitates personal dose adjustment for carbohydrate intake and physical activity, so concern about shift work on insulin treatment is reduced. However, because shift work can increase insulin resistance, careful consideration should be given to the continuation of shift work and adjustments to reduce the adverse effects on diabetes in those who struggle to achieve their BGL target.

It is important to adjust meal timings in accordance to the shift pattern. This may include more frequent meals or snacks within the shift, especially for long night shifts, to ensure a sufficient source of carbohydrate is available throughout the shift. This should be balanced with adequate insulin measured by the carbohydrate content and physical activity. Healthy food should be available throughout the shift, reducing reliance on fast food and unhealthy snacks. All employees, especially those with diabetes, should be encouraged to consume healthy foods while on shift.

The importance of adequate sleep should be reiterated to individuals with diabetes to counteract the disruptive impact of shift work on BGLs.

Adjustments

Work modifications should be based on individual assessment of functional limitation caused by diabetes, its complications, or treatment in the context of job requirements. Box 25.5 offers common work adjustments.

Box 25.5 Common work adjustment for those with diabetes

- Set and/or extra breaks, to allow regular eating and hydration, monitor BGL, administer insulin, and rest.

- Appropriate space to monitor BGL and inject insulin.

- Safe disposal system for sharps.

- Flexible working pattern or time off to attend diabetic review (ongoing) and educational courses (usually one-off).

- Adjusting shift pattern; avoiding rapidly changing shifts, reduce shift work or total removal from shift work if needed. In the UK this can be also supported under the Working Time Regulations 1998.

- Access to water and healthy food throughout the shift.

- Sensitive absence management to accommodate a higher rate of sickness absence.

- Preparedness to deal with emergencies; availability of trained first aider and hypoglycaemic kit including ketone testing equipment (if risk of DKA).

- Protective footwear for those with neuropathy.

- Extra breaks or adjusting work pattern for dialysis (in advanced nephropathy).

- Avoidance of isolated or safety-critical work proportionate to history of diabetic control.

Legal considerations

In the UK, the Health and Safety at Work etc. Act 1974 requires employers to ensure the health and safety of the employees and others. In the context of diabetes, sudden incapacity caused by severe hypoglycaemia can impact safety, and therefore requires risk assessment and mitigation.

The UK Equality Act 2010 is likely to apply to many people with diabetes. Importantly, the effect of treatment should be discounted so even if their condition is well controlled by medication, people with diabetes can still be classed as disabled, because without treatment their condition would have a substantial impact on day-to-day activities.

Diabetes of any type is not automatically a disability, but it is very likely that someone with diabetes on medical treatment (e.g. insulin) would be considered disabled within the meaning of the Act. The application of the Act to those who are diet controlled is debatable and depends on the circumstances.

Other endocrine conditions

There are numerous endocrine conditions other than diabetes for which a detailed description is beyond the scope of this chapter. Examples are outlined in Table 25.9.

Fitness to work and work adjustments depend on the functional limitation caused by any specific endocrine abnormality and its treatment. Common symptoms include

Table 25.9 Common endocrine diseases

	Condition	Treatment
Adrenal	Hypoadrenalism (e.g. Addison's disease)	Steroid replacement
Thyroid	Thyrotoxicosis (e.g. Graves' disease)	Antithyroid agents (carbimazole, propylthiouracil) Radioactive iodine
	Hypothyroidism	Thyroxine replacement
Pituitary	Prolactinoma	Dopamine agonist (e.g. cabergoline) Surgical excision
	Acromegaly	Medical suppression of growth hormone Surgical excision
	Cushing's syndrome	Surgical excision or radiotherapy

tiredness and loss of stamina. Work modification should therefore focus on exercise tolerance, pace, and shift pattern. In particular conditions such as Addison's disease, the timing of medication (oral steroid replacement) is important, especially for shift workers. A recent study suggested that night work may disrupt the secretion of thyroid-stimulating hormone[52] although the clinical impact is unclear.

Workers on steroid replacement may carry a vial of hydrocortisone for emergency use. The workplace should be prepared for this, including training for first aiders, facilities for storage and administration of hydrocortisone, and sharps disposal.

Occupational exposure and endocrine disorders

The main work exposures that are known to cause endocrine disruption are lead[53,54] (usually >50 micrograms/dL) and pesticides.[55] Both are associated with disruption of thyroid and sex hormones. Ionizing radiation can affect the thyroid and reproductive systems but occupational exposures are well below the danger limits.

Key points

- Diabetes is very common. Prevalence, especially of T2DM, is increasing.
- A healthy lifestyle including physical activity and healthy diet should be promoted.
- Diabetes can adversely affect employment including a higher rate of unemployment and early retirement and reduced productivity.
- Most people with good glycaemic control have no functional limitation and are capable of performing most work types. Work adjustments may be required to facilitate employment.
- Safety-critical and shift work require special consideration in the context of diabetes.

Useful websites

National Institute for Health and Care Excellence guidelines

T1DM	https://www.nice.org.uk/guidance/ng17
T2DM	https://www.nice.org.uk/guidance/ng28
GDM	https://www.nice.org.uk/guidance/ng3
Obesity	https://www.nice.org.uk/guidance/cg43

Patient information

Diabetes UK	https://www.diabetes.org.uk/
NHS Digital. 'Diabetes'	https://www.nhs.uk/conditions/diabetes/

Legislation

Health and Safety at Work etc. Act 1974	http://www.legislation.gov.uk/ukpga/1974/37
Equality Act 2010	http://www.legislation.gov.uk/ukpga/2010/15/contents

Guidance for safety-critical work

DVLA. 'Assessing fitness to drive – a guide for medical professionals'	https://www.gov.uk/government/uploads/system/uploads/attachment_data/file/652720/assessing-fitness-to-drive-a-guide-for-medical-professionals.pdf
Civil Aviation Authority	https://www.caa.co.uk

References

1. **American Diabetes Association**. Diagnosis and classification of diabetes mellitus. 2014, Diabetes Care 2014;**37**(Suppl. 1);S81–90.
2. **Diabetes UK**. Diabetes prevalence 2016 (November 2016). Available at: https://www.diabetes.org.uk/professionals/position-statements-reports/statistics/diabetes-prevalence-2016.
3. **International Diabetes Federation**. Diabetes atlas, 7th edn. 2015. Available at: http://www.diabetesatlas.org/.
4. **National Institute for Health and Care Excellence**. Type 1 diabetes in adults: diagnosis and management. NICE guideline [NG17]. 2015. Available at: https://www.nice.org.uk/guidance/ng17.
5. **The InterAct Consortium**. Long-term risk of incident type 2 diabetes and measures of overall and regional obesity: the EPIC-InterAct Case-Cohort Study. *PLoS Med* 2012;**9**:e1001230.
6. **Gray LJ, Davies MJ, Hiles S, et al.** Detection of impaired glucose regulation and/or type 2 diabetes mellitus, using primary care electronic data, in a multiethnic UK community setting. *Diabetalogia* 2012;**55**:959–66.
7. **World Health Organization**. Use of glycated haemoglobin (HbA1c) in the diagnosis of diabetes mellitus: abbreviated report of a WHO consultation. 2011. Available at http://www.who.int/diabetes/publications/report-hba1c_2011.pdf.
8. **Gaede P, Lund-Andersen H, Parving HH, Pedersen O**. Effect of multifactorial intervention on mortality in type 2 diabetes. *N Engl J Med* 2008;**358**:580–91.

9. **Steinsbekk A, Rygg LØ, Lisulo M, Rise MB, Fretheim A.** Group based diabetes self-management education compared to routine treatment for people with type 2 diabetes mellitus. A systematic review with meta-analysis. *BMC Health Serv Res* 2012;**12**;213.

10. **National Institute for Health and Care Excellence.** Continuous subcutaneous insulin infusion for the treatment of diabetes mellitus. Technology appraisal guidance [TA151]. 2008. Available at: https://www.nice.org.uk/guidance/ta151.

11. **Steinbeck I, Cederholm J, Eliasson B, et al.** Insulin pump therapy, multiple daily injections, and cardiovascular mortality in 18 168 people with type 1 diabetes: observational study. *BMJ* 2015;**350**:h3234.

12. **National Institute for Health and Care Excellence.** Type 2 diabetes in adults: management. NICE guideline [NG28]. 2015. Available at: https://www.nice.org.uk/guidance/ng28.

13. **Nauck M, Stöckmann F, Ebert R, Creutzfeldt W.** Reduced incretin effect in type 2 (non-insulin-dependent) diabetes. *Diabetalogia* 1986;**29**:46–52.

14. **Marso S, Daniels G, Brown-Frandsen K, et al.** Liraglutide and cardiovascular outcomes in type 2 diabetes. *N Engl J Med* 2016;**375**:311–22.

15. **Fralick M.** Risk of diabetic ketoacidosis after initiation of an SGLT2 inhibitor. *N Engl J Med* 2017;**376**:2300–2.

16. **Zinman B, Wanner C, Lachin JM, et al.** Empagliflozin, cardiovascular outcomes and mortality in type 2 diabetes. *N Engl J Med* 2015;**373**:2117–28.

17. **The Diabetes Control and Complications Trial Research Group.** The effect of intensive treatment of diabetes on the development and progression of long-term complications in insulin-dependent diabetes mellitus. *N Engl J Med* 1993;**329**:977–86.

18. **UK Prospective Diabetes Study (UKPDS) Group.** Intensive blood-glucose control with sulphonylureas or insulin compared with conventional treatment and risk of complications in patients with type 2 diabetes (UKPDS 33). *Lancet* 1998;**352**:837–53.

19. **The Action to Control Cardiovascular Risk in Diabetes Study Group.** Effects of intensive glucose lowering in type 2 diabetes. *N Eng J Med* 2008;**358**:2545–59.

20. **The ADVANCE Collaborative Group.** Intensive blood glucose control and vascular outcomes in patients with type 2 diabetes. *N Engl J Med* 2008;**358**:2560–72.

21. **Hippisley-Cox J, Coupland C, Vinogradova Y, Robson J, Brindle P.** Performance of the QRISK cardiovascular risk prediction algorithm in an independent UK sample of patients from general practice: a validation study. *Heart* 2008;**94**:34–9.

22. **Joint British Diabetes Societies – Inpatient Care Group.** The hospital management of hypoglycaemia in adults with diabetes mellitus (revised September 2013). Available at: http://www.diabetologists-abcd.org.uk/subsite/JBDS_IP_Hypo_Adults_Revised.pdf.

23. **Donnelly LA, Morris AD, Frier BM, et al.** Frequency and predictors of hypoglycaemia in type 1 and insulin-treated type 2 diabetes in a population-based study. *Diabet Med* 2005;**22**:749–55.

24. **Elliott J, Heller S.** Hypoglycaemia unawareness. *Pract Diabet Int* 2011;**28**:227–32.

25. **Lobmann R, Smid HG, Pottag G, et al.** Impairment and recovery of elementary cognitive function induced by hypoglycemia in type-1 diabetic patients and healthy controls. *J Clin Endocrinol Metab* 2000;**85**:2758–66.

26. **Holmes CS, Hayford JT, Gonzalez JL, et al.** A survey of cognitive functioning at different glucose levels in diabetic persons. *Diabetes Care* 1983;**6**:180–5.

27. **Cox DJ, Gonder-Frederick L, Clarke W.** Driving decrements in type I diabetes during moderate hypoglycemia. *Diabetes* 1993;**42**:239–43.

28. **Weinger K, Kinsley BT, Levy CJ, et al.** The perception of safe driving ability during hypoglycemia in patients with type 1 diabetes mellitus. *Am Am J Med* 1999;**107**:246–53.

29. **Hussein Z, Kamaruddin NA, Chan SP, et al.** Hypoglycemia awareness among insulin-treated patients with diabetes in Malaysia: a cohort subanalysis of the HAT study. *Diabetes Res Clin Pract* 2017;**133**:40–9.

30. **Leckie AM, Ritchie PJ, Graham MK, et al.** Frequency, severity and morbidity of hypoglycaemia in the workplace in people with insulin-treated diabetes. *Diabetes Care* 2005;**28**:1333–8.

31. **McNay EC, Cotero VE.** Mini-review: impact of recurrent hypoglycemia on cognitive and brain function. *Physiol Behav* 2010;**100**:234–8.

32. **Diabetes Control and Complications Trial Research Group.** Effects of intensive diabetes therapy on neuropsychological function in adults in the Diabetes Control and Complications Trial. *Ann Intern Med* 1996;**124**:379–88.

33. **Wang F, Zhao M, Han Z, et al.** Long-term subclinical hyperglycemia and hypoglycemia as independent risk factors for mild cognitive impairment in elderly people. *Tohoku J Exp Med* 2017;**242**:121–8.

34. **Northam EA, Rankins D, Lin A, et al.** Central nervous system function in youth with type 1 diabetes 12 years after disease onset. *Diabetes Care* 2009;**32**:445–50.

35. **Xiang Q, Zhang J, Li CY, et al.** Insulin resistance-induced hyperglycemia decreased the activation of Akt/CREB in hippocampus neurons: molecular evidence for mechanism of diabetes-induced cognitive dysfunction. *Neuropeptides* 2015;**54**:9–15.

36. **Geijselaers SLC, Sep SJS, Claessens D, et al.** The role of hyperglycemia, insulin resistance, and blood pressure in diabetes-associated differences in cognitive performance – The Maastricht Study. *Diabetes Care* 2017;**40**:1537–47.

37. **Ardran M, MacFarlane I, Robinson C.** Educational achievements, employment and social class of insulin-dependent diabetics: a survey of a young adult clinic in Liverpool. *Diabet Med* 1987;**4**:546–8.

38. **Yassin AS, Beckles GL, Messonnier ML.** Disability and its economic impact among adults with diabetes. *J Occup Environ Med* 2002;**44**:136–42.

39. **Latif E.** The impact of diabetes on employment in Canada. *Health Econ* 2009;**18**:577–89.

40. **Mayfield JA, Deb P, Whitecotton L.** Work disability and diabetes. *Diabetes Care* 1999;**22**:1105–9.

41. **Cawley J, Rizzo JA, Haas K.** The association of diabetes with job absenteeism costs among obese and morbidly obese workers. *J Occup Environ Med* 2008;**50**:527–34.

42. **Dray-Spira R, Herquelot E, Bonenfant S, et al.** Impact of diabetes mellitus onset on sickness absence from work – a 15-year follow-up of the GAZEL Occupational Cohort Study. *Diabet Med* 2013;**30**:549–56.

43. **Vamos EP, Mucsi I, Keszei A, et al.** Comorbid depression is associated with increased healthcare utilization and lost productivity in persons with diabetes: a large nationally representative Hungarian population survey. *Psychosom Med* 2009;**71**:501–7.

44. **Alavinia SM, Burdorf A.** Unemployment and retirement and ill-health: a cross sectional analysis across European countries. *Int Arch Occup Environ Health* 2008;**82**:39–45.

45. **Herquelot E, Guéguen A, Bonenfant S, et al.** Impact of diabetes on work cessation: data from the GAZEL cohort study. *Diabetes Care* 2011;**34**:1344–9.

46. **Gan Y, Yang C, Tong X, et al.** Shift work and diabetes mellitus: a meta-analysis of observational studies. *Occup Environ Med* 2015;**72**:72–8.

47. **Kivimäki M, Virtanen M, Kawachi I, et al.** Long working hours, socioeconomic status, and the risk of incident type 2 diabetes: a meta-analysis of published and unpublished data from 222 120 individuals. *Lancet Diabetes Endocrinol* 2015;**3**:27–34.

48. **Young J, Waclawski E, Young JA, Spencer J.** Control of type 1 diabetes mellitus and shift work. *Occup Med (Lond)* 2013;**63**:70–2.

49. **Manodpitipong A, Saetung S, Nimitphong H, et al.** Night-shift work is associated with poorer glycaemic control in patients with type 2 diabetes. *J Sleep Res* 2017;**26**:764–72.

50. **Annor FB, Roblin DW, Okosun IS, Goodman M.** Work-related psychosocial stress and glycemic control among working adults with diabetes mellitus. *Diabetes Metab Syndr* 2015;**9**:85–90.

51. **Civil Aviation Authority.** UK CAA policy for the medical certification of pilots and ATCOs with diabetes. 2015. Available at: https://www.caa.co.uk/WorkArea/DownloadAsset.aspx?id=4294973794/.

52. **Moon SH, Lee BJ, Kim SJ, et al.** Relationship between thyroid stimulating hormone and night shift work *Ann Occup Environ Med* 2016;**28**:53.

53. **Tuppurainen M, Wagar G, Kurppa K, et al.** Thyroid function as assessed by routine laboratory tests of workers with long-term lead exposure. *Scand J Work Environ Health* 1988;**14**:175–80.

54. **Winker R.** Reproductive toxicology in occupational settings: an update. *Int Arch Occup Environ Health* 2006;**79**:1.

55. **Mnif W, Hassine AI, Bouaziz A, et al.** Effect of endocrine disruptor pesticides: a review. *Int J Environ Res Public Health.* 2011;**8**:2265–303.

Chapter 26

Cardiovascular diseases

Joseph De Bono and Anli Yue Zhou

Introduction

Cardiovascular diseases (CVDs) remain one of the commonest causes of ill health and death but their incidence and mortality rates in the UK have declined since 1980.[1] CVDs affect fitness to work in a number of ways. First, through disabling symptoms that limit working capacity, which can often be quantified and partially alleviated by effective treatment. The second, less common but more difficult, problem is the risk of sudden incapacity, especially in apparently well individuals. This includes the risk of sudden cardiac death following ventricular fibrillation, which is the most common cause of cardiac arrest, and while the risk of sudden incapacity is very small, the consequences can be unacceptable. Assessment of risk and its impact is possible, but explaining this concept to a bus driver who has lost his job is not easy. Finally, treatment for a patient's cardiac condition such as a pacemaker or implantable cardiac defibrillator may preclude working in certain environments.

Limitation of working capacity and the risk of sudden incapacity can be well judged in populations by specialist opinion. For the individual, this must be backed up by objective data, usually derived from the results of non-invasive tests such as electrocardiography (ECG) and exercise testing, and imaging such as echocardiography and cardiac magnetic resonance imaging (MRI). While disease progression can be unpredictable, objective data can ensure individuals are not unfairly excluded from work they can safely do.

Sometimes cardiovascular symptoms are not proportionate to the objective evidence of disease. This could be due to psychological co-morbidity, which is also an independent risk factor for CVD onset, progression, and recurrence.[2] The negative psychological impact of a myocardial infarction (MI) could prevent return to work despite prompt treatment, a full cardiac recovery, and only modest residual disease. The occupational physician needs to recognize the psychological co-morbidity associated with CVDs and ensure holistic management plans are considered to facilitate workplace rehabilitation.

Epidemiology

CVD is the collective term for all disease affecting the heart and blood vessels such as coronary heart disease (CHD), hypertension, stroke, and non-CHD such as congenital heart disease, valvular disease, and atrial fibrillation (AF).[3]

CVD is more common in older populations (>65 years); however, the prevalence of CVD in Great Britain for those in the 45–65 years age group has been found to be as high as 8–10% of the population, and £9 billion is spent annually on treating CVD. This is not surprising considering CVD account for almost 10% of all 2017 hospital admissions. The prevalence of CHD has reduced, whereas other CVDs such as AF and stroke have been increasing.[1,3] In 2018, over 7 million people were living with CVD. Over 1.2 million live with stroke, 9.25 million have hypertension, 920,000 have heart failure, and 1.3 million have AF.

Although CVD is no longer the leading cause of UK deaths, it is still responsible for 152,465 deaths in 2016, of which 70% were caused by CHD and stroke.[3] CVDs account for 26% of deaths in the UK, of which 12% were due to CHD (which is caused by atherosclerosis and is also known as ischaemic heart disease). CHD was responsible for 66,076 UK deaths in 2016 and is responsible for 34% per cent of deaths before the age of 75 years.

The prevalence of CVDs caused or made worse by work according to self-reported work-related illness surveys in 2016 was 18,000[4] and subsequent productivity losses due to CVD morbidity equate to nearly £2.3 billion.[5]

Coronary heart disease

Clinical features

CHD (also known as ischaemic heart disease and coronary artery disease) represents a spectrum of conditions associated with atherosclerosis within the coronary arteries. Acute coronary syndromes (ACSs) occur when CHD is associated with the sudden rupture of plaque inside the coronary artery and can consist of unstable angina, non-ST-segment elevation MI (NSTEMI), and ST-segment elevation MI (STEMI). CHD can present with silent ischaemia (especially in diabetes mellitus). However, CHD usually presents as chest pain due to an ACS, but it may also present with symptoms resulting from arrhythmia or heart failure, or be detected incidentally by ECG. Anyone with cardiac-sounding chest pain should summon help urgently because prompt treatment can save lives. After recovery, the risk of further cardiac events (sudden death, recurrent MI, or need for myocardial revascularization) is assessed by clinical history and simple investigations. Despite the improvement in treatment, survivors of acute MIs are at a high risk of recurrence as well as other complications such as stroke compared to the general population. Heart failure is a frequent complication of MI and increases the mortality risk by up to four-fold. Approximately 40% of MIs are associated with left ventricular systolic dysfunction.[6] ECGs, echocardiograms, and serum natriuretic peptide levels can be used to assess heart failure and can contribute to diagnosis, monitoring, and prognosis.

Assessment

Cardiologists grade symptom limitation from stable angina and heart failure using the Canadian Cardiovascular Society (CCS) and the New York Heart Association (NYHA)

Table 26.1 Canadian Cardiovascular Society grading of angina

Class	Symptoms
I	Angina only during strenuous or prolonged physical activity
II	Slight limitation with angina only during vigorous physical activity
III	Symptoms with everyday living activities (i.e. moderate limitation)
IV	Inability to perform any activity without angina or angina at rest (i.e. severe limitation)

Source: data from Canadian Cardiovascular Society, https://www.ccs.ca/en/. Copyright © 2012 Canadian Cardiovascular Society.

systems respectively (Tables 26.1 and 26.2). Although there is a relationship between symptoms and survival, studies have demonstrated that even those with mild symptoms may still have a higher risk of hospitalization and death.[7] The NYHA classification has also been used to provide guidance for heart failure treatment, and those with class II or higher are recommended to commence pharmacological treatment.[7] The CCS classification (Table 26.1) can also provide information to contribute to the overall management plan including investigations and pharmacological treatment.[8]

Approximately 50% of CHD-related deaths are due to sudden cardiac death, which is death that occurs within 1 hour of symptom onset.[9] The personal risk predictions of sudden disability and death through ventricular tachyarrhythmias are currently limited; however, a family history of sudden cardiac death can contribute to risk profiling. The risk is greatest in the early days following an ACS event, and may remain raised for months to years. Those with severe myocardial damage and/or continuing ischaemia form a high-risk group. The extent of ventricular damage may be judged by the presence of heart failure, gallop rhythm, and poor left ventricular function on ECG.

Residual myocardial ischaemia may be judged by recurrent angina and can be confirmed by exercise testing, ischaemia imaging, and coronary computed tomography (CT) angiography.[8] An exercise test may also reveal cardiovascular incapacity in other ways, namely exhaustion, inappropriate heart rate, and blood pressure (BP) responses, arrhythmia, and ECG change, especially ST segment shift. In practice, the exercise

Table 26.2 New York Heart Association grading of heart failure

Class	Symptoms
I	No limitation of physical activities and no shortness of breath when walking or climbing stairs
II	Mild symptoms of shortness of breath and slight limitation during ordinary activity
III	Marked symptoms and shortness of breath during less than ordinary activity (e.g. walking 20–100 yards). Comfortable only at rest
IV	Severe limitation of activity with symptoms at rest

Source: data from The Criteria Committee of the New York Heart Association. *Nomenclature and Criteria for Diagnosis of Diseases of the Heart and Great Vessels*, 9th Edition. Copyright © 1994 Wolters Kluwer Health.

test and the opinion of an accredited specialist are generally sufficient to assess fitness for work. This is reflected in the guidance material for vocational drivers (see Chapter 15). Individuals who are asymptomatic and can achieve a good workload without adverse features have a very low risk of further cardiac events. This applies particularly to younger individuals and employers should little hesitation in taking them back to work.

An individual who reaches stage 4 of the Bruce protocol on a treadmill is at such low risk of further cardiac events that vocational driving may be permitted. The carefully considered Driver and Vehicle Licensing Agency (DVLA) guidelines are now being applied more widely to other groups of workers whose occupation involves an element of risk to themselves and others in the event of cardiovascular collapse. Most employees, however, are not required to demonstrate such high levels of cardiovascular fitness.

Those whose early investigations are inconclusive will require further tests, often including MRI or radionuclide imaging to assess ventricular function and myocardial perfusion. Those who have continuing symptoms, or whose non-invasive investigations are unsatisfactory will be recommended to undergo coronary angiography with a view to myocardial revascularization. This is mildly unpleasant and hazardous with a risk of local complication of 1 in 500, and of catastrophe (including stroke and death) of 1 in 1000. Facilities for angiography are now widely available. Most angiograms are undertaken as day case procedures.

Management strategies: medical

Lifestyle management and drug therapy have transformed the management of CHD. Smoking, diabetes mellitus, hyperlipidaemia, and hypertension have been identified as independent predictors of CHD and previous studies have shown that over 80% of those with CHD have at least one of these four risk factors.[10] Employers therefore should support and reinforce community measures by discouraging smoking, encouraging healthy activities including alcohol intake, and by providing a healthy diet at work.

The prognosis of patients following MI is improved by intervention and drug treatment. Aspirin improves prognosis in all patients with CHD. Nitrates, beta-adrenergic antagonists, and calcium antagonists alleviate the symptoms of myocardial ischaemia. Beta-adrenergic antagonists and angiotensin-converting enzyme inhibitors improve symptoms and survival in patients with heart failure. Statins also improve prognosis and reduce the risk of subsequent events in all groups of patients with CHD. These and other cardiovascular drugs are generally well tolerated and remarkably free from long-term side effects. Many owe their efficacy to their vasodilating action; hence, hypotension and faintness are possible complications. All patients will require lifelong medication, with aspirin and a statin as a minimum.

For primary prevention, the QRISK®2 assessment tool is recommended by the National Institute for Health and Care Excellence guidelines and it estimates the 10-year cardiovascular risk in individuals.[11] It includes age, ethnicity, sex, cholesterol level, body mass index (BMI), smoking status, and the presence of diabetes, AF, chronic kidney disease, angina, hypertension, and rheumatoid arthritis.[12] Atorvastatin 20 mg is currently offered for primary prevention to people who have greater than a 10% 10-year risk of developing CHD. Lifestyle advice regarding smoking and alcohol, exercise, weight management, and a cardioprotective diet that consists of reducing saturated fats and sugar and increasing mono-unsaturated fat, fruit, and vegetable intake should be given.[11] Currently, there is no National Institute for Health and Care Excellence recommendation regarding ramipril and aspirin treatment for primary prevention of CHD.

Coronary angioplasty and stenting (percutaneous coronary intervention)

For years, balloon angioplasty was bedevilled by a high recurrence rate. The development of the coronary stent led to a substantial reduction in the restenosis rate. A stent is a tubular metal mesh that is delivered on the balloon in a collapsed state, down the artery, and subsequently deployed at high pressure (e.g. 16 atmospheres) into the arterial wall. The angiographic results are remarkable and relief of symptoms can be equally dramatic. Complex, distal, and multiple stenoses can be safely treated. The introduction of drug-eluting stents for selected cases—usually smaller arteries and long lesions—has reduced the restenosis risk to almost zero.

Primary percutaneous coronary intervention (PCI) has replaced thrombolysis as the treatment of choice for MI with ST segment elevation. Almost invariably the blocked artery can be opened up and stented. Those who receive this treatment make a speedy and dramatic recovery, often returning home after 3 days in hospital. Some people doubt that they have had a heart attack. Rehabilitation with early ECG and echocardiography is becoming the norm; return to work may be accelerated.

Urgent angiography proceeding to PCI has become a standard approach for most confirmed ACSs. Elective PCIs constitute the minority of cases in cardiac centres. Success rates are of the order of 97%. Disasters necessitating surgery occur in about 1 in 700 procedures. Groin haematomas are an unusual but well-recognized complication of the femoral approach, which has led to most cases being performed via the radial artery. Return to work within 1 week is commonplace after elective PCI.

Coronary artery bypass grafting

Coronary artery bypass grafting (CABG) is a more complex method of achieving myocardial revascularization and nowadays is undertaken less commonly than PCI. It is also remarkably safe, with mortality rates of about 1% for elective operations. Recovery is rapid and most patients resume work within 2–3 months and most are relieved of their angina. Patients who were working before surgery generally do so afterwards, and restrictions that may have been appropriate previously should no longer be relevant.

Although CABG has been associated with a delay in returning to work compared to PCI, no significant difference was found between PCI and CABG for returning to work, quality of life, or staying in long-term employment.[13] No special restrictions are necessary after return to work. Coronary graft stenosis and occlusion leads to a recurrence rate of angina of about 4% per year. This is generally less severe than previously but may affect long-term job placement. CABG for left main stem or three-vessel disease improves prognosis. Rehabilitation programmes are now well established in many hospitals. These enable many patients to make a full recovery following a cardiac event such as MI or CABG.

Return to work after developing coronary heart disease

Studies on return to work after the onset of heart disease have shown that several different considerations apply.

The nature of the original cardiovascular event that led to the individual stopping work. Whichever form CHD takes, the important factors influencing return to work include the persistence of chest pain during exercise, the risk of arrhythmia, and the level of left ventricular function. Additionally, the possibility of silent ischaemia needs consideration for high-risk individuals. While angioplasty ensures a speedier return to work than CABG, long-term employment prospects are similar in both treatment groups.[13]

The residual loss of function following the cardiac event. The individual's functional capacity should be assessed prior to return to work. For cardiac disease, an exercise stress test will give the required information, while those with cardiac failure may need further investigation. Cardiac failure formerly meant that a return to work was unlikely, but improvements in treatment of the underlying cause mean now that more people with heart failure can return to work. Using the NYHA criteria for heart failure, individuals with functional capacity I and II are likely to return to their previous role. Those with NYHA functional capacity III and IV or those returning to a very strenuous job may require additional functional testing and cardiological opinion.

Recurrent cardiac events. Those who experienced arrhythmias and recurrent cardiac event (requiring hospital admission and treatment) were less likely to be at work 12 months after the ACS event.[14]

The prognosis of the causative CVD. Prognostic indicators are well documented for most cardiovascular problems. Where the prognosis is poor and the risk of recurrence high, return to work may be unrealistic. Where there are other co-morbid conditions, the impact of these conditions will affect function and return to work. A recent occupational study found that co-morbid conditions such as depression, migraine, and chronic bronchitis are common in those with angina; co-morbidity strongly predicts functional status, mortality, hospitalization, number of days in hospital, and medical care costs.[15]

Individual factors. Psychological factors may play a bigger part in whether an individual returns to work than physical factors. Depression has been found to be an important predictor of poorer return to work after a cardiac event.[16] Some other factors which make return to work less likely following a cardiac event are summarized in Table 26.3.

Table 26.3 Factors reducing likelihood of return to work

Individual factors	Increasing duration of absence independent of the prognosis of the CVD
	If the cardiac event happened at work
	Increasing age
	Fear of recurrence
	Poor motivation
	Poor understanding of the condition
	Secondary gain from the 'sick role'
	Where the job is perceived as unrewarding, dangerous or damaging to health
	When redeployment/retraining is difficult to achieve due to certain individual factors such as education, adaptability, or even personality
	Perception that it is a long-term illness
Employment factors	Employer's fear of further illness at work and subsequent litigation
	Reluctance to consider redeployment
	Demanding work environment
Other factors	Sickness benefits
	Overcautious standards
	Low acceptability of risk by regulatory authorities

Cardiac rehabilitation

Cardiac rehabilitation programmes are successful at facilitating return to normal life including work and are remarkably safe. A 12-week programme has been shown to improve quality of life, but programmes may vary according to the country and individual. They are structured in three phases. The aim of the programme is to develop a functional capacity of 8 metabolic equivalents (METs). However, this level is only rarely reached as heavy work is defined as activity requiring 6–8 METs and maximal work includes any activity that requires greater than 9 METs (Table 26.4). A recent Cochrane review of cardiac rehabilitation programmes showed this intervention reduced cardiovascular mortality and hospital admissions, but did not reduce the risk of MIs.[17]

Return to work

It is estimated that up to 80% of patients with uncomplicated MI will return to work. When work is resumed, the levels and duration of activity should be increased progressively. In general, physical activity is good for the heart but the degree of physical activity must take into account previous fitness and the results of exercise testing. Patients with stable angina can safely work within their limitations of fitness but should not be put in situations where their angina may be readily provoked. Patients with persistent angina or an abnormal exercise test should be assessed for myocardial revascularization. Following an acute coronary event, those with no complications and good exercise tolerance may return to work in 4–6 weeks.

Fatigue usually resolves over time. It may be helpful to arrange reduced hours or other temporary restrictions, but these should be defined and not left open-ended. A recent systematic review investigating older workers with cardiac disease has suggested that

Table 26.4 Phases of cardiac rehabilitation

Phase	Aims
1. Acute/inpatient	◆ Determine exercise capacity ◆ Provide patient education about necessary supervision ◆ Start exercise programme under medical supervision
2. Reconditioning outpatient supervised	◆ Improve exercise capacity and strengthen ◆ Continue lifestyle changes ◆ Monitor exercise programme as an outpatient in a supervised fashion
3. Maintenance outpatient unsupervised	◆ Emphasize long-term lifestyle changes ◆ Exercise programmes three to five times per week without medical supervision ◆ Monitoring in outpatient setting

multicomponent interventions could be of benefit for those returning to work.[18] This could include a structured return to work plan, job-simulated cardiac rehabilitation and education.[18]

Psychological factors

Depression and anxiety are common in CHD and are both a causal factor and poor prognostic indicator for mortality.[19,20] A recent study has found that CHD patients who screen positive on the Hospital Anxiety and Depression Scale were more likely to incur higher healthcare costs and lower quality of life over a 3-year period, which suggests psychological factors can persist over long periods.[21] Psychosocial work characteristics such as job strain could also be aetiological and prognostic factors for CHD and social support could potentially buffer these effects.[20] A recent Cochrane review showed that psychological treatments did reduce the cardiac mortality rate and alleviate psychological symptoms.[22]

Screening for coronary disease

Those populations at high risk of sudden incapacity can be identified once their disease has become manifest, but silent coronary disease is extremely common. Sudden death may be the first manifestation of CHD. Many cardiac events will therefore occur in those who appear to be fit—approximately one-quarter in studies of road traffic accidents, for example. One solution to this problem may be to screen employees by clinical examination and exercise testing for 'silent' myocardial ischaemia. This may be justifiable in certain groups and has been adopted by the United States Air Force. Exercise-induced ECG ST-segment change in an asymptomatic individual has several causes; using the criterion of 1 mm ST-segment depression, however, only about one-third will turn out to have coronary disease on angiography. Screening for asymptomatic CHD in this way cannot therefore be recommended routinely because of the high incidence of false-positive results. Simple clinical features such as age, male sex, history of chest pain, smoking habit, or a strong family history of premature CHD, and physical examination are better methods of assessing seemingly healthy individuals. The development of fast multislice CT scanners has encouraged commercial screening organizations to offer this as a means of detecting silent coronary disease. Two methods are advertised—a coronary calcium score, which is cheap and easy, and CT angiography. The former commonly leads to the latter, which carries a small radiation risk and requires careful interpretation by an experienced specialist. The place of this investigation in screening is uncertain, mainly because there are no long-term follow-up studies of prognosis by lesion type. Coronary CT can be very helpful in cardiac centres in two particular circumstances—to rule out coronary disease in patients with acute chest pain, where it has the merit of enabling other diagnoses such as aortic dissection and pulmonary embolism to be made; and in patients with complex coronary anatomy, particularly after CABG.

Valvular disease

Accurate anatomical and physiological diagnosis of valvular heart disease in young people can now be carried out by non-invasive methods such as echocardiography and MRI. Acquired valvular disease—usually degenerative aortic stenosis or mitral regurgitation—is mostly seen now in those beyond working age, but mitral valve prolapse deserves emphasis as it affects some 2% of the population and carries an excellent prognosis. Aortic stenosis may also require surgery in patients of working age particularly where there is an underlying bicuspid valve. It often presents as an auscultatory finding at a pre-employment medical examination, may be associated with ECG change, and may sometimes lead to a false diagnosis of significant heart disease.

The satisfactory results of valve surgery have led to the practice of early surgery, before left ventricular function declines. Many mitral valves can be repaired nowadays, leading to a full functional drug-free recovery. Percutaneous balloon valvotomy is now the treatment of choice for pulmonary stenosis in rheumatic mitral stenosis and children. Transcutaneous aortic valve replacement is possible although it is generally reserved for elderly patients deemed at too high risk for surgery. Finally, younger patients may require emergency valve replacement surgery having developed endocarditis.

Following replacement of the aortic or mitral valves by mechanical or biological prostheses, patients generally recover rapidly and resume work fully 2–3 months after surgery. Those with mechanical valves need to take anticoagulants indefinitely and are therefore at a slightly increased risk of bleeding, with serious events occurring at a rate of about 2% per annum. Biological valves undergo slow deterioration, can fail suddenly some years after implantation, and are rarely used in people of working age. However, in specific roles such as fire fighters, their use may be considered to avoid the need for ongoing anticoagulants.

Congenital heart disease

About 9 in 1000 babies are born with a congenital heart defect.[23] Over the last 70 years there have been spectacular advances in the surgical treatment of these patients. The majority now survive until adulthood even with the most serious conditions.[24]

Congenital heart disease is classified as simple, moderate, or complex (Table 26.5). Most patients with simple or moderate disease will function at a normal or near normal level (NHYA class I), lead a normal life, and are capable of full-time employment.[25] They usually require only intermittent clinical review. Some of these patients will function at a high level for the majority of the time with occasional periods of ill health reflecting deterioration in their cardiac conduction. This can often be treated by intervention, either surgical or percutaneous, following which their functional levels may return to near normal. In contrast, patients with more severe congenital disease still have a significantly reduced life expectancy. They usually have impaired functional status (NYHA class >I) with ongoing decline throughout their early to mid-adult years. Many will die while still of working age. In 1986, the American Heart Association recommended that patients with adult congenital heart disease should not exceed light work (2.6–4.9 cal/min), but despite significant advances in the management of congenital heart disease since then no new guidelines have been produced.[26] The majority of patients (70%) with simple or moderate disease are in active employment.[25] Although more limited physically, a significant proportion of patients with complex disease are still able to work (>40%). All patients with moderate or severe congenital heart disease should be under regular follow-up

Table 26.5 Classification of congenital heart disease

Simple	Moderate	Complex
Native	Atrioventricular canal defects	Eisenmenger syndrome
Isolated congenital aortic or mitral valve disease	Coarctation of the aorta	Fontan procedure
Isolated PFO or ASD	Ebstein's anomaly	Double outlet ventricle
Mild pulmonic stenosis	Tetralogy of Fallot	Mitral or tricuspid atresia
Isolated small VSD	Patent ductus arteriosus or unrepaired sinus venosus ASD	Single ventricle
Repaired	VSD with other associated malformations	Pulmonary atresia
Repaired ductus arteriosus	Infundibular right ventricular outflow obstruction	Transposition of the great arteries (L or D type)
Repaired secundum or sinus venosus ASD	Pulmonary valve stenosis or regurgitation (moderate or severe)	
Repaired VSD	Subvalvular or supravalvular aortic stenosis	
	Aorto-left ventricular fistula	
	Anomalous pulmonary venous drainage	

ASD, atrial septal defect; PFO, patent foramen ovale; VSD, ventricular septal defect.

Source: data from Webb, G. and Williams, RG. 32nd Bethesda Conference: care of the adult with congenital heart disease. *Journal of the American College of Cardiology*. 37(5), 1161–98. Copyright © American College of Cardiology.

by a specialist in adult congenital heart disease who would be able to provide detailed information to occupational health services about an individual's functional status and limitations.

Cardiac arrhythmias

Transient cardiac arrhythmias (e.g. extrasystoles) are common and do not usually indicate heart disease. They may be provoked by alcohol and coffee. Assessment by a specialist is recommended if symptoms persist. A few individuals suffer recurrent arrhythmias. The commonest is AF, which affects 2% of the population and tends to be paroxysmal in individuals of working age. Drug treatment is sometimes required and individuals need to withdraw from work and rest for a short period. Many patients with AF are asymptomatic, particularly when it is persistent and it is only detected incidentally. AF may complicate CHD or valve disease; for those with no apparent underlying heart disease, research has shown that the focus for the arrhythmia lies in the sleeves of muscle that extend from the left atrium backwards into the pulmonary veins. This has led to the development of an increasingly popular and successful ablation technique known as pulmonary vein isolation which has a high chance of successfully treating the symptoms of particularly paroxysmal AF. AF is associated with an increased risk of stroke. Patients who have AF and an additional risk factor for stroke (congestive heart failure, hypertension, diabetes, age >65, previous stroke or embolic event, known ischaemic heart disease or peripheral vascular disease, or significant valvular heart disease) should be considered for anticoagulation. Patients with no additional risk factors do not require anticoagulation unless they are undergoing either an ablation or a cardioversion.

Ventricular arrhythmias are more problematic. Isolated ventricular extrasystoles in otherwise healthy hearts can be ignored. Patients with an otherwise normal heart may develop a very high ectopic burden or sustained runs of ventricular arrhythmia arising from the outflow tracts. This can usually be treated successfully with ablation or medication. The prognosis for individuals with ventricular arrhythmias depends on the underlying disease and ventricular function. Patients with poor underlying left ventricular function or a cardiomyopathy will usually require treatment with an implantable defibrillator with ablation reserved for treating ongoing symptoms.

Syncope

Syncope, other than a simple faint, requires specialist evaluation, which may include neurological as well as cardiovascular review. Following unexplained syncope, provocation testing and investigation for arrhythmia must be undertaken. If no major problem is found, return to work is recommended, including re-licensing for vocational drivers after 3 months (if the trigger can be avoided or it has been established the syncope was vasovagal). If the syncope is unexplained, vocational licences will be revoked for 12 months.[27] Careful follow-up is essential.

Increasingly, implantable loop recorders are being used to identify the cause for syncope. These small devices are implanted under the skin and continuously record the cardiac rhythm on a loop. They will automatically store evidence of dangerous rhythms, but can also be activated by patients when they have an attack. The devices can be remotely monitored. Strong electromagnetic fields may cause artefactual recordings or potentially delete the stored electrograms but are unlikely to present any significant risk to the patient.

Pacemakers and implantable devices

Pacemakers

The presence of an implanted cardiac pacemaker to maintain regular heart action is entirely compatible with normal life, including strenuous work. The underlying heart condition for which the pacemaker was implanted may, however, impose its own restrictions.

The indications for cardiac pacing have broadened, given the sophistication of modern pacemaker technology which allows pacing of atria and ventricles, variation in the output of the generator, and facilities for telemetry.

Virtually all pacemakers have the capacity to sense and can be inhibited by the patient's own heart rhythm. Somatic muscle action potentials and electromagnetic fields can in theory interfere with the pacemaker, causing temporary cessation of pacing. Usually the interference will be brief and the pacemaker will revert to a fixed-rate mode so that symptoms will be minimal although there is a small risk of this provoking ventricular arrhythmia.

Biventricular pacing (cardiac resynchronization therapy) involves the insertion of leads into both ventricles. This can be extremely helpful in patients with refractory heart failure and a dyssynchronous cardiac contraction which usually manifests as a prolonged QRS complex. Generally the severity of the underlying heart failure precludes work.

Implantable cardioverter defibrillators

The implantable cardioverter defibrillator (ICD) is now the preferred treatment for individuals with haemodynamically significant ventricular tachycardia and/or fibrillation whose arrhythmia is refractory to drugs or myocardial revascularization; the ICD device often has cardiac resynchronization therapy capacity.

ICDs are implanted in two groups of patients. Secondary prevention devices are implanted in patients who have already suffered a significant ventricular arrhythmia or who have been resuscitated from ventricular tachycardia. Usually, although not always, these patients have evidence of significant underlying cardiac disease. Primary prevention ICDs are implanted in patients with a high risk of sudden cardiac death. The majority have ischaemic cardiomyopathy with impaired left ventricular function. Primary prevention ICDs are also implanted in patients with impaired left ventricular function for other reasons and in patients with inherited cardiomyopathies such as Brugada syndrome, hypertrophic cardiomyopathy, and arrhythmogenic right ventricular dysplasia. The majority of patients with inherited cardiomyopathies do not require ICDs.

The ICD is implanted by a cardiologist under local anaesthetic. Both ventricular tachycardia and ventricular fibrillation can be detected and treated, the former by antitachycardia pacing and the latter by a DC shock. In either event, transient impairment of consciousness is possible, so jobs such as vocational driving are not permitted. A shock from an ICD is very painful and patients can have significant long-term psychological symptoms following a shock particularly when they have received multiple shocks as a result of a ventricular tachycardia storm or device failure.

Working following implantation of a cardiac device

Most cardiac devices are implanted in a left pre-pectoral position. Occasionally they will be implanted on the right-hand side, usually because of difficulty accessing the heart from the left, but occasionally because of patient preference. Following implantation of a pacemaker, patients should avoid lifting heavy objects with the arm on the side of the pacemaker or ICD and avoid lifting this arm above the shoulder for 1 month. Usually they will have their device checked in outpatients at this point after which, if all is well, they can resume normal activities. Patients implanted with a standard or biventricular pacemaker usually have a significant improvement in symptoms following implantation with increased exercise tolerance or reduced syncopal episodes, depending on the reason for implantation. Implantation of an ICD usually does not result in any improvement in function and can be associated with a significant psychological impact.

Electromagnetic fields and implantable devices

Electromagnetic field is the term to describe the combination of electric and magnetic fields. Electromagnetic interference can occur due to conducted or radiated electromagnetic energy.[28] Industrial electrical sources such as arc welding, faulty domestic equipment, engines, antitheft devices, airport weapon detectors, radar, and citizen-band radio, all generate electromagnetic fields that can, in theory, affect pacemakers and ICDs. Any pacemaker abnormality is usually confined to one or two missed beats or reversion to the fixed mode. ICD discharges are equally rare.

However, both pacemakers and ICDs have been designed to have a high degree of tolerance to electrical and magnetic interference fields, and special filtering components have been incorporated to minimize the effects.

If pacemaker patients are expected to work in the vicinity of high-energy electromagnetic fields capable of producing signals at a rate and pattern similar to a QRS complex (e.g. on some electrical generating and transmission equipment and welding) then formal testing is recommended. The employee's responsible cardiac centre will usually provide a technical service for this purpose, enabling the risk of interference to be defined precisely. The cardiac physiology department at the implanting centre will also be able to give specific advice depending on the exact types of device and lead used and the patients underlying cardiac condition. Patients with implanted devices carry cards that identify the type of pacemaker and the supervising cardiac centre. Persons with implanted devices are generally advised to avoid work that may bring them into close contact with strong magnetic fields, which includes MRI machines in radiology departments. If patients experience untoward symptoms or collapse while near electrical apparatus then they should move or be moved away, but the likely cause of the symptoms will be unrelated to the device. There is little data on exactly what strength of electromagnetic field is likely to cause a problem. Data from Sweden suggests that overhead power cables, electronic commuter trains, and mobile phone base stations are highly unlikely to cause a problem for modern bipolar pacemakers.[29] Further evidence[30] suggests that electromagnetic fields within the limits of the 2004 European Guidelines on occupational exposure (electric field <10 kV/m, magnetic field <0.5 mt) do not cause any problems to a modern ICD programmed to nominal settings.[31] In contrast, higher strength fields falling within the 2002 American National Standards Institute occupational recommendations (electric field 20 kv/m, magnetic field 1 mt) may cause problems.[32]

There has been interest in the possibility that mobile telephones might interfere with pacemakers and ICDs. A review article in 2013 identified studies that showed minimal or clinically insignificant interference with mobile phones and implantable cardiac devices.[28] In practice, no clinically significant interference has yet been reported, but individuals are advised to use the hand and ear furthest from the pacemaker, not to dial with the telephone near to the pacemaker, and not to keep the phone in a pocket near the device.

Hypertension

Hypertension affects over 25% of the UK adult population and prevalence increases with age.[33] Hypertension can be defined into stages (Box 26.1).

Treatment is initiated at stage 1 if there is evidence of target organ damage, established CVD, renal disease, diabetes, or a 10-year cardiovascular risk equivalent to 20% or greater. Treatment is offered to all patients with stage 2 hypertension. Hypertension can also be classified into two types: primary, which is not associated with a definite cause; and secondary hypertension, which is due to other diseases (e.g. endocrine and renal disease) and could be a cause of resistant hypertension (Box 26.1).

Box 26.1 Hypertension

- Stage 1: BP 140/90 mmHg or greater and subsequent ambulatory BP monitoring (ABPM) daytime average or home BP monitoring (HBPM) average BP 135/85 mmHg or greater.
- Stage 2: clinic BP 160/100 mmHg or greater and subsequent ABPM daytime average or HBPM average 150/95 mmHg or greater.
- Severe hypertension: clinic systolic BP 180 mmHg or greater, or clinic diastolic BP 110 mmHg or greater.

There are few contraindications to employment in the hypertensive person. Side effects of antihypertensives could potentially lead to hypotension with resultant giddiness and fatigue. Furthermore, hypotension can affect judgement and the performance of skilled tasks.

Patients with controlled hypertension can expect to manage most work. Occasionally, frequent postural changes prove troublesome, due to altered central and peripheral vascular responses. Very heavy physical work and exposure to very hot conditions with high humidity may result in postural hypotension. Group 2 vehicle driving is allowed provided that the BP is under satisfactory control. However, drivers must not drive if systolic BP is 180 mmHg or greater, or diastolic BP is 100 mmHg or greater. The licence can be reinstated as long as the BP is controlled and there are no side effects from the medication that may affect safe driving.[27]

The presence of resistant hypertension may be first noted as part of health surveillance or on routine medical examination (Box 26.2). This needs communicating to the primary care provider.

Those with hypertensive crisis (which is defined as a systolic BP ≥180 or diastolic BP ≥110 mmHg) are not fit to work and should not be considered so until the underlying cause has been treated and BP is controlled. Untreated hypertensive crisis can lead to

Box 26.2 Causes of resistant hypertension

- Poor adherence to therapeutic plan/non-compliance with medication.
- Failure to modify lifestyle—weight gain or alcohol misuse (especially binge drinking).
- Continued use of pharmacological substances and toxins: alcohol, liquorice, ginseng, cocaine, steroids, non-steroidal anti-inflammatory drugs, oral contraceptive pill, amphetamines, ciclosporin, tacrolimus, erythropoietin, or decongestants containing ephedrine
- Unsuspected secondary causes: renal—systemic sclerosis, glomerulonephritis, polycystic kidney disease, or renovascular disease; endocrine—Cushing's syndrome, Conn's syndrome, acromegaly, hyperparathyroidism, phaeochromocytoma, or thyroid disease; coarctation of aorta; obstructive sleep apnoea.
- Irreversible end organ damage (e.g. renal).
- Volume overload due to inadequate diuretic therapy.
- Progressive renal insufficiency.
- High sodium intake.
- 'Spurious' resistant hypertension—inappropriate cuff size.
- 'White coat' hypertension.

encephalopathy, left ventricular failure, MI, unstable angina, or dissection of the aorta. Rare causes of crisis include phaeochromocytoma, severe preeclampsia/eclampsia, and severe hypertension associated with subarachnoid haemorrhage or cerebrovascular accident. Hypertensive emergencies can also be associated with recreational drugs.

Lifestyle factors have been indicated in the management of hypertension such as weight reduction, smoking cessation, diet, alcohol, and salt restriction.[8] The association of hypertension and stress has also been explored but has not been identified as a lifestyle factor by the European Arterial Hypertension Guidelines.[34] Previous studies however, have suggested that BP fluctuations due to psychological stress contribute to developing hypertension in later life.[35] The relationship between stress and CVD is well established[36] and interventions to manage occupational psychological stress could potentially contribute to reducing the risk of CVD in employees (see 'Work stress').

Special work issues

Physical activity

As a general rule, activities that cause no symptoms can be undertaken safely. Careful history taking will identify what activities are possible, initially by eliciting activities of daily living then matching these with equivalent work activities (Table 26.4). A useful model to quantify what individual workers are capable of in terms of physical activity is that of METs. This can also be compared with the results of exercise testing in that stage 1 of the Bruce protocol approximates to 4.6 METs, stage 2 is 7.0 METs, stage 3 is 10.1 METs, and stage 4 is 12.9 METs. Jobs that may require extreme physical effort, for example, those in the emergency services, may be unsuitable for workers with CHD. Each case must be judged on its individual merits, however, and specialist advice taken as required (Box 26.3).

Firefighters and sudden cardiac death

Firefighting is a physically demanding occupation. Sudden cardiac death is the leading cause of death in firefighters while operational or on the training ground, with 45% of causes due to heart disease.[37,38] The risk of CHD events occurring is highest during emergency call outs and the increased cardiovascular demand of fire suppression as well as factors such as poor physical fitness, underlying cardiovascular factors, raised BMI, and low level of fitness increases the risk of CHD events.[38,39] Other studies have found that sudden cardiac death in firefighters less than 45 years of age were primarily due to lifestyle factors such as obesity, smoking, hypertension, and previous history of CHD. Furthermore, fire fighters may be exposed to chemical hazards (carbon monoxide, fine particulate matter, and other cardiac toxins), which may increase the risk of sudden MIs.[40]

Lifting weights

Only the very fit might reasonably attempt heavy work, when defined as lifting 23–45 kg (40–100 lb). Many employees quite comfortably manage medium work, such as lifting 11–23 kg (25–50 lb) at the rate of once a minute, providing they do not have other physical limitations. If weights are supported or kept at waist height, the effort is considerably

Box 26.3 Some metabolic equivalents

1–2 METs

- Doing seated activities of daily living (ADLs) (eating, performing facial hygiene, resting).
- Doing seated recreation (sewing, playing cards, painting).
- Doing seated occupational activities (writing, typing, doing clerical work).

2–3 METs

- Standing ADLs (dressing, showering, shaving, doing light housework).
- Standing occupation (mechanic, bartender, auto repair).
- Standing recreation (fishing, playing billiards, shuffleboard).
- Walking (2.5 mph).

4–5 METs

- Doing heavy housework (scrubbing floor, hanging out washing).
- Canoeing, golfing, playing softball, tennis (doubles).
- Social dancing, cross country hiking.
- Swimming (20 yards/min).
- Walking 4 mph (level), 3 mph (5% gradient).
- Bike ride 10 mph.

6–7 METs

- Heavy gardening (digging, manual lawn mowing, hoeing)
- Skating, water skiing, playing tennis (singles)
- Stair climbing (<27 feet/min)
- Swimming (25 yards/min)
- Jogging 5 mph (level), 3.5 mph (5% gradient)

8–9 METs

- Active occupation (sawing wood, digging ditches, shovelling snow).
- Active recreation (downhill skiing, playing ice hockey, paddleball).
- Bike riding (12–14 mph).
- Stair climbing (more than 27 feet/min).
- Swimming 35 yards/min.
- Running 10 mph (level), 3 mph (15% gradient).

reduced, and if the task only requires them to be slid along benches or roller tracks, then the effective strain will be reduced by some 50%. Those with continuing symptoms as defined by NYHA class II or CCS class III may need more specific assessment including exercise testing to confirm fitness for the proposed roles. Symptoms will help define capability.

Driving

The DVLA provides readily accessible guidance on fitness to drive. These are regularly updated for both group 1 and group 2 licences and can be readily accessed on the DVLA website online.[27] Drivers with group 2 licences should notify the DVLA if they develop any CVD or have undertaken any CVD-related procedures. Guidance can also be sought from the DVLA directly for complex cases. The DVLA guidelines are regularly updated and it is important to ensure that guidelines are checked before advising for both group 1 and group 2 licences.

Work stress

There is considerable evidence to support the role of job strain (a combination of high work demands and low job control) as a risk factor for CHD.[41–43] Previous research suggests an average 50% excess cardiovascular risk among employees with work stress[17] and job strain causes a 1.8 times higher age-adjusted risk of incident ischaemic heart disease (particularly in younger male populations between 19–55 years of age).[44] Where an individual reports the feeling of being dealt with unfairly at work, recent research suggests that this is an independent risk factor for increased coronary events and impaired health.[44] Furthermore, organizational downsizing has been associated with increased CHD risk.[45]

The presence of work stress cannot be completely removed but utilization of the Health and Safety Executive 'Stress Management Standards' for work-related stress is a helpful tool to address such issues objectively and consider risk minimization strategies.[46] In most individuals, the presence of stress will not prevent return to work after a cardiovascular event. However, risk reduction strategies in relation to the source of stress are likely to make a return to work more successful and help the individual adopt lifestyle strategies to prevent recurrence of the underlying cardiac problem, thereby maintaining attendance and performance at work.

The INTERHEART case–control study included 11,119 cases from 52 different countries and examined the link between psychosocial risk factors and risk of acute MI.[47] Stress at home or at work and the incidence of major life events in the preceding year showed a significant correlation with the risk of MI. A third more cases experienced several periods of work stress than controls (odds ratio (OR) 1.38; 99% confidence interval (CI) 1.19–1.61), while the exposure OR for permanent work stress was doubled (OR 2.14; 99% CI 1.73–2.64). The population attributable risk (i.e. the proportion of all cases in the population attributable to the relevant risk factor if causality were proven) was calculated as 9% for both stress at work and depression, 11% for financial stress, and 16% for low locus of control. A caveat is that exposures were self-reported in retrospect, with the potential that cases may have relatively over-reported exposures widely supposed to aggravate heart disease. A meta-analysis of 197,473 participants also confirmed the association between job strain and CHD events (hazard ratio 1.23; 95% CI 1.10–1.37).[42] Although managing workplace stress could potentially decrease the risk of CHD, it is important to consider other factors that may also contribute to CHD besides job strain. Other studies have found non-occupational stress may also contribute to CHD risk, such as bereavement of a child or caring for a sick spouse.[48,49]

Shift work

Nearly 20% of the working population in the UK engages in shift work.[50] In addition, there is a growing number of workers with more than one job. Shift work may affect the cardiovascular system through the desynchronization of cardiovascular rhythms due to altered sleep patterns, which predisposes to heart disease by provoking hypertension, dyslipidaemia, insulin resistance, and obesity.[51] Shift working may thus confer a risk of CVD, but assessment of this is complicated because shift workers tend to differ from non-shift workers in their general risk profile for CVD (e.g. smoking habits, diet, weight, alcohol intake, and uptake of preventive medical services), therefore potentially confounding study results. There may also be issues surrounding selection bias and the difference in defining shift work within the studies.[52] Although shift work has been found to be associated with an increased risk of CVD in employees, the observational studies on shift work research cannot definitely prove causality.[53,54] A substantial body of studies in different countries using different methodologies suggest that risks of CVD in shift workers, if increased, are elevated only slightly.[51,55] Further research is required to confirm shift work as a causative factor for CHD, to identify vulnerable groups as well as shift modifying strategies,[53] before informing policy and guidance regarding CHD risk and shift work.

Most observational studies on shift work focus on new cases of CVD and few have included past CHD as a variable.[56] Those that have included past CHD as a variable have removed these cases from analyses,[57] have looked at specific sexes,[57,58] or explored a specific shift pattern.[59]

Shift work can also involve working beyond the 40-hour working week and a recent systematic and meta-analysis on overtime and CVD has found a 40% excess risk of CVD in those who work overtime.[60]

Shift work may need to be restricted on the basis of specific clinical features such as severe night/early morning chest pain in an otherwise stable clinical situation, but this is advice to minimize continuing symptoms and not to prevent recurrence. The potential effects of shift work can be counteracted through health promotion and education for shift workers from the occupational health team to look at risk minimization strategies and early identification of reversible risk factors, in particular the metabolic syndrome, hypertension, and dyslipidaemia.

Hazardous substances

Work involving exposure to certain hazardous substances may aggravate pre-existing CHD and careful consideration should be given to patients who are returning to work involving exposure to chemical, gases, and pollutants. Methylene chloride, an ingredient of many commonly used paint removers, is rapidly metabolized to carbon monoxide in the body; in poorly ventilated areas, blood levels of carboxyhaemoglobin can become high enough to precipitate angina or even MI (impairment of cardiovascular function begins at a blood carboxyhaemoglobin level of 2–4%). Careful assessment taking account of the total exposure to carbon monoxide (active/passive smoking, air pollutants/chemicals) and correlation against symptoms of chest pain will allow a pragmatic approach to risk assessment in these rare cases.

Smokers, especially pipe smokers, will have an elevated blood carboxyhaemoglobin, which is additive to carbon monoxide in the workplace, potentially increasing their risk of adverse cardiac events.

The World Health Organization (WHO) recommends a maximum carboxyhaemoglobin level of 5% for healthy industrial workers and a maximum of 2.5% for susceptible persons in the general population exposed to ambient air pollution.[61] This level may also be applied to workers whose jobs entail exposure to carbon monoxide (e.g. car park attendants and furnace workers). There is a good correlation between carbon monoxide levels in air and blood carboxyhaemoglobin levels, in accordance with the Coburn equation. To ensure that the 2.5% carboxyhaemoglobin level is not exceeded, the ambient carbon monoxide concentration should not be higher than 10 ppm over an 8-hour working day—equivalent to exposure at 50 ppm for no more than 30 minutes. Occupational exposure to carbon disulphide in the viscose rayon manufacturing industry is a recognized causal factor of CHD but the mechanism remains unclear.

Solvents, such as trichloroethylene or 1,1,1-trichloroethane, may sensitize the myocardium to the action of endogenous catecholamines resulting in ventricular fibrillation and sudden death in workers with high exposure.[62] Chlorofluorocarbons (CFCs) have been used as propellants in aerosol cans and as refrigerants. CFC-113 has been implicated in sudden cardiac deaths and CFC-22 has been reported to cause arrhythmias in laboratory workers using aerosols. Where an individual has poorly controlled arrhythmia and is awaiting more definitive treatment such as ablation therapy, exclusion from work where there is known exposure to solvents/CFCs may be appropriate.

There are no formal medical standards for workers who have to enter confined spaces where there may be hazards of oxygen deficiency or a build-up of toxic gases. However, workers with heart disease or severe hypertension may need to be excluded. Certain occupations may require the use of special breathing apparatus either routinely (e.g. asbestos removal workers), or in emergencies (e.g. water workers handling chlorine cylinders). The additional cardiorespiratory effort required while wearing a respirator, combined with the general physical exertion that may be required, should be factored in to any risk assessment undertaken and may require specialized input from the treating cardiologist to confirm exercise capability appropriate to the demands of the role.

Hot conditions

The law does not state a minimum or maximum working temperature; however, the temperature in workrooms should be at least 16°C or 13°C if rigorous physical effort is involved.[63] Work in hot conditions may prove difficult for some patients with heart disease. High ambient temperatures or significant heat radiation from hot surfaces or liquid metal, added to the physical strain of heavy work, will produce profound vaso-dilatation of muscle and skin vessels. Work environments such as bakeries, mines, foundries, compressed air tunnels, and smelting may expose employees to high temperatures. Compensatory vascular and cardiac reactions to maintain central BP may be inadequate and lead to reduced cerebral or coronary artery blood flow. The resulting weakness or giddiness could prove dangerous. As many cardioactive drugs have vaso-dilating and negative inotropic actions, some reduction in dosage may be necessary. Careful risk assessment will be required, taking account of the work conditions, the nature of the cardiac condition, how well it is managed, and the impact of medication side effects (Box 26.4).

The risk of cardiac ischaemia in employees with CHD seems to be related to the level of heat stress[64] and therefore the workplace should try and ensure the risk of heat stress to employees are minimized. The Health and Safety Executive recommends careful risk assessment to explore the work rate, working climate, and employee clothing as well as any protective equipment (Box 26.5).[65]

Travel

Following a cardiac event, individuals should convalesce at home and not travel. A specialist should then assess them at 4–6 weeks. Those with no evidence of continuing myocardial ischaemia or cardiac pump failure can then travel freely within the UK for pleasure. Business and overseas travel is more problematical because the physical and psychological demands are greater. Additional difficulties for the overseas traveller include the uncertain provision of coronary care facilities in some countries and the reluctance of insurance companies to provide health cover. Such travel is best deferred until

---

Box 26.4 Potential measures to reduce the sources of heat

1. Controlling the temperature.
2. Providing mechanical aids to reduce work rate.
3. Preventing dehydration.
4. Providing suitable protective equipment.
5. Providing training.
6. Identifying staff who are fit and who are at risk (e.g. those with CHD).
7. Monitor health of workers at risk.

Box 26.5 Cold conditions

Cold is a notorious trigger of myocardial ischaemia and caution must therefore be exercised in placing individuals with CHD in cold working environments. Impaired circulation to the limbs will result in an increased risk of claudication, risk of damage to skin (frostbite), and poor recovery from accidental injury to skin and deeper structures. Clear work procedures that include short periods spent in the cold, provision of appropriate cold weather clothing and regular hot drinks, coupled with clear safety guidelines may reduce risk sufficiently to allow the individual to continue working in those conditions.

3 months have elapsed and any necessary further investigations and treatment have been carried out to ensure cardiovascular fitness.

Overseas travel for those with continuing cardiovascular symptoms need not be ruled out. Clear guidelines exist regarding fitness to fly for commercial travellers (Table 26.6). Airport services for disabled travellers can ease the journey and modern aircraft can be very comfortable. The cabins are kept at a pressure equivalent to 6000 feet (2000 m) so that those with angina are not likely to experience symptoms; most developed countries have an excellent coronary care service. Business people with continuing cardiac disorders may therefore fly to Europe and North America with very little risk. Flights in unpressurized aircraft, work in undeveloped countries or in remote areas of the world, and work in a hostile environment (both climatic and political) is best avoided. Aircrew are subject to European Aviation Safety Agency Medical Standards and advice should always be sought from the Civil Aviation Authority (see Chapter 15). Continuing medication is key for individuals with cardiac conditions. The traveller should ensure access to their medications for the whole of their trip.

Cardiac deaths are uncommon in trekkers or workers at high altitude (8000–15,000 feet/2440–4570 m). The increase in cardiac output at altitude will exacerbate symptoms in those who already experience symptoms at sea level, but asymptomatic individuals with CHD are unlikely to be at special risk.

Although evidence is minimal, ICD follow-up has shown electrical resets of ICDs during air travel.[67] The reset can trigger an audible alert to the patient but effects are unlikely to affect the functioning of the ICD. A sensible approach is to warn the patient with an ICD of the possible effects of cosmic radiation on the device but to reassure them that it is unlikely to affect the ability of the device to detect and treat life-threatening arrhythmias.

Vibration can affect pacemakers and ICDs (used to match pacing rate to activity levels). In fixed-wing aircraft, this is not problematic but in helicopters, vibration levels are high throughout the flight and sustained raised levels of pacing rates are seen, which may cause problems for some individuals. Specific advice from the pacemaker clinic may be needed where helicopter travel is required.

Table 26.6 Fitness to fly for passengers with cardiovascular disease

Condition	Functional status	Restriction/guidance
Angina	CCS angina I–II	No restriction
	CCS angina III	Consider airport assistance and possible in-flight oxygen
	CCS angina IV	Defer travel until stable or travel with medical escort and in-flight oxygen available Unstable angina is a contraindication
Post-STEMI and NSTEMI	Uncomplicated MI	Fly after 7 to 10 days
	Complicated MI	Consider delaying travel for at least 4 to 6 week and until condition is stable.
Elective PCI uncomplicated		Fly after 3 days but individual risk assessment is essential
Elective CABG uncomplicated	Allow for intrathoracic gas resorption. If complicated or symptomatic, *see* Heart failure	Fly after 10–14 days if no complications. If symptomatic, follow guidance for specific symptoms
Acute heart failure		Fly after 6 weeks if stabilized (*see* Chronic heart failure)
Chronic heart failure	NYHA I and II	No restrictions
	NYHA III	May require in-flight oxygen
	NYHA IV	Advised not to fly without in-flight oxygen and medical assistance
	Severe symptomatic valvular diseases and decompensated congestive heart failure	Contraindicated
Cyanotic congenital heart disease	NYHA I and II	May require in-flight oxygen[a]
	NYHA III	Consider airport assistance and may require in-flight oxygen advisable[a]
	NYHA IV	Advised not to fly without in-flight oxygen and airport assistance available[a]
Valve disease (*see* Heart failure)		
Following pacemaker implantation		once medically stable
Following ICD implantation		The same advice as for pacemakers but, in addition, rhythm instability should be treated
Arrhythmia	Stable	No restrictions
	Uncontrolled arrhythmia	

(continued)

Condition	Functional status	Restriction/guidance
Ablation therapy		Fly after 2 days[a]
Hypertension	Controlled hypertension	No restrictions
	Uncontrolled hypertension	Contraindicated

[a] Consider at high risk of deep vein thrombosis.

Source: data from Smith, D. et al. on behalf of the British Cardiovascular Society. Fitness To Fly For Passengers With Cardiovascular Disease. *Heart* 2010: 96, 1–16. Copyright © British Cardiovascular Society.

Anticoagulation in the workplace

Workers requiring long-term anticoagulation may need careful risk assessment in terms of potential injuries at work and also access to regular monitoring to ensure adequate anticoagulation. Multiple anticoagulants exist on the market such as warfarin and direct oral anticoagulants (DOAC) (e.g. dabigatran, rivaroxaban, and apixaban). The intracranial bleeding risk with DOACs has been found to be lower than warfarin and they do not require frequent coagulation monitoring.[68] Common uses for anticoagulation include AF, deep vein thrombosis, pulmonary embolism, valvular heart disease, and thrombotic disorders. In certain occupations (e.g. firefighting), use of anticoagulants may be considered a contraindication to operational roles. Nearly 1% of contraindications for anticoagulation were due to occupational risks; however, the authors did not specify the types of occupational risks within their study.[69] Bleeding risk increases during the initial phase of warfarin treatment and during inter-current illnesses that may affect warfarin intake absorption or metabolism, such as diarrhoea, fever, heart failure, and liver failure, which are known risk factors for bleeding.[70] Other considerations need to be taken into account such as risk of trauma, alcohol intake, previous CVD and gastrointestinal disorders, age, history of bleeding, and polypharmacy.[71]

Anticoagulation near-patient testing and self-monitoring is increasing in use, particularly for the person at work. In cases of warfarin-related bleeding, management depends on the value of the international normalized ratio. Those with serious or life-threatening bleeding require rapid full reversal of warfarin effect with vitamin K or four-factor prothrombin complex concentrate in a secondary care setting, whereas those with minor bleeding may benefit from intravenous vitamin K.[72]

DOACs do not require as regular monitoring and have fewer restrictions on lifestyle such as alcohol intake; however, only dabigatran has a reversal agent if bleeding occurs. Doses are adjusted according to renal function. Serious bleeding requires admission for investigations and treatment such as transfusion prothrombin complex concentrate and antifibrinolytic therapy such as tranexamic acid. Those with minor bleeding may also benefit from admission if bleeding cannot be controlled with simple measures.[73]

Combining clinical assessment alongside individual risk assessments of the workplace and of the individual's job role will help identify any hazards and identify any adjustments that are required. Those in heavy physical roles, or work associated with injury (e.g. sharp equipment, working at height, confined spaces, and safety-critical roles) may need work adjustments, personal protective equipment, or reassignment of job roles if they are anticoagulated and at risk of bleeding. Employees working with moving machinery and sharps should be provided with training to ensure they have the correct skills, knowledge, and experiences, as well as supervision and appropriate safety equipment. Furthermore, safety guards alongside jigs, holders, and push sticks can be used to prevent access to dangerous parts. Machinery maintenance, good record-keeping, and regular risk assessments can reduce the risk.

The Health and Safety (First-Aid) Regulations 1981 require employers to provide adequate and appropriate first-aid equipment and facilities, making sure that employees receive immediate attention if they are taken ill.

The Equality Act 2010

The Equality Act 2010 will apply to many cardiovascular conditions. Some useful pointers include conditions where activities of daily living are unlikely to be affected. These include angina which is defined as CCS class I or II, heart failure defined as NYHA class I or II, cardiac arrhythmias with minimal impact, and conditions that relate to incidental findings or investigations, for example, ECG or ultrasound scan findings that do not translate into current symptoms. Importantly, assessment of whether an individual is legally disabled should be done after discounting the benefit of any treatment they are receiving or have received (including angioplasty or surgery).

Key points

- CVDs are one of the most common causes of morbidity and mortality in the UK.
- Multiple considerations should be taken into account when assessing return to work, including psychosocial factors.
- Cardiac risk factors should be addressed as part of the return-to-work assessment in those with cardiac disease.
- There is strict guidance regarding flying and driving and guidelines should be reviewed for updates.
- There is little data on exactly what strength of electromagnetic field is likely to cause a problem; however, persons with implanted devices are generally advised to avoid work that may bring them into close contact with strong magnetic fields, which includes MRI machines in radiology departments.

References

1. **Bhatnagar P, Wickramasinghe K, Wilkins E, Townsend N.** Trends in the epidemiology of cardiovascular disease in the UK. *Heart* 2016;**102**:1945–52.
2. **Rugulies R.** Depression as a predictor for coronary heart disease. A review and meta-analysis. *Am J Prev Med* 2002;**23**:51–61.

3. **British Heart Foundation**. Cardiovascular disease statistics. 2018. Available at: https://www.bhf.org.uk/what-we-do/our-research/heart-statistics/heart-statistics-publications/cardiovascular-disease-statistics-2018.

4. **Health and Safety Executive**. LFS - Labour Force Survey - Self-reported work-related ill health and workplace injuries: index of LFS tables. Available at: http://www.hse.gov.uk/statistics/lfs/index.htm.

5. **European Heart Network**. European Cardiovascular Disease Statistics. 2017. Available at: http://www.ehnheart.org/component/downloads/downloads/2452.

6. **Minicucci MF, Azevedo PS, Polegato BF, Paiva SA, Zornoff LA**. Heart failure after myocardial infarction: clinical implications and treatment. *Clin Cardiol* 2011;**34**:410–4.

7. **Ponikowski P, Voors AA, Anker SD, et al.** 2016 ESC Guidelines for the diagnosis and treatment of acute and chronic heart failure: The Task Force for the diagnosis and treatment of acute and chronic heart failure of the European Society of Cardiology (ESC). Developed with the special contribution of the Heart Failure Association (HFA) of the ESC. *Eur J Heart Fail* 2016;**18**:891–975.

8. **Task Force Members, Montalescot G, Sechtem U, et al.** ESC guidelines on the management of stable coronary artery disease: the Task Force on the management of stable coronary artery disease of the European Society of Cardiology. *Eur Heart J* 2013;**34**:2949–3003.

9. **Myerburg RJ, Junttila MJ.** Sudden cardiac death caused by coronary heart disease. *Circulation* 2012;**125**:1043–52.

10. **Khot UN, Khot MB, Bajzer CT, et al.** Prevalence of conventional risk factors in patients with coronary heart disease. *JAMA* 2003;**290**:898–904.

11. **National Institute for Health and Care Excellence**. Cardiovascular disease: risk assessment and reduction, including lipid modification. Clinical guideline [CG181]. 2014. Available at: https://www.nice.org.uk/guidance/cg181/chapter/1-Recommendations#identifying-and-assessing-cardiovascular-disease-cvd-risk-2.

12. **QRISK®**. QRISK®2-2017 risk calculator. Available at: https://www.qrisk.org/2017/.

13. **Maznyczka AM, Howard JP, Banning AS, Gershlick AH.** A propensity matched comparison of return to work and quality of life after stenting or coronary artery bypass surgery. *Open Heart* 2016;**3**:e000322.

14. **Bhattacharyya MR, Perkins-Porras L, Whitehead DL, Steptoe A.** Psychological and clinical predictors of return to work after acute coronary syndrome. *Eur Heart J* 2007;**28**:160–5.

15. **Hemingway H, Vahtera J, Virtanen M, Pentti J, Kivimaki M.** Outcome of stable angina in a working population: the burden of sickness absence. *Eur J Cardiov Prev Rehabil* 2007;**14**:373–9.

16. **O'Neil A, Sanderson K, Oldenburg B.** Depression as a predictor of work resumption following myocardial infarction (MI): a review of recent research evidence. *Health Qual Life Outcomes* 2010;**8**:95.

17. **Anderson L, Oldridge N, Thompson DR, et al.** Exercise-based cardiac rehabilitation for coronary heart disease: Cochrane systematic review and meta-analysis. *J Am Coll Cardiol* 2016;**67**:1–12.

18. **Steenstra I, Cullen K, Irvin E, Van Eerd D.** A systematic review of interventions to promote work participation in older workers. *J Safety Res* 2017;**60**:93–102.

19. **Watkins LL, Koch GG, Sherwood A, et al.** Association of anxiety and depression with all-cause mortality in individuals with coronary heart disease. *J Am Heart Assoc* 2013;**2**:e000068.

20. **Hemingway H, Marmot M.** Clinical evidence: psychosocial factors in the etiology and prognosis of coronary heart disease: systematic review of prospective cohort studies. *West J Med* 1999;**171**:342–50.

21. **Palacios JE, Khondoker M, Achilla E, Tylee A, Hotopf M.** A single, one-off measure of depression and anxiety predicts future symptoms, higher healthcare costs, and lower quality of life in coronary heart disease patients: analysis from a multi-wave, primary care cohort study. *PloS One* 2016;**11**e0158163.

22. **Richards SH, Anderson L, Jenkinson CE, et al.** Psychological interventions for coronary heart disease. *Cochrane Database Syst Rev* 2017;**4**:CD002902.

23. **van der Linde D, Konings EE, Slager MA, et al.** Birth prevalence of congenital heart disease worldwide: a systematic review and meta-analysis. *J Am Coll Cardiol* 2011;**58**:2241–7.

24. **Khairy P, Ionescu-Ittu R, Mackie AS, Abrahamowicz M, Pilote L, Marelli AJ.** Changing mortality in congenital heart disease. *J Am Coll Cardiol* 2010;**56**:1149–57.

25. **Karsenty C, Maury P, Blot-Souletie N, et al.** The medical history of adults with complex congenital heart disease affects their social development and professional activity. *Arch Cardiovasc Dis* 2015;**108**:589–97.

26. **Gutgesell HP, Gessner IH, Vetter VL, Yabek SM, Norton JB.** Recreational and occupational recommendations for young patients with heart disease. A Statement for Physicians by the Committee on Congenital Cardiac Defects of the Council on Cardiovascular Disease in the Young, American Heart Association. *Circulation* 1986;**74**:1195–8A.

27. **Driving and Vehicle Licensing Agency.** Cardiovascular disorders: assessing fitness to drive. Available at: https://www.gov.uk/guidance/cardiovascular-disorders-assessing-fitness-to-drive.

28. **Beinart R, Nazarian S.** Effects of external electrical and magnetic fields on pacemakers and defibrillators: from engineering principles to clinical practice. *Circulation* 2013;**128**:2799–809.

29. **Tiikkaja M, Aro AL, Alanko T, et al.** Testing of common electromagnetic environments for risk of interference with cardiac pacemaker function. *Saf Health Work* 2013;**4**:156–9.

30. **Napp A, Joosten S, Stunder D, et al.** Electromagnetic interference with implantable cardioverter-defibrillators at power frequency: an in vivo study. *Circulation* 2014;**129**:441–50.

31. **European Union.** Corrigendum to Directive 2004/40/EC of the European Parliament and of the Council of 29 April 2004 on the minimum health and safety requirements regarding the exposure of workers to the risks arising from physical agents (electromagnetic fields) (18th individual Directive within the meaning of Article 16(1) of Directive 89/391/EEC). *OJ* 2004;**184**:1–9.

32. **IEEE Standards association (IEEE-SA).** *IEEE Standard for Safety Levels with Respect to Human Exposure to Electromagnetic Fields 0-3k Hz.* New York: The Institute of Electrical and Electonics Engineers; 2002.

33. **Kennard L, O'Shaughnessy KM.** Treating hypertension in patients with medical comorbidities. *BMJ* 2016;**352**:i101.

34. **Mancia G, Fagard R, Narkiewicz K, et al.** 2013 ESH/ESC Guidelines for the management of arterial hypertension: the Task Force for the management of arterial hypertension of the European Society of Hypertension (ESH) and of the European Society of Cardiology (ESC). *J Hyperten* 2013;**31**:1281–357.

35. **Carroll D, Phillips AC, Der G, Hunt K, Benzeval M.** Blood pressure reactions to acute mental stress and future blood pressure status: data from the 12-year follow-up of the West of Scotland Study. *Psychosom Med* 2011;**73**:737–42.

36. **Cohen S, Janicki-Deverts D, Miller GE.** Psychological stress and disease. *JAMA* 2007;**298**:1685–7.

37. **Yang J, Teehan D, Farioli A, Baur DM, Smith D, Kales SN.** Sudden cardiac death among firefighters ≤45 years of age in the United States. *Am J Cardiol* 2013;**112**:1962–7.

38. **Kales SN, Soteriades ES, Christophi CA, Christiani DC.** Emergency duties and deaths from heart disease among firefighters in the United States. *N Engl J Med* 2007;**356**:1207–15.

39. **Rosenstock L, Olsen J.** Firefighting and death from cardiovascular causes. *N Engl J Med* 2007;**356**:1261–3.

40. **Burgess JL, Nanson CJ, Bolstad-Johnson DM, et al.** Adverse respiratory effects following overhaul in firefighters. *J Occup Environ Med* 2001;**43**:467–73.

41. **Kivimaki M, Virtanen M, Elovainio M, Kouvonen A, Vaananen A, Vahtera J.** Work stress in the etiology of coronary heart disease – a meta-analysis. *Scand J Work Environ Health* 2006;**32**:431–42.

42. **Kivimaki M, Nyberg ST, Batty GD, et al.** Job strain as a risk factor for coronary heart disease: a collaborative meta-analysis of individual participant data. *Lancet* 2012;**380**:1491–7.

43. **Theorell T, Jood K, Jarvholm LS, et al.** A systematic review of studies in the contributions of the work environment to ischaemic heart disease development. *Eur J Public Health* 2016;**26**:470–7.

44. **Kivimaki M, Theorell T, Westerlund H, Vahtera J, Alfredsson L.** Job strain and ischaemic disease: does the inclusion of older employees in the cohort dilute the association? The WOLF Stockholm Study. *J Epidemiol Community Health* 2008;**62**:372–4.

45. **Vahtera J, Kivimaki M, Pentti J, et al.** Organisational downsizing, sickness absence, and mortality: 10-town prospective cohort study. *BMJ* 2004;**328**:555.

46. **Health and Safety Executive.** What are the management standards for work-related stress? Available at: http://www.hse.gov.uk/stress/standards/.

47. **Rosengren A, Hawken S, Ounpuu S, et al.** Association of psychosocial risk factors with risk of acute myocardial infarction in 11119 cases and 13 648 controls from 52 countries (the INTERHEART study): case-control study. *Lancet* 2004;**364**:953–62.

48. **Li J, Hansen D, Mortensen PB, Olsen J.** Myocardial infarction in parents who lost a child: a nationwide prospective cohort study in Denmark. *Circulation* 2002;**106**:1634–9.

49. **Lee S, Colditz GA, Berkman LF, Kawachi I.** Caregiving and risk of coronary heart disease in US women: a prospective study. *Am J Prev Med* 2003;**24**:113–9.

50. **Health and Safety Executive.** Changes in shift work patterns over the last ten years (1999 to 2009). Available at: http://www.hse.gov.uk/research/rrpdf/rr887.pdf.

51. **The Industrial Injuries Advisory Council.** Position paper 25. The Association between shift working and (i) breast cancer and (ii) ischaemic heart disease. 2009. Available at: https://assets.publishing.service.gov.uk/government/uploads/system/uploads/attachment_data/file/328536/iiac-pp25.pdf.

52. **Stevens RG, Hansen J, Costa G, et al.** Considerations of circadian impact for defining 'shift work' in cancer studies: IARC Working Group Report. *Occup Environ Med* 2011;**68**:154–62.

53. **Vyas MV, Garg AX, Iansavichus AV, et al.** Shift work and vascular events: systematic review and meta-analysis. *BMJ* 2012,**345**:e4800.

54. **Frost P, Kolstad HA, Bonde JP.** Shift work and the risk of ischemic heart disease – a systematic review of the epidemiologic evidence. *Scand J Work Environ Health* 2009;**35**:163–79.

55. **Vetter C, Devore EE, Wegrzyn LR, et al.** Association between rotating night shift work and risk of coronary heart disease among women. *JAMA* 2016;**315**:1726–34.

56. **Huang KL, Su TP, Chen TJ, Chou YH, Bai YM.** Comorbidity of cardiovascular diseases with mood and anxiety disorder: a population based 4-year study. *Psychiatry Clin Neurosci* 2009;**63**:401–9.

57. **Kawachi I, Colditz GA, Stampfer MJ, et al.** Prospective study of shift work and risk of coronary heart disease in women. *Circulation* 1995;**92**:3178–82.

58. **Fujino Y, Iso H, Tamakoshi A, et al.** A prospective cohort study of shift work and risk of ischemic heart disease in Japanese male workers. *Am J Epidemiol* 2006;**164**:128–35.

59. **Wang A, Arah OA, Kauhanen J, Krause N.** Shift work and 20-year incidence of acute myocardial infarction: results from the Kuopio Ischemic Heart Disease Risk Factor Study. *Occup Environ Med* 2016;**73**:588–94.

60. **Virtanen M, Heikkila K, Jokela M, et al.** Long working hours and coronary heart disease: a systematic review and meta-analysis. *Am J Epidemiol* 2012;**176**:586–96.

61. **World Health Organization.** *Environmental Health Criteria 213: Carbon Monoxide.* 2nd edn. Geneva: World Health Organization; 2004.

62. **Boon NA.** Solvent abuse and the heart. *BMJ* 1987;**294**:722.

63. **Health and Safety Executive.** Workplace temperatures. 2017. Available at: https://www.gov.uk/workplace-temperatures.

64. **Price AE.** Heart disease and work. *Heart* 2004;**90**;1077–84.

65. **Health and Safety Executive.** Heat stress. 2017. Available at: http://www.hse.gov.uk/temperature/heatstress/index.htm.

66. **Smith D, Toff W, Joy M, et al.** Fitness to fly for passengers with cardiovascular disease. *Heart* 2010;**96**(Suppl 2):ii1–16.

67. **Bhakta D, Foreman LD.** Cosmic radiation: not science fiction, but clinical reality. *Heart Rhythm* 2008;**5**:1204–5.

68. **Sharma M, Cornelius VR, Patel JP, Davies JG, Molokhia M.** Efficacy and harms of direct oral anticoagulants in the elderly for stroke prevention in atrial fibrillation and secondary prevention of venous thromboembolism systematic review and meta-analysis. *Circulation* 2015;**132**:194–204.

69. **O'Brien EC, Holmes DN, Ansell JE, et al.** Physician practices regarding contraindications to oral anticoagulation in atrial fibrillation: findings from the Outcomes Registry for Better Informed Treatment of Atrial Fibrillation (ORBIT-AF) registry. *Am Heart J* 2014;**167**:601–9.

70. **Penning-van Beest FJA, van Meegen E, Rosendaal FR, Stricker BHC.** Characteristics of anticoagulant therapy and comorbidity related to overanticoagulation. *Thromb Haemostasis*2001;**86**:569–74.

71. **National Institute for Health and Care Excellence.** Anticoagulation – oral. Clinical Knowledge Summaries. 2016. Available at: https://cks.nice.org.uk/anticoagulation-oral.

72. **Keeling D, Baglin T, Tait C, et al.** Guidelines on oral anticoagulation with warfarin - fourth edition. *Brit J Haematol* 2011;**154**:311–24.

73. **Raval AN, Cigarroa JE, Chung MK, et al.** Management of patients on non-vitamin K antagonist oral anticoagulants in the acute care and periprocedural setting: a scientific statement from the American Heart Association. *Circulation* 2017;**135**:E604–E33.

Chapter 27

Respiratory disorders

Kaveh Asanati and Paul Cullinan

Introduction

Respiratory diseases commonly cause sickness absence, unemployment, medical attendance, illness, and handicap.[1] Collectively, in the UK, these disorders cause 19 million days/year of certified sickness absence in men and 9 million days/year in women (with substantial additional lost time from short term self-certified illness) and, among adults of working age, a general practitioner consultation rate of between 21 and 43 per 1000/year with more than 240,000 hospital admissions/year. Prescriptions for bronchodilator inhalers run at some 24 million/year, and mortality from respiratory disease causes an estimated loss of 164,000 working years by the age of 64 and an estimated annual production loss of £1.6 billion.

Respiratory diseases may be caused, and pre-existing disease may be exacerbated, by the occupational environment. More commonly, respiratory disease limits work capacity and the ability to undertake particular duties. Finally, individual respiratory fitness in 'safety-critical' jobs can have implications for work colleagues and the public. Within this broad picture, different clinical illnesses pose different problems. For example, acute respiratory illness commonly causes short-term sickness absence, whereas chronic respiratory diseases—in particular asthma and chronic obstructive pulmonary disease (COPD)—have a greater impact on long-term absence and work limitation. Occupational causes of respiratory disease represent a small proportion of the total burden, except in some specialized work settings where specific exposures give rise to particular disease excesses. Consequently, the common fitness decisions on placement, return to work, and rehabilitation more often involve non-occupational illnesses than occupational ones. By contrast, statutory programmes of health surveillance focus on specific occupational risks (e.g. exposure to silica) or specific occupational health (OH) outcomes (e.g. occupational asthma). In assessing the individual, it is important to remember that respiratory problems are often aggravated by other illnesses, particularly disorders of the cardiovascular and musculoskeletal systems and by obesity and low levels of general fitness.

Prevalence of respiratory disease

Table 27.1 displays estimates of the contemporary prevalence and incidence—at all ages—of the more common, chronic respiratory diseases.

Table 27.1 Estimated prevalence and incidence of the more common chronic respiratory diseases in the UK; all ages

	Asthma	Bronchiectasis	COPD	IPF	Lung cancer	Mesothelioma	OSA	Sarcoidosis
Estimated prevalence in 2013								
Overall	8,028,741	211,598	1,201,685	32,479	85,796	5419	201,411	107,824
Male	3,873,724	88,993	627,019	19,450	45,329	4255	152,074	52,514
Female	4,155,017	122,606	574,666	13,028	40,467	1164	49,337	55,310
New diagnoses in 2012								
Overall	160,090	19,177	114,219	7865	32,226	2319	18,998	4579
Male	75,378	8322	61,448	4968	17,168	1892	13,810	2175
Female	84,712	10,855	52,771	2897	15,058	427	5187	2404

COPD, chronic obstructive pulmonary disease; IPF, idiopathic pulmonary fibrosis; OSA, obstructive sleep apnoea.

Source: data from British Lung Foundation. *Lung Disease in the UK: big picture statistics.* Copyright © 2016 British Lung Foundation. Available at: https://statistics.blf.org.uk/lung-disease-uk-big-picture.

Methods of assessing respiratory disability

General considerations

OH professionals in the UK have responsibilities under the Health and Safety at Work etc. Act 1974 (to place people in safe employment) and the Equality Act 2010 (to ensure that disabled workers are not discriminated against unfairly on health grounds). The dual requirements of these Acts challenge OH professionals to weigh matters carefully. They need to consider the likely duration of respiratory illness and its prognosis; the weight of evidence for incapacity on the one hand and risk on the other; and the scope for reasonable accommodation by the employer.

When assessing fitness in patients with respiratory disease, OH professionals should consider the following:

◆ Many aspects of lung function can be measured objectively but, except at the lower extremes, a poor correlation exists between measurements and symptoms (general fitness and motivation may be more important).

◆ Assessment of workplace demands and risks quite often varies according to individual circumstances.

◆ Many respiratory conditions improve given sufficient time, appropriate treatment, proper environmental control, or work modification.

An employer's failure to control potentially modifiable respiratory hazards (dusts, fumes, etc.) may be construed not only as a failure of control (under Regulation 6 of the Control of Substances Hazardous to Health (COSHH) Regulations 1994), but a failure to make a reasonable accommodation under the Equality Act 2010.

Historically, some organizations and public services have applied predefined fitness standards; many others have conducted routine measures of respiratory function, and applied predetermined protocols and decision algorithms. However, the provisions of the Equality Act 2010 make it increasingly appropriate to tailor risk assessments to each individual's needs.

Measurements of lung function

Respiratory disease may produce impairment in lung function which, if severe enough, will impair the ability to perform some work tasks. Whether a given loss of lung function causes difficulty at work depends on the nature of the job and the presence or absence of coexisting disease. The duration, intensity, and pattern of work, the environmental conditions (e.g. temperature, humidity, dust and fume content, and sometimes altitude), and the attitude and personality of the individual all play a part. Pulmonary function testing is, therefore, only one component in the process of assessing fitness for work.

In an occupational setting, lung function tests are used routinely in one of two ways. First, as a single set of measurements performed at a point in time (typically the pre-placement assessment, or during or following illness) to assess lung function in relation to accepted norms; and second, as serial measurements over time, to detect adverse occupational effects at an early stage or monitor disease control or progression.

Standard lung function tests are conveniently classified into measurements of airway function, static lung volume, and gas exchange. Measurements of *airway function* (e.g. spirometry and peak expiratory flow (PEF)) should be routinely available in occupational healthcare, and can be augmented, under medical supervision, by trials of response to bronchodilator medication; the other tests, as well as measurements of bronchial responsiveness to inhaled histamine or similar, require specialist facilities, and are generally used in secondary care and research settings.

In the workplace setting, *spirometry* is performed by taking a maximal inspiration and then blowing as hard as possible into the spirometer until the lungs are empty. Modern spirometers produce a short list of measurements including: forced expiratory volume (FEV_1), the volume of gas expired in the first second as a measure of the speed of airflow through larger airways; forced vital capacity (FVC), the total volume of expired gas; and a set of measurements at different points of exhalation (variously described as $FEF_{25/50/75}$ or $MEF_{25/50/75}$) indicative of flow through smaller airways. Measurements of peak flow are recorded but are unreliable when made during forced spirometry and often differ from measurements made with a peak flow meter. The absolute volumes obtained during spirometry depend upon age, height, sex, and racial origin, and values need to be compared with appropriate 'predicted normal values' of which several are available.

Most spirometers will also produce two graphical depictions of the forced manoeuvre (Figure 27.1). The first, a spirogram, is a plot of the volume of gas expired against time. The trace should be a smooth curve with a final 'plateau'. The second, the expiratory flow–volume curve or 'loop', plots flow against expired volume between maximal inspiration

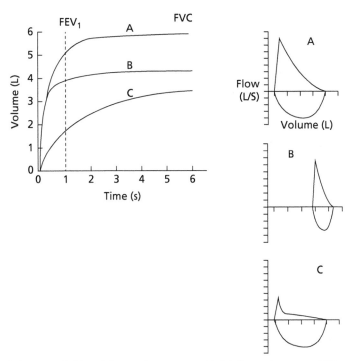

Figure 27.1 Spirograms (left) and flow–volume curves (right) illustrating normal (A) restrictive (B) and obstructive (C) patterns of abnormal ventilation.

(total lung capacity) and maximal expiration (residual volume). A normal 'loop' has a steep up-curve, a sharp angle, and a flat downward slope to the end of expiration.

Spirometry requires training, which is likely to become mandatory in the UK. A number of basic points of technique need to be observed to minimize measurement errors. Spirometry equipment should be calibrated regularly and checked for leaks, wear and tear, and blockages. Spuriously low results can occur if inspiration is incomplete, if partial leakage occurs (around the mouthpiece or in the tubing), or if expiratory effort is submaximal. The FVC is commonly underestimated because the blow is finished early, as is apparent in tracings that fail to attain a plateau. Variable effort is indicated by wobbly curves and poor reproducibility. Other factors that need to be considered include recent infections, irritant exposures (including smoking) and exercise, and variation between observers, between machines, and between reference values. Subjects should be encouraged to repeat the procedure until three acceptable manoeuvres are achieved (the best two FVCs should be within 5% or 0.1 L of one another). The documented values should be the highest values from any of the acceptable curves. Sometimes, despite encouragement and multiple attempts, subjects are unable to produce acceptable tracings. This commonly results from an inability to master the technique, but in some of these cases, so-called test failure is a marker of incipient health problems. Benchmark standards have been provided by national and international respiratory societies but these focus on measurements made in secondary or primary healthcare and a more useful guide for OH professionals is that produced by the American College of Occupational and Environmental Medicine.[3]

When interpreting lung function tests it is helpful to consider the pretest probability of disease. In most healthy non-smokers this probability is low and abnormal spirometry (especially that interpreted as 'restrictive') is usually attributable to poor technique. In addition, it needs to be remembered that the range of normal values is large, two standard deviations being approximately 20% of the average value. This means that a healthy individual can appear to have deficient lung function simply because their lung function lies in the lower tail of the normal Gaussian distribution; or that an individual with impaired lung function can still produce values within the normal range. In the latter case, if measurements have moved from the top of the predicted normal range for a particular parameter to the bottom, the fall will represent 40% of the population mean. Hence, serial patterns are more informative than a single snapshot. While the common practice of relating measurements proportionately to reference values ('per cent predicted') is widely criticized, in clinical practice it rarely makes any significant difference from the more technically correct use of comparison with '(lower) limits of normal'.[4]

Measurements of airflow such as FEV_1 and PEF are influenced most by disease in the larger airways, where most of the resistance to flow lies. The cross-sectional area of the bronchial tree increases exponentially with distance from the trachea as the bronchi divide, and resistance to flow falls concomitantly. Narrowing in the peripheral airways of less than 2 mm in diameter has little effect on FEV_1 and PEF unless damage is extensive. This means that early disease in small airways, such as that caused by smoking or other toxic fumes, is poorly reflected in these measurements.

Two main patterns of ventilatory abnormality can generally be defined, namely obstructive and restrictive. Obstruction is evident in some cases of asthma and is integral to the diagnosis of COPD, producing a diminution in FEV_1 greater than that in FVC. The ratio of FEV_1 to FVC should normally be greater than 0.7 (70%), but in airflow obstruction lower values arise accompanied by a reduction in FEV_1. Early obstruction may be evident in measures of low flow (such as FEF_{25-75}), although these measurements are less reproducible than FEV_1 and their reference ranges less precise. Restrictive lung changes are uncommon and caused by diffuse inflammatory and fibrotic diseases of the lung parenchyma, such as fibrosing alveolitis and asbestosis, by pleural disease, and by respiratory muscle weakness. In this case FEV_1 is reduced but so too is FVC, so that the ratio of FEV_1 to FVC is preserved and often increased.

PEF measurements are usually made serially over time, and used in one of two ways: to assess the degree of control achieved in patients with established asthma; and to look for work-related changes in situations where occupational asthma is suspected (the later section on asthma describes this last application more fully). PEF measures the highest flow recorded during a forced expiratory manoeuvre and is best measured with a peak flow meter. The subject must perform a short, sharp, hard blow into the meter; the best of three attempts is taken, providing the readings are reproducible. As with simple spirometry, a number of errors are possible, particularly variable subject effort, errors in reading PEFs and transcribing them to a diary, and incomplete returns. A great deal of instruction and encouragement are required to obtain adequate data. Meters that automatically record and store measurements are available but are still relatively expensive; applications ('apps') for use on smartphones are becoming available and are likely to be used increasingly. Self-treatment with bronchodilators and corticosteroids may affect PEF records; the influence of the first of these factors can be minimized by making recordings before drug delivery.

Measurements of static lung volumes, such as total lung capacity (TLC) and residual volume (RV), involve advanced techniques including inert gas dilution and body plethysmography; they require a specialized pulmonary function laboratory, but may be useful in clarifying diagnoses. Thus, in airflow obstruction, all static lung volumes are increased, but the increase in RV is proportionately greater than in TLC because of gas trapping; while in restrictive lung disease all lung volumes are reduced. An algorithm for best predicting true restriction from spirometry findings is available.[5]

Measurements of gas exchange such as oxygen consumption (VO_2) during incremental exercise, CO_2 production (VCO_2), and arterial blood gases, may be useful in assessing disability, especially in those with interstitial lung disease or emphysema. However, the findings reflect total cardiorespiratory function as well as peripheral muscle deconditioning, require sophisticated equipment, and are time-consuming to perform. Simpler tests of exercise capacity such as shuttle walk tests, step tests, and 6- or 12-minute walks are easier to use in the field, but still require skilled technical help and time. Carbon monoxide diffusion, expressed as transfer factor (TLCO), or gas transfer coefficient (KCO), measures the uptake of CO from the lung to the blood. CO is of similar molecular weight to oxygen, and is bound to haemoglobin, so its uptake provides a measure of oxygen diffusion. It is reduced in interstitial lung disease and in emphysema, but it is also affected by other factors such as smoking habits, haemoglobin levels, and resting cardiac output. Again, its measurement requires a dedicated lung function laboratory. In the clinical setting, the portable pulse oximeter provides a simple inexpensive guide to diffusion, and can be used to detect desaturation of haemoglobin at rest and during exercise.

Several other tests are used as adjuncts to diagnosis. Immunological responsiveness (sensitization) to workplace agents may be detected by the serological identification of specific immunoglobulin (Ig)-E antibodies, or by the response to a specific challenge to the skin (skin prick testing) or airways (bronchial provocation testing). The usefulness of these investigations varies from one agent to another. It also depends on accurate identification of the suspected agent, and in the case of skin prick and provocation tests, may depend on obtaining a correct formulation of the material, or achieving a representative challenge. The subject is more fully discussed later.

Screening questionnaires

In OH practice, screening questionnaires are commonly used at pre-placement and in routine surveillance programmes. The best known is the Medical Research Council

Table 27.2 The Medical Research Council breathlessness scale (1986 version)

1	Troublesome shortness of breath when hurrying on level ground or walking up a slight hill
2	Shortness of breath when walking with other people of own age on level ground
3	Have to stop for breath when walking at own pace on level ground

standardized questionnaire on respiratory symptoms.[6] This was devised for the epidemiological investigation of chronic bronchitis, but has since been adapted to assess respiratory symptoms in groups working with silica, asbestos, or other hazardous agents (for examples, see reference[7]).

There are no validated questionnaires for the screening of occupational asthma but questions, such as those in Table 27.2, that directly enquire into any relationship between symptoms and work are useful. Questions on respiratory symptoms are usefully supplemented by enquiry into nasal and ocular symptoms since occupational asthma is frequently accompanied by (occupational) rhinitis and conjunctivitis (Box 27.1).

Box 27.1 Outline questionnaire for employees exposed to respiratory sensitizing agents.

1. Since starting work at [x] (or over the past 12 months), has your chest ever felt tight or your breathing become difficult?
2. Since starting work at [x] (or over the past 12 months), has your chest ever sounded wheezy or whistling?
3. If 'yes' to 1 *or* 2, in what year (month) did you first notice this?
   a. What happens to this on days off or on holidays of 2 days or more?
   b. Do you get this on contact with anything at work?
   c. Do you get this on contact with anything at home?
4. Since starting work at [x] (or over the past 12 months), has your nose been blocked, itchy, runny, or sneezing? (Do not count the times you were ill with colds or 'flu.)
5. Since starting work at [x] (or over the past 12 months), have your eyes been itchy or runny?
If 'Yes' to 4 or 5, in what year (month) did you first notice this?
   a. What happens to this on days off or on holidays of 2 days or more?
   b. Do you get this on contact with anything at work?
   c. Do you get this on contact with anything at home?

Chest radiography

Chest radiography, and in particular the use of computed tomography (CT) scanning, plays a clinical role in assessing those with lengthy exposure to fibrogenic dusts such as asbestos and silica (see 'Interstitial lung disease') and may be valuable in the assessment of workers exposed to tuberculosis (TB) who develop suggestive respiratory symptoms. However, the routine application of chest radiography in most employment situations has fallen into disfavour. For example, a former requirement for routine radiography in commercial divers has been lifted, with investigation dictated rather by clinical need. Radiography is no longer considered helpful in routine surveillance of asymptomatic healthcare workers with potential TB exposure; and for the common round of health problems (upper respiratory tract infections, asthma, and COPD), decisions on fitness for work seldom rest upon the outcome of radiography.

An exception, in many jurisdictions, is the use of chest radiography in the routine surveillance of workers exposed to respirable crystalline silica. In the UK, for example,[8] employers are required to provide chest X-rays for their workers after a total of 15 years' exposure and then 3-yearly thereafter while exposure continues.

Clinical conditions and capacity for work

Asthma

Asthma affects about 5% of the adult population although the condition is often misdiagnosed.[9] It is a condition of variable airflow obstruction associated with bronchial hyper-responsiveness and symptoms of cough, breathlessness, and chest tightness. The predominant physical sign is wheeze. Onset in childhood or early adult life is frequently associated with the syndrome of atopy, characterized by elevated IgE antibody levels and positive skin prick tests to common inhaled antigens, and an increased incidence of eczema and allergic rhinitis. Childhood symptoms often remit in early adult life, but may recur in middle age. New-onset disease in middle life is not usually associated with manifestations of atopy, and the condition tends to be more persistent and more likely to progress in severity.

There are some difficulties in defining asthma. Wheeze is a highly prevalent symptom in the community, and many people with occasional wheeze do not have asthma. Conversely, subjects with bronchoconstriction do not recognize the symptom as often as might be supposed. A further difficulty, in middle-aged employees, arises in distinguishing between chronic asthma and COPD, as there may be an overlap between the classical features of asthma (wheeze and reversibility) and those of COPD (sputum, dyspnoea, and irreversible airflow obstruction). It is important for doctors making a fitness assessment to decide whether the diagnosis is truly asthma and whether some response to (further) treatment is likely. A more detailed history, including smoking habits, periodicity, currency and remission of symptoms, and precipitating factors is helpful. Ideally, the history should be supported by serial, diurnal measurements of PEF and evidence of responsiveness to bronchodilators. Due to asthma's variable nature, simple screening questions and a single measurement of lung function and bronchodilator responsiveness may prove misleading. The most usual pattern on spirometry is to observe an obstructive deficit (low FEV_1 with an abnormal FEV_1/FVC ratio), but these measurements, though specific, have a relatively low sensitivity[10] in a disorder characterized by variable airflow obstruction. Another common mistake is to confuse asthma with recurrent chest infection, especially in those who smoke. One unfortunate consequence of this mislabelling is to undertreat asthma and to limit employment opportunities thereby. Recent advances in better controlling disease, for example, the introduction of targeted 'biological' therapies, has enabled patients even with severe asthma to maximize their functional capacity and remain at work.

In the worker with established asthma, fitness and placement judgements may hinge on a number of important questions:

How severe is the condition?

Hyper-responsive airways represent a biological continuum and policies that refer in blanket terms to 'asthma' without distinction fail to encompass the spectrum of its severity. Asthma varies from mild disease with intermittent symptoms, through mild to moderate persistent disease requiring regular prophylactic treatment, to severe disease requiring regular high-dose inhaled steroids, or more rarely, continuous oral steroids or biological therapy. As a general rule, people with asthma run 'true to form' and there is far less variation within than between patients; the label 'asthmatic' can be unhelpful, leading simply to misinformed and prejudicial decisions on work fitness.

In the common situation where asthma is mild, infrequent, or amenable to simple treatment, job placement decisions are straightforward. Adequate control may require only occasional use of a bronchodilator at times of unusual exertion or intercurrent infection; simple work modifications may be helpful. Disease at the moderate to severe end of the spectrum poses more concern and at the extreme end, asthma may be severe and life-threatening. A particular worry arises if the workplace is far removed from medical care facilities and emergency transfer is expensive, disruptive, or technically difficult but it is worth noting that serious, unexpected attacks are rare.

A broad indication of disease activity can be gained from the frequency of bronchodilator use and the degree of sleep disturbance. In more severe disease, it is essential to know whether, when, and how often a patient has been admitted to hospital with asthma; whether or not they have required ventilation because of asthma; or have been prescribed oral steroid medication. A number of guidelines on assessing disease severity have been produced by specialist societies, such as those regularly published by the British Thoracic Society and Scottish Intercollegiate Guidelines Network.[11] An alternative approach, particularly in physically demanding jobs, is to measure changes in lung function during representative work tasks. Exercise tests are difficult to standardize and seldom specific enough to be used routinely in pre-placement screening, but in subjects with active, troublesome disease a fall in FEV_1 greater than 15% may indicate current work handicap.

Are there any work factors that are liable to aggravate constitutional asthma?

Asthmatic airways can be hyper-responsive to a wide range of non-specific irritants that are commonly encountered at work, as well as many highly prevalent environmental irritants and allergens. Extremes of temperature or humidity; irritant dusts or fumes, pollens, and house dust or pet allergens; heavy physical exertion; and even shift patterns may all provoke constitutional asthma. Such 'work-exacerbated' asthma can pose temporary or enduring employment problems to employees with asthma in a wide range of occupations, from cold store workers in refrigeration plants through to outdoor workers in construction and farming. A useful summary of the available literature has been published by the American Thoracic Society,[12] but it is likely to overestimate the true prevalence of the condition which in practice seldom causes major work-fitness issues that cannot be ameliorated.

Can the principal aggravating factors be removed or limited?

Can irritant fumes or dusts be better controlled by exhaust ventilation or different work practices? Can less irritating materials be used? Can the process be enclosed? Can respiratory protection be used to limit exposure? If physical exertion is a limiting factor, can the effort of the work be reduced (e.g. by providing a lifting aid)? These are areas in which OH professionals need to be particularly influential.

Has optimum treatment been offered, or could disease control be improved?

Asthma is often undertreated, with insufficient use made of long-term prophylactic treatment. Regular use of inhaled corticosteroids has a beneficial effect on attack frequency, sleep disturbance, and hospital admission rates. The well-informed patient should be able to self-monitor, self-medicate, and self-refer but poor adherence to treatment is common. Deteriorating serial peak flow and worsening nocturnal symptoms should trigger an increase in medication and early medical consultation attendance; while in severe asthma, a home supply of oral steroids has enabled earlier treatment in those most in need. Current UK guidelines[11] provide a detailed stepwise approach to the treatment of asthma and it is important to determine, if needed, whether better control is possible at an early stage.

Might the patient have occupational (sensitization) asthma?

This is an important question to consider when asthma begins or recurs in adulthood, and a vital question in industries from which most case reports arise (Table 27.3). The possibility is suggested if symptoms are worse on work days, are better when away from work (at weekends and on holiday), and deteriorate upon return to work; and when work-related eye and nose symptoms are also present. In this setting, questionnaires and history taking, while very important, do not confirm or exclude the diagnosis of occupational asthma; the existing evidence suggests that their negative predictive value is better than their positive predictive value.[13,14] Moreover, there is evidence that in some settings

Table 27.3 Agents frequently reported to cause occupational asthma and occupations that often give rise to such reports

Agents	Occupations
Diisocyanates	Paint spraying, foam manufacture, industrial gluing, other chemical processing
Flour and grain dust	Baking, pastry making, dock work
Colophony and fluxes	Electronic assembly
Animal proteins	Laboratory animal work, animal handling
Wood dusts (some)	Woodwork, timber handling
Enzymes	Baking, food processing, detergent manufacture
Persulphate salts	Hairdressing, circuit board manufacture
Complex platinum salts	Precious metal refining

workers with occupational asthma may choose not to disclose symptoms,[15] presumably through concern over the potential implications for their employment.

A similar asthmatic picture can arise from a non-specific response to irritant conditions, as described earlier, and the distinction between these possibilities is important. Sensitized workers may react to amounts of material so small that workplace controls cannot be guaranteed to afford reliable protection; and occupational asthma may (rarely) result in severe bronchospasm. By contrast, it is more realistic to achieve the control measures that ease the problems of aggravated ('work-exacerbated') non-occupational asthma, so the prospects for continued healthy employment are correspondingly brighter.

In practice, it may be difficult to distinguish between the two diagnoses: irritant industrial exposures often coexist with the presence of a workplace sensitizer, and workers with pre-existing asthma are not immune to occupational sensitization. A separate diagnostic problem arises in sensitized workers who manifest late asthmatic reactions, rather than immediate ones. Symptoms often arise at night-time, and thereby mimic the pattern of constitutional asthma. In difficult cases, assistance in diagnosis from a respiratory specialist with an interest in occupational lung disease is recommended.[16]

A single measurement of FEV_1 is an insensitive indicator of occupational asthma and alternative investigations are required to secure a diagnosis. Agents that cause occupational asthma can be classified broadly into those that sensitize with the induction of specific IgE antibodies, and those such as diisocyanates, colophony, and most wood dusts that sensitize by other poorly understood means, and have mute or inconsistent antibody responses. Hence, for some causes of occupational asthma the detection of specific IgE antibodies may serve as an indicator of sensitization, as may a positive skin prick test. Examples include sensitivity to flour and enzymes in bakery workers, to animal products in exposed workers, or to latex in those who wear (powdered) latex gloves. These specific tests can be relatively sensitive for some agents,[17] and can be used in case investigation. In some settings, such as the detergent industry, they are used in routine surveillance as an adjunct to exposure controls. The distinction between sensitization and frank occupational asthma is an important one to draw; skin prick and serological tests do not in themselves indicate work-limiting disease and corroborative evidence is required before making placement decisions.

It is rarely necessary for an employee to be removed from their work while undergoing investigation for occupational asthma. If they are still exposed, and fit for further exposure, the standard investigative tool is serial measurement of PEF.[18] A pattern is sought of exaggerated PEF variability and a fall in mean PEF level around times of exposure (see Figure 27.2). Normally, several readings a day (at work and away) will be required over a 3–4-week period—at least four per day to ensure adequate sensitivity and specificity. The record must cover a period in which exposure occurs which may require some pre-planning if exposures are intermittent. It is helpful to keep to the same broad pattern of measurement at work and on rest days.

Interpretation of serial PEF measurements has traditionally been based on pattern recognition by an experienced physician, but rule-based quantitative approaches have been suggested and computerized diagnostic algorithms have been developed with some success.[19] Serial PEF measurement, if conducted correctly, is dependable, with good agreement on interpretation between experts and few false-positive results, but it may fail to identify about 20% of cases.[17]

The 'gold standard' for diagnosis is a specific bronchial provocation test (BPT; or specific inhalation challenge) with the suspected sensitizer: a simulated industrial exposure conducted in hospital under controlled conditions, with FEV_1 and responsiveness to histamine or methacholine measured serially. A late response, in particular, is taken as evidence of an allergic response; bronchial hyper-reactivity can also be demonstrated for 2–3 days after the challenge. The procedure entails a small risk of severe bronchospasm, and needs to be undertaken as an inpatient in a specialist unit. Due to its risk and cost, BPT is usually reserved for special circumstances, which include the investigation of mixed exposures and novel agents, and situations of significant diagnostic uncertainty. Although it is often assumed that BPT is always correct, false negatives can arise if testing is conducted with the wrong material, too low an exposure, or if the patient has been unexposed to the sensitizing agent for a long period.

Occupational asthma is important and comparatively common; over 400 causal agents have been identified and several hundred new cases are diagnosed annually by UK specialists. It can result in acute severe bronchospasm in the workplace and chronic ill health during employment. For some sensitizing agents, such as isocyanates, non-specific bronchial hyper-responsiveness is known to persist for several years after leaving employment. There is reasonable research evidence that early redeployment away from exposure can mitigate against the risk of continuing symptoms, and thus improve the long-term prognosis.[20] A comprehensive systematic review of this and other issues in occupational asthma draws attention to the benefits of early withdrawal from exposure (Box 27.2).

In the UK, the COSHH Regulations 1994 require health surveillance programmes to be conducted where there is a risk of occupational asthma. Guidance on the

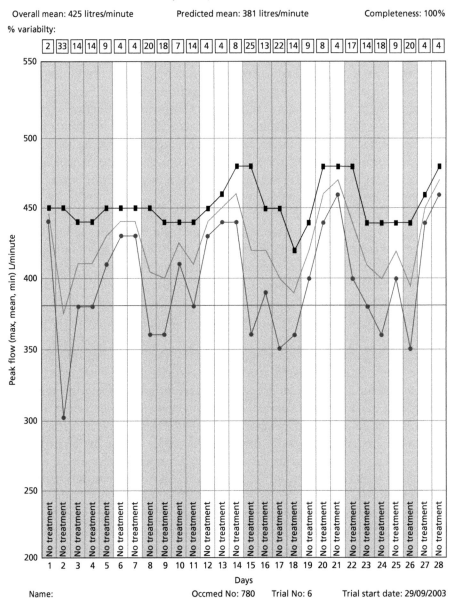

Figure 27.2 Plot of serial peak flow measurements made over a 28-day period by a baker with occupational asthma. Each column represents a day, those shaded are work days. The three lines indicate, from the top respectively, the maximum, mean, and minimum measurements of the day. The figures in the small boxes above each column are a measure of diurnal variability.

> ## Box 27.2 Evidence-based guidelines relating to the need to withdraw from causal exposures in subjects with occupational asthma; statements and strength of evidence
>
> The likelihood of improvement or resolution of symptoms or of preventing deterioration is greater in workers who:
>
> - avoid further exposure to the causative agent (2+)
> - have relatively normal lung function at the time of diagnosis (2+)
> - have a shorter duration of symptoms prior to diagnosis (2+)
> - have a shorter duration of symptoms prior to removal from exposure (2+).
>
> Redeployment to a low-exposure area may lead to improvement or resolution of symptoms or prevent deterioration in some workers, but is not always effective (3).
>
> Where clinical considerations permit, reduction of exposure may be a useful alternative associated with fewer socioeconomic consequences to complete removal from exposure (2+).
>
> Air-fed helmet respirators may improve or prevent symptoms but not for all workers who continue to be exposed to the causative agent (3).
>
> 2+: evidence from well-conducted case–control or cohort studies with a low risk of confounding or bias and a moderate chance of causality.
>
> 3: evidence only from non-analytic studies (e.g. case reports).
>
> Source: data from Nicholson, PJ et al. (2010) *Occupational asthma: prevention, identification, and management: systematic review and recommendations.* Copyright © 2010 The British Occupational Health Research Foundation (BOHRF).

ingredients of suitable programmes is available through the UK Health and Safety Executive (HSE).[21] Periodic symptom enquiries (including nasal symptoms, an important precursor of occupational asthma) and review of sickness absence reports are advised, the exact schedule being based on an assessment of risk. The effectiveness of health surveillance, in detecting early reversible disease, has not been rigorously established, and the elements that have the most impact are not well defined. Nonetheless, screening, early detection of symptoms, and prompt action are seen as vital ingredients in fitness assessment of workers from high-risk industries. The strong presumption is that those with occupational asthma should be protected from further exposure to the sensitizing agent that caused their asthma, a policy for which there is persuasive evidence.[20]

Nonetheless, some doctors perceive a difficulty with employees who develop mild occupational asthma with normal pulmonary function when exposures are low or occasional. The pressure to continue in work (and preserve earning power) has to be balanced against the longer-term risks of deterioration, chronicity of symptoms, and fixed airflow limitation. With respiratory protection, modification of their job to reduce exposure, and effective treatment, many workers with occupational asthma have continued to work successfully. Under these circumstances close supervision is essential, and the ever-present risk of control failures should be borne in mind. Every effort should be made to explore work and process modifications that minimize the risk. Ideally, patients should withdraw permanently from all further exposures; but if not, they should be aware that progression of symptoms can and sometimes does occur despite great care and redeployment to work areas of lower exposure.[22]

Some authorities have recommended policies that restrict the placement of workers perceived to be at greater risk of developing occupational asthma. Atopic individuals appear to be at increased relative risk when working with agents that induce specific IgE antibodies such as animal or bakery proteins, while smokers are at greater risk of asthma from diisocyanates, complex platinum salts, and seafood proteins. In general, these risk factors are too common and too poorly discriminating to form a rational basis for health-based pre-placement selection. However, prudence dictates that careful consideration should be made of persons with very poorly controlled asthma before they are newly placed in environments known to contain respiratory sensitizers, since any supervening occupational asthma will be more troublesome.

Chronic obstructive pulmonary disease

COPD is a common diagnosis, made in about 900 000 adults in the UK although it is estimated that a further 2 million (10% of those aged 18–65) have the condition unrecognized.[23] Smoking leads to a syndrome of chronic mucus production with goblet cell hyperplasia (simple chronic bronchitis), and also to chronic airflow limitation with airways narrowing and emphysema. Exposure to industrial dust and fumes may contribute to both syndromes but the association between occupational exposures and COPD is complex.[24] COPD often coexists with other diseases that share tobacco smoking as a risk factor, of which the most common are heart disease and lung cancer.

The principal symptoms in COPD are cough, sputum, and breathlessness on effort; the symptoms and signs are non-specific and detection of latent airflow limitation is delayed until disease is more advanced. In assessing the fitness for work of a person with COPD for employment, a number of matters need to be considered:

Is the problem primarily one of mucus hypersecretion or of airflow limitation?

Mucus hypersecretion by itself does not limit capacity to work, and in the absence of airflow limitation simple chronic bronchitis is compatible with a wide range of normal employment. Infective exacerbations and sickness absence may be more frequent, although a programme of winter influenza vaccinations may ameliorate the problem. In these circumstances, a medical label may be unhelpful and prejudicial to employment prospects. Frequently, however, mucus hypersecretion coexists with airflow limitation, which can be a real cause of disability.

If airflow limitation is present, how severe is it and what is its functional effect?

Emphysema and airflow limitation are defined, respectively, in pathological and functional terms but their presence can be presumed when there is an obstructive pattern on spirometry with evidence of increased static lung volumes (TLC), gas trapping (disproportionate increase in RV with reduced RV/TLC ratio), and impaired gas transfer (TLCO). Although FEV_1 may be normal despite significant small airways disease, there is a broad correlation in COPD between FEV_1 and breathlessness. Spirometry predicts prognosis in COPD; for example, ventilatory failure (hypercapnia) is unusual if the FEV_1 is greater than 1.5 L. More comprehensive measures, such as the 'BODE' index (comprising body mass index (BMI), FEV_1, dyspnoea, and exercise tolerance) may provide better prognostic value than FEV_1, a reflection probably that breathlessness in COPD is multifactorial.[25]

Measurements of lung function should, in principle, provide a fair guide to work capability in patients with airflow limitation, and spirometric findings can be banded according to their likely impact on function (Table 27.4). However, the energy demands of work vary through time as the component activities of a task vary; individuals also vary in their oxygen requirements for a given task, because of personal and job-related factors; and resting lung function tests explain only a small part of the variance in VO_{2max}. The subjective appreciation of breathlessness usually proves to be the limiting factor. Hence, 'objective' measurements of disability provide no more than a rough guide to work capacity. Crudely speaking, those with 'mild' impairment (Table 27.4) can manage most ordinary work, whereas those with 'moderate' impairment fail to meet the physical demands of many jobs, and those with 'severe' or 'very severe' impairment struggle to cope in most jobs. However, given wide individual variation and scope for job modification, fitness decisions still depend on subjective medical judgements.

Has optimum treatment been offered, or could disease control be improved?

In individuals with airflow limitation due to COPD, there is limited scope for therapeutic improvement, and certainly less than for asthma. Detailed guidance on the stepped

Table 27.4 Spirometric criteria for the diagnosis of chronic obstructive pulmonary disease

Post bronchodilator measurements		Diagnosis
FEV$_1$/FVC ratio	FEV$_1$% predicted	
<0.7	≥80	Mild
<0.7	50–79	Moderate
<0.7	30–49	Severe
<0.7	<30	Very severe

Symptoms should be present to diagnose COPD in people with mild airflow obstruction.

treatment of COPD is to be found in evidence-based guidelines.[26] Inhaled beta agonists, both short and long acting, are less effective than in asthma but may improve breathlessness and exercise tolerance, even in the absence of measurable bronchodilation. Anticholinergic agents, such as ipratropium bromide or the longer-acting tiotropium, may be more effective, and in disease of moderate severity either or both may be employed on a regular basis with long-acting beta agonists substituted for shorter-acting ones. The existing evidence suggests that inhaled steroids decrease exacerbations and modestly slow the progression of respiratory symptoms, but appear to have little impact on lung function and mortality. In COPD, inhaled steroids are used as part of a combined regimen, but should not be used as sole therapy for COPD (i.e. without long-acting bronchodilators).[27]

Theophyllines have only a modest bronchodilatory effect, but may modify small airways function and gas trapping and can be used in combination with other bronchodilators. Beneficial effects on exercise tolerance have been reported, but not consistently. Plasma theophylline levels should be monitored in view of their narrow therapeutic range and propensity to cause side effects and drug interactions. Mucolytic drugs have no effect on lung function, but may reduce the volume of expectorated sputum, the number of exacerbations, and the number of days of COPD illness.

Formal exercise programmes ('pulmonary rehabilitation') increase functional and maximal exercise tolerance in symptomatic patients with moderately severe COPD. Programmes of rehabilitation should be tailored to individual needs; ingredients include disease education, including smoking cessation, a review of medication, and an assessment of psychological and nutritional needs. Patients should be encouraged to commit to an ongoing exercise programme.

It is essential to encourage COPD sufferers to stop smoking. In people with smoking-induced COPD, the rate of decline in FEV_1 is increased from the average value of 20–30 mL per year seen in non-smokers to a value of around 60–80 mL per year or more. In smokers with moderate impairment of lung function, the rate of loss of function returns to normal upon smoking cessation, but the benefit in severe COPD and in industrial disease is less certain. Thus, an important preventive role for the OH service is to educate and to provide support for attempts to stop smoking, especially in employees with COPD. Guidance on smoking cessation in workplaces has been published by the National Institute for Health and Care Excellence.[28]

Finally, intercurrent infections require prompt treatment to prevent acute deteriorations and chronic airways damage. Annual vaccination against influenza (and a one-off vaccination against pneumococcal infection) is generally recommended.

Are there any work factors that are liable to aggravate COPD?

In workers who develop troublesome progressive airflow limitation, continuing employment may still be possible in more sedentary work, or under a modified work schedule. One possible strategy may be to conduct less arduous work spread over a longer time period. Better process control (dust and fume control at source, assisted mechanical lifting, etc.) may also extend the range of employment possibilities and these measures should all be considered before declaring the worker unfit.

Are there special work problems for COPD sufferers?

The wearing of respiratory protective equipment may increase the effort of work. Some respiratory protective equipment, such as self-contained breathing apparatus, can be bulky, heavy, or awkward; while some systems, such as canister respirators and half-face masks, increase the work of breathing, requiring the wearer to inspire air against the resistance of a filter. It may be possible, instead, to provide a filter free 'active' system such as an air fed respirator which blows a stream of fresh air across the face behind a visor, the positive pressure generated preventing the ingress of hazardous fumes. However even these require extra weight to be carried around while physically active and the choice of system may be limited by the circumstances. The need to attain very high degrees of protection may necessitate self-contained breathing apparatus, and work in oxygen-deficient atmospheres may necessitate the carriage of gas cylinders. Fitness decisions need to be made in the light of residual lung capacity, the work in question, and the options for process control over and above respiratory protective equipment use.

The presence of emphysema, particularly bullous disease, increases the risk of spontaneous pneumothorax and is thus a bar to employment in certain occupations that involve changes in barometric pressure such as diving (see Chapter 16).

Interstitial lung diseases

The important diseases in this group include interstitial fibrosis, chronic pulmonary sarcoidosis, and hypersensitivity pneumonitis (known also as extrinsic allergic alveolitis). All these conditions can produce pulmonary fibrosis. In functional terms, they reduce pulmonary compliance, reduce static lung volumes, and impair gas transfer. $FEV_1/FVC\%$ is usually preserved, but airflow limitation may be present in addition to fibrosis. These conditions are all associated with radiological abnormalities; high-resolution CT scanning is more sensitive than plain radiography in assessing their extent.

Pulmonary fibrosis is frequently 'idiopathic', but may be secondary to other clinical disorders (such as rheumatoid arthritis, systemic sclerosis, inflammatory bowel disease, and sarcoidosis), or due to occupational contact with fibrogenic dusts (pneumoconiosis). A number of professional groups, including miners and quarrymen, stonemasons, foundry fettlers, and some construction workers, are at special risk, although this fact may go unrecognized.

Established fibrosis from any cause frequently progresses, although the rate of progression can be very variable. In the case of fibrogenic dust disease, progression may occur despite removal from the industry. Early identification and withdrawal from exposure may result in a better long-term outcome. It seems prudent therefore to identify pneumoconiosis at an early stage and to recommend avoidance of further exposure. Unfortunately, there are no unique symptoms or signs and disease onset is insidious (over a decade or longer) and may even postdate employment. Gradually progressive dyspnoea may be attributed erroneously to ageing or smoking.

A programme of regular surveillance in high-risk professions helps to obviate this problem. The elements of surveillance programmes for workers exposed to silica or asbestos all include symptom questionnaires and spirometry but vary in their requirements for regular radiography. Tests of pulmonary function are not diagnostically specific and their longitudinal assessment requires care to detect a pattern of decline against the 'noise' created by errors in spirometry; the National Institute for Occupational Safety and Health in the US provides free software ('SPIROLA') which is helpful in this respect (see 'Useful websites'). Chest radiography is more sensitive than either questionnaires or spirometry and detects fibrosis in about 80% of cases of asbestosis and silicosis; in some countries, the use of high-resolution CT, which is more sensitive (but entails a higher dose of radiation) is applied to exposed workforces.

Table 27.5 summarizes two model surveillance programmes advocated by the World Health Organization[29] alongside the current requirements set by the HSE in the UK.[8,30] Note that the programmes suggested by the WHO (only) are intended to be lifelong.

Ideally, chest radiographs are scored against a standard set of International Labour Office films, based on the presence, profusion, size, and shape of opacities.[31] Category 1 changes can occur without evidence of impaired lung function. Category 2 change and above is associated with increasing impairment of lung function, and warrants removal from further contact with fibrogenic dust.

Silica-exposed workers are at increased risk of TB, including reactivation of old disease. Questionnaires should include relevant items but in the UK routine immunological surveillance for TB is not currently recommended.

A number of new treatments are available for established fibrotic lung disease and appear to slow the natural decline in pulmonary function although their effect on longevity is more uncertain. The principal disability is breathlessness on effort, which is often accompanied by significant falls in arterial oxygen levels. Spirometry and measurements of oxygen saturation during representative exercise provide a basis for fitness assessment;

Table 27.5 Suggested surveillance programmes for workers exposed to asbestos or silica

	Asbestos		Silica	
	WHO	**HSE**	**WHO**	**HSE**
Questionnaire	Annually	≤2 yearly	Annually	Annually
Spirometry	Annually	≤2 yearly	Annually	Annually
Chest X-ray	Baseline then according to duration of exposure: <10 years: 3–5 yearly 10–20 years: 1–2 yearly >20: annually	At discretion	Baseline after 2–3 years' exposure then 2–5 yearly	±Baseline after 15 years' exposure then 3 yearly

the general considerations are the same as those for COPD with airflow limitation. Portable oxygen may help to alleviate some symptoms and pulmonary rehabilitation may, at least in the short term, be similarly helpful. Affected workers may remain gainfully employed in less manual work, but disability tends to progress with time, and a periodic medical review is appropriate. Many forms of pulmonary fibrosis are associated with an increased risk of bronchogenic carcinoma.

Hypersensitivity pneumonitis (synonymous with extrinsic allergic alveolitis) is often provoked by allergens such as moulds or bird excreta although the commonest occupational cause in the UK now is contaminated metal working fluid.[32] In its acute form it produces a systemic 'flu-like illness, with fever, aches and pains, malaise, weight loss, and dry cough; symptoms develop within a few hours of exposure. Mild attacks resolve spontaneously once exposure ceases, but severe attacks may require corticosteroid therapy. Chronic exposure can cause pulmonary fibrosis and permanent respiratory disability. Established fibrosis is unresponsive to treatment, so regular surveillance (through a symptoms questionnaire and lung function testing, with chest radiography as clinically indicated) is appropriate for those with continuing potential for exposure.

Respiratory infections

Respiratory tract infections

These are very common. Occupational environments which are enclosed with little natural ventilation favour the spread of prevalent (particularly viral) upper respiratory infections. These contribute importantly to short-term sickness absence, but are self-limiting and pose no special difficulties in fitness assessment. More serious are a range of viral upper respiratory tract infections that may be complicated by chest problems or protracted debility. Influenza is a highly infectious condition that involves a longer period of sickness and a greater risk of complicating illness (tracheobronchitis, pneumonia, and exacerbated COPD). Some occupational groups such as healthcare workers and teachers, are at particular risk, and may benefit from prophylaxis with influenza vaccine. Vaccination in these worker groups is important in limiting risk to clients,[33] and is also recommended in those with pre-existing lung diseases such as asthma and COPD, irrespective of occupation.

Glandular fever and the other infectious mononucleoses are relatively common in young adults. Although they are self-limiting, it is not uncommon to feel tired and fatigued for 3–6 months after the acute stage of illness. Sufferers who lack their normal stamina are often signed off as unfit to attend work, although a modified work programme with phased rehabilitation is a more constructive approach. Ideally, this would encourage the individual to work their normal duties, but only for a part of the week to begin with, the hours gradually increasing as their stamina improves.

Some respiratory infections may be occupationally acquired (e.g. Q fever in slaughterhouse workers and veterinary surgeons and *Legionella* pneumonia in industries using humidification and water cooling plants), but these are uncommon occurrences. Welders have an increased risk of contracting pneumococcal pneumonia and it is advisable to offer them specific vaccination.

Tuberculosis

TB is a respiratory infection spread by infected droplets from person to person. In the UK, after 1950, the number of cases fell tenfold from around 50,000 per year, but this decline has reversed and the number of annual cases has risen to about 9000; the rise has been especially steep since 2000 and most prominent in English cities, in particular in parts of London. Worldwide, 9 million new cases occur each year, 95% of which arise in low-income countries. Migrants from these countries bring with them an increased risk of TB. Among people born in the UK the annual incidence of TB is about 4/100,000 but rates in those born in other parts of the world, and especially Africa or the Indian subcontinent, are over 20 times higher so that 75% of new cases reported in the UK occur in immigrants.

In countries with a high prevalence of TB, the advent of HIV disease is promoting the disease in working-aged people. In the UK, where the reservoir of tuberculous infection has traditionally been in elderly people, HIV has been less of a factor but this is now changing with increasing numbers of HIV-positive cases of TB being diagnosed in patients arriving from high-risk countries. Worldwide, about 2 million people die from TB each year of whom one in seven also has HIV infection. Rates of TB are also high in other vulnerable groups such as homeless people, asylum seekers, prisoners, and substance misusers.

Cross-infectivity in TB arises principally in the close (domestic) contacts of patients with smear-positive sputum; the risk with non-respiratory TB is very low. Most occupational contacts are considered to be 'casual' rather than 'close'. Screening of workplace contacts is only necessary if the index case is smear positive and contacts are unusually susceptible—for example, immunocompromised adults—or the index case is considered highly infectious as shown by transmission to more than 10% of close contacts. In the UK, cases of TB must be notified by the physician making or suspecting the diagnosis to the Health Protection Agency, which will institute screening of people at risk.

While it is uncommon for healthcare staff to acquire TB from patients, there is a duty of care to reduce the risks of transmission from staff to patients. Employees new to the NHS who will be working with patients or clinical specimens should not start work until they have completed a TB screen or health check, or documentary evidence is provided of such screening having taken place within the preceding 12 months. Health checks for employees who will have contact with patients or clinical materials should include[34]:

- assessment of personal or family history of TB
- asking about symptoms and signs, possibly by questionnaire
- documentary evidence of TB skin testing (or interferon-gamma release assay (IGRA)) within the past 5 years and/or bacillus Calmette–Guérin (BCG) scar check by an OH professional, not relying on the applicant's personal assessment.

If a new employee from the UK or other low-incidence setting, who has not had a BCG vaccination, has a positive Mantoux test and a positive IGRA, they should have a medical assessment and a chest X-ray. They should be referred to a TB clinic to determine whether they need TB treatment if the chest X-ray is abnormal, or to determine whether they need treatment of latent TB infection if the chest X-ray is normal.

Vaccination has been shown to reduce the risk of active TB by 70–80%. It is not necessary to inspect the site after the vaccination unless as a means of quality control of the technique of administering the BCG vaccine. BCG vaccination is contraindicated in HIV-positive individuals. Potential employees from countries or groups with a high prevalence of HIV infection who are Mantoux negative (<6 mm) should be considered for HIV testing before BCG vaccination.

Since there is a UK shortage of BCG vaccine, the current practice in the UK is to offer it to eligible healthcare workers when the vaccine becomes available. As it is uncommon to have patients with unidentified infectious TB in the hospital and also the risk of infection normally requires prolonged period of exposure, it is considered that the likelihood of an unvaccinated healthcare worker acquiring TB from a patient is low, particularly with strict adherence to infection control policies and procedures. Therefore, the eligible healthcare workers for BCG vaccination are able to commence working without vaccination.

Healthcare workers who are found to be HIV positive during employment should have medical and occupational assessments of their TB risk, and may need to modify their work to reduce exposure; HIV-positive healthcare workers should not be employed in areas where there is a risk of contracting active TB.

Similar guidance is provided for healthcare workers who care for prisoners and remand centre detainees; and for prison service staff and others who have regular contact with prisoners, for example, probation officers and education and social workers. Routine pre-placement screening is no longer required for schoolteachers and others working with children but it is important that these groups are aware of how TB presents.

During employment, routine periodic chest radiography is neither necessary nor effective in screening. Awareness and early reporting of suspicious symptoms is the mainstay of detection. If a worker contracts TB, treatment should be started and supervised by an experienced physician. In fully sensitive infections (the majority in the UK), the patient is non-infectious after 2 weeks of treatment, and it is not usually necessary to restrict work after 2–3 weeks of treatment. Caution may be appropriate, however, where there is reason to suspect drug resistance, and in healthcare workers who deal with vulnerable patient groups (such as the immunosuppressed and young children). An infectious risk should be assumed until drug sensitivities are known or the sputum is known to be negative on culture. Drug resistance should be suspected in patients who have relapsed from earlier treatment, and those who come from areas where drug resistance is common (e.g. Africa and the Indian subcontinent). HIV infection is a risk factor for drug-resistant TB. Problems may also arise in patients who comply poorly with treatment.

Disorders of sleep

Sleep and attendance at work

It is generally recommended that adults aged 18–64 years should sleep 7–9 hours and those 65 years of age or older 7–8 hours in 24 hours. Poor sleep may have an impact on attendance at work; for example, women with insomnia and men who use sleeping tablets have higher rates of sickness absence.[35] Shift workers are prone to sleepiness, difficulties with cognition and with psychomotor function, and affective instability.[36] Indeed, performance after a lengthy on-call medical shift is reported to be equivalent or worse than alcohol sufficient to produce a blood level of 0.04–0.05g%.[37]

Obstructive sleep apnoea

Obstructive sleep apnoea (OSA) is the most common sleep-related breathing disorder, affecting 4% of middle-aged men; in younger women, the prevalence is approximately half this but it rises to a similar level after the menopause. Obesity is the strongest risk factor but others include older age, craniofacial abnormalities, and upper airway soft tissue abnormalities. Individuals with acromegaly, congestive heart failure, stroke, hypothyroidism, Marfan syndrome, and ankylosing spondylitis have an increased risk of OSA.

Patients usually present with snoring and daytime sleepiness which are symptoms that are relatively sensitive but of low specificity. Sleepiness can be quantitated by the Epworth sleepiness score or the STOP-BANG questionnaire (see 'Useful websites'). In OSA, the physical examination can be normal, although obesity, elevated blood pressure, a narrow airway, and a large neck circumference are common. The diagnosis is confirmed by in-laboratory polysomnography or home sleep apnoea testing (for those who do not have medical co-morbidities, e.g. heart failure). Patients with OSA benefit from behaviour modifications including weight loss, and OSA-specific therapies such as positive airway pressure, oral appliances, or surgery. OSA, especially when severe and untreated, is associated with cardiovascular morbidities and an increased risk for all-cause mortality.

Excessive daytime sleepiness, which is closely linked to OSA, appears to increase the risk of industrial accidents twofold although the risk can be ameliorated by appropriate management. Shift or night work, endured by around 20% of the working population, may incur a similar risk,[38] although this may be explained by a relative lack of supervision, under-reporting, and other factors that potentially confound variations in working times.

Driving implications

The UK Driver and Vehicle Licensing Agency (DVLA) has an in-depth guide for medical professionals who are making assessments of fitness to drive and OH professionals should refer to the latest guidelines on the DVLA website (see 'Useful websites').

The American Academy of Sleep Medicine has released recommendations for commercial drivers.[39] These recommend that drivers meeting any of the following high-risk criteria be referred to a sleep medicine specialist for evaluation:

- BMI greater or equal to 40 kg/m².
- Fatigue or sleepiness during the duty period or involvement in a sleepiness-related crash or accident.
- BMI greater or equal to 33 kg/m² *and* either hypertension requiring two or more medications to control *or* type 2 diabetes.

Neoplastic disease

Lung cancer

In men, lung cancer is the leading cause of cancer deaths worldwide; in women, it is second only to breast cancer. In both sexes it causes an estimated 1.6 million deaths annually.[40] The most important risk factor is smoking. The relative risk of lung cancer in the long-term smoker compared with the lifetime non-smoker is between 10 and 30. The cumulative lung cancer risk among heavy smokers may be as high as 30%, compared with a lifetime risk of 1% or less in never-smokers.[41]

A number of occupational risk factors are also well recognized, asbestos exposure being numerically the most important. For asbestos-induced lung cancer, the risks multiply with those of smoking. Occupationally related lung cancers may also arise in the extraction of chromium from its ore, the manufacture of chromates, nickel refining, and exposure to polycyclic aromatic hydrocarbons, cadmium compounds, arsenic (in mining, smelting, and pesticide production), diesel exhaust, and bis-chloromethyl and chloromethyl methyl ethers. Silica is probably also a lung carcinogen, albeit a relatively weak one.

The different histological types of lung cancer vary in their growth rate. In the absence of treatment, a patient with adenocarcinoma is likely to survive for about 2 years from diagnosis, a patient with a squamous cell tumour for about 1 year, and a patient with a small cell tumour for about 4 months. Small cell tumours metastasize early, and are rarely amenable to surgical cure but 85% respond to combination chemotherapy. The median survival is thus extended to about 8 months in patients with extensive disease, and to about 14 months in patients with limited disease; but a minority survive longer (10% for 2 years, 4% for 5 years). During this period, patients often enjoy a good quality of life and can sometimes continue in light work.

For non-small cell lung cancer (adenocarcinoma, squamous carcinoma, and undifferentiated tumours), chemotherapy is much less successful, and the preferred treatment is surgical resection. Radiotherapy is usually used as an adjunct to surgery, or for the palliation of specific problems, such as haemoptysis and localized bone pain. Unfortunately, most tumours present when advanced, and other smoking-related lung disease often limits resectability. About 25% of patients are suitable for surgery. Of these, about a third survive for 5 years (65–85% in the absence of lymph node, chest wall, and metastatic involvement; but only around 25–35% when there is ipsilateral mediastinal lymph node involvement). Employees who undergo successful resection may well be able to return to work, though the choice of employment will depend on the physical demands of the job and their residual lung function.

Mesothelioma

Mesothelioma is a rare tumour in the absence of asbestos exposure. It is a malignant condition affecting the pleura, or less often the peritoneum. The tumour arises after a long latent period—rarely less than 20 years from first exposure, and typically 35–40 years. Thus, most cases arise after retirement.

The incidence of the tumour continues to rise in the UK, reflecting the greater use of asbestos (especially amphibole types) after the 1960s. Currently there are about 2000 cases/year, 80% of them in men, and the great majority attributable to occupational asbestos exposure, but there has been a shift from those employed in industries with primary exposure such as asbestos manufacture and lagging to those with secondary exposures such as carpenters, plumbers, and other crafts trades.[42] The disease has a long latency and occupational exposures before the age of 30 pose the highest risk. Amphibole fibre types (crocidolite and amosite) are in this respect more toxic than chrysotile although this is seldom helpful in the UK where fibre mixtures were widely used. Rates of mesothelioma in the UK are as high as anywhere in the world and are expected to increase until 2020.

Mesothelioma presents with chest wall pain, breathlessness, and pleural effusion. It progresses mainly by local invasion, although distant metastases can sometimes occur. Involvement of the chest wall, diaphragm, mediastinum, and neck root is common, and results in local pain, restricted chest movement, dysphagia, obstruction of the great veins, and pericardial involvement. The condition is incurable and most patients die within 2 years of presentation. It is rare for a patient with mesothelioma to be able to continue for long in active employment. In the UK, individuals with this condition can claim Industrial Injuries Disablement Benefit if they were employed in a job or were on an approved employment training scheme or course that caused their disease.

Other diseases of the pleura

A common manifestation of pleural disease is *pleural effusion*. Effusions that result from inflammatory processes are exudates, with a high protein content (>30 g/L). Underlying causes include infection, collagen vascular disease, malignancy, and pulmonary infarction. Pleural malignancy, pulmonary infarction, and asbestotic pleurisy can also produce blood-stained effusions. Effusions of low protein content (transudates, protein <25 g/L) may arise in cardiac failure and low protein states such as nephrotic syndrome and cirrhosis of the liver.

Fitness decisions require accurate information on the cause of the effusion and its prognosis. When inflammatory effusions resolve, they frequently leave behind an area of pleural thickening, and adhesions that obliterate the pleural space. If extensive, this thickening can restrict lung movement and produce chest discomfort and breathlessness on exertion.

A *pneumothorax* may be a primary, 'spontaneous' event or a complication of trauma or of other, serious lung disease such as emphysema, pulmonary fibrosis, or cystic fibrosis. The incidence of primary pneumothorax is five times higher in men; it characteristically afflicts young, tall men and causes symptoms of breathlessness and chest pain commensurate with its size; a tension pneumothorax is potentially lethal. Treatment depends on the extent of the air leak and ranges from simple observation to intrapleural drainage. The natural incidence of recurrence after spontaneous pneumothorax is about 50% over 4 years; but is virtually eliminated by surgical pleurodesis. The occurrence (and recurrence) of pneumothorax is of concern in certain occupations where sudden changes in ambient air pressure are expected; specific guidance is available (see 'Special work problems and restrictions').

At work, asbestos exposure frequently causes *pleural plaques*, which are circumscribed areas of hyaline fibrosis on the parietal pleura that may gradually calcify. Plaques are discovered radiographically (and seldom become evident within 15 years of first exposure) and produce no impairment of lung function or other disability. Their presence does not correlate well with that of pulmonary fibrosis (asbestosis), nor do they predicate the occurrence of mesothelioma (which is related to levels of exposure, but is no more common in those who develop plaques than in those who do not). They tend to be discovered accidentally and do not require work restriction or redeployment. In contrast, *diffuse pleural thickening*, which may follow a pleural effusion induced by heavy exposure to asbestos, can cause restriction of lung expansion, dyspnoea, and work limitation. The condition is increasingly rare in UK men of working age.

Smoking

Smoking is a major cause of respiratory disability, being the principal cause of both COPD and lung cancer, the two conditions that together account for the majority of deaths from primary respiratory disease; the heavier the smoking, the greater the risk. It is clearly good preventive practice to offer help and support to those who want to stop smoking and to make the workforce generally aware of the risks. The benefits of smoking cessation in COPD have already been discussed. A review of smoking cessation interventions in the workplace[43] concluded that measures directed towards individual smokers, including counselling and pharmacological treatment of nicotine addiction, all increase the likelihood of quitting (the effects being similar to those when offered outside the workplace). Self-help interventions and social support seem to be less effective. There is only limited evidence that participation in cessation programmes can be increased by competitions and incentives organized by the employer.

In the past, some 600 premature deaths annually in the UK could be attributed to passive workplace smoking,[44] a figure about three times higher than the annual number of deaths from industrial accidents. Legislation in the UK no longer permits smoking in any wholly or substantially enclosed workplace used by more than one person, or in any vehicle used for business purposes; employers are not obliged to provide an outside smoking area.

Special work problems and restrictions

Sometimes work is conducted in adverse environments, or in safety-critical roles characterized by a requirement for high standards of respiratory fitness. Such is the case for airline pilots and cabin crew, commercial and military divers, caisson workers, and members of the armed forces, security, and rescue services. A number of these work activities involve changes in gas pressure and composition, and the use of breathing apparatus to extend the range of hostile environments in which work can be conducted; and all require a general level of fitness that transcends simple respiratory health.

Recommended minimum fitness standards for workers in the UK armed services are laid down in a Joint Services System of Medical Classification (JSP 950). New applicants with certain respiratory diseases such as active TB or bronchiectasis are normally rejected, but if disease appears for the first time in service the worker is individually assessed. Current asthma, or recurrent wheeze requiring recent treatment (within the past 4 years), is treated similarly; while those with a more distant history are tested for exercise-induced decrements of FEV_1. The occurrence of pneumothorax requires individual assessment, and depends on the nature of the work and the success or otherwise of surgical treatment.

Each of the UK's armed services uses the 'PULHHEEMS' system to rank fitness for a number of physical and mental attributes against an eight-point scale of descriptors. Respiratory fitness is not separately identified in the rubric, although the P scale (physical fitness) encompasses cardiorespiratory fitness. Between services and between jobs there may be some differences; for example, the fitness standards in RAF air crew are more stringent than for ground personnel, such as engineers and technicians. However, for many jobs the minimum standard (fit with training for heavy manual work, including lifting and climbing, but not to endure severe or prolonged strain) precludes sufferers of significant respiratory disease.

Firefighters are required to operate in very adverse environments, to wear breathing apparatus, and to perform physically arduous tasks. Due to the potential to be exposed to asbestos during or after a fire, a doctor should perform asbestos medicals on firefighters at intervals of not more than 3 years. UK standards also require them to have their FEV_1 and FVC measured by a doctor, and to have their aerobic capacity measured in a step test prior to employment. The regulations stipulate that a duly qualified medical practitioner must be satisfied that these measurements are compatible with the fitness requirements of firefighting. The Fire and Rescue Services Act 2004 has permitted an individual approach to fitness assessment in fire service personnel, matching the requirements of the Equality Act 2010. Approximate standards have evolved on the basis of careful job analysis and the separation of operational from other roles. However, current guidance recognizes that individuals with the same diagnosis may differ considerably in the severity of their condition, and advice on respiratory restrictions (still evolving) is less prescriptive than hitherto. Rescue workers may encounter irritant or more occasionally sensitizing fumes and the many products of combustion; some of these will exacerbate asthma, and some, including products of PVC combustion, may incite new asthma (reactive airways dysfunction syndrome). Poorly controlled asthma on application often leads to rejection; if there is a prior history, or disease develops during employment, the circumstances should be individually assessed, but recurrent, severe, or refractory symptoms may precipitate medical retirement. Most firefighters with well-controlled asthma, however, are able to function effectively, including when wearing breathing apparatus. Severe reductions in FEV_1 and FEV_1/FVC ratio in firefighters with COPD may be incompatible with active firefighting, and close monitoring is advocated in the case, for example, of restrictive lung disease. The occurrence of pneumothorax should trigger individual review, but a successful pleurodesis may enable active duties to continue. Finally, the development of lung cancer would lead to rejection or retirement, but a successfully resected benign tumour is not a definite bar.

The fitness standards of pilots and divers, and the physiological demands of their work are described in Chapters 15 and 16. In new entrants, a history of spontaneous pneumothorax (untreated by pleurodesis), poorly controlled asthma, or other obstructive respiratory disease may be a bar to employment. In established workers who develop chest disease, the criteria are slightly less stringent: it may, for example, be possible for well-controlled asthmatics, or patients with a pleurectomy or pleurodesis, to continue as members of an air crew.

Key points

- Occupational lung diseases occur as a direct result of workplace exposure to metals, dusts, fumes, smoke, or biological agents. These disorders include asthma, bronchitis, interstitial lung disease (pneumoconiosis and occupational hypersensitivity pneumonitis), and tumours.
- Occupational asthma begins during adulthood and can be caused by immunological (latency period between exposure and symptoms) or non-immunological stimuli (absence of a latency period and following exposure to a high level of an irritant agent). As it is estimated that 5–25% of all adult-onset asthma cases are occupationally related, occupational asthma should be suspected and evaluated in every patient with adult-onset asthma.
- COPD is a common condition with a high mortality. It results from complex interactions between genetic and clinical risk factors. Some of the clinical risk factors for COPD can be modified, thereby reducing the rate of lung function decline. Smoking cessation is the most important way to reduce the rate of lung function decline and the risk of developing COPD. Influenza and pneumococcal vaccination can help reduce infections and exacerbations. Whenever possible, occupational exposure to particulate matter, dusts, gases, and fumes should be avoided or reduced.
- Pneumoconiosis results from inhalation and deposition of inorganic particles and mineral dust with subsequent reactions of the lung (e.g. silica, coal, talc, asbestos, iron, tin, barium, beryllium, and cobalt). This is usually diagnosed by a positive exposure history and suggestive radiographic presentation. A programme of regular surveillance in high-risk professions helps to obviate this problem. Occupational exposure to certain organic dusts, moulds, and chemicals can lead to hypersensitivity pneumonitis, an inflammatory reaction that is reversible if exposure is stopped in the acute or subacute phases.
- There is a clear association with occupational exposure to asbestos and the subsequent development of lung cancer. Tobacco smokers exposed to asbestos have a greatly increased risk of lung cancer, in addition to mesothelioma. In the context of lung cancer, chromium and arsenic are the other commonly associated toxins. Occupationally related lung cancers may also arise in nickel refining, exposure to polycyclic aromatic hydrocarbons, cadmium compounds, diesel exhaust, bis-chloromethyl, and chloromethyl methyl ethers. Silica is probably also a lung carcinogen, albeit a relatively weak one.

Useful websites

Health and Safety Executive (HSE). Asbestos regulations	http://www.hse.gov.uk/asbestos/mslw1-licensed.pdf http://www.hse.gov.uk/pubns/ms31.pdf
HSE. Asthma	http://www.hse.gov.uk/pubns/guidance/g402.pdf
HSE. Health surveillance	http://www.hse.gov.uk/pubns/priced/healthsurveillance.pdf
The National Institute for Occupational Safety and Health (NIOSH). Spirometry software	https://www.cdc.gov/niosh/topics/spirometry/spirola-software.html
Epworth sleepiness score	http://epworthsleepinessscale.com/about-the-ess/
STOP-BANG questionnaire	http://www.stopbang.ca/osa/screening.php
National Institute for Health and Care Excellence (NICE). Guidelines	https://www.nice.org.uk/guidance
Driver and Vehicle Licensing Agency (DVLA). Assessing fitness to drive	https://www.gov.uk/government/uploads/system/uploads/attachment_data/file/652720/assessing-fitness-to-drive-a-guide-for-medical-professionals.pdf

References

1. **British Thoracic Society**. The burden of lung disease: a statistics report from the British Thoracic Society. 2006. Available at: http://www.brit-thoracic.org.uk/Portals/0/Library/BTS%20Publications/burden_of_lung_disease.pdf.
2. **British Lung Foundation**. Lung Disease in the UK; big picture statistics. 2016. Available at: https://statistics.blf.org.uk/lung-disease-uk-big-picture.
3. **Townsend MC, Occupational and Environmental Lung Disorders Committee**. Spirometry in the occupational health setting – 2011 update (ACOEM guidance statement). *J Occup Environ Med* 2011;**53**:569–84.
4. **Culver BH.** How should the lower limit of the normal range be defined? *Respir Care* 2012;**57**:136–45.
5. **De Matteis S, Iridoy-Zulet AA, Aaron S, Swann A, Cullinan P.** A new spirometry-based algorithm to predict occupational pulmonary restrictive impairment. *Occup Med (Lond)* 2016;**66**:50–3.
6. **Medical Research Council on the Aetiology of Chronic Bronchitis**. Standardized questionnaires on respiratory symptoms. *Br Med J* 1960;**ii**:665.
7. **Occupational Safety and Health Administration**. Standards. Available at: https://www.osha.gov/pls/oshaweb/owadisp.show_document?p_table=STANDARDS&p_id=10055.
8. **Health and Safety Executive**. Health surveillance for those exposed to respirable crystalline silica (RCS). Supplementary guidance for occupational health professionals. 2015 (amended January 2016). Available at: http://www.hse.gov.uk/pubns/books/healthsurveillance.htm.
9. **Aaron SD, Vandemheen KL, FitzGerald JM, et al.** Reevaluation of diagnosis in adults with physician-diagnosed asthma. *JAMA* 2017;**317**:269–79.

10. **Stenton SC, Beach JR, Avery AJ, Hendrick DJ.** The value of questionnaires and spirometry in asthma surveillance programmes in the workplace. *Occup Med (Lond)* 1993;**43**:203–6.

11. **Scottish Intercollegiate Guidelines Network, British Thoracic Society.** British guideline on the management of asthma: a national clinical guideline. Revised 2016. Available at: https://www.brit-thoracic.org.uk/document-library/clinical-information/asthma/btssign-asthma-guideline-2016.

12. **Henneberger PK, Redlich CA, Callahan DB, et al.** An official American Thoracic Society Statement: work-exacerbated asthma. *Am J Respir Crit Care Med* 2011;**184**:368–78.

13. **Baur X, Huber H, Degens PO, Allmers H, Ammon J.** Relation between occupational asthma case history, bronchial methacholine challenge, and specific challenge test in patients with suspected occupational asthma. *Am J Ind Med* 1998;**33**:114–22.

14. **Malo JL, Ghezzo H, L'Archeveque J, Lagier F, Perrin B, Cartier A.** Is the clinical history a satisfactory means of diagnosing occupational asthma? *Am Rev Respir Dis* 1991;**143**:528–32.

15. **Brant A, Nightingale S, Berriman J, et al.** Supermarket baker's asthma: how accurate is routine health surveillance? *Occup Environ Med* 2005;**62**:395–9.

16. **Fishwick D, Barber CM, Bradshaw LM, et al.** Standards of care for occupational asthma: an update. *Thorax* 2012;**67**:278–80.

17. **Nicholson P, Cullinan P, Burge P, Boyle C.** *Occupational Asthma: Prevention, Identification, and Management: Systematic Review and Recommendations.* London: British Occupational Health Research Foundation; 2010. Available at: http://www.bohrf.org.uk/downloads/OccupationalAsthmaEvidenceReview-Mar2010.pdf.

18. **Moore VC, Jaakkola MS, Burge PS.** A systematic review of serial peak expiratory flow measurements in the diagnosis of occupational asthma. *Ann Respir Med* 2010;**1**:31–44.

19. **Moore VC, Jaakkola MS, Burge CB, et al.** A new diagnostic score for occupational asthma: the area between the curves (ABC score) of peak expiratory flow on days at and away from work. *Chest* 2009;**135**:307–14.

20. **de Groene GJ, Pal TM, Beach J, et al.** Workplace interventions for treatment of occupational asthma. *Cochrane Database Syst Rev* 2011;**5**:CD006308.

21. **Health and Safety Executive.** Health surveillance for occupational asthma. G402. Available at: http://www.hse.gov.uk/pubns/guidance/g402.pdf.

22. **Merget R, Pham N, Schmidtke M, et al.** Medical surveillance and long-term prognosis of occupational allergy due to platinum salts. *Int Arch Occup Environ Health* 2017;**90**:73–81.

23. **National Institute for Health and Care Excellence.** Chronic obstructive pulmonary disease in adults. Quality standard [QS10]. 2016. Available at: https://www.nice.org.uk/guidance/qs10/chapter/introduction.

24. **Cullinan P.** Occupation and chronic obstructive pulmonary disease (COPD). *Br Med Bull* 2012;**104**:143–61.

25. **Celli BR, Cote CG, Marin JM, et al.** The body-mass index, airflow obstruction, dyspnea, and exercise capacity index in chronic obstructive pulmonary disease. *N Engl J Med* 2004;**350**:1005–12.

26. **National Institute for Health and Care Excellence.** Chronic obstructive pulmonary disease. Clinical guideline [CG101]. 2010. Available at: http://www.nice.org.uk/nicemedia/live/13029/49397/49397.pdf.

27. **Global Initiative for Chronic Obstructive Lung Disease (GOLD).** Global Strategy for the Diagnosis, Management, and Prevention of COPD. 2017. Available at: www.goldcopd.org.

28. **National Institute for Health and Care Excellence.** Stop smoking interventions and services. NICE guideline [NG92]. 2018. Available at: https://www.nice.org.uk/guidance/ng92.

29. **Wagner GR.** Asbestosis and silicosis. *Lancet* 1997;**349**:1311–5.

30. **Health and Safety Executive**. *Guidance for Appointed Doctors on the Control of Asbestos Regulations*. London: HSE Books; 2011.

31. **International Labour Office**. *Guidelines for the Use of ILO International Classification of Radiographs of Pneumoconioses*. Geneva: International Labour Office; 1980.

32. **Barber CM, Wiggans RE, Carder M, Agius R.** Epidemiology of occupational hypersensitivity pneumonitis; reports from the SWORD scheme in the UK from 1996 to 2015. *Occup Environ Med* 2017;**74**:528–30.

33. **Public Health England**. Healthcare worker vaccination: clinical evidence (updated August 2016). Available at: http://www.nhsemployers.org/~/media/Employers/Publications/Flu%20Fighter/flu%20 fighter%20clinical%20evidence%20Aug%202016.pdf.

34. **National Institute for Health and Care Excellence**. Tuberculosis. NICE guideline [NG33]. 2016. Available at: https://www.nice.org.uk/guidance/ng33/chapter/Recommendations#preventing-tb.

35. **Lallukka T, Kaikkonen R, Harkanen T, et al.** Sleep and sickness absence: a nationally representative register-based follow-up study. *Sleep* 2014;**37**:1413–25.

36. **Simonds AK.** Abnormal sleep conditions and work. In: Newman Taylor AJ, Cullinan P, Blanc A, Pickering A (eds), *Parkes' Occupational Lung Disorders*, 4th edn, pp. 495–506. Boca Raton, FL: CRC Press; 2016.

37. **Arndt JT, Owens J, Crouch M, Stahl J, Carskadon MA.** Neurobehavioral performance of residents after heavy night call vs after alcohol ingestion. *JAMA* 2005;**294**:1025–33.

38. **Salminen S, Oksanen T, Vahtera J, et al.** Sleep disturbances as a predictor of occupational injuries among public sector workers. *J Sleep Res* 2010;**19**:207–13.

39. **Gurubhagavatula I, Sullivan S, Meoli A, et al.** Management of obstructive sleep apnea in commercial motor vehicle operators: recommendations of the AASM Sleep and Transportation Safety Awareness Task Force. *J Clin Sleep Med* 2017;**13**:745–58.

40. **Brambilla E, Travis WD.** Lung cancer. In: Stewart BW, Wild CP (eds), *World Cancer Report*, pp. 489–508. Lyon: World Health Organization; 2014.

41. **Samet JM.** Health benefits of smoking cessation. *Clin Chest Med* 1991;**12**:669–79.

42. **Rake C, Gilham C, Hatch J, Darnton A, Hodgson J, Peto J.** Occupational, domestic and environmental mesothelioma risks in the British population: a case-control study. *Br J Cancer* 2009;**100**:1175–83.

43. **Cahill K, Lancaster T.** Workplace interventions for smoking cessation. *Cochrane Database Syst Rev* 2014;**2**:CD003440.

44. **Jamrozik K.** Estimate of deaths attributable to passive smoking among UK adults: database analysis. *BMJ* 2005;**330**:812.

Chapter 28

Dermatological disorders

Hanaa Sayed and John English

Introduction

The skin acts as a protective barrier against a number of hazards within our environment. These hazards can be *chemical* (e.g. acids, alkalis, solvents, or oils), *biological* (e.g. bacteria, plant allergens, or raw food), or *physical* (e.g. ultraviolet (UV) light or mechanical shearing forces). In some situations, the defensive properties of the skin are exceeded, resulting in cuts, grazes, inflammation, ulceration, infection, and occasionally malignant change. Exposure to hazardous substances at work can cause harm in several ways. Substances absorbed by the skin can cause systemic diseases. Other substances can cause 'local effects': corrosive substances causing burns, irritant substances causing irritant contact dermatitis, and sensitizing substances causing allergic contact dermatitis.[1] The risk factors for breakdown of skin defences can be categorized as (i) *occupational*—common at-risk groups are cleaners, food handlers, hairdressers, and workers in contact with cutting fluids; and (ii) *non-occupational*—where genetic predisposition to skin disorders is an important factor. Workers with non-occupational skin disorders can suffer exacerbations of their underlying dermatological condition in workplaces where the environment is hot and humid or extremely cold or dry.

Prevalence

During 2013–2016, the Labour Force Survey estimated that 6000 new cases of skin problems annually were caused or made worse by work. Prevalence has been declining since the late 1990s, but has plateaued in recent years.[1] Among 1579 new cases of skin disease reported by dermatologists to the EPIDERM scheme (part of The Health and Occupation Reporting (THOR) network) in 2015[1]:

- 80% were contact dermatitis (equally caused by allergens and irritants)
- 4% were non-cancerous dermatoses (mainly contact urticaria and nail conditions)
- 16% were skin cancers.

In 2015, 45 cases of skin disease were assessed for Industrial Injuries Disablement Benefit. Based on reporting to the THOR general practitioners scheme (2013–2015), skin diseases accounted for around 1% of total sickness absence days certified due to occupational illnesses. For contact dermatitis cases specifically (2006–2012), a sickness

Table 28.1 Occupations with the highest rate of dermatitis

Occupation	Rate of dermatitis (cases per 100,000 workers per year) in 2015–2016
Florists	109
Hairdressers and barbers	81
Beauticians	73
Cooks	61
Metal working operatives	54

Source: data from EPIDERM (2016). *Work-related skin diseases in Great Britain*. London, UK: EPIDERM. Copyright © EPIDERM 2016. Available at: http://www.hse.gov.uk/statistics/causdis/dermatitis/skin.pdf?pdf=skin.

certificate was issued in 9%, and 16% were referred to a hospital specialist or other health practitioner.[1]

Contact with soaps and detergents and working with wet hands are the most common causes of occupational contact dermatitis (Table 28.1).

Dermatitis

Occupational dermatitis can be defined as an inflammation of the skin caused by work, and is classified into allergic or irritant contact dermatitis. These may be indistinguishable by clinical history and examination alone, and investigation usually requires skin patch testing. If an occupational cause is identified, a reduction in exposure to irritants or allergens in the workplace is needed to control symptoms. Contact dermatitis is treated with moisturizers and topical steroids.

Eczema

Atopic eczema affects one in five children. In later life, it can render an employee more susceptible to the effects of skin irritants. If the condition was severe in childhood, and particularly if the hands were involved, then the risk for developing (non-allergic) dermatitis in employment with irritants is significant. This should not preclude employment, however it should be considered in the risk assessment at pre-placement.[2] Atopics with a history only of asthma or hay fever do not have an increased susceptibility. There is no evidence that atopics are at increased risk of allergic contact reactions, and clinical experience suggests that they are less likely to develop sensitization to contact allergens than non-atopics. However, all atopics are more likely to develop contact urticaria, asthma, and anaphylaxis from natural rubber latex, and preventative measures must be considered.[3] Provided they are closely monitored and the use of personal protective equipment (PPE) renders the worker symptom free, it is sometimes reasonable to allow workers with allergic contact dermatitis to continue working with the sensitizer.

Many organizations, particularly those in healthcare, have policies to limit glove-wearing at work for specific tasks. Latex-free gloves should replace latex where possible. The requirement for hand washing between patients has increased, to reduce methicillin-resistant *Staphylococcus aureus* (MRSA) infections, and this has increased the risk of dermatitis. Trainee healthcare workers with active skin involvement or a past history of severe eczema should receive a supervised programme of hand care and be followed up if symptoms occur.

Other occupations at risk from irritant contact dermatitis are domestic cleaning, bar work, printing, construction work, motor vehicle maintenance, horticulture, and agriculture. Extremes of temperature and low humidity can also aggravate atopic eczema (Box 28.1).

In certain occupations, hand involvement can also pose a risk of *bacterial* contamination. Eczematous skin is more prone than normal skin to be colonized with *Staph. aureus* and/or *Streptococcus pyogenes*. In one study, 43% of nurses with occupational skin diseases were colonized with MRSA.[4] Atopic dermatitis and severe hand eczema are the main risk factors for colonization. Densities of *Staph. aureus* may exceed $10^6/cm^2$, leading to clinically apparent infection (impetigo); non-involved skin is colonized in up to 90% of individuals. Organisms that colonize or contaminate the skin surface are dispersed into the environment during the natural shedding of skin scales. This can have serious implications in healthcare (risk of patient infection), catering (food poisoning), and the pharmaceutical industry (product contamination). Active eczema in these occupations therefore carries a risk of infective spread and requires individual assessment. However, providing adequate hand hygiene measures can be performed, this risk is negated.[5]

Box 28.1 Advice to avoid irritant contact dermatitis

- Wash hands with lukewarm water.
- Rinse and dry hands thoroughly.
- Alcohol gel is preferable (less irritant) to soap.
- Use protective gloves. Ensure they are intact, clean, and dry.
- Wear gloves for shortest possible time.
- Wear inner cotton gloves when occlusive gloves are needed for more than 10 minutes.
- Apply lipid-rich moisturizers during and after work to the entire hand.
- Avoid hand products with fragrance and preservatives.
- Follow the same advice at home.

It has been shown that, even where the occupation provides no hazard to the skin, around half of those with a previous history of atopic eczema may develop new or exacerbations of pre-existing hand eczema. When hand eczema develops in an atopic person exposed to a skin irritant, it is often difficult for the patient, their trade union, and insurers to accept that the condition may not be occupational. In claims for compensation, industrial injury assessors and expert witnesses will often allow patients the benefit of the doubt.[6]

Irritants can be chemical, biological, mechanical, or physical. Repeated and prolonged contact with water, *wet work* (e.g. more than 20 hand washes or having wet hands for more than 2 hours per shift), is likely to lead to irritant contact dermatitis. Wet work can cause the skin to overhydrate. Dermatitis from wet work is common in hairdressing, metal machining, catering, cleaning, and healthcare.[7]

Seborrhoeic eczema may be aggravated by exposure to chemical irritants, but hot environments will contribute most to the risk of flare-ups. As the hands are unaffected, restrictions for occupations involving wet work are not required. The main problem is shedding of skin scales, with risks of bacterial contamination similar to those found in atopics.

Stasis (varicose) eczema, which may be associated with varicose ulceration, can be aggravated by prolonged standing. Clinical management requires extra support compression for the legs. Work adjustments include the following:

◆ Encourage walking regularly to increase venous return.

◆ Leg elevation may be required during rest periods.

◆ Avoid prolonged standing.

◆ Allow frequent change of posture.

Discoid (nummular) eczema carries few implications for employment. It is treatable with topical therapies and rarely aggravated by the work environment. Sometimes it can present as a feature of chromate dermatitis and soluble oil dermatitis, albeit usually associated with coexisting hand dermatitis.

Asteatotic eczema (eczema craquelé) is caused by drying of the skin. It commonly affects the lower limbs. Low humidity (air conditioning, vehicle heaters), frequent showering, and use of degreasing chemicals (soaps, shampoos) cause skin to dry and crack. It can be prevented or treated by minimizing the causative factors (Table 28.2 and Table 28.3).

Other non-cancerous skin disorders

Chronic urticaria can be aggravated by temperature (heat and rarely cold) and emotional stresses. Cholinergic urticaria is specifically triggered by exercise. Most forms of urticaria can be controlled by adequate doses (sometimes greater than the licensed amount) of non-sedating antihistamines during the daytime. Short-acting sedative antihistamines (e.g. chlorpheniramine) may be added at night. Sedative antihistamines are contraindicated

Table 28.2 Examples of skin irritants and sensitizers, and associated occupations

Example occupations	Examples of irritants
General manufacturing, healthcare	Alcohols
General manufacturing, engineering	Degreasers
Engineering	Cutting oils, coolants
Food, cleaning, beauty, healthcare	Disinfectants
Motor vehicle repair, petrochemical industry, chemical production	Petroleum products
Food, cleaning, beauty, healthcare	Soaps, cleaning products
Food, cleaning, beauty, healthcare	Wet work
Example occupations	**Examples of sensitizers**
Engineering, manufacture of hard metal, foundries	Cobalt
Plating, engineering	Chromium, chromates
Hair and beauty, product manufacture	Cosmetics, fragrances
Construction	Epoxy resins
Plating, hair and beauty, engineering	Nickel
Florists, horticulture, agriculture	Plants
Product manufacture	Preservatives
Construction, healthcare	Resins, acrylates

where alertness is required (e.g. operating machinery or driving). Where urticaria is associated with natural rubber latex, the provision of a latex-free environment is needed to prevent anaphylaxis.

Photosensitive dermatoses and, to a lesser extent, *vitiligo* may make outdoor work inadvisable. Up to 80% of available UV light penetrates through cloud cover. Sufficient

Table 28.3 Examples of causes of contact urticaria and associated occupations

Example of occupations	Agents
Animal husbandry, farmers, vets	Cow dander
Cooks, food preparation workers, kitchen workers	Food, animal products
Kitchen workers, bakers, millers	Flour, grains
Healthcare, animal husbandry, vets, laboratory workers	Natural rubber latex

protection in the form of clothing and high-factor sunscreens are needed. The latter should be applied frequently around the middle of the day (e.g. 10 a.m., noon, and 2 p.m.). Many medications (e.g. tetracyclines, amiodarone) can increase the risk of photosensitivity.

Acne, if severe and nodulocystic, contraindicates work in hot, humid environments as severe exacerbations can occur. There is no evidence that pre-existing acne increases the risk of oil-induced acne, which is caused by occlusion of the pilosebaceous units in the skin. Acne responds slowly to treatment. Even the most resistant cases can be treated with systemic isotretinoin. Being an office worker versus being unemployed or being a house-wife was associated with acne (odds ratio 2.24; 95% confidence interval 1.24–4.09) in one multicentre study in females.[10]

Viral warts have a predilection for the hands and are a source of cosmetic embarrassment. Most involute spontaneously over time. They pose little risk to fellow workers as adults typically acquire immunity in childhood. In occupations involving food handling, patient care, and public contact, pressure often exists to actively treat the condition. Butchers and abattoir workers are at special risk of hand warts (the causative papillomavirus can in-fect meat and poultry). These occupations are associated with repeated minor trauma to the skin of the hands, so spread and cross-contamination occur easily. Active treatment is justified for these groups. *Verrucas* (also papillomaviruses) pose little risk to others. Restrictions are not required for swimming pool attendants, divers, and workers sharing showering facilities.

Fungal skin infections are common. The antifungal action of sebum discourages fungal growth in adults. Therefore, ringworm in the scalp (tinea capitis) from cats and dogs (*Microsporum canis*) is rare in adults. More aggressive fungi found on cattle and hedge-hogs can grow in the presence of sebum, leading to hair loss (alopecia) and secondary bacterial infections (kerion).

The common fungus *Trichophyton rubrum* thrives in warm moist body locations (e.g. between the toes (tinea pedis) and in the groin (tinea cruris). It spreads easily in oc-cupations that require communal showering or the use of occlusive footwear. Infected individuals should not be excluded from work, but diagnosis and treatment should be initiated. Athlete's foot (tinea pedis) is commonly misdiagnosed. One-third of suspected cases arise from other causes. Unresponsive cases may be due to occlusive maceration be-tween the toes, with overgrowth of commensal bacteria (*Staph. pyogenes*). This disorder can be treated with appropriate footwear, wedging toes apart with cotton wool rolls, and adequate drying. Ringworm on the body (tinea corporis) is overdiagnosed and confused with other skin conditions (e.g. psoriasis, granuloma annulare).

Although *zoonoses* can be acquired by humans from animals, they cannot be trans-ferred between humans. No restrictions are required for infected employees.

Bacterial skin infections are transmissible to other employees. The commonest, im-petigo (usually caused by *Staph. aureus*) requires prompt local treatment. Widespread infections may require temporary exclusion from the workplace, although the risk of cross-contamination becomes minimal after 2 days of treatment. Boils (carbuncles) are also usually caused by *Staph. aureus*, but the potential for contamination is less than for impetigo. Staphylococci can grow in foods, releasing endotoxins that cause serious food poisoning. Therefore, occupations involving food handling require exclusion pending clinical resolution.

Hyperhidrosis affecting the hands may cause problems in engineering, as sweat can corrode ferrous metalwork (these employees are known as 'rusters'). Hyperhidrosis may be disadvantageous in public relation jobs that require frequent hand shaking. Botulinum toxin has revolutionized treatment.

Psoriasis is present in 1 in 20 persons. Most cases are minor and not apparent even to the sufferer. Psoriasis may be aggravated occupationally by physical or chemical trauma (Köebner phenomenon). The commonest presentation is with psoriatic knuckle pads. The disease can be unpredictable, with sudden extensive flare-ups. Rarely, this can involve the entire body surface. Psoriasis typically develops in the early teens and twenties, but can start at any age. With adequate treatment and compliance it is possible to control most cases. Psoriasis may undergo spontaneous remission. Individuals with psoriasis from early childhood and with more than 40% of the surface skin affected are the most difficult to control.

Psoriasis affecting the palms and soles can be particularly troublesome at work. Affected individuals are unable to wear protective shoes and have difficulty with work involving heavy manual handling, the construction and service industries. Cosmetic embarrassment can compromise emotional and social well-being.[11,12] Some chemicals and solvents can exacerbate existing psoriasis. Solvents (e.g. trichloroethylene) degrease the skin, causing drying, cracking, and Köebner phenomenon. Soap, detergents, washing-up liquids, and shampoos also have a degreasing effect. However, friction is the main perpetuating factor in the hands and feet. It is widely accepted that stressful work can be associated with exacerbations. Disease-modifying drugs have little impact on occupational psoriasis which is usually localized to the hands due to friction and they are reserved for severe widespread psoriasis.

Psoriatic arthropathy can affect mobility, and pain can increase sickness absence. Although psoriatic lesions can become infected, work in catering or nursing is generally tolerated (with monitoring by the occupational health (OH) department).

Alopecia, particularly in women, can cause mental anguish that affects attendance at work. Treatable causes (e.g. endocrine disorders, drugs, or iron deficiency) should be excluded. Wearing a wig sometimes aids return to work.

Disorders of pigmentation, particularly on the face (vitiligo or hyperpigmentation), can cause embarrassment, especially in people of Asian or African descent. Cosmetic camouflage can be helpful.

Skin cancer

In 2014, 15,419 new cases of melanoma and 132,000 new cases of non-melanoma skin cancer were recorded in the UK.[13] Few arise from occupational causes. Epithelioma of the scrotum due to contact with mineral oils is now rare, although cases have been reported at other anatomical sites (arms and hands). UV radiation from excessive exposure to sunlight is currently a major cause of skin cancer. Others include X-rays, arsenic, tar products, and industrial burns (Table 28.4).[14] UV radiation from welding is a potential risk factor for non-melanotic skin cancer among welders. Exposure to nickel and hexavalent chromium in welding fumes is associated with increased cancer risk.[15]

Basal cell carcinoma, or rodent ulcer, is the commonest skin cancer. It is frequently found on the face and is associated with exposure to sunlight. Fair-skinned expatriates working in sunny climates are at particular risk.

Squamous cell carcinomas commonly occur on hands, ears, and lips. Sunlight, chronic trauma, and chronic inflammation are aetiological factors.

Malignant melanoma is one of the most aggressive skin cancers. Its incidence has increased dramatically over the last few decades (over 11,000 cases annually in the UK), probably due to greater sunlight exposure. Some reports indicate a higher prevalence in aircrew, possibly because of cosmic radiation, but high sunlight exposure may also contribute.[16]

The estimated total attributable fraction for cutaneous malignant melanoma in one study was 2% (48 deaths (in 2012) and 241 registrations (in 2011) attributable to occupational exposure to solar radiation in Britain). Higher exposure of larger numbers of men increases risk compared to women. Industries of concern are construction, agriculture, public administration, defence, and land transport.[17]

Common primary cancers that metastasize to skin are breast, lung, and leukaemia. Surgical excision is the most effective treatment for primary skin cancer. Return to work is normally possible after excision and wound healing. A poor cosmetic result occasionally affects the outcome.

Table 28.4 Examples of agents that cause skin cancer and associated occupations.

Agents	Type of work
UV rays from the sun	Outdoor work
Coal tar and derivatives	Coal tar handling, coal gasification, coal tar distillation
Polycyclic aromatic hydrocarbons (PAHs)	Petroleum refining, coal tar distillation
Ionizing radiation	Radiation-related work
Arsenic	Metal ore handling and smelting, pesticide manufacturing
Coke	Coke processing
Soot	Chimney cleaning

General considerations

Many myths surround skin disorders. One of the commonest is that eczema is contagious. Bacterial contamination can occur, but the risk to work colleagues is small. However, individuals are sometimes shunned and excluded from communal activities. Health education should be provided to line manager and colleagues.

During an outbreak of dermatitis in the workforce, cases may be falsely attributed to scabies, athlete's foot, psoriasis, constitutional eczema, symptomatic dermographism, and rosacea. If unions are involved or new work practices have been introduced then an emotionally charged situation can develop which requires skill to resolve. Intervention by an occupational physician or a dermatologist may alleviate concerns

Investigations

Patch testing, to identify delayed type IV hypersensitivity, is important in the investigation of persistent dermatitis. No employee should be advised to give up their work without the benefit of detailed patch test investigations at a regional centre. Patch testing will identify causes of acquired sensitization, facilitating avoidance/substitution of contact allergens, and preserving employment for most. However, it has no role in pre-placement screening, unless (pre-)existing dermatitis is incompletely investigated.

Prick testing pre-placement has little value apart from confirming atopy. If assessment for type 1 hypersensitivity is necessary, immunoglobulin E and radioallergosorbent test (RAST) blood tests are useful to confirm atopic tendency. However, only people with active atopic eczema carry a risk of developing dermatitis from irritants. So these tests add little to a good medical history and examination. RAST tests are also not 100% specific. In particular, some atopics have a strong positive reaction to latex and yet can handle latex with impunity, whereas some with negative antibodies develop anaphylaxis with minimal latex exposure. In this situation, a prick test can be more reliable, but in view of the risk of anaphylaxis, full resuscitation measures must be accessible.

Managing the worker with a skin condition

Rehabilitation of employees with skin ailments is usually possible even if s/he is working with a known irritant or sensitizer. If workplace adjustments or temporary redeployment can exclude exposure to the offending agent, a return to work can usually be effected prior to the complete resolution of the skin condition. Flexible or home working may minimize stigmatization in workers with skin disfigurements, preserving their psychosocial well-being and employment. However, some occupations with special safety needs may be considered unsuitable. Secondary skin infection may preclude employment in healthcare, food handling, and in the pharmaceutical industry. Individuals with widespread skin lesions may not be suitable for work in some industries because of a heightened personal risk. In the nuclear industry, extensive skin disease could reduce the protective barrier of the skin, provide a portal of entry, and make decontamination more difficult. In the sewage or waste disposal industry, there is a greater risk of exposure to infection.

A dermatology opinion is essential if employment is at risk because of a skin condition. Close collaboration between the OH professional, dermatologist, general practitioner, employer, and employee may achieve successful rehabilitation and return to work. Many individuals can be retained with adjustments or redeployment despite chronic skin disorders.

Prevention of occupational dermatoses starts by avoiding or reducing contact with causative materials using the hierarchy of control (elimination, substitution, engineering control, administrative controls, and PPE). PPE has a number of limitations: it can only protect the wearer, it has to be the right material and the right size and used properly, and it may limit the wearer's mobility. The continued effectiveness of PPE will depend on proper cleaning, maintenance, training, and supervision.

Natural rubber latex protein gloves can cause irritation and type I and type IV allergic reaction. Natural rubber latex proteins are substances hazardous to health under the Control of Substances Hazardous to Health (COSHH) Regulations 2002. Employers should provide non-latex gloves where possible.[18] Protection of the skin is mainly by using skincare products to maintain a stable and adequately hydrated barrier layer, including pre-work creams, cleansers, and moisturizers. Employees should be encouraged to examine their own skin and report all changes.

Management and prevention of occupational skin diseases

Following skin exposure to hazardous substances, visual checks for 'local effects' should be carried out, by the employee, their manager, or responsible person. Regular skin checks help to identify early skin effects, and demonstrate the adequacy of controls.[2] Health surveillance and skin checks can be carried out by an OH professional or a Responsible Person. Health surveillance should assess the condition of a new employee's skin before, or as soon as possible after, they start work and there should be periodic checks for the early signs of skin disease. Records must be kept securely and the employer should be informed of surveillance results.

At pre-placement assessment of occupations where the prevalence of occupational dermatitis is high, prospective employees should be made aware of the potential risks of the work and individuals with pre-existing skin problems encouraged to seek advice from the OH department.

Most alcohol-based hand rubs contain emollients which help prevent drying. Some studies report that nurses who routinely use alcohol rubs have less skin irritation and dryness than those using soap and water.[13] Alcohol hand rubs will sting if applied on broken skin. Such areas should be covered with waterproof plasters. Allergic contact dermatitis due to alcohol-based hand rubs is very rare.

Legal considerations

The COSHH Regulations and the Management of Health and Safety Regulations 1999 require that all employers assess risks, provide adequate controls, information, training, and (where appropriate), health surveillance.[19] It should be recognized that the risk of irritation or sensitization may be understated on health and safety data sheets. Training should include the characteristic features of the particular dermatoses and arrangements should exist to identify new cases. Employees should follow their training and cooperate with their employer. Health surveillance includes checking the skin for early signs of disease.[19]

Occupational dermatitis is reportable under the Reporting of Injuries, Diseases and Dangerous Occurrences Regulations (RIDDOR) 2013 when a registered medical practitioner confirms it is attributable to or exacerbated by work activity that involves significant exposure to a known skin sensitizer or irritant.[20] Where the skin condition causes impairment that has a 'substantial' and 'long-term' negative effect on the worker's ability to do normal daily activities, they will be considered disabled as defined in the Equality Act 2010. This includes disfigurement caused by skin disease.

Key points

♦ Irritant contact dermatitis is the commonest occupational skin disease in the UK.

♦ The distinction between allergic and irritant contact dermatitis is not always straightforward.

♦ Most skin conditions in the workplace are neither infectious nor contagious.

♦ Health surveillance under the COSHH Regulations includes control of exposure using the hierarchy of control and requires regular skin checks.

Useful websites

Health and Safety Executive. 'Skin at work' http://www.hse.gov.uk/skin

Health and Safety Executive. 'Packaging and labelling' http://www.hse.gov.uk/chemical-classification/labelling-packaging

Health and Safety Executive. 'Control of Substances Hazardous to Health (COSHH). Essentials guidance publications' http://www.hse.gov.uk/pubns/guidance/index.htm

Health and Safety Executive. The Control of Substances Hazardous to Health Regulations 2002. 'Approved Code of Practice and guidance (sixth edition)', 2013 http://www.hse.gov.uk/pubns/books/l5.htm

Health and Safety Executive. 'EH40/2005 Workplace exposure limits: Containing the list of workplace exposure limits for use with the Control of Substances Hazardous to Health Regulations (as amended)', 2018 http://www.hse.gov.uk/pUbns/priced/eh40.pdf

Health and Safety Executive. 'Preventing contact dermatitis and urticaria at work', 2015	http://www.hse.gov.uk/pubns/indg233.htm
Health and Safety Executive. 'Choosing the right gloves to protect skin: a guide for employers'	http://www.hse.gov.uk/skin/employ/gloves.htm
World Health Organization. 'Alcohol-based handrub risks/hazards'	http://www.who.int/gpsc/tools/faqs/abhr2/en/
Cancer Research UK. 'Melanoma skin cancer incidence'	http://www.cancerresearchuk.org/health-professional/cancer-statistics/statistics-by-cancer-type/skin-cancer#heading-Zero

References

1. **Health and Safety Executive**. Work-related skin diseases in Great Britain 2016. Available at: http://www.hse.gov.uk/statistics/causdis/dermatitis/skin.pdf?pdf=skin Last updated.
2. **Rystedt I.** Factors influencing the occurrence of hand eczema in adults with a history of atopic dermatitis in childhood. *Contact Dermatitis* 1985;**12**:185–91.
3. **Posch A, Chen Z, Raulf-Heimsoth M, et al.** Latex allergens. *Clin Exp Allergy* 1998;**28**:134–40.
4. **Brans R, Kolomanski K, Mentzel F, Vollmer U, Kaup O, John SM.** Colonisation with methicillin-resistant Staphylococcus aureus and associated factors among nurses with occupational skin diseases. *Occup Environ Med* 2016;**73**:670–5.
5. **Smedley J, Williams S, Peel P, Pedersen K, Dermatitis Guideline Development Group.** Management of occupational dermatitis in healthcare workers: a systematic review. *Occup Environ Med* 2012;**69**:276–9.
6. **Rystedt I.** Work related hand eczema in atopics. *Contact Dermatitis* 1985;**12**:164–71.
7. **Health and Safety Executive.** Dermatitis. Available at: http://www.hse.gov.uk/skin/employ/dermatitis.htm.
8. **Health and Safety Executive.** Examples of skin irritants and sensitisers, together with occupations where they occur. Available at: http://www.hse.gov.uk/skin/professional/causes/agentstable1.htm.
9. **Health and Safety Executive.** Examples of causes of contact urticaria and occupations where they occur. Available at: http://www.hse.gov.uk/skin/professional/causes/agentstable2.htm.
10. **Di Landro A, Cazzaniga S, Cusano F, et al.** Adult female acne and associated risk factors: results of a multicenter case-control study in Italy. *J Am Acad Dermatol* 2016;**75**:1134–41.
11. **Krueger G, Koo J, Lebwohl M, et al.** The impact of psoriasis on quality of life: results of a National Psoriasis Foundation patient-membership survey. *Arch Dermatol* 2001;**137**:280–4.
12. **Ginsburg IH, Link BG.** Psychosocial consequences of rejection and stigma feelings in psoriasis patients. *Int J Dermatol* 1993;**32**:587–91.
13. **World Health Organization.** Alcohol-based handrub risks/hazards. Available at: http://www.who.int/gpsc/tools/faqs/abhr2/en/.
14. **Health and Safety Executive.** Examples of agents that cause skin cancer and occupations where they occur. Available at: http://www.hse.gov.uk/skin/professional/causes/agentstable3.htm.
15. **Barkhordari A, Zare Sakhvidi MJ, Zare Sakhvidi F, Halvani G, Firoozichahak A, Shirali G.** Cancer risk assessment in welder's under different exposure scenarios. *Iran J Public Health* 2014;**43**:666–73.
16. **Sanlorenzo M, Wehner MR, Linos E, et al.** The risk of melanoma in airline pilots and cabin crew: a meta-analysis. *JAMA Dermatol* 2015;**151**:51–8.

17. **Rushton L, Hutchings SJ.** The burden of occupationally-related cutaneous malignant melanoma in Britain due to solar radiation. *Br J Cancer* 2017;**116**:536–9.

18. **Royal College of Physician, NHS Plus.** *Latex Allergy: Occupational Aspects of Management.* London: The Health and Work Development Unit; 2008. Available at: https://www.rcplondon.ac.uk/guidelines-policy/latex-allergy-occupational-aspects-management-2008.

19. **Health and Safety Executive.** Managing skin exposure risks at work. 2015. Available at: http://www.hse.gov.uk/pubns/priced/hsg262.pdf.

20. **Health and Safety Executive.** Reporting injuries, diseases and dangerous occurrences in health and social care: guidance for employers. 2013. Available at: http://www.hse.gov.uk/pubns/hsis1.pdf.

Chapter 29

Cancer survivorship and work

Philip Wynn and Elizabeth Murphy

Introduction

The overall cancer burden due to workplace exposures in the UK is estimated to be 5%.[1] Consequently, occupational health (OH) professionals are more likely to provide advice relating to the workplace impact of the common, non-work related, cancers. The average annual incidence of cancer in the UK between 2012 and 2014 for people aged between 20 and 64 years was over 121,000[2] with survival rates of more than 10 years in 50% of adults and 5 years in 82% of children.[3] There are currently 2 million people living with cancer in the UK and this number is predicted to increase by 3% annually, reflecting an increase in the incidence of cancer and improved survival rates.[4] UK clinical support services have been reconfigured to support the survivors of cancer with active lives for extended periods.[5] Returning to employment is a part of this strategy, and OH professionals are very likely to see adults seeking work after cancer treatment. As cancer is an age-related disorder, the increasing age of retirement in the UK may lead to an increase in the number of cancer survivors seeking advice. The psychological and social impact on employees with care responsibilities for relatives with cancer may also increase.[6] This chapter presents the published evidence regarding cancer survivorship and work capability, treatment and complications, rehabilitation, and occupational risk assessments for adult cancer survivors. (Specific cancers are addressed under the relevant systems chapters within this book.)

Cancer survivorship

Significant advances in cancer diagnosis and treatment over recent decades have led to better outcomes and an improved survival rate among both children and adults with cancer (Table 29.1)

Set against these improvements in clinical outcome and support for cancer survivors, evidence suggests that many encounter financial and occupational difficulties, including loss of income. Unemployment rates among adult cancer survivors who were employed at the time of diagnosis are higher at follow-up than the general population.[7] Although most working adults diagnosed with primary cancer return to work, a significant minority do not. Cancer survivorship is considered to encompass people who are

Table 29.1 Numbers of people living in the UK who have had a cancer diagnosis[4]

	UK	% of total
Total	2,080,000	100
Male	850,000	41
Female	1,230,000	59
Breast	570,000	27
Colorectal	243,000	12
Prostate	255,000	12
Lung	65,000	3
Other	946,000	46

Source: data from Maddams, J. et al. Projections of cancer prevalence in the United Kingdom, 2010–2040. *British Journal of Cancer*. 107, 1195–1202. Copyright © 2007 Springer Nature.

undergoing primary treatment, are in remission following treatment, show no symptoms of the disease following treatment, or are living with active or advanced cancer (Figure 29.1).

Employers will usually seek guidance from OH on how to manage employees who have developed a serious illness. Therefore, OH professionals are in a key position to coordinate the vocational rehabilitation of cancer survivors (Box 29.1).[8] Cancer can be treated effectively, but functional outcomes vary considerably (Box 29.2).

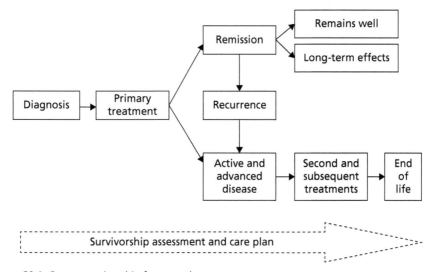

Figure 29.1 Cancer survivorship framework.

Box 29.1 Roles of OH professionals in relation to cancer survivors

◆ On commencement, assessment of applicants who have survived cancer in adult or childhood.
◆ Guidance on duration of cancer-related sickness absence.
◆ Vocational rehabilitation of employees newly diagnosed with cancer.
◆ Advice on long-term adjustments for employees returning to work after diagnosis and treatment, or affected by one of the long-term sequelae of cancer or its treatment.
◆ Advice on health and safety implications of cancer diagnosis and treatment.
◆ Advice on whether the ill health retirement provisions of occupational pensions are met.

Box 29.2 Outcomes after primary cancer diagnosis

◆ All evidence of cancer eliminated following primary treatment, have a period of remission, and are not affected by the illness for the rest of their lives (e.g. the majority of people diagnosed with breast cancer, colorectal cancer, and many other cancers).
◆ Treated successfully but giving rise to long-term side effects:
  • Problems with urination, bowel control, and sexuality in survivors of cancers of the uterus, bladder, or prostate.
  • Problems with insufficient hormone production in patients who survive cancers of the lymph glands or the brain.
  • An increased incidence of heart disease following breast or prostate cancer.
◆ Live with active cancer following treatment—for example, patients with lung and pancreatic cancer. Others will develop active and advanced cancer after a period of remission. Some of these enter further periods of remission after secondary or subsequent treatment. Typically, however, cancers become less responsive to treatment over time.
◆ Diagnosed with active or advanced cancer—may die from their illness within a matter of weeks or months.
◆ Live with cancer for many years without developing significant symptoms—they might die 'with' cancer but 'from' another cause.

Work capability

On average, long-term survivors of cancer report poorer health and well-being than the general population. Many are significantly affected, even among those who do return to work.[9–11] The long-term effects of cancer or cancer treatment can be defined as symptoms or changes to physical, psychological, or social function. These include a broad range of problems, which depend upon factors such as the primary site of the cancer and treatments administered. Approximately 25% of people treated for cancer experience a late effect that reduces their quality of life.[10] Of childhood cancer survivors, 67% go on to develop one or more late morbidities.[11] Survey data suggest that awareness of these late effects is low in patients surviving initial treatment and in their treating doctors.[12]

Estimates of the proportion of cancer survivors who return to work vary widely. A summary of the likelihood of return to work, based on a systematic review of the literature, is given in Table 29.2. Overall, this study found an unemployment rate higher in cancer survivors than healthy controls, with a relative risk of 1.4.[7]

Table 29.2 Employment rate and relative risk of being employed after a cancer diagnosis

Cancer type	% of cancer survivors unemployed at follow-up	% of cancer controls unemployed at follow-up	Range of mean periods of follow-up (years)	Relative Risk (95% CI) of unemployment
Breast	36	32	1–9	1.28 (1.11–1.49)
Blood	31	24	2–14	1.41 (0.95–2.09)
Gastrointestinal	49	33	2–3	1.44 (1.02–2.05)
Female reproductive system	49	38	2–11	1.28 (1.17–1.40)
Testicular	18	18	1–11	0.94 (0.74–1.20)
Prostate	39	27	1–4	
Melanoma	*	*	2–3	0.94 (0.82–1.08)
Nervous system	*	*	2–3	1.78 (1.58–1.99)
Thyroid	*	*	2–3	1.00 (0.84–1.18)
Sarcoma	*	*	15	1.33 (0.53–3.35)
Nasopharyngeal	*	*	7	2.47 (1.67–3.66)
Overall rate of unemployment	34	15		1.37 (1.21–1.55)

* Single study only.

Source: data from de Boer, AG. Et al. Cancer survivors and unemployment: A meta-analysis and meta-regression. *JAMA*. 301(7), 753–762.Copyright © 2009 American Medical Association.

The overall percentage of cancer survivors who return to work has been estimated at 63% (range 24–100%). On average, 40% have returned to work by 6 months, 62% at 12 months, and 89% at 24 months post diagnosis.[13]

A number of associations between biopsychosocial factors and return to work have been reported (Box 29.3). The design and quality of the underlying studies is limited. However, one review looked at studies that took self-reported 'workability' as the outcome measure, defined as 'how able is a worker to do his or her job with respect to the work demands, health and mental resources rather than the ability to enter or return to employment'.[14] Only studies involving subjects who had continued to work during treatment or returned after treatment were included. This study found that workability in cancer survivors (on average, living 2 years after diagnosis) was lower than in non-affected working adults. Workability for a range of common cancers improves over time

---

Box 29.3 Associations between biopsychosocial factors and return to work

Modifiable and non-modifiable factors significantly associated with return to work by a cancer survivor:

◆ Sociodemographic:
  • Younger age.
  • Male gender.
  • Higher education and income.
◆ Cancer and treatment related:
  • Cancer type (more likely for cancers of younger age groups, e.g. Hodgkin's disease, melanoma, and genitourinary cancers).
  • Earlier stage.
  • Type of treatment: absence of surgery.
  • Fewer symptoms.
  • Advice on work from doctor.
◆ Work-related:
  • Type, sector, and job demands.
  • Employers' and colleagues support.
◆ Personal and subjective:
  • The (new) meaning of work.

Reproduced from Kiasu, MR et al. Barriers and opportunities for return to work of cancer survivors: time for action-rapid review and expert consultation. *Systematic Reviews*. 24(5):35–39. Copyright © BioMed Central.

(usually for at least 18 months), irrespective of age, although the average workability of people with cancer tends to remain lower than in comparison groups and lower than in people with other chronic conditions such as heart disease, stroke, major depression, or panic disorder.[14] Those with lung and gastrointestinal cancers are reported to have the greatest reduction in workability, and patients with testicular cancer are the least affected. The work productivity of cancer survivors has also been found to be lower, and in some reports cancer survivors worked fewer hours. Irrespective of cancer type, chemotherapy has consistently been associated with impaired workability compared to other treatment modalities. Employers managing employees with a cancer diagnosis describe understandable difficulties in exploring work-related issues while respecting privacy and managing prognostic uncertainty and the emotional upset of the diagnosis.[15]

In one survey, more than 50% of cancer patients declared their diagnosis to their employer, but fewer than 50% reported any subsequent workplace adaptation or support being implemented, irrespective of cancer type. Those who continued to work during treatment were more likely to report modified work arrangements and paid time off when attending medical appointments. Overall, the survey did not provide good evidence of the impact of workplace support or illness disclosure on future workability.[17] Increasing evidence that therapeutic work is associated with improved return-to-work rates should encourage OH professionals to help overcome these communication barriers in the workplace.[18]

Treatment and complications

Adjuvant treatment refers to radiotherapy, chemotherapy, hormonal therapy, or other pharmacotherapy for cancer. It can be administered prior to (neoadjuvant) or after (adjuvant) primary surgery and given with curative, life-prolonging, or palliative intent. Each treatment has well-recognized acute and long-term side effects that can affect a patient's functional status. Long-term health and functional consequences can also arise directly as a result of surgery for cancer or the nature of the underlying cancer itself.

Lymphoedema

Lymphoedema is an accumulation of protein-rich lymph fluid in the interstitial space arising from the interruption of lymph vessel drainage. This may result from cancers such as uterine, vulval, or prostate cancer, melanoma, or lymphoma. The prevalence following gynaecological cancers is estimated at 28–47%.[19]

Lymphoedema after breast cancer occurs in 16–28% of patients who have had axillary lymph node dissection (approximately one-third of women at presentation), and 75% of those who develop lymphoedema will do so within 12 months of surgery, 90% within 3 years, and 1% per year thereafter. Where only sentinel node biopsy is required, 5–7% develop lymphoedema[19]. Advice on upper limb exercise after the onset of upper limb lymphoedema can be conflicting, and access to vocational assistance and counselling has been rated highly as an unmet need by women with lymphoedema.[20]

Infection in the limb ipsilateral to the tumour may precipitate lymphoedema.[21] Occupational risk assessment should aim to minimize the risk of trauma to the limb, and should be discussed with the patient and employer when OH advice is provided. Generic advice on good skin care is also available (see Macmillan Cancer Support website in 'Useful websites').

Suspicion that exercising the arm after axillary surgery may cause lymphoedema has led to advice to avoid lifting children or other heavy objects with the affected arm. However, a recent major literature review concluded that non-fatiguing exercise does not increase the risk of upper limb lymphoedema following breast cancer surgery.[19] Moreover, survivors of breast cancer with stable lymphoedema of the arm who were unrestricted in their manual handling activities experienced no significant increase in limb swelling. The unrestricted group had fewer exacerbations of lymphoedema, better upper and lower body strength, and reported less severe symptoms than women advised not to lift. No limit was placed on resistance exercise in the non-restricted group.[23] Subsequently, national advice in the UK to those who have or who are at risk of breast-cancer related lymphoedema states there is no indication that exercise prevents, causes, or worsens lymphoedema.[24]

Where upper limb lymphoedema has already developed, consensus holds that a degree of physical activity is beneficial. However, an individual risk assessment may be necessary and advice obtained from treating specialists if an employee undertakes repetitive tasks involving isometric exercise or heavy manual handling. In such circumstances, the patient may benefit from a schedule of graded non-fatiguing activity on their return to work.

There is less evidence on how exercise and manual handling affect lower limb lymphoedema. However, specific specialist lymphoedema services provide advice, support, and physical therapies for patients affected by lymphoedema from any cause and are widely available within the UK.

There are no established pharmacotherapeutic options for the treatment of lymphoedema. Surgical treatment for lymphoedema is rarely performed and is limited to severe and refractory cases.[25]

Fatigue

Cancer-related fatigue has been defined as 'a distressing persistent subjective sense of physical, emotional and/or cognitive tiredness or exhaustion related to cancer or cancer treatment that is not proportional to recent activity and interferes with usual functioning'.[26] Fatigue is the most common side effect of cancer treatment, and is reported in 14–96% of patients undergoing cancer treatment and in 19–82% of patients post treatment.[27] Fatigue can be functionally debilitating, particularly in combination with the distress of diagnosis, and other symptoms associated with cancer and its treatment.

Box 29.4 provides guidance on history taking in cases of cancer-related fatigue. Fatigue often runs a predictable course, arising prior to diagnosis, increasing with treatment, then improving but with a higher baseline thereafter. If fatigue is associated with chemotherapy, symptoms frequently arise a few days after each cycle, although fatigue is often a result of cumulative treatment over a number of months. If associated with fractionated

Box 29.4 Causes of cancer-related fatigue

- Malignancy itself: possibly immune mediated.
- Nausea and vomiting: causes include chemotherapy and radiotherapy, with their associated complications.
- Anaemia: causes include gastrointestinal malignancy with bleeding, nutritional deficiency, and myelosuppression from chemotherapy.
- Anorexia.
- Disturbed sleep: causes include pain, anxiety, depression, and other emotional problems, not meeting the criteria for formal psychiatric diagnosis.
- Pre-existing co-morbidities such as chronic obstructive pulmonary disease.
- Side effects of medication.

radiotherapy, a cumulative effect can also be seen, with symptoms increasing towards the end of treatment. Cancer survivors report fatigue as being more distressing and having a greater functional impact than other cancer-related symptoms, including pain and depression.[28]

Virtually all long-term treatment modalities for cancer, including hormonal and biological treatments and stem cell transplantation, have been associated with fatigue. One survey of breast cancer patients indicated that up to 21% of survivors had persistent fatigue 5–10 years after diagnosis.[29]

Treatment approaches for fatigue include the pacing of activities; overt advice to rest may be inadvisable as it may prolong symptoms. By contrast, there is good evidence suggesting that patients should be encouraged to remain as active as possible with benefits for physical, functional, and emotional status of patients.[27]

Recent guidance from the National Institute for Health and Care Excellence recommends that all patients should have access to an exercise programme if they are experiencing cancer-related fatigue.[24]

Given the subjectivity of fatigue, it is not possible to provide prescriptive advice on whether an employee with cancer is fit to work when experiencing this symptom. However, awareness that a graded return to appropriate work should not prove harmful for those with moderate or mild fatigue, and may prove therapeutic, should be encouraged. It can also help to inform clinical assessment and the development of vocational rehabilitation plans with the employee and treating clinicians.

Immunosuppression

Employers may ask for advice from OH about the risk of a cancer survivor acquiring a work-related infection but there is no definitive evidence on how specific cancers or work activities may increase susceptibility to a work-related infection. Cytotoxic chemotherapy is widely used in the treatment of many common cancers. Virtually all cytotoxic drugs can lead to immunosuppression, a global term that describes both the quantitative and qualitative effects of chemotherapy on immune function, not all of which can be routinely measured. Leucopenia is easily measurable; the specific type of leucopenia (neutropenia vs lymphopenia) is noteworthy as the spectrum of infection risk varies.

Neutropenia is readily quantifiable, forming a component of overall immunosuppression, during which any infection, especially bacterial, can be life-threatening. Neutropenia typically occurs 7–10 days after the administration of chemotherapy in patients who are undergoing cycles of treatment every 3 weeks. The risk of the development of chemotherapy-induced neutropenia is reported to be highest during the first cycle of treatment.[30] These timings are unpredictable and should not be relied upon in risk assessment. All patients receiving chemotherapy are given guidance on what to do in the event of neutropenic fever. The incidence of chemotherapy-induced neutropenia leading to hospital admission has been estimated at 3.4% of cancer patients receiving chemotherapy, with lower rates in non-haematological cancers (2%) compared to haematological cancers (4.3% for all such tumours and 10% in those treated with chemotherapy).[31] In part, this increased risk is secondary to the profound immunosuppressive effects of intensive chemotherapy regimens such as those used to combat haematological cancers. In particular, the high chemotherapy doses in the treatment of non-Hodgkin's lymphoma have been associated with a risk of neutropenia. This can lead to periods of immunocompromise lasting months to years and these patients may require antibiotic, antifungal, and antiviral prophylaxis over this period.[32]

Febrile neutropenia carries an overall mortality rate of approximately 5%.[32] Fever in a neutropenic patient (usually defined as a neutrophil count of <0.5 cells $\times$ 10^9/L) requires immediate admission for broad-spectrum intravenous antibacterial therapy.[33] Neutropenic sepsis can occur at neutrophil counts above these levels, but this is likely to be associated with superadded immunocompromise such as arises from concomitant high-dose steroids, hypogammaglobulinaemia (a common accompaniment of the haematological malignancies such as myeloma and chronic lymphocytic leukaemia), or poor marrow reserve due to disease infiltration.

Although evidence is lacking on specific risks in the workplace, those at risk of neutropenia at some point during chemotherapy are generally counselled to reduce their potential exposure to microbes by avoiding work with young children or roles involving high levels of contact with other people.

Immunomodulatory therapies such as thalidomide, lenalidomide, and the proteasome inhibitor bortezomib, typically used in conjunction with high-dose steroids, can also contribute to immunosuppression and low blood counts.

Monoclonal antibodies, such as the anti-CD20 antibody rituximab, which have an increasing role in cancer therapy, particularly for the haematological cancers, can cause neutropenia months after therapy, rather than in the cyclical way seen with conventional chemotherapy.

Patients receiving chemotherapy or other immunosuppressive treatments are normally considered to be at greater risk of community-acquired infection than average, even with normal neutrophil counts, leading to current UK guidance that those receiving treatment or likely to remain immunosuppressed after treatment ends should receive the seasonal influenza vaccine.[34]

Radiotherapy

Radiotherapy rarely leads to immunosuppression and neutropenia, unless a large volume of active marrow is included in the field. The likelihood of this depends on the total radiation dose and treatment volume, the radiotherapy fractionation schedule, and the body area being irradiated. Severe immunosuppression occurs after total body irradiation, which is used in stem cell transplant settings, but patients typically remain under specialist care until there is an improvement. Radiotherapy schedules for primary treatment involve 3–8 weeks of daily fractionated doses delivered every weekday at tertiary treatment centres. The incidence of acute side effects is limited by using such schedules and by the localized nature of most treatments. However, depending on the size of the field, inclusion of mucous membranes, and number of fractions, many patients do experience significant side effects, including skin or mucous membrane breakdown with resultant pain or nausea and vomiting and significant fatigue. In the event of skin or mucous membrane breakdown, the extent of microbiological exposures in the workplace should be considered. In most cases, the intrusiveness of the treatment schedule and ongoing side effects make it impractical to work during treatment.

Hormonal adjuvant treatment

Employees returning to work after a cancer diagnosis may continue on long-term adjuvant treatment, particularly when affected by hormone-driven cancers such as breast and prostate cancers. Adjuvants can lead to side effects or involve treatment schedules that impact functional capacity and work. The following section outlines some of the most common adjuvant treatments and their effects.

Trastuzumab (Herceptin®) is a chemotherapeutic agent that specifically targets a subset of 15–20% of breast cancers that have the HER2 receptor. It is used in adjuvant and palliative treatment which can last up to a year and is commonly administered for 18 cycles that take place every 3 weeks, following the primary chemotherapy/radiotherapy regimen for breast cancer. The drug is administered by intravenous infusion in an outpatient setting; it takes 30 minutes to complete the infusion. It does not have the immunosuppressive effects of traditional non-targeted chemotherapeutic regimens. Trastuzumab is typically well tolerated, the most common side effects being chills and fevers during the course of infusion. Echocardiograms are carried out every 3 months during treatment, as the drug can reduce left ventricular ejection fraction. If this occurs, the drug may need to be discontinued or delayed to allow recovery, so increasing the overall duration of therapy.

Once the side effects have begun to abate, patients who have been absent from work may contemplate a return to work at which point OH advice should reflect the ongoing demands that treatment will have on an employee's time.

Two-thirds of breast cancers contain receptors for the female hormones oestrogen and progesterone ('hormone receptor positive'). Tamoxifen and the aromatase inhibitors are long-term oral hormone antagonists that are typically well tolerated, although they can cause menopausal symptoms and fatigue. The product characteristics of individual treatments are available from the websites of pharmaceutical manufacturers.

Pain

Pain symptoms are estimated to affect up to one-third of patients with cancer and 75% of those with advanced cancer.[35] Pain can arise from the cancer itself, such as bone or brain metastatic cancer; the long-term effects of treatment, for example, neuropathic pain from chemotherapy (particularly platinum-containing therapies and the proteasome inhibitor, bortezomib), brachial or sacral plexopathy caused by radiotherapy to these areas; or phantom limb pain or post-mastectomy pain after surgery.

The application of the World Health Organization's analgesia three-step 'ladder' has been found to improve pain in 85% of cancer patients, although breakthrough pain still arises in up to 50%. Additionally, the further physical, behavioural, cognitive, emotional, spiritual, and interpersonal effects pain has on a person are well-recognized and have been subject to detailed appraisal.[36] Where pain affects the workability of employees with cancer, the OH assessment should consider the adequacy of symptomatic support before commenting on the likely long-term functional impact.

Organ effects

OH professionals should be aware of the late effects of treatment on other organ systems (Box 29.5).

Musculoskeletal

Upper limb function can be impaired in the long term as a result of surgery and/or radiotherapy for breast cancer. However, while upper limb symptoms are common in patients treated for breast cancer, long-term symptoms do not appear to have a major impact on quality of life provided that the disease does not involve axillary node clearance or axillary radiotherapy.

Even in the absence of lymphoedema, patients who have undergone axillary node clearance or axillary radiotherapy are at risk of long-term upper limb morbidity. The impact on shoulder function can range from minor to substantial and is thought to arise from surgical and radiotherapy-induced fibrosis. One study found that the impact of radiotherapy on upper limb function can manifest over 4 years after treatment has ended.[39,40]

Box 29.5 Late effects of cancer treatment

- Cardiovascular disease, such as premature coronary artery disease or cardiomyopathy (from radiotherapy to the mediastinum or anthracycline use).

- Respiratory disease (radiotherapy to the chest, or certain agents such as bleomycin).

- Osteoporosis (gonadotropin-releasing hormone analogues for prostate cancer, aromatase inhibitors for breast cancers, and prolonged steroid usage).

- Endocrine effects such as hypothyroidism (radiotherapy to the neck, or hypogonadism) and infertility (due to intensive chemotherapy).

- Increased risk of secondary or subsequent malignancies.

- Pelvic radiotherapy can lead to later bowel and/or bladder dysfunction. For 50% of patients, the effects are severe, including diarrhoea and incontinence. Rates of moderate or severe late gastrointestinal toxicity from external beam radiotherapy have been estimated at 17%.[37] In one study, 19% of patients undergoing radiotherapy for rectal cancer reported having to toilet more than eight times a day, although patients affected in this way may not say so when asked.[38]

Psychological impact of cancer

A diagnosis of cancer usually has a significant psychological impact, and can undermine self-image and self-confidence. It can lead to persistent intrusive thoughts of recurrence years after successful treatment and precipitate fear, anxiety, and anger.

Although these symptoms may not fulfil the criteria of a formal psychiatric diagnosis, they may impair well-being and functioning significantly. The psychosocial impact of a diagnosis may change over the course of treatment and recovery and into the longer term, possibly requiring a re-evaluation of the support required over time.[41]

When addressing the workability and potential to return to work of an employee with psychological distress, a clinical assessment approach adopting illness representation theory may help to elicit the nature of any barriers to work.[42] This approach may also inform what practical support is needed within the workplace.

Studies have reported significant psychosocial distress in up to 50% of cancer patients, with up to 25% developing major depression. Significant anxiety and/or depression affects approximately 50% of breast cancer patients in the first year after diagnosis, 25% in the second to fourth years, and 15% in the fifth year.[43]

Long-term psychological symptoms were associated with pre-cancer psychological treatment, younger age, and experience of severe non-cancer-related life stressors. However, anxiety and depression were not related to any clinical factors.

In a recent comparison study of women on hormonal therapy for breast cancer, 11% in the aromatase inhibitor group had moderate to severe depressive syndrome versus 37.5% in the control group. [44]

Health professionals commonly underestimate the psychological impact of cancer and significant psychiatric morbidity is underdiagnosed.[45] There is some evidence that psychological support can ease the distress arising from a breast cancer diagnosis, and access to such services is recommended in UK clinical management guidelines. [23]

The role of psychological stressors in the onset of primary and recurrent breast cancer has been researched. However, a meta-analysis of the few well-designed studies in this area reported no reliable evidence of a link,[46] and a prospective cohort study that followed women under 60 years of age for the 5 years following primary breast cancer diagnosis, found no increase in incidence of stressful life events among those who relapsed.[47] A link between psychosocial stress and prostate cancer has also been proposed but evidence is inconclusive.

Vocational rehabilitation

For cancer survivors, survey data suggest that work ranks only behind personal health and the well-being of their families in order of importance.[48,49] Work can be a significant part of the individual's identity and a source of self-esteem. Many people who return to work do so without medical or rehabilitation advice.[47] While cancer survivors often experience long-term reduced physical and mental abilities, many who do return to work (90% in one study) report they coped well with the demands of their work roles.[50] However studies have identified that there is a lack of services to support individuals experiencing long-term effects to remain in or return to work.[48] The experiences of cancer survivors in the workplace are typically recorded only in small cross-sectional surveys, with little control for confounding factors. Within these limits, patient surveys suggest that timely support in relation to work is desired and appreciated by many, while poor employer understanding of the significance and implications of the diagnosis in relation to work continue to be reported.[51] Current international research into cancer survivors includes a focus on establishing reliable screening tools to identify those 'at risk' of work loss, and the development of interventions which effectively support employment.[52,53]

There is some general evidence to suggest that vocational rehabilitation is more effective with early intervention and good communication between the key players.[54] However, a 2011 Cochrane review of the evidence for the effectiveness of support to improve return to work found no randomized control trials exploring interventions after cancer diagnosis where return to work was a primary outcome.[54] Over recent years there has been an increase in research interest relating to effective interventions to improve work outcomes in cancer survivors. These have explored psychological, physical, pharmacological, and multidisciplinary interventions to support return to work.[50] Delivery models include clinical specialist (typically oncology) outpatient or inpatient support; provision of self-management materials for employees; OH services-based support (either alone or in collaboration with specialist oncology services); employer/manager training; and multidisciplinary interventions. Study groups have included those off work due to ill health, the unemployed, and young adults entering the workplace after childhood cancers.[55] While research is still developing, there remain few robust randomized control studies evaluating effectiveness on which to base guidance on evidence-based models of support to enhance rates of return to work.

Occupational risk assessment and recommendations for work adjustments

Immunosuppression

It is not appropriate to make specific overarching recommendations regarding the infective risks in individual patients with cancer who work with varying degrees of immunosuppression across a range of occupations. It is important that each individual receives information and is informed of the reasons for the avoidance of infection and the actions to take if infection is suspected. Box 29.6 provides a summary of risk management advice provided by medical and charitable bodies in this context, which may inform the OH professional's guidance regarding microbiological risks at work.

Box 29.6 Reducing infection risk in patients with cancer undergoing treatment

- Avoid large crowds.
- Avoid contact with anyone with a fever, flu, or other infection.
- Wear thick gloves for gardening and wash hands afterwards.
- Use moist cleaning wipes to clean surfaces used by other people, such as door handles and keypads.
- Do not wade or swim in ponds, lakes, or rivers.
- Wear shoes at all times.
- Perform prompt first aid for cuts and abrasions to the skin.
- Avoid contact with animal or human faeces (especially the nappies of children who have been recently vaccinated).
- Wash your hands after handling animals, fresh flowers, or pot plants.
- Do not share towels or drinking vessels with others.
- Avoid inorganic dusts (e.g. farms and construction sites).
- Discuss foreign travel with your doctor.

Immunization

Immune response to vaccines is likely to be reduced in immunocompromised patients. There may be a risk of generalized infection with live vaccines in patients with severe immunosuppression (e.g. bacillus Calmette–Guérin (BCG), measles, mumps, and varicella zoster vaccines).

Corticosteroids are often used in the treatment of haematological cancers and in end-stage malignant disease. Specialist advice should be sought regarding the appropriateness of live vaccination if patients are receiving 40 mg daily dose equivalents of prednisolone (or lower doses if other immunosuppressive factors are present) for more than 1 week, other immunosuppressive drugs, chemotherapy, or wide-field radiotherapy.

Patients should not receive live vaccines until at least 3 months after stopping high-dose systemic steroids and at least 6 months after they have discontinued other immunosuppressants or radiotherapy. The *British National Formulary* recommends that there should be at least a 12-month delay before administering live vaccines to a person who has stopped taking immunosuppressants following a stem cell transplant. However, immunosuppression can be severe and prolonged following such procedures and it is essential to clarify fitness for live vaccines with the treating specialist.

Inactivated vaccines are safe to administer to immunosuppressed patients, but may elicit a lower immunological response than in immunocompetent individuals. Ideally, where immunization is warranted, this should be administered 2 weeks before commencement of the immunosuppressive treatment. The same advice applies following splenectomy. In severely immunosuppressed patients, consideration should be given to repeat immunizations after completion of treatment and recovery. In particular, after stem cell transplantation, patients are likely to lose both natural and immunization-derived antibodies from most vaccine-preventable diseases. Current advice is for such patients to be offered re-immunization, having sought confirmation from the treating physician or an immunologist. See Chapter 35 for an example re-immunization regimen post stem cell transplant.

Workplace adjustments

Temporary or permanent changes to the working conditions of the employee with a cancer diagnosis may facilitate and maintain return to work (see Box 29.7). Such changes may impact the employee's terms of employment and it should be ensured that employee and employer are clear on this issue before substantial changes are agreed.

The US National Cancer Initiative publish patient guidance on a wide range of conditions and the side effects of treatment that may necessitate workplace adaptation, which can be a useful basis for discussion in the clinical settings.[56]

Legal considerations

The employment provisions of the UK Equality Act 2010 apply to all cancer patients from the point of diagnosis. The Act gives people living with cancer protection from discrimination in a range of areas, including employment and education. There is a requirement for the employer to consider reasonable adjustments to the employee's role that may

Box 29.7 Examples of possible workplace adjustments to be considered

- Changes to and/or flexibility in working hours/days.
- Changes to start/finish times to reduce travel at peak commuting times.
- Help with travel (e.g. designated parking space or taxi through Access to Work).
- Home working to reduce travel demands.
- Provision of additional breaks.
- Changes to work duties (e.g. redistribution of duties).
- Redeployment.
- Physical adaptations or reorganization of the working environment.
- Additional equipment, aids, and adaptations (e.g. communication aids/software).
- Advice on specific symptom management, e.g. fatigue.
- Advice on the use of coping strategies (e.g. for cognitive impairment).
- Job coaching/support worker.
- Additional training, supervision and/or support (e.g. mentoring, advocacy, etc.).
- Education for supervisor, manager, and colleagues about the condition and its effects.
- Advice/support for supervisor, manager, and colleagues.
- Regular reviews with the employee and supervisor/manager to plan and prioritize future work.
- Support from outside work (e.g. from a rehabilitation service or vocational practitioner).
- Flexibility for employees to attend outpatient appointments if they fall within working hours.

overcome the functional impact of enduring health issues on their work capability (potential examples of which are described above).

Surveys suggest that only one in five employers were aware that the Disability Discrimination Act 1995 (the predecessor of the Equality Act 2010) covered cancer survivors.[57,58] Support from employers is variable, with 50% of employees stating their employers did not inform them of their statutory rights and less than half were offered flexible working arrangements.

Cancer survivorship care plans

Medical follow-up has been designed to 'screen' individuals for signs of cancer at regular intervals after the completion of treatment. The usual follow-up is not designed to manage the immediate after-effects of cancer treatment, when symptoms such as fatigue can persist for many months. It may not always provide adequate support to individuals who have experienced recurrent cancer or had to repeat treatment over several years.

Engaging patients to take interest in their health and self-management is widely recognized as crucial to improving care and outcomes for people with long-term conditions. This belief is reflected in a move towards 'personalized care plans' supported by a survivorship information prescription tailored to individual needs. This shift towards information and support raises patients' awareness of the signs of recurrent or progressive illness and what they should do if they believe they are affected. In the context of OH, clinical screening is usually not relevant and any follow-up is focused on vocational rehabilitation. Review should only be necessary if occupational difficulties arise, while ensuring the employee is aware of the range of support services available.

Fitness to drive

For all patients who have cancer, fitness to drive depends largely upon intracranial (primary or secondary) involvement and the subsequent secondary risk of a seizure or visual impairment. If a person has been affected, a decision on their fitness to drive would be made by the Driver and Vehicle Licensing Agency (DVLA) (see 'Useful websites'). Where there is no intracerebral involvement, there is no consistent evidence that a cancer diagnosis affects a person's fitness to drive (Box 29.8).

Shift work and breast cancer

The impact of shift work on the incidence and recurrence of breast cancer has been subject to research. Following a review, the International Agency for Research on Cancer

Box 29.8 Factors to consider in fitness to drive in patients with cancer

- General state of health: this includes the impact of treatment such as chemotherapy or radiotherapy.
- Specific limb impairment (e.g. from primary or secondary bone cancer or surgery).
- Advanced malignancy causing symptoms (e.g. general weakness or cachexia to such an extent that safe driving would be comprised).
- Strong analgesics: any impact of strong analgesics on cognitive functioning (the use of the World Health Organization's analgesic three-step 'ladder' and adjuvant analgesia involves the use of many drugs with potential cognitive effects).

(IARC) concluded that overnight shift work is a 'probable' carcinogen to humans (Grade 2A) (see 'Useful websites'). However, the IARC identified the possibility of bias, chance, and confounding in epidemiological studies and recognized that it had not been proven conclusively. Most recently, a study involving 1.4 million women, the largest such study to date, found no link between shift work and cancer.[60]

Health promotion

Evidence is emerging that lifestyle factors including physical activity and diet can influence the rate of cancer progression, improve quality of life, reduce side effects during treatment, reduce the incidence of relapse, and improve overall survival.[61] Breast cancer survivors and colon cancer survivors who exercised after their diagnosis had improved survival rates compared with more sedentary survivors although caution in drawing firm conclusions regarding physical activity and cancer survival is warranted.[62] (See also the National Cancer Institute website in 'Useful websites'.)

Prognosis

Cancer Research UK provides the latest UK cancer incidence, mortality, and survival statistics, as well as information on the causes, diagnosis, treatment, screening, and molecular biology and genetics of cancer. Several validated prognostic indices for the common cancers are available, such as the NHS Predict tool for breast cancer and nomograms for prostate cancer (see 'Useful websites'). Awareness of the approaches taken to grade the severity of cancers, and sources of the most up-to-date survival data, is essential in informing decisions to ensure that an employee diagnosed with advanced cancer has access to the benefits they are entitled to through their occupational pension scheme.

Key points

- Improvements in detection and treatment are anticipated to increase the number of cancer survivors in the UK by 3% per year.
- Changes in the age profile of the workforce from increasing retirement ages will increase the prevalence of common cancers among employees, and lead to greater disruption of work–life balance from their roles as informal carers of family members affected by cancer.
- Most employees remain at work, or return shortly after treatment, without formal OH advice. However, a significant minority of working age adults have long-term or late effects of diagnosis and/or treatment for which workplace support may be required. Research is ongoing to aid early identification of those who require workplace support.
- There is evidence that adjustments and vocational rehabilitation can facilitate return to work after treatment, but more research is needed on the effectiveness of interventions.

Useful websites

Health and Safety Executive. 'The burden of occupational cancer in Great Britain'	http://www.hse.gov.uk/research/rrhtm/rr595.htm
Cancer Research UK. 'Cancer incidence by age – UK statistics'	http://www.cancerresearchuk.org/health-professional/cancer-statistics
National Cancer Institute. 'Late effects of treatment for childhood cancers'	https://www.cancer.gov/types/childhood-cancers/late-effects-hp-pdq
National Cancer Institute. 'Lymphedema (PDQ®)–Health Professional Version'	http://www.cancer.gov/cancertopics/pdq/supportivecare/lymphedema/healthprofessional
National Cancer Institute. 'Prognostic nomograms for prostate cancer'	https://www.cancer.gov/types/prostate/hp/prostate-treatment-pdq#link/_2097_toc
National Cancer Institute. 'Fatigue (PDQ®)–Patient Version'	http://www.cancer.gov/about-cancer/treatment/side-effects/fatigue/fatigue-pdq
National Cancer Institute. 'Physical activity and cancer'	https://www.cancer.gov/about-cancer/causes-prevention/risk/obesity/physical-activity-fact-sheet#q9
Macmillan Cancer Support. Skin care and lymphoedema	https://www.macmillan.org.uk/information-and-support/coping/side-effects-and-symptoms/lymphoedema
NHS. Predict tool	http://www.predict.nhs.uk/predict_v2.0.html
The British Pain Society. 'Cancer pain management—a perspective from the British Pain Society, supported by the Association for Palliative Medicine and the Royal College of General Practitioners'	http://britishpainsociety.org/book_cancer_pain.pdf
National Comprehensive Cancer Network. Distress management	http://www.nccn.org/professionals/physician_gls/PDF/distress.pdf
Driver and Vehicle Licensing Agency (DVLA). Assessing fitness to drive	https://www.gov.uk/guidance/assessing-fitness-to-drive-a-guide-for-medical-professionals
International Agency for Research on Cancer. 'Shiftwork', 2010	http://monographs.iarc.fr/ENG/Monographs/vol98/mono98-8.pdf
National Institute for Clinical Excellence. 'Advanced breast cancer: diagnosis and treatment'	http://guidance.nice.org.uk/CG81

References

1. **Health and Safety Executive**. The burden of occupational cancer in Great Britain. Available at: http://www.hse.gov.uk/research/rrhtm/rr595.htm.
2. **Cancer Research UK**. Cancer incidence by age – UK statistics. Available at: http://www.cancerresearchuk.org/health-professional/cancer-statistics.
3. **Cancer Research UK**. Children's cancer statistics. Available at: http://www.cancerresearchuk.org/health-professional/cancer-statistics/childrens-cancers.
4. **Maddams J. Utley M, Miller H.** Projections of cancer prevalence in the United Kingdom, 2010–2040. *Br J Cancer* 2012;**107**:1195–202.
5. **Cancer Research UK**. Cancer Research UK's strategy 2009–2014. Available at: http://www.cancerresearchuk.org/prod_consump/groups/cr_common/@abt/@gen/documents/generalcontent/cr_043314.pdf.
6. **Romito F, Goldzweig G, Cormio C, et al.** Informal caregiving for cancer patients. *Cancer* 2013;**119**(Suppl. 11):2160–9.
7. **de Boer AGEM, Taskila T, Ojajarvi A, van Dijk FJ, Verbeek JH.** Cancer survivors and unemployment: a meta-analysis and meta-regression. *JAMA* 2009;**301**:753–62.
8. **Young V, Bhaumik C.** *Health and Well-Being at Work: A Survey of Employees.* Research Report No. 751. London: Department for Work and Pensions; 2011.
9. **Carlsen K, Jensen AJ, Rugulies R, et al.** Self-reported work ability in long-term breast cancer survivors. A population-based questionnaire study in Denmark. *Acta Oncol* 2013;**52**:423–9.
10. **Armes J, Crowe M, Colbourne L, et al.** Patients' supportive care needs beyond the end of cancer treatment: a prospective, longitudinal survey. *J Clin Oncol* 2009;**27**:6172–9.
11. **National Cancer Institute**. Late effects of treatment for childhood cancers. Available at: https://www.cancer.gov/types/childhood-cancers/late-effects-hp-pdq.
12. **Macmillan Cancer Support**. *Macmillan Study of the Health and Well-Being of Cancer Survivors – Follow-Up Survey of Awareness of Late Effects and Use of Health Services for Ongoing Health Problems.* London: Macmillan Cancer Support; 2008.
13. **Mehnert A.** Employment and work-related issues in cancer survivors. *Crit Rev Oncol Hematol* 2011;**77**:109–30.
14. **Munir F, Yarker J, McDermott H.** Employment and the common cancers: correlates of work ability during or following cancer treatment. *Occup Med (Lond)* 2009;**59**:381–9.
15. **Tiedtke C, Donceel P, de Rijk A, et al.** Return to work following breast cancer treatment: the employers' side. *J Occup Rehabil* 2014;**24**:399–409.
16. **Kiasuwa Mbengi R, Otter R, Mortelmans K, et al.** Barriers and opportunities for return to work of cancer survivors: time for action-rapid review and expert consultation. *Syst Rev* 2016;**5**:35.
17. **Pryce J, Munir F, Haslam C.** Cancer survivorship and work: symptoms, supervisor response, co-worker disclosure and work adjustments. *J Occup Rehab* 2007;**17**:83–92.
18. **van Egmond MP, Duijts SF, van Muijen P, et al.** Therapeutic work as a facilitator for return to paid work in cancer survivors *J Occup Rehabil* 2017;**27**:148–55.
19. **National Cancer Institute**. Lymphedema (PDQ®). Available at: http://www.cancer.gov/cancertopics/pdq/supportivecare/lymphedema/healthprofessional.
20. **Girgis A, Stacey F, Lee T, et al.** Priorities for women with lymphoedema after treatment for breast cancer: population based cohort study. *BMJ* 2011;**342**:d3442.
21. **National Institute for Health and Care Excellence (NICE)**. *Guidelines for Early and Locally Advanced Breast Cancer: Full Guideline.* Clinical guideline [CG80]. London: NICE; revised 2017. Available at:https://www.nice.org.uk/guidance/cg80.

22. **Schmitz KH, Ahmed RL, Troxel AB, et al.** Weight lifting in women with breast-cancer-related lymphedema. *N Engl J Med* 2009;**361**:664–731.

23. **National Institute for Health and Care Excellence (NICE).** *Advanced Breast Cancer: Diagnosis and Treatment.* Clinical guideline [CG81]. London: NICE; revised 2017. Available at: https://www.nice.org.uk/guidance/cg81.

24. **National Institute for Health and Care Excellence (NICE).** *Liposuction for Chronic Lymphoedema.* London: NICE; 2017. Available at: https://www.nice.org.uk/guidance/ipg588.

25. **Cormier JN, Rourke L, Crosby M, Chang D.** The surgical treatment of lymphedema: a systematic review of the contemporary literature (2004–2010). Armer J Ann Surg Oncol 2012;**19**:642–51.

26. **Ahlberg K, Ekman T, Gaston-Johansson F, et al.** Assessment and management of cancer-related fatigue in adults. *Lancet* 2003;**362**:640–50.

27. **Morrow GR.** Cancer-related fatigue: causes, consequences, and management. *Oncologist* 2007;**12**(Suppl. 1):1–3.

28. **Hofman M, Ryan JL, Figueroa-Moseley CD, Jean-Pierre P, Morrow GR.** Cancer-related fatigue: the scale of the problem. *Oncologist* 2007;**12**(Suppl. 1):4–10.

29. **Bower JE, Ganz PA, Desmond KA, et al.** Fatigue in long-term breast carcinoma survivors: a longitudinal investigation. *Cancer* 2006;**106**:751–8.

30. **Dale DC.** Advances in the treatment of neutropenia. *Curr Opin Support Palliat Care* 2009;**3**:207–12.

31. **Caggiano V, Weiss RV, Rickert TS, Linde-Zwirble WT.** Incidence, cost, and mortality of neutropenia hospitalisation associated with chemotherapy. *Cancer* 2005;**103**;1916–24.

32. **Naik JD, Sathiyaseelan SR, Vasudev NS.** Febrile neutropenia. *BMJ* 2010;**341**:c6981.

33. **National Institute for Health and Care Excellence (NICE).** *Neutropenic Sepsis: Prevention and Management in People with Cancer.* Clinical guideline [CG151]. London: NICE; 2012. Available at: https://www.nice.org.uk/guidance/cg151.

34. **National Institute for Health and Care Excellence.** Immunization seasonal influenza. 2018. Available at: https://cks.nice.org.uk/immunizations-seasonal-influenza#!scenario.

35. **NHS Quality Improvement Scotland.** *The Management of Pain in Patients with Cancer: Best Practice Statement.* Edinburgh: NHS Quality Improvement Scotland; 2009.

36. **Peach MS, Showalter TN, Ohri N.** Systematic review of the relationship between acute and late gastrointestinal toxicity after radiotherapy for prostate cancer. *Prostate Cancer* 2015;**2015**:624736.

37. **Bruheim K, Guren MG, Skovlund E, et al.** Late side effects and quality of life after radiotherapy for rectal cancer. *Int J Radiat Oncol Biol Phys* 2010;**76**:1005–11.

38. **Pinkawa M, Holy R, Piroth MD, et al.** Consequential late effects after radiotherapy for prostate cancer – a prospective longitudinal quality of life study. *Radiat Oncol* 2010;**5**:27.

39. **Levangie PK, Droin J.** Magnitude of late effects of breast cancer treatments on shoulder function: a systematic review. *Breast Cancer Res Treat* 2009;**116**:1–15.

40. **Hidding JT, Beurskens C, van der Wees PJ, et al.** Treatment related impairments in arm and shoulder in patients with breast cancer: a systematic review: *PLoS One* 2014;**9**:e96748.

41. **National Cancer Institute.** *Adjustment to Cancer: Anxiety and Distress (PDQ®)–Health Professional Version.* Bethesda, MD: National Cancer Institute. Available at: https://www.cancer.gov/about-cancer/coping/feelings/anxiety-distress-hp-pdq.

42. **Diefenbach MA.** Illness representations. National Cancer Institute. Available at: https://cancercontrol.cancer.gov/brp/research/constructs/illness_representations.pdf.

43. **Burgess B, Cornelius V, Love S, et al.** Depression and anxiety in women with early breast cancer: five year observational cohort study. *BMJ* 2005;**330**:702–5.

44. **Couillet A, Tredan O, Oussaid N, et al.** Prevalence of depressive syndrome in patients with breast cancer treated with or without aromatase inhibitors. *Oncologie* 2015;**17**:587.

45. **Fallowfield L, Ratcliffe D, Jenkins V, et al.** Psychiatric morbidity and its recognition by doctors in patients with cancer. *Br J Cancer* 2001;**84**:1011–5.

46. **Heikkila K, Nyberg ST, Theorell T, et al.** Work stress and risk of cancer: meta-analysis of 5700 incident cancer events in 116 000 European men and women. *BMJ* 2013;**346**:f165.

47. **Graham J, Ramirez A, Love S, Richards M, Burgess C.** Stressful life experiences and risk of relapse of breast cancer: observational cohort study. *BMJ* 2002;**324**:1420.

48. **Spelten E, Spragers M, Verbeek J.** Factors reported to influence the return to work of cancer survivors: a literature review. *Psychooncology* 2002;**11**:124–31.

49. **Amir Z, Neary D, Luker K.** Cancer survivors' views of work 3 years post diagnosis – a UK perspective. *Eur J Oncol Nurs* 2008;**12**:190–7.

50. **Torp S, Nielsen RA, Gudbergsson SB, Dahl AA.** Worksite adjustments and work ability among employed cancer survivors. *Support Care Cancer* 2012;**20**:2149–56.

51. **Pryce J, Munir F, Haslam C.** Cancer survivorship and work. *J Occup Rehabil* 2007;**17**:83–92.

52. **de Boer AG.** The European Cancer and Work Network: CANWON. *J Occup Rehabil* 2014;**24**:393–8.

53. **Waddell G, Burton AK, Kendall NAS.** *Vocational Rehabilitation: What Works, for Whom and When?* Commissioned by the Vocational Rehabilitation Group in association with the Industrial Injuries Advisory Council. London: The Stationary Office; 2008.

54. **De Boer AGEM, Taskila T, Tamminga SJ, Frings-Dresen MH, Feuerstein M, Verbeek JH.** Interventions to enhance return-to-work for cancer patients. *Cochrane Database Syst Rev* 2011;**2**:CD007569.

55. **Mehnert A, de Boer A, Feurstein M.** Employment challenges for cancer survivors. *Cancer* 2013;**119**(Suppl 11):2151–9.

56. **National Cancer Institute.** Side effects of cancer treatment. 2018. Available at: https://www.cancer.gov/about-cancer/treatment/side-effects.

57. **Nieuwenhuijsen K, Bos-Ransdorp B, Uitterhoeve LL, Sprangers MA, Verbeek JH.** Enhanced provider communication and patient education regarding return to work in cancer survivors following curative treatment: a pilot study. *J Occup Rehabil* 2006;**16**:647–57.

58. **de Boer AGEM, Fring-Dresen MHW.** Employment and the common cancers: return to work of cancer survivors. *Occup Med* 2009;**59**:378–80.

59. **Simm C, Aston J, Williams C, Hill D, Bellis A, Meager N.** *Organisations' Responses to the Disability Discrimination Act.* DWP Research Report 410. London: Department for Work and Pensions; 2007.

60. **Travis RC, Balkwill A, Fensom GK, et al.** Night shift work and breast cancer incidence: three prospective studies and meta-analysis of published studies. *J Natl Cancer Inst* 2016;**108**:djw169.

61. **Amir Z, Brocky J.** Employment and the common cancers: epidemiology. *Occup Med* 2009;**59**:373–7.

62. **Thijs KM, de Boer AG, Vreugdenhil G.** Rehabilitation using high-intensity physical training and long-term return-to-work in cancer survivors. *J Occup Rehabil* 2012;**22**:220–9.

Chapter 30

Vision and eye disorders

Stuart J. Mitchell and John Pitts

Introduction

This chapter is arranged in six sections. The first sets out the effect of vision impairment on work and the effect of work on the health of the visual system. The second introduces the main symptoms and functional effects of vision disorders. The third reviews the main categories of ocular disease and uses a tabular approach to link the symptoms of visual dysfunction to their effect on work—and the adjustments that have to be made as a result. The fourth takes a brief look at workplace design—including lighting, display screen equipment (DSE), visual fatigue, and the employment of people with visual impairment. The fifth introduces the commonest ocular hazards found in the workplace and reviews the types of eye protection. The sixth is a brief introduction to ocular first aid in the workplace.

The effect of vision impairment on work and the effect of work on the health of the visual system

The important aspects of vision for work are distance, intermediate and near visual acuity (VA), visual field, colour vision, and stereopsis. Diseases of the eye or nervous system result in varying degrees of disturbance of these parameters. Work can affect the visual system in ways that are temporary, such as visual fatigue, or permanent, such as ocular injuries. Most workplace injuries are preventable, so eye protection is a vital component of workplace assessment.

Perception is more than simply vision.[1] It is affected by neural processing, which modifies the meaning of a stimulus on the basis of previous experience. As a result, neuropsychological adaptation can sometimes compensate for visual dysfunction; for example, a colour-impaired worker might use contrast instead of hue to differentiate colours. In corollary, errors can also result from visual illusions that trick central information-processing mechanisms, not just from defects in vision.[2] Such perceptual errors occur more frequently with fatigue and high workload.

To minimize such errors, good displays are designed to respect the physiological and psychological limitations of the human visual system. Displays should present information in a legible, coherent manner, without crowding, and with intelligent use of iconography and colour to convey meaning. Likewise, controls should be labelled such that the function of levers, knobs, and switches is conveyed unambiguously.

Optical correction should be optimized for the task at hand, whether the worker has normal or impaired vision. Attention to this and aspects of workplace design should enable visually impaired people to function safely in appropriate roles in the workplace.

Matching visual capability to the task required

A sound knowledge of the workplace is of fundamental importance in occupational health.[3] Any eye care professional (ophthalmologist, optometrist, or orthoptist) who is asked to advise on occupational medical issues should therefore become familiar with the workplace, the tasks performed there, and their demands on the employee.

In addition, an assessment of the individual is required to determine whether their visual abilities match the requirements of the job. If a mismatch exists, there are two possible courses of action:

- The task can be adjusted where possible. If the Equality Act 2010 is likely to apply, the employer should make 'reasonable adjustments'.
- The visual capabilities of the individual can be enhanced by spectacles or other visual aids.

Many occupations have historically prescribed visual standards that are neither evidence-based nor task-related.[4] There are signs that this is now changing. In aviation, for example, the simulator can be used to investigate task proficiency with different degrees of colour vision deficiency.[5]

Vision and work involving driving

The DVLA requirements are published online (see 'Useful websites'). The numerical parameters are not given here, as these are subject to periodic updates. Driving simulators and functional driving tests are an option in cases where clinical vision measurements are borderline.

The main symptoms and functional effects of vision disorders

The main symptoms and signs of eye disease are given in Box 30.1.

Disturbed visual acuity

Central visual function is measured clinically as a VA. In measuring Snellen VA, the patient is asked to stand 6 m from the test chart: 6/6 vision means that the individual can see at 6 m what they ought to be able to see at 6 m; 6/60 vision means they can see at 6 m what they ought to be able to see at 60 m. In some countries, such as the US, feet are used instead of metres, and so the VA will be expressed as a fraction with numerator 20 (20/20 being normal, 20/200 being equivalent to 6/60, and so on). Care should be taken

Box 30.1 Main symptoms and functional effects of vision disorders

- Disturbed visual acuity.
- Disturbed colour vision.
- Disturbed visual field.
- Disturbed night vision.
- Disturbed contrast sensitivity.
- Disturbed binocularity.
- Visual discomfort/glare.
- Somatosensory discomfort/pain.

with such values, as there are a variety of different systems for recording VA (decimal, logMAR, ETDRS, etc.)

Near VA is measured by using standard printers' font sizes at the standard working distance of 33 cm. It is important to realize that the actual working distance may be greater than 33 cm (e.g. 50, 75, or 100 cm), in which case near VA should be measured at these distances as well.

These methods assess static VA. Specialized tests of dynamic VA may be better at predicting performance at certain tasks. In occupational health (OH) settings, devices known as optometers are often used to screen employees. While these may be better at assessing function in certain industrial tasks such as inspection of mechanical parts, the 6 m test of VA is more reproducible.

Disturbed colour vision

There are three types of cone present in the retina, and each type senses light optimally over different regions of the visual spectrum. Red (R) and green (G) cones detect and compare light over the middle- and long-wavelength regions of the visual spectrum. Blue (B) cones cover the short-wavelength region of the spectrum. It is the comparison of R and G cone signals that gives rise to the perception of R and G, and the comparison of R plus G and B cone signals that gives rise to the perception of yellow (Y) and B.

The pigments in R and G cones are genetically (X-linked) determined, and the absence of one pigment class or the presence of a variant pigment give rise to partial or complete RG colour deficiencies. Up to 8% of males and 0.4% of females exhibit congenital colour deficiency. This causes reduced RG colour discrimination and the subsequent potential confusion of Rs, Gs, and sometimes even white lights.

All of these are frequently used as signal lights in many transport environments and are consequently employed in many lantern tests to assess colour safety. Y/B colours are becoming more popular in visual displays and as signal lights at night, but congenital loss of YB colour vision is very rare and is not therefore a problem. Acquired loss of YB colour vision, on the other hand, can be significant in older subjects due to systemic diseases such as diabetes or the use of medications (e.g. ethambutol and phosphodiesterase inhibitors) and this is likely to become more important as Y/B becomes commoner in visual displays.

There are a number of occupations in which normal or close to normal colour vision is a safety requirement. This is particularly the case where no other visual cues to identify an object or signal information exist. For example, electricians have to discriminate between differently coloured wires; and in the transport industries (particularly railway, maritime, and aviation), the 'solo' discrimination of coloured signal lights is safety-critical.

Assessment of colour vision

Colour vision can be assessed by a variety of techniques. The commonest screening test is the use of 'pseudoisochromatic' Ishihara plates consisting of patterned coloured dots against a background of other coloured dots which vary randomly in luminance contrast. This technique isolates the use of RG colour signals and detects the commonest form of inherited colour deficiency: R/G confusion. Care should be taken in the exact choice of test (i.e. there are a number of different versions available with varying number of plates), and different statistical outcomes. In general, the plates should be illuminated with daylight and the plates should be shown in random order to prevent subjects from passing the test by simply learning the sequence or using other cues. The result judged to constitute a 'pass' should be defined for each particular occupation, as it is not uncommon for subjects with severe loss of RG colour vision to pass some of the Ishihara-based protocols.[6]

The anomaloscope test (e.g. Oculus) is available commercially and requires the subject to match a monochromatic Y field with a similar field illuminated with a mixture of R and G lights. Anomaloscopes exhibit great variability in the R/G matching range and cannot be used reliably to quantify the severity of colour vision loss; they do, however, provide a useful way of confirming colour deficiency and differentiating between deutan and protan deficiencies. Care must be taken with the conduct of the tests and the interpretation of the results. Realistically, these tests can only discriminate between those who have normal trichromatic vision and those who do not.

The various lantern tests (e.g. Holmes-Wright, Beyne, and Spectrolux), originally developed for maritime work and previously commonly used in aviation, and matching tests used historically in the textiles industry, were developed for particular occupations. It is very important to follow the manufacturers' protocols exactly and take care when extrapolating between work-colour environments. In general, they all exhibit large intra- and inter-subject variability and cannot be used to provide a reliable measure of the severity of RG colour vision loss. This is particularly true in mild to moderate deficiency. Lantern and matching tests are now being superseded by computer-based tests such as the City University CAD (colour assessment and diagnosis) test. This is very sensitive at detecting the smallest RG and YB colour deficiencies, and also quantifies the severity of loss. It is therefore particularly useful in occupations where some degree of colour deficiency can be tolerated without compromising performance or safety.[7]

There are now numerous online colour vision screening sites and patients may refer to these in evidence of normality. Any reliance on such tests should be cautious and a check should be made that these are validated to a particular occupation. It cannot be overemphasized that the results of colour vision testing are not valid unless the protocols are followed properly and consistently.

Disturbed visual fields

Visual fields are nowadays routinely measured by static techniques, using multiple targets that blink on and off with varying intensity, generating an accurate map that includes relative as well as absolute defects.

Vision towards the periphery of the field is dominated by the rod photoreceptors. These are part of the *magnocellular system*, which is concerned with movement and balance. Severe visual field defects are therefore commonly associated with disturbed balance; workers so affected should be individually assessed with regard to working at heights.

Disturbed night vision

Worse-than-normal vision in low illumination is a non-specific feature of myopia, cataract, glaucoma, and presbyopia. True *nyctalopia* is a feature of retinitis pigmentosa and vitamin A deficiency.[8] The diagnosis should be ascertained and, where possible, the condition treated. Retinitis pigmentosa is a genetic degeneration of the photoreceptors, particularly the rods. It can present with nyctalopia, but progresses to loss of visual field and daytime acuity. Its onset is typically early in the working lifetime, in the third decade of life,[9] and so workplace adjustments (day shifts, optimal illumination, etc.) are important.

Disturbed contrast sensitivity

Snellen acuities are measured using high-contrast icons and optimal illumination. Measuring contrast sensitivity utilizes icons of variable contrast and illumination to perform a more subtle, 'real-world' assessment of visual performance. Contrast sensitivity defines the threshold between the visible and the invisible[10] and is 1% across a wide range of targets and illumination. It is conceptually similar to an audiogram, and measures a threshold at various different spatial frequencies.

Clinically, it is far less widely-used than Snellen acuity, probably because it is more time-consuming. It is useful in the diagnosis of early disease, in monitoring disease in clinical trials, and in situations where patients complain of poor vision but have normal acuity. A vast array of vision charts and computer-based tests are used to measure contrast sensitivity, so standardization is important and test results must be accompanied by a description of the process and the particular test's normal ranges.

Disturbed binocularity

Stereopsis enables three-dimensional vision. It can be measured, and is expressed in seconds of arc. Stereopsis of 120 seconds of arc gives a stereoscopic range of 120 m, 60 seconds gives 240 m, and 30 seconds gives 480 m. Stereopsis is only important for visual tasks relatively close to the subject and in certain specific workers such as forklift drivers. This is because it is not the brain's only mechanism for depth perception.

Beyond approximately 0.5 km, the use of monocular (psychological) cues assumes greater importance in judging depth. These monocular cues are relative size, perspective, overlapping, position in field, washout due to atmospheric scattering of light (Rayleigh scattering), and parallax. Monocular workers, by definition, do not have stereopsis, and these people use psychological clues to judge depth perception at all distances.

Notably, some 4% of the general population have amblyopia[11] and an additional 32% without amblyopia have poor stereoscopic vision.[12] The reason for this is unclear, and many people with reduced vision in one eye are unaware of these problems and can only be identified by testing the VA in each eye separately.

Increasing age reduces stereopsis; by the age of 65 it is normal in only 27% of the population.[13]

Visual discomfort/glare

Visual discomfort can occur as asthenopia, eye strain, or glare. Asthenopia is due to an imbalance between accommodation and convergence, and glare is due to scattering of light inside the eye. Discomfort glare by definition does not degrade VA, instead causing distraction, aversion, and fatigue. Disability glare reduces VA, and this can be measured clinically[14] (See Box 30.2).

Somatosensory discomfort/pain

Sensation in the eyes is served by the ophthalmic branch of the trigeminal nerve, and so referred pain (e.g. from a dental origin) and neurological disorders (e.g. trigeminal neuralgia) must be considered as possible causes of apparent ocular pain.

Box 30.2 Types of glare

- *Veiling glare* (e.g. due to windscreen reflections) results from a diffuse light source being superimposed on a retinal image, thus reducing contrast.
- *Dazzle glare* (e.g. due to the headlights of oncoming vehicles) occurs because the rays from a bright light source reduce contrast at the fovea.
- *Scotomatic glare* (e.g. due to arc welding) is caused by a particularly intense light source temporarily bleaching the photoreceptors.

Because the eyes have such a rich supply of sensory nerves and such a large area of representation in the somatosensory cortex, discomfort and pain in ocular disease can be extremely severe. Discomfort varies from mild foreign body sensation of tear deficiency to the excruciating pain of scleritis. Such severe ocular pain cannot be ignored, and distracts from any occupational task, even if safety critical.

The main categories of ocular disease and their effect on work

The OH professional must avoid making assumptions about an individual's ability to work based on a disease label, since a particular diagnosis may have a vast range of functional effects depending on factors such as disease severity, personality, and the level of support in the work environment.

Refractive errors and their correction

In *myopia* (short-sightedness), the eye is relatively long or the cornea is relatively steeply curved, so rays of light are brought into focus short of the retina. This is corrected by a concave (minus) lens. Myopia is not simply an optical state.[15] It is associated with degeneration of the vitreous gel and peripheral retina, an increased risk of retinal detachment, and a higher risk of early-onset macular degeneration.

In *hyperopia* (long-sightedness), the eye is relatively short or the cornea has a relatively flat curvature, such that rays of light have a virtual focus behind the retina. This is corrected by a convex (positive) lens. Hyperopia is associated with an increased risk of squint and amblyopia in childhood and with angle closure glaucoma in later life.

In *astigmatism*, the cornea has different radii of curvature in different axes and is sometimes described as being shaped like a spoon or a rugby ball. Astigmatism may be myopic, hyperopic, or be a mixture of both.

Presbyopia is loss of reading vision associated with progressive age-related loss of flexibility of the natural lens and accommodative function (flexibility of focus). Because hyperopic people are already using some of their accommodative reserve to focus in the distance, they are affected by loss of near vision earlier in life. Presbyopia is easily corrected with a plus lens in spectacles or contact lenses, but accurate correction critically depends on determination of the individual's working distance. Presbyopic symptoms may initially only occur in poor light.

Where spectacles are used to correct refractive errors, they must be compatible with any necessary personal protective equipment (PPE). Contact lenses have the advantages of a more physiological retinal image and almost universal compatibility with PPE. However, they may be impractical in dry, dusty, or contaminated work environments, where contact lens care is difficult and there is an increased risk of potentially sight-threatening complications such as keratitis (infection of the cornea).

Refractive surgery

Modern techniques of refractive eye surgery, including laser, are safer than contact lens wear—but not without risk.

Photorefractive keratectomy uses an excimer laser to reshape the corneal curvature. In low myopia, it typically removes 10% of the corneal thickness. A subepithelial haze peaks at 2–3 months and gradually disappears at 12 months. The refraction stabilizes at 6 months. With modern techniques, regression (a tendency to return to the original refraction) is less likely.

Modern laser-assisted *in situ* keratomilieusis (LASIK) uses two lasers to raise a flap of cornea with air bubbles and then reshape the underlying cornea. Because surgery is carried out under an intact epithelial surface, haze, scar formation, and pain are minimal. Modern LASIK also uses wavefront-guided technology, which has been shown to produce less optical aberration and better night vision. Wavefront-guided LASIK can also treat astigmatism and hyperopia.

Surgical techniques are now emerging for the treatment of presbyopia, such as refractive lens exchange, multifocal LASIK, and femtosecond laser reshaping of the posterior cornea.

Another common surgical strategy is to use conventional LASIK to render one eye optimum for distance and the other optimum for near. The resulting visual status is known as monovision. Even if this uses the technique of micro-monovision (<2 dioptres of difference between the eyes), it is *specifically banned* in some occupations such as civil aviation (unless reversed by spectacles, which then have to be worn on task).

Suggestions for disposition of refractive errors at work are given in Table 30.1.

External eye diseases

Dry eye

Reduction in the amount of aqueous tears or, much more commonly, degradation in the quality and stability of the tear film accompanied by Meibomian gland dysfunction causes gritty discomfort and comprises a group of problems with the eye surface which are bundled together as 'dry eyes'.

Some working environments exacerbate the symptoms of dry eye. When investigating complaints of dry eyes, it is important to measure the relative humidity in the workplace. Some workplaces cannot be humidified, and redeployment will be necessary if lubricant eye drops don't control symptoms adequately.

Allergy

Allergic conjunctivitis, the most common allergic eye disease, is characterized by itching, redness, burning, and lachrymation. Based on the aeroallergen, it can present with either seasonal or perennial symptoms. In allergy, conjunctivitis rarely presents without associated allergic rhinitis.

Table 30.1 Refractive errors and their management at work

Condition	Symptoms and signs	Workplace adjustment	Other medical actions
Myopia	Reduced acuity		Optometry
Hyperopia	Reduced acuity Asthenopia discomfort		Optometry
Astigmatism	Reduced acuity		Optometry
Presbyopia	Reduced acuity (near only)	Test luminance of workplace	Optometry
Photorefractive keratectomy	Discomfort/glare up to 1 year		Glare testing
LASIK	Discomfort/glare up to 3 months		Glare testing
Monovision		Banned in some occupations, e.g. pilots.	Check occupational requirements

In northern Europe, sensitization is predominantly to the house dust mite species *Dermatophagoides pteronyssinus* (median prevalence of 22%). House dust mite allergy usually causes perennial symptoms. Grass pollen sensitization occurs in 17% of patients, usually to Timothy grass or *Phleum pratense*[16] and results in seasonal symptoms.

There are two main approaches to treating allergic conjunctivitis.[17] Allergen avoidance can help but it is rarely practical. Occasionally, avoidable occupational causes of allergic conjunctivitis can be found, so an occupational history is mandatory.

Treatment with an intranasal steroid is essential to decrease priming of the nasal-ocular reflex. Combining an intranasal steroid such as fluticasone propionate with an intranasal antihistamine spray (e.g. azelastine hydrochloride in Dymista®) is very effective. Oral antihistamines can help, but a better option may be a topical ocular mast cell-stabilizing approach.

Ocular steroids should only be used in the short term, due to the risk of cataract and glaucoma induction. Immunotherapy (desensitization to the provoking aeroallergen supervised by an experienced allergist) can be effective long term.

Allergic contact dermatitis can occur on the eyelids, particularly due to secondary contact with sensitizing agents on the hands (or gloves). Contact dermatitis presents with erythema, itch, and scaling or eczema of the periorbital and eyelid skin. It requires patch testing to define the culprit allergen (e.g. wheat germ protein in bakers).

Infection

Infective conjunctivitis can be bacterial, viral, or chlamydial. Viral conjunctivitis can cause workplace epidemics ('shipyard eye').[18] Affected subjects must be sent home promptly until their conjunctivitis has recovered.

Infective keratitis is inflammation of the cornea, commonly in the form of a corneal ulcer. Inflammation may spread into the eye, causing hypopyon (pus in the anterior chamber), and can rapidly result in blindness.

Soft contact lens wear is a risk factor for keratitis. Workers should not swim, shower, or sleep in contact lenses, and should use daily disposable lenses where possible in order to reduce the risk of serious infection.

Fungal keratitis is seen in agricultural workers, and is sight-threatening.[19] Workers must be referred urgently for an eye opinion when they complain of red eye with blurred vision after an injury involving a tree branch or contact with other organic material or animals. The key predisposing factor is trauma with implantation of spores into a corneal abrasion (by vegetation, for example, or an animal's tail). Eye protection for agricultural workers should not be neglected[20] (Table 30.2).

Cataract

This term describes opacification of the lens, either pathological or a normal ageing phenomenon. Visible lens changes are almost universal from the age of 40, but cataract can be accelerated by various factors including diabetes, trauma, and steroids.

Surgery is indicated when the vision deteriorates such that the individual patient is disabled for desired visual tasks. Modern phacoemulsification surgery is carried out as a day case through a small incision under local anaesthesia and heals very rapidly with a minimum of astigmatism and time off work.

Table 30.2 External eye disorders and their management at work

Condition	Symptoms and signs	Workplace adjustment	Other medical actions
Dry eye	Mild discomfort Reduced acuity rarely	Measure relative humidity Adjust humidity. Remove from unavoidably dry or dusty workplace	Ophthalmological assessment (tear drops)
Allergy	Moderate discomfort and/or itch; discomfort/glare less commonly	Remove from workplace source of allergen Discourage working at height or operating machinery if requires antihistamines	Ophthalmological and/or allergist assessment. Try to identify allergen Consider replacing antihistamine with steroid nasal sprays
Infective conjunctivitis	Moderate discomfort	Remove from workplace as may be infectious (via droplets or fomites)	Ophthalmological assessment
Infective keratitis	Severe discomfort/ glare/pain Severely reduced acuity	Consider whether other employees at risk When resolved, re-employ depending on degree of visual disability	Urgent ophthalmological assessment (these patients may need hospital admission)

The glaucomas

This family of diseases is characterized by the triad of raised intraocular pressure, optic nerve damage, and visual field loss.

Intraocular pressure is maintained by the balance of production and drainage of aqueous humour. As the pressure rises, perfusion of the optic nerve head falls. This results in ischaemic and direct pressure damage to the fibres serving the visual field, which appears clinically as increased cupping of the optic disc.

Ocular hypertension

In this condition, intraocular pressure is raised above 22 mmHg but there is no optic nerve damage or visual field loss. Approximately 9% of patients with ocular hypertension progress to primary open-angle glaucoma (POAG) in 5 years.[21] The risk is greater where other glaucoma risk factors are present.

Primary open-angle glaucoma

In POAG, the rise in intraocular pressure is insidious, intermittent, and asymptomatic. POAG is more common in myopes and those with a family history. Pressure may show a circadian variation, with spikes in the early morning.

Asymptomatic visual loss starts as an expansion of the physiological blind spot. Detection of POAG therefore depends on screening of visual fields, intraocular pressure, and optic discs. Ideally, everyone would be screened but resource-limited screening is targeted to high-risk groups such as myopes, people with a family history, and ethnic groups such as African-Caribbean and Asian.

POAG was traditionally treated with eye drops, and surgery was reserved for late-stage disease. However, poor results generated a bad reputation for glaucoma surgery. Nowadays, surgery is offered earlier in the disease and the techniques are less disruptive to the eye. Newer micro-invasive glaucoma surgery (placing tiny stents in the drainage angle)[22] permit shorter periods of time off work but still require long-term follow up studies.

Normal-tension glaucoma

In normal-tension glaucoma, the disc and field features are identical but the pressure is low or normal. Normal-tension glaucoma is due to axonal dropout in the optic nerve head, from impaired perfusion or primary neuronal degeneration. The disease is more difficult to treat. This has generated the concept of target intraocular pressure, which states an aim for a reduction of 40% of the pressure at diagnosis.

More recently, some glaucoma specialists have challenged this paradigm and emphasized that 'lower is better', that is, that the target pressure should only reflect the upper limit of acceptable glaucoma control.[23] Some glaucoma medications are claimed to be neuroprotective. There is some evidence that statin use is associated with a reduced incidence of glaucoma. The effect on progression is less certain.[24]

Angle-closure glaucoma

In angle-closure glaucoma, the outflow of aqueous is blocked by contact between the iris root and the peripheral cornea. This is an extremely painful condition, which produces blurred vision, red eye, headache, and vomiting.

Table 30.3 Anterior segment disorders and their management at work

Condition	Symptoms and signs	Workplace adjustment	Other medical actions
Cataract	Reduced acuity Glare	Usually none necessary as cataract surgery is widely available and has a high success rate. Could increase luminance and contrast while waiting for surgery or in the very rare inoperable case	Ophthalmological assessment Time off after cataract surgery, depending on type of operation and type of job[a]
Ocular hypertension	None	None	Ophthalmological assessment
Primary open-angle and normal-tension glaucoma (POAG and NTG)	Visual field defects Reduced acuity (in very late disease)	Ophthalmological assessment	Assess risks based on the residual visual field defect
Angle-closure glaucoma (ACG)	Severe discomfort Reduced acuity Visual field defects	Ophthalmological assessment	Urgent ophthalmological assessment Assess risks based on residual visual field defect

[a] In all cases of eye surgery in safety-critical occupations, such as aviation, a report must be obtained from the treating clinician that there are no complications and the patient has recovered. The patient must meet the visual requirements of the appropriate regulatory authority.

Sometimes angle-closure glaucoma occurs in a more insidious, chronic form as recurrent headaches. Angle closure is more common in hyperopia, or when early cataract causes the lens to swell. Treatment uses surgery or the YAG (yttrium aluminium garnet) laser to make a small hole in the periphery of the iris (a peripheral iridotomy) to allow the aqueous to bypass the pupil block (Table 30.3).

Squint

In this family of conditions, the visual axes of the eyes are not aligned. This may produce double vision if the squint is of recent onset. If the squint is of gradual onset (or present since childhood), the brain will adapt such that the image from the squinting eye is suppressed and thus diplopia is prevented. In these circumstances, of course, binocular vision is impossible and stereopsis is absent.

Childhood-onset squint results in amblyopia (lazy eye) if it goes undetected before the age of 5 years. Since there are other non-strabismic causes of amblyopia, some people who have reached adulthood with amblyopia do not have an obvious squint.

Squint can often be treated with surgery to lengthen or shorten the extraocular muscles. There is considerable evidence that people with squints are subject to discrimination in the recruitment process and in the workplace.[25] Despite this, there is direct evidence that people with squints do as well as orthophoric (straight-eyed) people in complex tasks such as flying.[26]

Table 30.4 Strabismus and its management at work

Condition	Symptoms and signs	Workplace adjustment	Other medical actions
Amblyopia	Reduced acuity in one eye Reduced binocularity	None after original diagnosis	Assess for role not requiring stereopsis
Long-standing squint since childhood	Visible strabismus Reduced binocularity	None after original diagnosis	Do not place in a role requiring stereopsis
Recent-onset adult squint	Visible strabismus Reduced binocularity Diplopia Nausea Disorientation	Urgent neurological assessment (for cranial nerve palsy)	Placement depends on success of treatment for diplopia
Stable squint in particular directions of gaze, e.g. upwards	Reduced binocularity and/or diplopia in relevant direction of gaze	Assess direction of gaze where problem lies, e.g. upgaze for forklift drivers	Placement depends on success of treatment for diplopia. Consider work placement where the affected direction of gaze is not necessary on task

Adult-onset squint is more commonly due to muscular or neurological disorders and must be investigated. Double vision is disabling and can cause serious danger if, for example, the employee is involved in transport or in working at height.

Double vision occurs in the direction of action of the weak muscle. In the chronic situation, this may be occupationally relevant. Diplopia in upgaze (due to weakness of an elevator muscle), for example, would be disabling to a forklift driver but not to an office worker (Table 30.4).

Retinal disorders

Diabetes

Diabetes mellitus causes a spectrum of eye problems due to capillary closure and ischaemia. These problems are seen in both type 1 and type 2 diabetes.

Background retinopathy is characterized by dots and blots due to capillary microangiography. *Pre-proliferative retinopathy* is characterized by variation in venous calibre, deep cluster haemorrhages, and cotton wool spots (also called 'soft exudates', although they are, in fact, retinal infarcts). In *proliferative retinopathy*, new vessels grow from the venous side of the circulation, commonly from the disc or from the major vascular arcades. These are fragile and prone to bleed. Bleeding causes vitreous haemorrhage and subsequent organization can cause tractional retinal detachment.

The development of retinopathy is related to diabetic control and is strongly associated with nephropathy.

Retinal vein occlusion

Venous occlusion may be associated with systemic hypertension, diabetes, ocular hypertension, and hyperlipidaemia and hyperviscosity syndromes. These conditions must be excluded and the patient may need to be followed in the eye clinic for ischaemic retinal complications.

Retinal artery occlusion

Some patients with retinal artery occlusion have prodromal episodes of amaurosis fugax. Retinal artery occlusion may be due to emboli from the heart wall, the cardiac valves, or the great vessels. The patient must be adequately investigated in order to prevent stroke, as detailed in the following sections.

Posterior ciliary artery occlusion

This causes anterior ischaemic optic neuropathy, which is characterized by the clinical triad of reduced acuity, relative afferent pupillary defect, and milky swelling of the optic disc ('pale papilloedema'). Posterior ciliary artery occlusion is most commonly due to giant cell arteritis, so all patients should have their erythrocyte sedimentation rate and C-reactive protein measured and be considered for temporal artery biopsy or temporal artery ultrasound.[27]

Retinal detachment

Rhegmatogenous retinal detachment is caused by abnormal attachments of the vitreous in conjunction with thinning and degeneration in the peripheral retina. The vitreous gel undergoes focal liquefaction and becomes more mobile. In other areas, the vitreous forms degenerate fibres which have contractile properties. The vitreous pulls on the retina as it contracts, tearing holes in the degenerate area. The fluid vitreous passes through the holes, separating the retina from the underlying retinal pigment epithelium. When separation occurs for more than a few hours, the photoreceptors begin to undergo irreversible damage. 'Macula-on' detachments or recent 'macula-off' detachments are, therefore, regarded as surgical emergencies with potential for preserving or restoring central vision.

Fresh tears can be spot-welded with the argon laser. Very peripheral small detachments can sometimes be treated by injecting gas into the vitreous. Larger detachments require formal surgery, either external or internal to the globe. In external surgery, indentation pushes the sclera onto the hole in the retina, thus obtaining a seal. This is combined with localized laser or freezing to cause an adhesive scar. Internal surgery involves removing the detached vitreous (vitrectomy). Thereafter, a variety of procedures including laser and gas, fluid, or oil injection fix the retina back in place. As gas is subject to changes in atmospheric pressure, patients should not fly thereafter. The retinal surgeon will be able to advise on the gas that was used in the procedure, and how long it is likely to remain in the eye before it is absorbed. Some gases are chosen because they linger in the eye for several weeks (Table 30.5).

Table 30.5 Retinal disorders and their management at work

Condition	Symptoms and signs	Workplace adjustment	Other medical actions
Background diabetic retinopathy	None	None	None ophthalmologically. Optimize diabetic control and co-morbidity, e.g. hypertension
Pre-proliferative diabetic retinopathy	None	Depends on other (non-ocular) aspects of the diabetes diagnosis	None ophthalmologically. Optimize diabetic control and co-morbidity, e.g. hypertension
Proliferative diabetic retinopathy	Reduced acuity	Depends on other (non-ocular) aspects of the diabetes diagnosis	Urgent ophthalmological and medical assessment
Retinal vein occlusion	Reduced acuity Visual field defect	Depends on extent of visual recovery May be left with field defect or reduced VA if affecting the macula	Urgent ophthalmological and medical assessment[a]
Retinal artery and posterior cerebral artery occlusion	Reduced acuity Reduced colour vision	Depends on extent of visual recovery May be left with field defect or reduced VA if affecting the macula	Urgent ophthalmological and medical assessment
Retinal detachment	Visual field defect Reduced acuity	Depends on extent of visual recovery May be left with field defect or reduced VA if affecting the macula.	Urgent ophthalmological and medical assessment[c]

[a] Medical assessment should include blood pressure by 24-hour blood pressure recording if necessary, management of other cardiovascular risk factors, exercise ECG to the Bruce protocol, and thrombophilia screen.

[b] Medical assessment as per 'a' but also including full blood count and erythrocyte sedimentation rate; temporal artery biopsy if erythrocyte sedimentation rate raised or if otherwise indicated, carotid Doppler scan, and echocardiogram.

[c] Retinal detachment should be treated before it progresses to affect the macula.

Time off work after surgery

This will depend on the nature of the job and the surgeon's recommendations in the individual case; also on whether work is manual or sedentary, and whether it is hazardous or safety critical (Table 30.6).

Workplace design

Lighting and visibility

Visibility is affected by lighting, air clarity (often reduced in foundries and mining, for example), and glare from reflective surfaces. Lighting is extremely important for safety, since the more rapidly a hazard is seen, the more easily it can be avoided. Poor lighting can result in significant costs from accidents or reduced productivity.

Table 30.6 Time off work after common ophthalmic surgical procedures. Suggested times are guidelines for uncomplicated cases only; these may vary in the individual case depending on the clinical circumstances

Operation	Time off work			
	Manual	**Sedentary**	**Hazardous, e.g. working at height**	**Safety critical**[a]
Cataract (phacoemulsification)	2 weeks	1 day	2 weeks	6 weeks
Drainage surgery for glaucoma	1 month	1week	1month	3 months
Pterygium excision	2 weeks	1 week	1 month	4 weeks
Corneal transplant	2 months	2 weeks	2 months	3 months
Refractive surgery	1 week	1 day	2 weeks	3 months
Squint correction	2 weeks	1 week	1 month	3 months
Conventional retinal detachment repair	2 months	2 weeks	2 months	3 months
Vitrectomy retinal detachment repair	2 months	2 weeks	2 months	3 months

[a] In all cases of eye surgery in hazardous and safety-critical occupations, such as aviation, a report must be obtained from the treating clinician that there are no complications and the patient has recovered. The patient must meet the visual requirements of the appropriate regulatory authority.

Employers should provide lighting that is suitable and adequate to meet the requirements of the workplace. In cases of doubt, measurement should be made by a competent person using an appropriate light meter with variable light source settings including daylight, fluorescent, mercury, and tungsten. The luminance should be task related and, ideally, adjusted for the age of the employee. Due to age-related miosis, lens opacity, and reduced retinal sensitivity, older employees may require higher levels of luminance to achieve visual efficiency. In addition to general diffuse lighting, local lighting at each workstation should be under the control of the employee (but avoiding glare for adjacent colleagues). Emergency lighting is required where people may be exposed to danger.

Detailed recommendations are published by the Charted Institution of Building Services Engineers. Their Society of Light and Lighting publishes a Code of Practice and various useful lighting application standards and guides (see 'Useful websites').

Display screen equipment

There is no evidence that working with computer screens can harm employees' sight, although temporary phenomena have been described (Box 30.3).

Regular work breaks are advised, particularly with visually demanding or repetitive work. The relevant legislation can be found in the Health and Safety (Display Screen Equipment) Regulations as amended by the Health and Safety (Miscellaneous Amendments) Regulations 2002 (see 'Useful websites').

Equipment should be properly maintained to avoid flicker, glare, and reflection. There should also be flexibility in positioning of the screen, keyboard, and source material,

Box 30.3 Temporary visual phenomena with use of display screen equipment

- DSE images are inherently blurred; as blur is a stimulus to the accommodation reflex, the eyes may undergo a constant focusing search, causing eye strain.
- Ciliary spasm produces a measurable increase in the resting point of accommodation after DSE use.
- Concentrating on a display screen produces a reduction in blink rate, exacerbating dry eye symptoms.

allowing the operator to adjust the workstation to meet their visual requirements. Headaches attributed to eyestrain may arise from poor ergonomics causing postural and muscular strain. The Display Screen Regulations emphasize the importance of correct seating at workstations.

Presbyopic individuals may have difficulty because their reading spectacle correction is unsuitable for the DSE distance. Operators should be able to read N6 throughout the range 75–33 cm. Phorias at working distances should be corrected, unless they are well compensated or suppressed. The near point of convergence should be normal and any convergence insufficiency should be treated.

Periodic eye tests should be offered to 'DSE users', who:

- use DSE for continuous or near-continuous spells of an hour or more at a time
- use DSE in this way more or less daily
- transfer information quickly to or from the DSE.

Periodic eye tests may comprise software tests run on the DSE, and the results can be collated on the computer. The regulations make the employer responsible for the provision of an optical correction necessary for the DSE task at the appropriate working distance.

Visual fatigue

Visual fatigue is avoided by optimizing the working environment in terms of lighting, ergonomics, and task rotation. Uncorrected defects in refraction, accommodation, and convergence may cause asthenopia and should be treated. Spectacles should be optimized for the working distance of the individual employee.

Employment of people with visual impairment

Adjustments for visual disability are covered under the provisions of the Equality Act 2010. Visual disability is highly variable in terms of impact on the activities of day-to-day living and suitability and adjustments available in employment. Advice for employers is available online from the RNIB and the government's Access to Work scheme (see 'Useful websites'). Notably older workers have more difficulty adapting to visual loss (often due to macular degeneration and cataracts), as do those who experience sudden loss of vision. A bereavement reaction is often associated with loss of sight and employment, and this can be accompanied by depression. It is therefore vital that the OH professional facilitates job replacement and rehabilitation promptly.

Workplace ocular hazards and eye protection

Heat

Direct thermal burns to the ocular surface occur with sparks and molten metal injuries. Infrared radiation can cause damage to the anterior lens capsule, and is implicated in a form of occupational cataract in glassblowers.

Light

Light is hazardous to the eyes and the skin. The impact of photons in tissues damages cells both directly and indirectly through production of free radicals. Chronic exposure to sunlight causes skin damage such as solar elastosis and keratosis, basal cell carcinomas, and squamous carcinomas. These conditions are more common in outdoor workers.

Sunlight can cause an acute keratitis, particularly when it is reflected from sea or snow (Labrador keratopathy). The harmful wavelengths are ultraviolet (UV)-B (295–315 nm). Chronic surface exposure causes conjunctival elastosis and pterygium formation. Sunlight also causes damage within the lens and is cataractogenic; the harmful wavelengths are UVA (315–380 nm). Phototoxic damage to the retina by high-energy blue light of 400–500 nm is also thought to be a risk factor for macular degeneration.

Light causes glare. Good-quality sunglasses protect the eyes from the toxic effect of light by filtering out harmful wavelengths. The light intensity passing through the filters in sunglasses should have a transmittance of 18%, reducing luminance at the ocular surface to 1000 cd/m^2. Neutral grey filters allow the preservation of the spectral composition of light. The transmittance of harmful wavelengths such as UVA/UVB and blue should not be more than 1%.

UV light is a cause of acute keratitis (welder's flash), retinal damage, and maculopathy in arc welding.[28] This has been reported even with a short duration of exposure or when wearing eye protection, and has also been reported to be potentiated by photosensitizing drugs.[29] Welding UV exposure has been implicated as a risk factor for skin and ocular malignancy.

Lasers

Laser (light amplification by stimulated emission of radiation) is a monochromatic (single wavelength), collimated (parallel), and coherent (in-phase) beam of light, which delivers high energy over a small area. Applications include cutting and shaping materials, measurement, recording, displays, communications, holography, remote sensing, surveying, uranium enrichment, medical uses, and as weapons.

Lasers are classified according to their energy levels and the risk of injury. In general, laser bioeffects can be photochemical, thermal, or acoustic. Photochemical effects are generally transient and are a form of scotomatic disability glare. Thermal effects include retinal burns, which cause permanent scotomas.

The site of laser damage is in the posterior segment, where the light is converted to heat by absorption within the pigments of the retinal pigment epithelium and retina to produce a burn.[30] The burn has more functional effect if it is at the fovea (caused when the patient was looking directly at the discharging laser source). Acute eye injuries occur in medical and industrial settings with inadequate eye protection. There is some evidence of chronic damage in the form of diminished colour vision in workers using lasers over long periods.

Laser hazards are significantly reduced by proper safety procedures. Multiple types of filter protect against beam-related injuries, and these are not always easy to distinguish, particularly in a dark work environment. It is imperative that eye protection contains a filter appropriate to the wavelength of the laser being used. It is less straightforward to protect certain occupational groups such as pilots from deliberate, criminal assault with hand-held laser pointers, a dangerous occurrence which is reported to be on the increase worldwide.[31]

Non-beam hazards associated with lasers include thermal injury, fire, smoke plume, and electrical hazards. There should be a qualified laser safety officer whose responsibilities include regular inspection, maintenance, and staff training.

An evidence-based protocol should be established for the diagnosis and management of laser injuries. Retinal laser lesions that cause serious visual problems are readily apparent on ophthalmological examination, and do not cause chronic pain without physical signs. Alleged laser injuries can result in lengthy medico-legal claims and therefore a full assessment should be carried out on all such cases.[32]

Radiation

Ionizing radiation can damage the lens of the eye (cataract), the posterior segment (radiation retinopathy), and the visual pathways. Radiation retinopathy presents clinically as degenerative and proliferative vascular changes, mainly affecting the macula.[33] The mechanism is similar to that in diabetes, that is, it is due to damage to the retinal capillaries.

Although less common, microwave injury also causes lens and retinal damage.

Electrical shock

High-voltage shock can produce cataract amenable to standard surgical treatment.

Chemicals, particles, fibres, irritants and aeroallergens

Caustic chemicals (acids and alkalis), solvents (alcohols such as *n*-butanol, aldehydes, and ethers), anionic or cationic surfactants, methylating agents such as dimethyl sulphate, aniline dyes, and toxic vegetable products such as *Euphorbia* saps[19] can all cause damage to both corneal and conjunctival epithelium, and can result in late scarring and opacification.

Exposure may be in the form of a splash, but the conjunctiva of the eye is a mucous membrane and is affected by the same gases (e.g. ammonia) that cause respiratory embarrassment. The pathogenesis of ocular toxic reactions varies with the agent with, for example, surfactants causing emulsification of the cell membrane lipid layer.

Fibres and dust in the atmosphere also cause irritation. Part of the response to atmospheric irritants is lacrimation, and this reduces VA by a surface effect, as well as being distracting. This may compromise safety in situations such as mining and work at heights.

Glass fibres occasionally lodge under the lids or in the lacrimal puncta, where they can be very difficult to visualize due to their virtual transparency.

One study of chemical industry workers in South Africa showed an increased prevalence of ocular disorders including tear film disorders, dry eye conditions, allergic conjunctivitis, and conjunctival melanosis. Forty-one per cent of the ocular disorders in this study were thought to have resulted from occupational exposure.

One study of animal workers in 2014 found 36% had evidence of sensitization to animals against 10% of controls. About a third of the workers, who were predominantly veterinarians, reported allergic conjunctivitis.[34]

Adequate ventilation is more effective than eye protectors in these circumstances. The American Society of Heating, Refrigeration and Air-Conditioning Engineers has recommended environmental controls for animal rooms at 10–15 air changes per hour with 100% outdoor air, relative humidity of 30–60%, and a temperature of 16–29°C (61–84°F). Good workplace hygiene and PPE (lab coats, gloves, face shields, and respirators) reduce exposure to hair, dander, urine, and saliva. Emergency procedures should be in place for managing anaphylaxis, including staff training in resuscitation and availability of adrenaline.

Occupational injuries and eye protection

US statistics show that eye injuries at work account for 13% of all eye injuries, compared with 40% at home, 13% on the street, 13% playing a sport, 12% other, and 9% unknown.

Among all eye injuries over a 1-year period in Glasgow, 61% were due to work, the majority of which were due to buffing and grinding, and in 83% the required eye protection was not being worn.[35]

One study in Hong Kong showed that in 85% of eye injuries in the construction industry, no eye protection had been worn.[36] The following were associated with lower risk:

◆ Longer duration in the current job.

◆ Job safety training before employment.

- Regular repair and maintenance of machinery or equipment.
- Wearing safety glasses regularly.
- A requirement for wearing eye protection.

Injuries to the eyes can occur in isolation, but the more severe injuries occur in the setting of more widespread trauma, in which case the Advanced Trauma Life Support® (ATLS®) principles of rapid primary survey and detailed secondary survey apply.

In an industrial setting, the common eye injuries seen are corneal abrasion, corneal and subtarsal foreign bodies, superficial burns, and chemical burns. Severe blunt injury, penetrating eye injury, intraocular foreign body, and compressed air injuries are rare but serious. Management comprises rapid first aid and protecting the eye while the patient is transferred to a specialist unit.

Corneal abrasion

In this condition, the corneal epithelium is damaged by a scratch. The abrasion can be highlighted with fluorescein drops and blue light. Treatment is antibiotic ointment and padding of the eye. Healing is rapid and complications are rare, but these do include infection and impaired healing with recurrent spontaneous breakdown of the epithelium (recurrent corneal erosion syndrome).

Corneal foreign bodies

These are commonly seen where workers are under a raised platform, or in grinding incidents. The metal is embedded in the epithelium and superficial stroma of the cornea. It is easily removed, but this is best done at the slit-lamp. Metal ions pass into the cornea and oxidize, forming a semi-solid rust ring. This is best removed with a corneal burr, again at the slit-lamp. Removal of the rust ring is sometimes best deferred until the day after the primary foreign body is removed, and several sessions are sometimes necessary to allow the cornea, which is only 0.5–1.0 mm thick, to heal. After each session, the treatment is as for a corneal abrasion.

Subtarsal foreign bodies

There is a longitudinal ridge under the upper eyelid where loose foreign bodies become trapped, abrading the cornea with each blink. These can be removed with a cotton bud after everting the lid. The vertical corneal abrasions on the upper cornea are managed as for corneal foreign bodies.

Superficial burns

These are common in welders, and are known in the trade as *arc eye* or *welder's flash*. The injury is caused by UV light. The symptoms of surface cell death are delayed for several hours, and include lid swelling, blepharospasm, ocular pain, photophobia, and profuse lacrimation. Treatment is with topical analgesia, antibiotic ointment, and padding.

Chemical burns

Chemical injury causes direct cell death and ischaemic necrosis, followed by ingress of leucocytes and release of inflammatory mediators such as prostaglandins, cytokines, superoxide radicals, and lysosomal enzymes.

Acid burns, while serious, tend to be more superficial than alkali burns. Due to surface coagulation, the acid may not penetrate the eye. They consist of stromal haze and ischaemia affecting less than one-third of the corneal limbus and are associated with a better visual prognosis.

Alkalis cause more severe and deeper effects because the alkali penetrates the eye and the pH in the anterior chamber rises rapidly, damaging intraocular structures such as the iris, the drainage angle, and the lens. These injuries, often causing stromal opacity and ischaemia affecting more than one-half of the corneal limbus are associated with a poor visual prognosis.

Immediate and sustained irrigation is required (see 'Ocular first aid at work'). Upon transfer to a specialist centre, medical treatment includes further irrigation, steroids, antibiotics, and ascorbic acid. Surgery may be necessary for late complications, and secondary glaucoma is a real risk in severely damaged eyes.

Blunt injury

Haematoma (black eye) may conceal a severe eye injury until the swelling subsides.

Orbital apex fractures are associated with high-velocity injuries. These damage the optic nerve, which can only withstand ischaemia for about 2 hours, or pressure-induced disturbance of axoplasmic flow for about 8 hours. If such an injury is suspected, the current consensus favours systemic steroids and early neurosurgical decompression.

Orbital blowout fracture describes a situation where the eye is propelled backwards and the walls of the orbit fracture outwards into the ethmoid and maxillary sinuses, leaving the eye and the orbital rim intact. Clinical features are enophthalmos, diplopia, surgical emphysema, and infraorbital nerve anaesthesia. Radiology shows the *hanging drop sign* in the maxillary antrum, and a CT scan will help quantify the bony defect. Management is controversial, with equally vociferous proponents of early surgery and conservative management. Antibiotics are useful first aid because asymptomatic sinus infection is common. The patient should be instructed not to blow their nose as this can spread infection to the soft tissues of the orbit, and surgical emphysema compressing the optic nerve has been described.[37]

Contusion injuries of the globe cause damage at the point of impact and contrecoup injuries. These include hyphaema, iris damage, angle damage, lens damage, vitreous haemorrhage, retinal oedema (*commotio retinae*), retinal breaks and detachment, and traumatic optic neuropathy. Their management is best left to specialist centres, with first aid during transfer consisting of adequate analgesia and antiemesis and a Cartella eye shield to protect the eye.

Penetrating injury

This is often deceptively painless in the acute stage. Signs include a visible laceration, prolapse of intraocular contents (iris appearing as a dark knot of tissue, vitreous as a blob of gel), and a collapsed anterior chamber. Extreme caution should be exercised in examining the eye to avoid prolapsing the ocular contents.

The eye should be covered with a shield and antiemetics or sedation given as necessary while preparing for transfer. Some injured eyes do well with primary repair and secondary reconstruction, but there is some evidence that an eye damaged beyond repair should be removed within 2 weeks to prevent the development of sight-threatening autoimmune inflammatory disease in the fellow eye (sympathetic ophthalmitis).

Intraocular foreign body

This is a special type of penetrating eye injury, where a small metallic body lodges in the eye, leaving a tiny entry wound that may not be apparent on casual inspection. The diagnosis depends on accurate history taking, with the patient usually hammering metal on metal without eye protection. The diagnosis must be made early to prevent metal ions diffusing into the eye tissues causing late toxicity and blindness. A missed intraocular foreign body is a frequent cause of clinical negligence claims, and a negative orbital X-ray does not exclude the diagnosis.

Compressed air injuries

Surgical emphysema can compress the optic nerve.[38] In situations where the vision is deteriorating, emergency decompression of the orbit can be performed with an intravenous cannula or by dis-inserting the lateral margin of the lower eyelid (emergency cantholysis).

Time off work

This is determined by considering time to recovery of function, bearing in mind that this may be less than time to full recovery (i.e. time to full stability). Between these there is a window of risk of structural failure producing incapacitation or indeed further damage to the eye. This latter risk may be mitigated to some extent by eye protection. For this reason, the times in Table 30.7 should be treated as suggestions only. The time off work will vary between individual cases, depending on relevant testing before a return to work.

Eye protection

An element of workplace design and culture, eye protection follows logically from task analysis, and must be part of a programme of continuous staff safety awareness training.

PPE should comply with the European Union Personal Protective Equipment Directive, bear the 'CE' mark, and be appropriate to the actual hazards of the work

Table 30.7 A rough guide to time off work following recovery from occupational eye injuries

Injury	Time off work			
	Manual	**Sedentary**	**Hazardous, e.g. dusty, at height**	**Safety critical**
Welder's flash	1 day	–	–	–
Corneal abrasion	2 days	1 day	1 week	2 weeks
Corneal foreign body	2 days	1 day	1 week	2 weeks
Subtarsal foreign body	1 day	1 day	1 day	1 day
Chemical burns—mild, e.g. perfume	1 day–1 week	1 day–1 week	1 day–1 week	1 day–1 week
Chemical burns—acid	1–3 months	1–3 months	1–3 months	1–3 months
Chemical burns—alkali	1–6 months	1–6 months	2–6 months	May not be able to return to pre-injury work
Haematoma	1 day–1 week	1 day–1 week	1 day–1 week	1 week–1 month
Apical orbital fracture with optic nerve involvement	2–6 months	2–6 months	2–6 months	May not be able to return to pre-injury work
Blow-out fracture	1 month	2 weeks	2 months	3 months
Blunt trauma	Depends on actual injuries and severity	Depends on actual injuries and severity	Depends on actual injuries and severity	May not be able to return to work
Penetrating trauma	Depends on actual injuries and severity	Depends on actual injuries and severity	Depends on actual injuries and severity	May not be able to return to work
Intraocular foreign body	2 months	2 weeks	2 months	3 months
Compressed air injury	Depends on actual injuries and severity	Depends on actual injuries and severity	Depends on actual injuries and severity	May not be able to return to work

undertaken with regard to dimensions, lens quality, optical power, prescription, field of vision, transmittance of infrared and UV, luminous transmittance, signal recognition, frame requirements, mechanical strength, impact resistance, abrasion resistance, resistance to molten metal, and resistance to dust and gas.

A plethora of products and brands are available, and attention should be paid to the appropriate standards for situation. The reader is advised to consult the up-to-date *European Standards and Markings for Eye and Face Protection* available on the Health and Safety Executive website.[39] See Box 30.4 for criteria that should be used in selection of PPE.

Box 30.4 Criteria to be considered when selecting personal protective equipment

1. Type of hazard:
   a. Mechanical (flying debris, dust, or molten metal).
   b. Chemical (fumes, gas, or liquid splash).
   c. Radiation (heat, UV, or glare).
   d. Laser (over a wide spectrum of wavelengths).
2. Type of protector:
   a. A safety face shield protects face and eyes but does not keep out dust or gas. It can be comfortably worn for long period.
   b. Safety goggles provide protection for all hazards and may be worn over spectacles.
   c. Safety spectacles are comfortable but will not keep out dust, gas, or molten metal. Prescriptions are easily incorporated.
3. Type and shade of lens:
   a. Toughened and laminated glass is less impact resistant but more resistant to abrasion.
   b. Polymethylmethacrylate and polycarbonate offer high-impact resistance but are easily scratched.

Ocular first aid at work

Planning

Risk assessment should include the possibility of chemical splashes to the eyes, the number of employees likely to be affected, and the optimum sites for positioning of emergency eye wash stations.[40] Staff should be trained, and updated regularly, in the actions to be taken if they or their colleagues are injured.

In remote workplaces, a prearranged telemedicine service provides an invaluable source of information for the care of casualties including eye injuries.

Assessment

An adequate light with magnification and fluorescein eye drops are necessary to examine eye casualties. Local anaesthetic drops are invaluable in calming the situation down and enabling adequate examination. Proxymetacaine does not sting, but has to be stored in a refrigerator.

A vision chart should be at hand. The telephone number of the local eye unit should be available with printed and laminated protocols for injury management at the first-aid station, and an emergency management slate for record keeping.

Irrigation

Immediate irrigation is the priority, using water, saline, Ringer's lactate, and balanced salt solution or, in reality, whatever is available and safe. Ideally, irrigation is continued using an intravenous infusion set while holding the lids open with a speculum if necessary.

Eye shields

In suspected eye injury, a transparent Cartella shield can be taped over the eye while arranging transfer. Shields should be secured with suitable tape, and Friar's balsam is useful to keep the skin sticky for long transfers in patients who may be sweating profusely.

Medications

Prior to transfer of the casualty to a specialist centre, emergency medical treatment may include antibiotic drops as directed by the telemedicine service. A preparation such as chloramphenicol Minims should be at hand. Ointment should not be used in eye injury as it may enter the eye in penetrating injuries. Preservative-free drops will not cause problems in this situation.

> **Key points**
>
> - Ophthalmology is advancing rapidly although the principles of assessment remain the same. Expert advice should be sought particularly for those undergoing surgery.
> - Vision is far more complex than VA. People with impaired test results (e.g. VA or visual fields) should be properly assessed clinically so that results are assessed in context.
> - Visual fitness criteria for workers should be based on an occupational task analysis. Otherwise, people with temporary or permanent visual conditions may be inappropriately excluded from particular occupations.
> - Colour vision is important for safety-critical occupations when it is the sole reference for detection of particular objects. Colour discrimination should be assessed using appropriately validated tests of colour vision to identify unsafe applicants for particular occupations.
> - The DSE regulations are of more than theoretical importance. Failure to attend to workplace design issues can result in discomfort and reduced productivity in the absence of actual eye disease.

Useful websites

Driver and Vehicle Licensing Agency (DVLA). 'Assessing fitness to drive: a guide for medical professionals', 2018

https://www.gov.uk/government/publications/assessing-fitness-to-drive-a-guide-for-medical-professionals

Charted Institution of Building Services Engineers (CIBSE)	www.cibse.org/Society-of-Light-and-Lighting-SLL
Health and Safety Executive (HSE). Working with DSE	http://www.hse.gov.uk/pubns/indg36.pdf
HSE. DSE regulations	http://www.hse.gov.uk/pubns/books/l26.htm
RNIB	http://www.rnib.org.uk
Access to Work	https://www.gov.uk/access-to-work

Acknowledgements

The authors gratefully acknowledge the contribution of Bruce Allan, Steve Winder, Harsha Kariyawasam, and John Barbur.

References

1. **Dutton GN.** Cognitive vision, its disorders and differential diagnosis in adults and children: knowing where and what things are. *Eye* 2003;**17**:289–304.
2. **Gibb R, Gray R, Scharff L.** *Aviation Visual Perception: Research, Misperception and Mishaps.* Farnham: Ashgate; 2010.
3. **Felton JS.** The heritage of Bernardino Ramazzini. *Occup Med* 1997;**47**:167–79.
4. **Clare G, Pitts JA, Edgington K, et al.** From beach lifeguard to astronaut: occupational vision standards and the implications of refractive surgery. *Br J Ophthalmol* 2010;**94**:400–5.
5. **Rodriguez-Carmona M, O'Neill-Biba M, Barbur JL.** Assessing the severity of colour vision loss with implications for aviation and other occupational environments. *Aviat Space Environ Med* 2012;**83**:19–29.
6. **Barbur J, Rodriguez-Carmona M.** Colour vision requirements in visually demanding occupations. *Br Med Bull* 2017;**122**:51–77.
7. **Bailey KGH, Carter T.** Consistency of secondary colour vision tests in transport industries *Occup Med* 2016;**66**:268–75.
8. **Clifford L, Turnbull AMJ, Denning AM.** Reversible night blindness – a reminder of the increasing importance of vitamin A deficiency in the developed world. *J Optom* 2013;**6**:173–4.
9. **Kanski J.** *Clinical Ophthalmology: A systematic Approach*, 8th rev. edn. London: WB Saunders/Elsevier; 2015.
10. **Pelli D, Bex P.** Measuring contrast sensitivity. *Vis Res* 2013;**90**:10–14.
11. **Levi D, Knill DC, Bavelier D.** Stereopsis and amblyopia: a mini review. *Vis Res* 2015;**114**:17–30.
12. **Hess R, To L, Zhou J, Wang G, Cooperstock JR.** Stereo vision: the haves and have-nots. *iPerception* 2015;**6**:1–5.
13. **Wright L, Wormald R.** Stereopsis and ageing. *Eye* 1992;**6**:473–6.
14. **Aslam T, Haider D, Murray IJ.** Principles of disability glare assessment. *Acta Ophthalmol Scand* 2007;**85**:354–60.
15. **Orr J, Wolffsohn J.** Are we short-sighted about amblyopia? *Eye News* 2018;**24**:22–4.
16. **Bousquet P, Chinn S, Janson C, et al.** Geographical variation in the prevalence of positive skin tests to environmental aeroallergens in the European Community Respiratory Health Survey I. *Allergy* 2007;**62**:301–9.
17. **Scadding G, Kariyawasam HH, Scadding G, et al.** BSACI guideline for the diagnosis and management of allergic and non-allergic rhinitis (Revised Edition 2017; First edition 2007). *Clin Exp Allergy* 2017;**47**:856–89.

18. **Jawetz E.** The story of shipyard eye. *BMJ* 1959;1:873–6.

19. **Thomas PA.** Fungal infections of the cornea. *Eye* 2003;17:852–62.

20. **Pitts J, Barker NH, Gibbons DC, Jay JL.** Manchineel keratoconjunctivitis. *Br J Ophthalmol* 1993;77:284–8.

21. **Royal College of Ophthalmologists.** Glaucoma and ocular hypertension. Available at: https://www.rcophth.ac.uk/standards-publications-research/commissioning-in-ophthalmology/glaucoma-and-ocular-hypertension/.

22. **Pillunat L, Erb C, Jünemann AG, Kimmich F.** Micro-invasive glaucoma surgery (MIGS): a review of surgical procedures using stents. *Clin Ophthalmol* 2017;11:1583–600.

23. **Singh K, Shrivastava A.** Early aggressive intraocular pressure lowering, target intraocular pressure, and a novel concept for glaucoma care. *Surv Ophthalmol* 2008;53(Supp 11):33–8.

24. **McCann P.** The effect of statins on intraocular pressure and on the incidence and progression of glaucoma: a systematic review and meta-analysis. *Invest Ophthalmol Vis Sci* 2016;57:2729–48.

25. **Durnian J, Noonan CP, Marsh IB.** The psychosocial effects of adult strabismus: a review. *Br J Ophthalmol* 2011;95:450–3.

26. **Chorley A, Hunter R, Dance C.** Heterotropia and time to first solo in student pilots. *Medécine Aéronautique et Spatiale* 2011;52:74–9.

27. **Luqmani R, Lee E, Singh S, et al.** The role of ultrasound compared to biopsy of temporal arteries in the diagnosis and treatment of giant cell arteritis (TABUL): a diagnostic accuracy and cost-effectiveness study. *Health Technol Assess* 2016;20:1–238.

28. **Magnavita N.** Photoretinitis: an underestimated occupational injury? *Occup Med* 2002;52:223–5.

29. **Power W, Travers SP, Mooney DJ.** Welding arc maculopathy and fluphenazine. *Br J Ophthalmol* 1991;75:433–5.

30. **Barkana Y, Belkin M.** Laser eye injuries. *Surv Ophthalmol* 2000;44:459–78.

31. **Houston S.** Aircrew exposure to handheld laser pointers: the potential for retinal damage. *Aviat Space Environ Med* 2011;82:921–2.

32. **Mainster MA, Stuck BE, Brown J Jr.** Assessment of alleged laser injuries. *Arch Ophthalmol* 2004;122:1210–17.

33. **Archer D, Gardiner T.** Ionising radiation and the retina. *Curr Opin Ophthalmol* 1994;5:59–65.

34. **Moghtaderi M, Farjadian S, Abbaszadeh Hasiri M.** Animal allergen sensitization in veterinarians and laboratory animal workers. *Occup Med* 2014;64:516–20.

35. **MacEwan C.** Eye injuries: a prospective survey of 5671 cases. *Br J Ophthalmol* 1989;73:888–94.

36. **Yu T, Liu H, Hui K.** A case-control study of eye injuries in the workplace in Hong Kong. *Ophthalmology* 2004;111:70–4.

37. **Pitts J.** Orbital blow-out fractures. *Eye News* 1996;3:12–14.

38. **Caesar R, Gajus M, Davies R.** Compressed air injury of the orbit in the absence of external trauma. *Eye* 2003;17:661–2.

39. **Health and Safety Executive.** European Standards and Markings for Eye and Face Protection. 2013. Available at: http://www.hse.gov.uk/foi/internalops/oms/2009/03/om200903app3.pdf.

40. **Beaudoin A.** Comparing eyewash systems. *Occup Health Saf* 2003;72:50–6.

Chapter 31

Hearing and vestibular disorders

Julian Eyears and Kristian Hutson

Introduction

Hearing loss is common and, when severe, can seriously compromise an individual's ability to understand speech, perceive danger, and communicate. Profound hearing loss can affect the acquisition and development of spoken language, compromise educational attainment,[1] reduce employability,[2] and impair the individual's ability to work in a safety-critical environment.[3,4] Similarly, dizziness is a common cause of lost time from employment. Vestibular disorders can affect balance, increase the risk of falls,[5] and render the sufferer unfit to drive vehicles,[6] use machinery, and work at heights.[4] Safety is an important consideration where a stumble at work might have serious consequences, for example, on board ships.

Occupational noise is a significant cause of adult-onset hearing loss. The majority of this noise-induced hearing loss (NIHL) burden can be minimized by the use of engineering controls to reduce the generation of noise at its source and/or the effective use of hearing protection (ear plugs or muffs).[7] The occupational health (OH) professional should remain mindful that noise hazards may exist outside the traditional noisy industries: in workplaces such as orchestra pits, bars, dog homes, and jobs that are close to road traffic.

Hearing loss: classification and causes

Hearing loss can be classified as acquired or congenital, bilateral or unilateral, and can be further subdivided into conductive, sensorineural, and mixed losses. Severity or degree of hearing loss can be categorized with pure tone audiometry (PTA) (see Table 31.1).

Table 31.1 Hearing loss categorization

Degree of hearing loss	Hearing loss range (decibel hearing level)
Mild	20–40 dB HL
Moderate	41–70 dB HL
Severe	71–90 dB HL
Profound	>90 dB HL

Conductive hearing loss results from disruption of the normal passage of sound from the outer ear through to the cochlea, and can therefore result from a problem with the external auditory canal, tympanic membrane, or middle ear. Acquired causes of conductive hearing loss are numerous and include infection of the external auditory canal, suppuration in the middle ear cavity (otitis media), perforation or scarring (tympanosclerosis) of the tympanic membrane, and ossicular abnormalities. Ossicular diseases range from progressive fixation of the ossicular chain in otosclerosis to loss of normal ossicular articulation as a result of trauma or local destructive disease processes (e.g. cholesteatoma). Impacted cerumen and foreign bodies may at times cause a mild conductive hearing loss. Congenital causes of conductive hearing loss include the absence, malformation, or dysfunction of the outer or middle ears and may or may not form part of a wider genetic syndrome.

Certain causes of conductive hearing loss are amenable to surgical intervention whereas others may benefit from aiding alone. Surgery may include ventilation tubes in otitis media with effusion, tympanoplasty to repair tympanic membrane perforations, stapedectomy in otosclerosis, and ossicular reconstruction in cases of disarticulation. With most surgical procedures there remains no guarantee of hearing improvement and a small but potential risk of worsening hearing loss.

Sensorineural hearing loss (SNHL) results from dysfunction of the cochlea, auditory nerve (cranial nerve VIII), and/or central auditory pathways. The majority of acquired SNHL has no single identifiable cause; a large proportion results from environmental–genetic interaction as well as age-related changes (presbycusis) to the cochlea and auditory pathway.

NIHL accounts for the largest proportion of identifiable SNHL. Diagnosis of NIHL should not be made simply on a report of a 'noisy' working environment. It requires a thorough history and audiological assessment. There is a direct relationship between volume and duration of noise exposure. A cumulative exposure of 100 dB(A) or more (noise emission level) is sufficient to cause SNHL; this is equivalent to a continuous daily exposure to sound levels of 85 dB(A) or more for 8 or more hours a day over several years.[8] Typically the PTA will demonstrate a frequency loss over the 3–6 kHz range, often with a notch centred around 4 kHz. Lack of a classic 'notch' does not exclude NIHL as the presence of overlapping presbycusis can turn a 'notch' into a less obvious tapered bulge.[8] NIHL is typically bilateral but when loss occurs secondary to activities such as shooting, a unilateral loss in the ear closest to the barrel can be observed. Other identifiable causes of SNHL include ototoxicity (e.g. gentamicin, streptomycin, phenytoin, cisplatin, quinine, and loop diuretics) and infections, in particular mumps, measles, rubella, meningitis, and encephalitis.

Usher syndrome remains a leading cause of congenital deaf-blindness. There are three recognized types distinguished by age of presentation, involvement of the vestibular system, and degree of sensorineural deafness.[9]

Unilateral SNHL may arise post infection or traumatic fracture of the temporal bone and can be a symptom of an underlying cerebellopontine angle tumour such as a vestibular schwannoma. Individuals who present with unilateral tinnitus and/or SNHL, with or without balance disturbance, require further investigation (PTA and magnetic resonance imaging) to exclude a cerebellopontine angle lesion. The diagnostic yield is however low, with approximately 3–7.5% of those investigated being found to have a vestibular schwannoma. Patients with a cerebellopontine angle lesion often experience a slowly progressive unilateral hearing loss, but a minority (5%) suffer acute hearing loss. Similarly, those reporting acute-onset vertigo and SNHL in whom a cerebrovascular accident is suspected will require brain imaging.[10]

Non-organic hearing loss refers to the situation where audiological testing indicates a more severe hearing loss than can be explained by organic pathology of the auditory system, and can be categorized into malingering and psychogenic types.[11] In malingering, the individual is intentionally feigning hearing loss, often because of an underlying reason such as a compensation claim or desire for leaving a job. Malingering may be suspected on PTA when there is poor reproducibility of hearing thresholds and/or the hearing loss appears flat across all frequencies.[11] More objective investigations may be required including otoacoustic emissions and auditory evoked potentials. Aggravation refers to a situation where although a degree of organic hearing loss is present, the individual mimics a greater degree of hearing loss.

Epidemiology of hearing loss and tinnitus

Hearing loss affects almost 11 million people in the UK of whom at least 3.7 million are of working age. This headline figure is expected to rise as the population ages, to reach 15.6 million people with hearing loss by 2035 (see the Action on Hearing Loss website, in 'Useful websites'). Over 900,000 people are severely or profoundly deaf and they are four times more likely to be unemployed than the general population. Although over 6 million people in the UK would benefit from a hearing aid, only about 2 million people have an aid and, of these, only 1.4 million people use their aid regularly. Studies that analysed the latest labour force survey have found that people with hearing loss were less likely to be employed than those who had no long-term disability or health issue.[12]

Studies in the UK and US have found the prevalence of hearing impairment (a mild hearing loss of at least 25 dB across the speech frequencies 0.5, 1, 2, and 4 kHz) to be 16%.[13,14] The prevalence of hearing loss in the US study was increased among men, those with lower educational attainment, of Caucasian race, and older age. Exposure to occupational, firearm, and leisure noise increased the risk of hearing loss as did hypertension, diabetes mellitus, and smoking (>20 pack-years). Passive smoking has also been shown to be associated with hearing loss affecting the low/mid frequencies (0.5, 1, and 2 kHz) in those who have never smoked and who are exposed to second-hand tobacco smoke.

Tinnitus, the perception of sound in the absence of an external auditory stimulus, is extremely common and experienced transiently by most people at some point in their life. In 2015, an estimated 32,000 new cases of tinnitus were diagnosed in England with approximately 10% of the adult population affected at any one time.[15] Tinnitus can be classified as objective or subjective. Both require audiological assessment and some patients may require radiological imaging. Subjective tinnitus is thought to occur secondary to cochlea damage and may occur with or without SNHL. Unilateral subjective tinnitus should be investigated with magnetic resonance imaging for the possibility of an underlying vestibular schwannoma. Objective tinnitus may result from vascular abnormalities including arteriovenous malformations and benign intracranial hypertension or from myoclonus of nearby palatal or middle ear muscles.

Analysis of data from the 1999–2004 National Health and Nutrition Examination Survey (NHANES)[16] found that the prevalence of frequent tinnitus, which was defined as tinnitus occurring at least once a day, rose with increasing age up to 14% of the population aged 60–69 years. Tinnitus was associated with ageing, hearing loss, noise exposure, hypertension, history of smoking, and anxiety.

The majority of tinnitus is mild and patients often find their own ways to habituate; further treatment will depend on whether an underlying cause is identified. There remains no pharmacological therapy to modify or treat subjective tinnitus, the main treatments available include counselling, hearing aids (if coexisting hearing loss), and sound therapy with masking devices or white noise generators. Objective tinnitus may be open to surgical and medical therapy. Cochrane reviews have found no strong evidence for the beneficial effects of sound therapy and masking.[17] However, cognitive behavioural therapy has been found to improve quality of life and associated depressive symptoms.[18] The British Tinnitus Association provides useful advice on managing tinnitus (see 'Useful websites').

Methods of assessing hearing disability

Brief enquiry about hearing problems may alert the assessing clinician to an individual with possible hearing impairment requiring further investigation (see Table 31.2).[19,20]

Table 31.2 Screening questions for hearing loss

Question	Sensitivity	Specificity
Do you have a hearing problem now?[a]	71%	71%
Do you feel you have a hearing loss?[b]	80%	77%
In general, would you say your hearing is 'excellent', 'very good', 'good', 'fair', or 'poor'?[b]	67%	85%
Currently, do you think you can hear 'the same as before', 'less than before only in the right ear', 'less than before only in the left ear', or 'less than before in both ears'?[b]	81%	76%

[a] From a study that screened for disabling hearing loss in the elderly when compared with the gold standard of a 40 dB hearing loss at 1 and 2 kHz in one ear or at 1 or 2 kHz in both ears on screening audiometry.[19]

[b] From a study of people of working age when compared to the gold standard of PTA.[20]

Source: data from Gates, GA. et al. Screening for handicapping hearing loss in the elderly. *Journal of Family Practice*. 52(1), 56–62. Copyright © 2003 MD Edge; and Ferrite, S. et al. Validity of self-reported hearing loss in adults: performance of three single questions. *Revista de Saúde Pública*. 45(5), 824–30. Copyright © 2011 SciElo.

The whisper test is a simple screening test for hearing impairment. A number of techniques are employed for the whispered voice test and a standardized approach is necessary to avoid problems with reproducibility. However, the test–retest reliability and reproducibility of this test have been questioned[21] and the use of the whisper test is not recommended.

Speech recognition tests potentially offer a more robust assessment of the understanding of speech than whisper tests as they are not amenable to lip reading. The UK charity Action on Hearing Loss, the new name for the Royal National Institute for the Deaf, has developed the English-language version of a validated Dutch speech recognition test: the 'Hearing Check'.[22] This speech in noise screening test relies on the identification of a series of three digits, presented with varying degrees of masking using background white noise. The test can be conducted over the Internet[23] or over a phone line (see 'Useful websites'). The test takes 5 minutes and results are presented as: (a) unimpaired, (b) possibly impaired, or (c) definitely impaired.

Rinne and Weber tuning fork tests can be useful to distinguish between conductive and SNHL; however, they are not sufficiently discriminating to be useful in screening for hearing impairment.

Audioscopy is a screening tool used for identifying hearing impairment.[21] It is a combined otoscope and audiometer which generates 25–40 dB tones across a range of speech frequencies (0.5, 1, 2, and 4 kHz). This screening tool has been shown to have high sensitivity and good specificity when judged against the gold standard of audiometry.[21,24]

PTA is the standard test of hearing thresholds. To distinguish between conductive and sensorineural losses both air and bone conduction testing are required. Note that PTA is a subjective test and the results of PTA are dependent both on the individual's attention and motivation. Screening audiometry, widely used by OH professionals in hearing surveillance programmes (as required by the Control of Noise at Work Regulations 2005),[25] employs air conduction testing alone and so cannot be used for diagnostic purposes. Detailed information on audiometry and audiometric testing methods are available from the British Society of Audiology (see 'Useful websites').

Evoked otoacoustic emissions is a simple, non-invasive test of hearing, which provides an objective assessment of the integrity of the cochlea. Otoacoustic emissions may be evoked from the healthy cochlea by the generation of tones or clicks which elicit sound from the cochlea and which can be detected by an intra-aural microphone.

Auditory evoked potentials are an objective assessment of hearing thresholds and assess the integrity of the auditory system from cochlea to cortex. These specialist audiological tests are generally used for the assessment of hearing in those who are unable to cooperate or those in whom malingering or compensation is an issue. A series of clicks or tones are presented through headphones and the brain's responses are recorded using scalp electrodes. Sedation or a general anaesthetic may be required in those who are unable to cooperate with testing.

Clinical aspects affecting work capacity including accidents

There is some evidence that hearing loss increases the risk of both occupational accidents[26] and road traffic accidents in adult life.[27] It would seem likely that the inability to hear warnings, moving vehicles, or alarms might play a role in this increased burden of workplace accidents. However, while a systematic review identified 15 studies which had explored hearing loss as a risk factor for accidents, the overall quality of research in this area is limited.[28] One large, well-designed Canadian study of almost 53,000 workers, who were followed up for 5 years from last audiogram, found that those with greater than 15 dB(A) mean hearing loss across 3, 4, and 6 kHz in both ears were at increased risk of accidents.[26] Moreover, those with severe hearing loss who were employed in worksites with noise levels at, or above, 90 dB(A) were at three times the background risk of having more than three accidents.[29] An analysis of over 46,000 Quebec workers for whom audiometry data, occupational noise exposures, and road insurance claims were available, found that workers with hearing loss were at increased risk of road traffic crashes. Those with a mean hearing loss of more than 50 dB had a prevalence ratio of road crashes of 1.31 (95% confidence interval 1.2–1.42).[27]

Individuals with impaired hearing may experience difficulty with the spoken word, in face-to-face communication, and by telephone. While hearing thresholds are a guide to hearing ability, how well an individual will function for any given hearing loss is influenced by motivational factors (both of the individual and their colleagues), environmental factors (e.g. proximity of the speaker, visibility of the speaker, adequacy of lighting which facilitates lip reading, background noise levels, availability of an induction loop, and room acoustics), and the complexity and predictability of speech. Reports of communication difficulties by colleagues and managers are important evidence as to how well an individual may hear, but additional assessment beyond PTA is helpful and an objective measure of hearing is required if there is any issue with respect to an accident, noise exposure, or compensation. As indicated earlier, the whisper test has significant limitations both in terms of reliability and repeatability and instead the use of a validated speech recognition test is preferable. The Maritime and Coastguard Agency recommends that the Action on Hearing Loss speech recognition test (the 'Hearing Check') is used, in conjunction with the results of audiometry, when determining communication abilities in seafarers.[3] For group 2 drivers, 'paramount importance is placed on a proven ability to communicate in an emergency by speech or suitable alternative such as SMS text'.[6]

Management: hearing aids and other assistive technology

There is a wide range of assistive devices for those with hearing impairments and additional information is available on the Action on Hearing Loss website (see 'Useful websites'). Hearing aids are constructed of four general components: a battery, microphone, amplifier, and speaker. Traditional hearing aids can be categorized depending on how they are worn: behind the ear, in the ear, in the canal, or body worn. In general, two hearing aids will provide better hearing, better sound location, and improved understanding in noisy situations than a single hearing aid. Most hearing aids have a telecoil or T-setting for use with induction loops and phones with inductive couplers. Digital aids may offer automatic noise reduction to reduce constant background noise such as traffic, feedback suppression to reduce the annoying whistling familiar to those with analogue aids, and twin or multi-microphones to allow the listener to focus on sound in front of them. In addition, digital aids offer automatic gain control, which selectively amplifies soft sounds more than loud ones. This is an important feature for wearers who have a reduced dynamic range of hearing (e.g. those with cochlear hearing loss), as they will struggle to hear quiet sounds but perceive louder sounds as uncomfortably loud.

One drawback to traditional hearing aids is that they work via air conduction and are thus dependent on a functioning middle ear as well as the presence of a pinna or patent external auditory canal, or both. Bone conduction hearing aids are a useful alternative as they work through vibration of the skull, bypassing the middle ear and allowing sound to be picked up by the functioning cochlea. As the conductive component is bypassed much less amplification is required. Bone conduction aids can be worn simply on a soft band; however, a number of devices are now available for surgical implantation. The current indications for a bone-anchored hearing aid (BAHA') include conductive or mixed hearing loss (air–bone gap of more than 30 dB hearing loss (HL) where the bone conduction threshold and hence cochlear reserve is better than 45 dB HL), inability to wear conventional hearing aids, and single-sided deafness. BAHA' devices consist of a titanium screw implanted into the skull connected to either an abutment which protrudes through the skin or a subcutaneously sited magnet. A sound processor can then either clip onto the exposed abutment or via an external magnet simply sit on the skin, converting sound into vibration that will transmit through the skull. Both types of BAHA' procedure can be carried out as day case operations and can be performed under general or local anaesthetic. The BAHA'5 SuperPower is a more powerful option for moderate to severe mixed hearing loss and has a fitting range up to 65 dB HL. There are now numerous features available including Bluetooth and wireless technology and an ability to connect with loop systems.

For those with single-sided deafness, another alternative is a CROS (contralateral routing of signals) hearing aid where sound is wirelessly transferred from the microphone in the deaf ear across to the hearing amplified ear. BICROS (bilateral CROS) hearing aids are similar but also facilitate aiding of the non-deaf ear when there is a coexisting but aidable loss.

Middle ear implantable hearing aids may provide a solution for those people with moderate to severe sensorineural or mixed hearing losses who fail to benefit or are unable to use conventional hearing aids.[30] These devices work via a floating mass transducer or microdrive system whereby electrical signals from the sound processor are converted to mechanical vibrations of the ossicular chain or round window. Examples of these devices include the Vibrant' Soundbridge™ and the now fully implanted Carina' system.

The development of multichannel cochlear implants, initially for use in post-lingually deaf people, offers the prospect of speech perception in profoundly deaf individuals with SNHLs.[31] Cochlear implants directly stimulate the auditory nerve via an electrode array in the cochlea. Assessment for implantation suitability is via a multidisciplinary team and involves a trial of the hearing aid, detailed hearing assessments, and imaging for structural anomalies. Simultaneous bilateral cochlear implantation for adults in the NHS is reserved for those with dual sensory loss.[32]

Advice, and in some cases financial support, is available from the Access to Work scheme to assist hearing-impaired people in securing and retaining work (see 'Useful websites').

A range of assistive listening devices exist including wireless (radio or infrared) listening equipment, portable or fixed induction loops, and conference folders with a built-in induction loop and microphone. Sadly, there is evidence that some induction loop systems are poorly maintained and do not function as intended. One-third of hearing-impaired workers who need a hearing loop/infrared system have not been provided with it.[33] Telecommunications devices include textphones such as Minicom, telephones with an amplifier or an inductive coupler (for use with a hearing aid on the T-setting), and videophones. In addition, hearing-impaired people can make or receive phone calls via Text Relay, the national telephone relay service (see 'Useful websites'). Alternatively, smartphone 'texting' and email are increasingly utilized at work in lieu of a spoken call.

Assisting hearing in the workplace

In addition to specialized devices to assist hearing in the workplace, the OH professional should consider recommending basic assistance (see Box 31.1).

Box 31.1 Hearing assistance in the workplace

- Make other workers aware of the hearing impairment.
- Encourage co-workers to visibly speak in the line of sight of the impaired worker, not to the side or behind.
- Ask co-workers to speak clearly with sufficient volume and articulation during, for example, meetings and in the office.
- Allow the employee to signal when they have not heard clearly.
- Use email for office communication in preference to telephone or speaking across the office room.
- Transfer to another role where the hearing impairment is less disadvantageous (e.g. less phone work and more email) may be considered.
- Devise a personal evacuation plan in the event of fire or emergency. This may include 'buddying up' with other workers and a vibrating pager or flashing lights linked to the building's fire alarm. Both the Equality Act 2010 and fire regulations (regarding equipment) apply here.

More costly options are access to electronic note takers (a service where an operator produces a typed summary of a meeting or seminar), lip speakers (someone who silently repeats a speaker's words, using clearly intelligible lip movements/facial expressions and, if requested, fingerspelling, to facilitate lip reading by the deaf or hard of hearing person), speech-to-text reporters (who produce a verbatim record—in contrast, electronic notetakers will provide a précis), and registered British Sign Language/English interpreters, either face-to-face or online using a webcam.

This last group are registered with Signature, which runs the National Registers of Communication Professionals working with Deaf and Deafblind People (NRCPD). This is the main registration body for sign language interpreters, lip speakers, speech-to-text reporters, language service professional deaf-blind manual interpreters, and electronic notetakers in the UK. A register of sign language interpreters in Scotland is maintained by the Scottish Association of Sign Language Interpreters (SASLI). These schemes are voluntary except for those professionals undertaking court and police work, who must be registered.

Probably the most frequent hearing issue encountered by the OH professional is that of a partially hearing-impaired worker who must further compromise their hearing ability by wearing hearing protection in a noisy work environment. In this case, the OH professional must ensure:

- that the remaining hearing is not further impaired by noise exposure (by suitable advice, consideration of double hearing protection using ear plugs and ear muffs) or removal of the worker from the noise source altogether
- for their own safety, the individual also needs to be assessed for their ability to hear, for example, alarms and a shouting voice behind them.

The employer should be asked to perform a risk assessment that includes a practical test with observation that the worker can respond appropriately to warning sounds.

New active digital hearing muffs are available that both reduce, for example, machinery noise but enhance the passage of the human voice. These are particularly valuable for hearing aid users as hearing aids cannot normally be used within a muff. In areas where explosive gases or vapours may escape, all electronic devices must be intrinsically safe.

Workplace audiometry programmes

OH professionals who are responsible for serial audiometric screening programmes should be aware that the purpose of the programme is twofold:

- To prevent individual workers developing NIHL and take appropriate action where it is identified.
- To allow review of collated audiometric data to identify inadequately engineered noise controls or poor compliance with hearing protection in worker groups and communicate those findings to management.

Therefore, the examination of audiometric trends, not the single most recent audiogram(s), and correlation with deficits with worker groups is essential practice. The OH professional should be wary of the malpractice of supervised neglect where audiograms are regularly viewed (perhaps by a succession of OH professionals) but a clear adverse trend is not acted upon.

Epidemiology of balance disorders

Dizziness is a common, imprecise, and sometimes vaguely described symptom that requires a thorough history and neuro-otological examination to determine the underlying cause. The patient may report experiencing true rotatory vertigo, disequilibrium, imbalance, or symptoms indicative of a secondary cause including neurological (cerebellar), cardiovascular (pre-syncopal), and psychological conditions.

Normal balance requires input from a number of sensory modalities. Proprioceptive and visual information account for approximately 80% while the remainder is formed by peripheral vestibular and auditory systems. The paired vestibular apparatus (each comprising three semicircular canals, utricle, and saccule) provide information on head motion and position. Information is interpreted centrally where balance is maintained through a number of mechanisms including gaze stabilization (vestibulo-ocular reflex) and postural control (vestibulo-spinal reflex). Mismatch between relayed information and/or an over-reliance on one sensory input (e.g. vision) will result in the experience of dizziness. In the older population and those with multiple co-morbidities, it is not unusual for there to be a multifactorial cause to imbalance symptoms. The NHANES 1999–2004 study found that over one-third of those over 40 years of age had impaired balance on the basis that they were unable to maintain balance, with their eyes shut, while standing on a foam padded surface.[5] Poor balance was more common with increasing age, lower education, and diabetes mellitus.[5]

Neuro-otological examination should include otoscopy, cranial nerve, cerebellar, and gait assessment. Other examinations that can help to yield further diagnostic information include testing for corrective saccades with a head-thrust test, Romberg, Unterberger, and Dix–Hallpike tests. In patients describing symptoms of 'light headedness', it is helpful to check for postural hypotension, cardiac arrhythmias, and anaemia. Those patients who fail to improve or in whom there is diagnostic uncertainty should be referred for a specialist opinion. Assessment in secondary care may include more in-depth vestibular function tests such as electronystagmography, video head impulse testing, and vestibular evoked myogenic potentials which can in turn test each individual vestibular organ.

Vestibular causes of imbalance

The assessment and management of the patient complaining of dizziness has been extensively reviewed.[34] Vertigo is defined as an illusion of motion which is either subjective (the patient feels he is moving) or objective (the patient sees the world moving). An acute peripheral vestibular deficit is a common cause of vertigo and can occur secondary to labyrinthitis, vestibular neuritis, trauma (including labyrinthine concussion), and middle ear infection.

Ménière's disease remains poorly understood and as a consequence there remains no gold standard diagnostic test. It consists of relapsing remitting episodes of severe rotary vertigo lasting for more than 20 minutes duration but rarely persisting for more than 24 hours. Presentation can include varying degrees of hearing loss, aural fullness, and tinnitus. These symptoms can persist throughout the attack and in some patients will precede the attack itself. The American Academy of Otolaryngology Head and Neck Surgery (AAO-HNS) have devised four diagnostic categories. The diagnosis of Ménière's disease is regarded as 'definite' when there have been two or more spontaneous episodes of vertigo of more than 20 minutes duration with documented hearing loss, symptoms of tinnitus and/or aural fullness, and an exclusion of other underlying causes.[35] Over time, a progressive SNHL develops which often demonstrates a predilection for lower frequencies. The interval between attacks can vary considerably and a minority of patients may develop sudden drop attacks termed 'otolithic crises of Tumarkin'. These severe episodes and general unpredictability of attacks may significantly impact an individual's ability to work. The evidence for the efficacy of diuretics,[36] betahistine,[37] and intratympanic steroids[38] in Ménière's disease is limited and an updated Cochrane review has failed to find strong evidence to support surgery for Ménière's disease.[39]

Vestibular migraine is a common cause for imbalance that was previously underdiagnosed and/or misdiagnosed as Ménière's disease. A large number of Ménière's patients may, however, also suffer migraines. Vestibular migraine may present as imbalance or rotatory vertigo episodes which can last from 5 minutes to several days.[40] The International Bárány Society and International Headache Society have developed a consensus document[40] on diagnostic criteria for vestibular migraine; features suggestive of vestibular migraine include personal history of migraine, associated headache, and/or autonomic overactivity/sensory disturbance (photophobia/phonophobia) during the episodes.[40] Other symptoms such as hearing loss and tinnitus can occur but with variable degrees of presentation. Episodes may be associated with a specific trigger (including stress, diet, hormonal changes, and local environment such as fluorescent lighting) and may be followed by fatigue and tiredness. Neuro-otological examination can often be normal between attacks. Treatment involves dietary avoidance of potential triggers, sleep hygiene education, stress reduction, and vestibular rehabilitation to help the background disequilibrium. If patients continue to experience episodes of vestibular migraine, classic migraine medications such as beta blockers and triptans can be used alongside tricyclic antidepressants such as amitriptyline.

Benign paroxysmal positional vertigo (BPPV) is frequently idiopathic. However, it can follow previous even innocuous head trauma and may coexist with other vestibular pathology. Individuals suffering with BPPV will usually describe transient episodes (often <60 seconds) of intense rotatory vertigo that are brought on by a change in head position (e.g. looking up at the top shelf). BPPV is thought to result from detached otoconia crystals in the semicircular canals, with more than 90% of cases affecting the posterior and most dependent semicircular canal.[41] However, BPPV can affect the lateral and (rarely) the superior semicircular canals. Therefore, where examination is equivocal, all canals should be tested. The Dix–Hallpike test is particularly useful in assessing posterior BPPV and its use is described by the British Society of Audiology (see 'Useful websites'). Treatment for BPPV predominantly involves repositioning manoeuvres, including Brandt–Daroff exercises, Epley manoeuvre (for confirmed posterior canal BPPV), and the BBQ roll for lateral canal BPPV. A recent Cochrane analysis[42] has shown evidence that the Epley manoeuvre is both safe and superior to Brandt–Daroff exercises in treating posterior canal BPPV. It was noted, however, that there remains a recurrence rate following treatment of up to 36%.[42]

The term visual vertigo is used to describe symptoms of imbalance or disorientation (not usually rotatory vertigo) that are triggered and/or exacerbated by visually challenging environments. Situations that may precipitate such symptoms include scrolling computer screens or environments with bright lights and/or fast-moving visual information (supermarket aisles, vehicles moving at speed). It is thought these patients may have become visually dependent following a vestibular insult; relying more heavily on visual clues for postural control and spatial orientation.[43] When in a busy visual environment, patients demonstrate increased difficulty resolving conflict between visual and vestibulo-proprioceptive inputs resulting in dizziness and discomfort. Treatment consists of vestibular rehabilitation including visual motion desensitization—by stressing the visual system in a controlled manner, the patients begins to rely more on their vestibulo-proprioceptive cues.

Non-vestibular causes of imbalance

Dizziness and/or vertigo may be associated with common mental health problems (anxiety, panic disorder, depression), but the relationship is complex as vertigo may result in associated psychological symptoms or be consequent upon anxiety. Many drugs cause dizziness as a side effect, including cardiovascular agents, antiepileptics, sedatives, hypnotics, anxiolytics, and antidepressants.

Management: vestibular disorders

Many people with an acute vestibular disorder will compensate over time and so their symptoms will improve, usually within 3–6 months. In the acute phase (days 1–7 post insult), static recovery occurs; medication such as cinnarizine or prochlorperazine may be of benefit but should be limited to a few days of treatment as they can delay dynamic vestibular compensation.[34] A systematic review of the use of oral corticosteroids for the treatment of vestibular neuronitis found insufficient evidence of benefit for this treatment.[44]

Condition-specific treatment options have already been outlined. It remains important, however, that ordinary physical activity is maintained and vestibular rehabilitation (e.g. Cawthorne–Cooksey exercises or, if possible, customized vestibular retraining exercises) is emphasized. A Cochrane review concluded that there was moderate to strong evidence that vestibular rehabilitation is both safe and effective for the treatment of unilateral peripheral vestibular conditions, including labyrinthitis, BPPV, and unilateral Ménière's disease.[45]

Clinical aspects of vestibular disorders affecting work capacity

Balance disorders can affect the sufferer's employment, personal safety, attendance at work, and productivity. The propensity for increased falls will be of particular concern in some industries, particularly those with safety-critical roles. The OH professional should also not neglect consideration of the safety of both personal and work driving in relation to such impairment. Assessment of balance capability in the consulting room does not necessarily constitute an adequate risk assessment and an employer should be asked to conduct a job-specific assessment where safe and practicable.

Vestibular dysfunction in association with dizziness was found to increase the risk of falls 12-fold in one large, well-designed US study.[5] Another study, which was set in neurology clinics in London and Siena, Italy, explored disability associated with dizziness among 400 patients.[46] BPPV, labyrinthitis, and Ménière's disease accounted for 28% of cases in London and 51% of cases in Siena; work disability was not analysed by diagnostic group, but 27% of participants had changed jobs and 21% had given up work as a result of their dizziness.[46] That survey found that, on average, sufferers had taken just over 7 days of sickness absence in the previous 6 months due to dizziness and that over half reported reduced efficiency at work. A postal survey of 2064 adults, aged 18–64 years, found that, of those with dizziness who were in work ($n = 278$), 25% reported difficulty doing their job and of those not working ($n = 194$), more than one in five stated that this was due to dizziness (sometimes in combination with anxiety).[47]

Key points

- Hearing and balance disorders are common in those of working age and become more prevalent with increasing age.
- A worker with impaired hearing or a balance disorder may significantly underperform, feel side-lined or alienated in the workplace, and may be prone to more accidents by virtue of their disability.
- Many work environments are noisy and regulations require that this hazard is controlled and health surveillance is performed to prevent NIHL and identify noise control failures.
- OH professionals should have a good understanding of NIHL and audiometry programmes. They should also be able to assess and advise about the impact of hearing loss in the workplace.
- Adjustments for an employee with hearing impairment include guidance for other employees and purchase of assistive equipment such as telephone amplifiers, voice-to-text software, or induction loops. Specialist advice is available from hearing disability organizations or Access to Work.

Useful websites

British Tinnitus Association	https://www.tinnitus.org.uk/
Action on Hearing Loss. Hearing check	https://www.actiononhearingloss.org.uk/hearing-health/check-your-hearing/
Action on Hearing Loss. Information on all aspects of deafness, hearing loss, and tinnitus	http://www.actiononhearingloss.org.uk/supporting-you/factsheets-and-leaflets.aspx
British Society of Audiology. Surveillance audiometry	http://www.thebsa.org.uk/resources/surveillance-audiometry/
British Society of Audiology. The Dix–Hallpike test	http://www.thebsa.org.uk/docs/RecPro/HM.pdf
Access to Work	http://www.direct.gov.uk/en/DisabledPeople/Employmentsupport/WorkSchemesAndProgrammes/DG_4000347
Text Relay	http://www.textrelay.org/

References

1. **Woodcock K, Pole JD.** Educational attainment, labour force status and injury: a comparison of Canadians with and without deafness and hearing loss. *Int J Rehabil Res* 2008;**31**:297–304.
2. **Rydberg E, Gellerstedt LC, Danermark B.** The position of the deaf in the Swedish labor market. *Am Ann Deaf* 2010;**155**:68–77.
3. **Maritime and Coastguard Agency.** Guidance for approved doctors ADG 13—hearing, ear disease, disorders of speech and communication. Available at: https://assets.publishing.service.gov.uk/government/uploads/system/uploads/attachment_data/file/706914/February_2018_AD_Manual.pdf.
4. **Health and Safety Executive.** Safety critical workers. Available at: http://www.hse.gov.uk/research/rrpdf/rr584.pdf.
5. **Agrawal Y, Carey JP, Della Santina CC, et al.** Disorders of balance and vestibular function in US adults: data from the National Health and Nutrition Examination Survey, 2001–2004. *Arch Intern Med* 2009;**169**:938–44.
6. **Drivers Medical Group.** *At a Glance Guide to the Current Medical Standards of Fitness To Drive: A Guide for Medical Practitioners.* Swansea: Driver Vehicle Licensing Agency; 2016. Available at: http://www.dft.gov.uk/dvla/medical/ataglance.aspx.
7. **Nelson DI, Nelson RY, Concha-Barrientos M, Fingerhut M.** The global burden of occupational noise-induced hearing loss. *Am J Ind Med* 2005;**48**:446–58.
8. **Coles RRA, Lutman ME, Buffin JT.** Guidelines on the diagnosis of noise-induced hearing loss for medicolegal purposes. *Clin Otolaryngol* 2000;**25**:264–73.
9. **Cohen M, Bitner-Glindzicz M, Luxon L.** The changing face of Usher syndrome: clinical implications. *Int J Audiol* 2007;**46**:82–93.
10. **Swartz R, Longwell P.** Treatment of vertigo. *Am Fam Physician* 2005;**71**:1115–22.
11. **Holenweg A, Kompis M.** Non-organic hearing loss: new and confirmed findings. *Eur Arch Otorhinolaryngol* 2010;**267**:1213–19.

12. **Coleman N, Sykes W, Groom, C.** Barriers to employment and unfair treatment at work: a quantitative analysis of disabled people's experiences. 2013 Equality and Human Rights Commission: research report 88. Available at: https://www.equalityhumanrights.com/sites/default/files/research-report-88-barriers-to-employment-and-unfair-treatment-at-work-disabled-peoples-experiences.pdf.

13. **Davis AC.** The prevalence of hearing impairment and reported hearing disability among adults in Great Britain. *Int J Epidemiol* 1989;**18**:911–17.

14. **Agrawal Y, Platz EA, Niparko JK.** Prevalence of hearing loss and differences by demographic characteristics among US adults: data from the National Health and Nutrition Examination Survey, 1999–2004. *Arch Intern Med* 2008;**168**:1522–30.

15. **McFerran DJ, Phillips JS.** Tinnitus. *J Laryngol Otol* 2007;**121**:201–8.

16. **Shargorodsky J, Curhan GC, Farwell WR.** Prevalence and characteristics of tinnitus among US adults. *Am J Med* 2010;**123**:711–8.

17. **Hobson J, Chisholm E, El Refaie A.** Sound therapy (masking) in the management of tinnitus in adults. *Cochrane Database Syst Rev* 2012;**14**:CD006371.

18. **Martinez-Devesa P, Perera R, Theodoulou M, Waddell A.** Cognitive behavioural therapy for tinnitus. *Cochrane Database Syst Rev* 2010;**8**:CD005233.

19. **Gates GA, Murphy M, Rees TS, et al.** Screening for handicapping hearing loss in the elderly. *J Fam Pract* 2003;**52**:56–62.

20. **Ferrite S, Santana VS, Marshall SW.** Validity of self-reported hearing loss in adults: performance of three single questions. *Rev Saude Publica* 2011;**45**:824–30.

21. **Yueh B, Shapiro N, MacLean CH, et al.** Screening and management of adult hearing loss in primary care: scientific review. *JAMA* 2003;**289**:1976–85.

22. **Smits C, Kapteyn TS, Houtgast T.** Development and validation of an automatic speech-in-noise screening test by telephone. *Int J Audiol* 2004;**43**:15–28.

23. **Smits C, Merkus P, Houtgast T.** How we do it: the Dutch functional hearing screening tests by telephone and Internet. *Clin Otolaryngol* 2006;**31**:436–55.

24. **McBride WS, Mulrow CD, Aguilar C, et al.** Methods for screening for hearing loss in older adults. *Am J Med Sci* 1994;**307**:40–2.

25. **Health and Safety Executive.** *Controlling Noise at Work: Guidance on the Control of Noise at Work Regulations 2005.* L108. London: HSE Books; 2005.

26. **Picard M, Girard SA, Simard M, et al.** Association of work-related accidents with noise exposure in the workplace and noise-induced hearing loss based on the experience of some 240,000 person-years of observation. *Accid Anal Prev* 2008;**40**:1644–52.

27. **Picard M, Girard SA, Courteau M, et al.** Could driving safety be compromised by noise exposure at work and noise-induced hearing loss? *Traffic Inj Prev* 2008;**9**:489–99.

28. **Palmer KT, Harris EC, Coggon D.** Chronic health problems and risk of accidental injury in the workplace: a systematic literature review. *Occup Environ Med* 2008;**65**:757–64.

29. **Girard SA, Picard M, Davis AC, et al.** Multiple work-related accidents: tracing the role of hearing status and noise exposure. *Occup Environ Med* 2009;**66**:319–24.

30. **Bernardeschi D, Hoffman C, Benchaa T, et al.** Functional results of Vibrant Soundbridge middle ear implants in conductive and mixed hearing losses. *Audiol Neurootol* 2011;**16**:381–7.

31. **Bond M, Mealing S, Anderson R, et al.** The effectiveness and cost-effectiveness of cochlear implants for severe to profound deafness in children and adults: a systematic review and economic model. *Health Technol Assess* 2009;**13**:1–330.

32. **National Institute for Health and Care Excellence (NICE).** Cochlear implants for children and adults with severe to profound deafness. Technology Appraisal Guidance [TA166]. 2009. Available at: http://www.nice.org.uk/nicemedia/pdf/TA166Guidancev2.pdf.

33. **Royal National institute for the Deaf (RNID).** Opportunity blocked: the employment experiences of deaf and hard of hearing people. 2007. Available at: https://www.actiononhearingloss.org.uk/how-we-help/information-and-resources/publications/research-reports/opportunity-blocked-report/.

34. **Luxon LM.** Evaluation and management of the dizzy patient. *J Neurol Neurosurg Psychiatry* 2004;**75**(Suppl 4):45–52.

35. **American Academy of Otolaryngology-Head and Neck Foundation, Inc.** Committee on Hearing and Equilibrium guidelines for the diagnosis and evaluation of therapy in Ménière's disease. *Otolaryngol Head Neck Surg* 1995;**113**:181–5.

36. **Thirlwall AS, Kundu S.** Diuretics for Ménière's disease or syndrome. *Cochrane Database Syst Rev* 2006;**19**:CD003599.

37. **James AL, Burton MJ.** Betahistine for Ménière's disease or syndrome. *Cochrane Database Syst Rev* 2001;**1**:CD001873.

38. **Phillips JS, Westerberg B.** Intratympanic steroids for Ménière's disease or syndrome. *Cochrane Database Syst Rev* 2011;**6**:CD008514.

39. **Pullens B, Verschuur HP, van Benthem PP.** Surgery for Ménière's disease. *Cochrane Database Syst Rev* 2013;**28**:CD005395.

40. **Lempert T, Olesen J, Furman J, et al.** Vestibular migraine: diagnostic criteria. *J Vest Res* 2012;**22**:167–72.

41. **Lee SH, Kim JS.** Benign paroxysmal positional vertigo. *J Clin Neurol* 2010;**6**:51–63.

42. **Hilton MP, Pinder DK.** The Epley (canalith repositioning) manoeuvre for benign paroxysmal positional vertigo. *Cochrane Database Syst Rev* 2014;**8**:CD003162.

43. **Bronstein AM, Golding JF, Gresty MA.** Vertigo and dizziness from environmental motion: visual vertigo, motion sickness, and drivers' disorientation. *Semin Neurol* 2013;**33**:219–30.

44. **Fishman JM, Burgess C, Waddell A.** Corticosteroids for the treatment of idiopathic acute vestibular dysfunction (vestibular neuritis). *Cochrane Database Syst Rev* 2011;**11**:CD008607.

45. **Hillier SL, McDonnell M.** Vestibular rehabilitation for unilateral peripheral vestibular dysfunction. *Cochrane Database Syst Rev* 2011;**16**:CD005397.

46. **Bronstein AM, Golding JF, Gresty MA, et al.** The social impact of dizziness in London and Siena. *J Neurol* 2010;**257**:183–90.

47. **Yardley L, Owen N, Nazareth I, et al.** Prevalence and presentation of dizziness in a general practice community sample of working age people. *Br J Gen Pract* 1998;**48**:1131–5.

Chapter 32

Hidden impairments

Marios Adamou and John Hobson

Introduction

The neurodevelopmental disorders include autism spectrum disorders (ASDs) and at-tention deficit hyperactivity disorder (ADHD). They have a prevalence of around 3% for ADHD[1] and 1.5% for autism.[2] These conditions are highly co-morbid and chronic and their symptomatology overlaps with other conditions. They commonly present with specific learning disabilities such as dyspraxia and dyslexia, which are also neurodevelopmental disorders.[3] They are among a number of conditions known as hidden impairments[4] as they are often missed by clinicians. These disorders are costly to society and it has been es-timated that accommodation, treatment, loss of earnings, and healthcare for individuals over their lifespan will range between £0.92 million and £1.5 million (without or with an intellectual disability, respectively).[5]

With equality legislation and increasing diagnosis of neurodevelopmental disorders, occupational health (OH) professionals should be aware of the functional impact of these conditions and the behavioural and cognitive challenges to performance at work. OH professionals require an appreciation of how work can be designed and organized to en-able people with neurodevelopmental disorders obtain and retain suitable employment and to benefit from work.

Autism spectrum disorders

ASDs are among the most severe of the neurodevelopmental disorders regarding preva-lence, morbidity, and impact on society. They are characterized by impairments in social communication and social interaction in the presence of restricted, repetitive behaviours or interests.[6] ASD symptoms typically occur by the age of 3 years, although may not fully manifest until school age or later. Although the exact cause of ASDs is unknown, research suggests an interacting role of genetic and environmental factors[7] causing aberrant brain growth, neuronal development, and functional connectivity. The observed increase in the prevalence of ASDs is partly attributable to enhanced diagnostic tools.

Diagnosis of autism spectrum disorders

Making a diagnosis of an ASD is a multi-stage process. The UK National Institute for Health and Care Excellence (NICE) advocates a multidisciplinary diagnostic approach by a specialist professional team using validated instruments[8] such as the Autism Diagnostic Observation Schedule (ADOS),[9] Autism Diagnostic Interview, Revised (ADI-R),[10] and the Diagnostic Interview for Social and Communication Disorders (DISCO).[11]

Additional useful assessments

Assessment of cognitive ability

The cognitive ability of people with an ASD has been found to be impaired (in the context of normal intelligence) in the areas of executive function,[12] theory of mind, selective attention,[13] and abstraction.[14] In terms of theory of mind (the capacity to understand subjective mental states, including thoughts and desires, regardless of whether or not the circumstances involved are real[15]), significant impairments in integrating mental state information[16] have been found in people with ASDs. These deficits could explain the impairments in social behaviour and communication observed in ASDs. Theory of mind can be assessed using the Theory of Mind Assessment Scale (Th.o.m.a.s.)[17] and the Geneva Social Cognition Scale (GeSoCS).[18]

Assessment of functional ability

Functional assessment will acknowledge the extent of difficulties in a wide variety of areas, including everyday living skills, social relationships, communication (receptive and expressive), imagination, occupational function, and executive function. It also identifies areas for developing skill and talent. These attributes govern the extent to which individuals can look after themselves, manage independently, take up education, employment, or leisure activities, develop relationships, and cope with the social demands of other people. In one study, approximately half of the adolescents assessed had a deficit in daily living skills.[19] A valid assessment tool is the Vineland Adaptive Behavior Scale.[20]

Other elements of importance

The criteria for determining mental capacity are well established, but the characteristics of an individual with autism may be subtle, requiring careful review. Medical problems may be associated with autism (e.g. epilepsy, atopies, gastrointestinal problems, and infections), or masked by the presence of autism (e.g. obesity, cancer, and dementia).

Management of autism spectrum disorders

Overall, the evidence is currently too limited to support the routine use of medicines for the core symptoms of ASDs[21] but a number of psychological approaches can be used.

Social learning programmes

Social learning programmes aim to improve social interaction. Behavioural therapy techniques are applied within a social learning framework, such as using video modelling, peer/individual feedback, imitation, and reinforcement to teach conventions of social engagement. Observational studies in adults with ASDs suggest that social skills groups may be effective at improving social interaction.[22] However, the only randomized controlled trial of social skills training found no positive treatment effect of emotion recognition training on general emotion recognition,[23] suggesting that social interaction programmes may only be effective when they include a more general social learning component.

Behavioural and life-skills interventions

Adults with ASDs of all intellectual abilities who need help with activities of daily living can be offered a structured training programme based on behavioural principles. However, evidence of the effectiveness of these programmes is indirect and largely reliant on studies of adults with a learning disability.[24] In adults with an ASD without a learning disability or with a mild to moderate learning disability who are socially isolated or have restricted social contact, interventions should focus on the acquisition of life skills based on the specific need of the individual. These may be provided by occupational therapists.

Cognitive behavioural interventions

Cognitive behavioural therapy (CBT) can help adults with ASDs across a range of domains by treating anxiety and obsessive–compulsive disorder. CBT supports adults who have difficulties with victimization and obtaining or maintaining employment. The best evidence is for treating anxiety in ASDs[25] and anxiety management performs just as well as CBT in reducing symptoms of obsessive–compulsive disorder in individuals with ASDs.[26]

Autism spectrum disorders and work

Relatively little is yet known about employment readiness and elements that promote access to, and the retention of, employment for adults with ASDs. Longitudinal studies of adults with ASDs and without intellectual disability have shown consistent and persistent deficits across cognitive, social, and vocational domains, indicating a need for effective treatments of these functional disabilities that impact employment.[27]

In the US, adults with ASDs experience high rates of unemployment and underemployment compared to adults with other disabilities and the general population. Despite having the ability and desire to work,[28] it is estimated that approximately half of adults with ASDs are unemployed.[29]

Recruitment

Barriers to recruitment

Personal factors and symptoms associated with ASDs[30] and organization and interactional difficulties all adversely affect the seeking of employment[31] (Box 32.1). The use of language and the way people communicate can lead to disadvantages during recruitment. Other barriers include employers' understanding of autism, the need for qualifications, outsourced recruitment, and unconscious bias.

Enablers for recruitment

It is suggested that employment among those with ASDs is inextricably linked with broader community resources, family support, workplace capacity building (e.g. employer,

Box 32.1 Factors that inhibit employment in ASDs

Personal factors and symptoms

- Limited cognitive ability.
- Severity of the ASD.
- Psychiatric co-morbidity.
- Oppositional personality.
- Epilepsy.
- Female sex.
- Lower speech and language abilities.
- Maladaptive behaviours.
- Social impairments and lack of empathy.
- Lack of drive.
- Prior institutionalization.

Aspects of the job-seeking process

- Organizing the job process (knowing how to look for a job).
- Initiating job contact and following up after contact.
- Developing succinct resumes.
- Knowing what information to provide on the job application form or at interview.
- A chequered work history (frequent job terminations and long periods of unemployment).
- Interviews.

co-workers), and policy.[32] There is evidence that employer-based interventions increase the likelihood of successful employment[33] and that employing an adult with an ASD benefits employers without incurring additional costs.[34] People who disclosed their ASD diagnosis to their employer were more than three times more likely to be employed than those who did not disclose. Education level significantly predicted employment status.[35] It is recommended that applicants with ASDs should declare this once they have been offered an interview, to allow adjustments (if required) to be made at the interview.

Interviews

Interviews for people with ASDs are said to be one of the biggest barriers to employment. People with autism can experience heightened anxiety when meeting new people or visiting new places and can find shaking hands and making eye contact stressful. They may give monosyllabic answers to questions or not realize when they are being asked to talk about something in detail. They may have difficulty answering questions about hypothetical situations and often need more time to process information and questions than other candidates.

Employers can facilitate interviews by:

◆ asking specific and direct questions in a logical order

◆ avoiding open-ended questions

◆ making any competency-based questions concrete rather than abstract

◆ allowing a candidate time for processing (if an answer does not come within a minute, they may need to give an appropriate prompt)

◆ consider the use of an autism recruitment specialist who can act as a 'translator'.

Specialist support can help bridge the gap of communication between applicant and interviewer but does not necessarily mean communication support is needed once they are employed in a role.

Work trials

Work trials may aid the successful recruitment of people with ASDs. These do not necessarily need to be paid. An alternative would be to ask the applicant to carry out a task. Trials are an opportunity for the person to show their ability, and help the employer to understand the person as an individual.

Starting employment

Communication and socializing in the workplace can be particularly difficult for people with ASDs. The start of employment should be planned to allow an individual to integrate into the team and company. Managers and the wider team may need a briefing to ensure the employee is not judged unfairly on first impressions. The use of third-party specialists can also be considered to facilitate this process. The document 'Square Holes for Square Pegs' gives useful guidance on employment in ASDs (see 'Useful websites').

Line management

Line managers do not need a comprehensive knowledge of autism, but rather a general understanding of how the condition can be difficult to manage in the workplace and how tiring it can be for the individual. Useful educational resources for managers are available from the ASD charities (see 'Useful websites').

Good line managers will make adjustments and be flexible, tolerant, and understanding. A line manager can simply ask how autism affects the worker. If they struggle to retain verbal information then the line manager can write down tasks for the person to complete. Similarly, if an employee was to come into work 5 days in a row wearing the same shirt they may need a line manager to be clear and direct explaining that it is not appropriate.

Poor line management can challenge retention of workers with ASDs. Difficulties arise when line managers are inflexible or unwilling to make adjustments. Due to the nature of autism, line managers may struggle to engage or communicate with an affected worker and there may be a natural reaction to engage less through unconscious bias. Line managers should be helped to recognize this and make adjustments suitable for workers with ASDs.

Adjustments

Common adjustments include ensuring communication is accessible, providing clear plans, and changing the physical environment. Instructions should be clear and simple rather than using inferred meaning or unnecessary metaphors.

Employees should be given a clear plan of what they need to do and by when. This should be provided in written format, or work can be listed or coded using colour. A lack of clarity may lead to an employee focusing disproportionate effort or attention on one aspect or item of work. Employers should not assume that an employee understands things that have not been clearly explained, for example, working times, when to take breaks, or when to leave at the end of the working day.

It is important that managers explain to employees what is expected of them regarding performance. Any failure to perform to required standards should be raised and clarified as early as possible, making any required adjustments to assist improvement.

Agile working may be a challenge for some people with autism. Hot-desking can lead to additional stress. Working from home can prove difficult if the person struggles to transfer work habits into the home environment or they do not properly disengage from work.

Sensory stimulation differs between individuals and can either be heightened or reduced, including sensory experiences relating to heat, light, balance, or other senses. For example, the noise level or visual stimulus can be distracting and changes to working environments can help the person to focus on their work. A busy space may cause distractions and room dividers could be used to create a calmer environment. Having a place to withdraw and be alone to work is vital for some people.

Communication and translation

People with ASDs often interpret language very literally. Vague or ambiguous language should be avoided and communication should be clear, precise, and 'up-front'. Translating information between employer and employee can aid understanding, remove challenges, and help to retain employees. A work colleague may need to have autistic behaviour or barriers explained and the employee with ASD may need to be told why requests made of them are not unreasonable, and that employers do not have to make unreasonable adjustments.

Levels of support and specialist support in the workplace

Unexpected issues may arise during an individual's employment. When workplace difficulties escalate, they may reach a point where specialist support is required. This may mean resolving issues between line managers and employees or facilitating a conversation between them. Levels of support can be built within an organization. The first level of support would be a 'buddy' who could provide support or guidance to both employee and line manager. Ideally this person would have autism experience and skills in coaching or mentoring. The second level of support would be an external job coach who could work with the organization if there are difficulties. The third level would be someone who can provide clinical support when there are serious concerns.

Attention deficit hyperactivity disorder

Attention deficit hyperactivity disorder (ADHD) is a common neurodevelopmental disorder that persists into adulthood. Its symptoms cause impairments in a number of social domains, one of which is employment. ADHD is characterized by pervasive symptoms of hyperactivity, inattentiveness, and impulsivity. These symptoms surface relatively early in childhood and are fairly persistent over a life course.[36] ADHD translates itself as overt behavioural disturbances in preschool infants, school-age children, adolescents, and adults.

Prevalence estimates depend on three main factors: the population sampled, the method of ascertainment, and the diagnostic criteria applied. Most estimates lie between 5% and 10%.[37] Three studies of English populations have shown a prevalence rate of between 2% and 5%, depending on which diagnostic criteria were applied.[37] ADHD is seldom diagnosed as a single disorder[38] and co-morbid conditions often lead the person to present for help.[39] These include substance use disorders, depression,[40] anxiety disorders,[41] personality disorders,[42] and antisocial personality disorder.[43–45] Adults with ADHD may also present with ASDs, dyspraxia, dyslexia, and dyscalculia.

Research on the aetiology of ADHD has concentrated on three distinct strands: morphological differences, hereditary factors, and functional differences. Morphological differences have been reported in children with ADHD. The estimated heritability of ADHD from simple genetic analyses ranges from 0.6 to 0.9[46] and an association between dopamine system genes and ADHD has also been shown.[47]

Despite this evidence, the general public associates ADHD with a rampant child with rowdy and disobedient behaviour brought on by the consumption of chemical additives. ADHD has been under the spotlight of public scrutiny, some of which has resulted in defective and flawed representations of ADHD, and a disregard of adult ADHD by some practitioners.

Diagnosis of attention deficit hyperactivity disorder

The diagnosis of ADHD is clinical and based on the collection of relevant information through the psychiatric history and screening questionnaires but not psychological testing. ADHD symptom severity scales can identify current attentional impairment, but this impairment is not itself diagnostic of adult ADHD. The diagnosis is facilitated by the use of screening instruments such as Conner's Adult ADHD Rating Scale,[48] diagnostic interviews such as DIVA,[49] and tools of objective measurement such as the QBTest.[50]

Additional useful assessments

Patients with adult ADHD have cognitive problems, which can be attentional[51] and/or related to impairment in executive functioning.[52] These can be assessed by experts using neuropsychological batteries, which may reveal abnormalities in:

- matching of familiar figures (impulsivity)
- verbal fluency
- continuous performance tests/word-finding (sustained attention)
- set shifting (dividing and shifting attention)
- word recall (working memory).

More generalized cognitive impairment often occurs with abnormalities in attentional and working-memory areas and decision-making.[53]

Neuropsychological testing is not diagnostic but is useful in identifying the presence of isolated attentional and working-memory impairment compared with the normal population.

Management of attention deficit hyperactivity disorder

Where adult ADHD symptoms persist without co-morbid symptoms, the recommended initial treatment is with stimulant medication. Treatment lasts for as long as there is clinical benefit and the response can be monitored using a symptom rating scale (e.g. ADHD investigator symptom rating scale (AISRS)).[54]

Psychological therapy is recommended as an optional adjunct to medication. Core symptoms of ADHD (with the exception of hyperactivity/impulsivity) can respond to CBT, as combined psychopharmacological treatment, with long-term effects. Co-morbid features of depression, anxiety, antisocial behaviour, and social functioning may also respond.[55] Alternative psychological therapies include dialectic behaviour therapy and metacognitive therapy.[56]

ADHD and work

Functional abnormality in ADHD has been documented in multiple domains. Adults may experience motor coordination problems as well as impaired working memory, planning and anticipation,[57] verbal fluency, effort allocation, application of organizational strategies, and self-regulation of emotional arousal. These deficits are closely linked with function at work.[58] Adults with ADHD may struggle to work in 'organizations run by rules'.[59]

The majority of research on adult ADHD has been conducted in the US, and few studies have examined implications for social and occupational functioning. The association of ADHD with work-related problems in adulthood such as poor job performance, lower occupational status,[60] less job stability,[61] and increased absence days[62] has been documented. A few longitudinal studies following children with ADHD into adulthood have documented impairment in scholastic, occupational, relationship, and daily life functioning[63] and this impairment is similar between the sexes.[64]

As expected, outcomes from studies of adults diagnosed with ADHD in childhood and followed to adulthood, differ somewhat from findings with samples of clinic-referred adults,[65] with clinic-referred adults reporting greater functional impairment than controls. Clinic-referred adults with ADHD indicate increased psychiatric co-morbidity,[45] and may report even higher rates of internalizing symptoms than adults followed from childhood.[58] Additionally, clinic-referred adults with ADHD and adults reporting a prior ADHD diagnosis have more relationship and employment problems than controls[66] and describe themselves as less socially competent.[67]

Poor performance and work loss is likely to have profound economic implications for adults with ADHD. One study quantified this impact by estimating the excess costs related to work loss[68] based on employer payments for disability claims and imputed wages for medically related work absence days.[68] Another study estimated a 4–5% reduction in work performance, a 2.1 relative odds of sickness absence, and a 2.0 relative odds of workplace accidents-injuries.[69] The excess costs were $1.2 billion for women with ADHD and $2.26 billion for men with ADHD in this US study.[70] However, after controlling for substance abuse and history of depression or anxiety, stimulant therapy during childhood was the strongest predictor for being in work as adults (odds ratio = 3.2).[68] In this study, it was suggested that treatment of ADHD in childhood created a pathway to employment.

A survey undertaken by the World Health Organization in ten countries reported that 3.5% of workers suffered from ADHD resulting in 143 million days of lost production. They had an average of 8.4 excess sickness absence days per year and even higher annualized average excess numbers of work days associated with reduced work quantity (21.7 days) and quality (13.6 days). Only a small minority of these workers are treated for ADHD despite evidence that such treatment can improve function.[71]

Effects of attention deficit hyperactivity disorder at separate stages of employment

Adults with ADHDs experience difficulty in all aspects of employment, from the initial job search, to the interview, and then in employment itself.

The job application

When searching for a job, adults with ADHD are disorganized and sporadic and find it difficult to interact with employment advisers. This difficulty in creating a working alliance is probably because adults with ADHD are disenfranchised and disengaged from the system in general. For example, their attentional problems and poor understanding of social conventions result in them avoiding 'tedious' tasks such as writing detailed application forms, completing them by missing out items, and/or completing them without having read the question properly or reflecting on their answer.

The job interview

At the interview, the person with ADHD may come across as very friendly and chatty. They may be inaccurate about their past history, and may overstate their ability to fulfil the requirements of the job. An important problem, however, is the decision of whether to disclose their ADHD status on application forms or in interviews. Most employers do not understand ADHD and may have concerns that it is a profound and prolonged condition. They may lack awareness that it can be treated and that reasonable adjustments can improve occupational functioning.

The working environment

Once employed and initially in post, adults with ADHD may be highly motivated workers but symptoms may then begin to hamper their performance. Some people find functional employments that mask organizational problems (e.g. where they have secretarial or administrative support), or have employment that complements their symptoms (e.g. highly creative work or sports). Nevertheless, most skilled and unskilled occupations (e.g. administration posts) will be hampered by symptoms of inattention, impulsivity, and hyperactivity.

Employees may have difficulties with time management, organizing their schedule, keeping on top of their work load, and following instructions and they may exhibit emotional lability. These are important symptoms to explore when assessing the level of impairment. Individuals with ADHD may also be disadvantaged by poor social skills and procrastination, which make it hard for them to work effectively with colleagues, accept line management, and/or deal with the public. In trying to resolve the issue around lack of performance, a line manager may confront the employee which may be taken personally and lead to difficulty in remotivating the employee. Relationships with colleagues may become impulsive, abrasive, and volatile. Information relayed in job appraisals may not be acted on as they may be unable to adapt their behaviour. There is a high risk of resulting loss of employment.

Adults with ADHD can also become hyper-focused in activities, especially if they are incentivized by it, and there is potential for workaholism. An employer must harness the positives of ADHD and maintain the right balance, taking care to avoid burnout.

Occupational health perspective

Screening

ADHD has non-trivial prevalence among workers, high impairment, and a low rate of treatment despite the existence of cost-effective therapies that can improve some objective aspects of role performance.[72,73] The adult ADHD self-report scale (ASRS)[74] can be used to identify employees with potential ADHD. Management and human resources should refer people with ADHD to OH professionals, who should be able to recognize these needs and suggest reasonable adjustments.

Adjustments

Several adjustments can be considered for adults with ADHD.[75] Generally managers should implement regular meetings, reviews, and structured feedback for the individual.

Table 32.1 Potential workplace adjustments for adults with ADHD

Symptom	Possible adjustments
Attention and impulsivity	Private office/quieter room/positioning in office, flexitime arrangement, headphones, regular supervision, buddy system
Hyperactivity/restlessness	Allowing productive movements at work, encouraging activity, structured breaks in long meetings
Disorganization, time management, and memory problems	Provide beepers/alarms, structured notes, agendas, regular supervision with frequent feedback, mentoring, delegating tedious tasks, incentive/reward systems, regularly introducing change, breaking down targets and goals, supplement verbal information with written material

Verbal information should be supplemented in written format with clear, concise instructions. More specific adjustments are summarized in Table 32.1.

Specific learning disorders

These are neurodevelopmental disorders which begin by school age although may not be recognized until later. They involve ongoing problems with learning and using key academic skills (including reading, writing, and arithmetic), which form the foundation for other academic learning. A key feature is that performance in a particular area is well below normal average for age, often at least 1.5 standard deviations below, within the domain of difficulty on standardized achievement tests.

To assign a diagnosis, the difficulties must not be due to:

◆ intellectual disability
◆ external factors, such as economic or environmental disadvantage or lack of instruction
◆ vision or hearing problems, a neurological condition (e.g. paediatric stroke), or motor disorders
◆ limited English language proficiency.

The generic term 'learning difficulties' refers to the 20–25% of students who exhibit problems acquiring academic skills due to a range of causes. These include intellectual disability, physical or sensory deficits (e.g. hearing impairment), emotional or behavioural difficulties, and inadequate environmental experiences.

A specific learning disorder (SLD) is a clinical diagnosis that is not necessarily synonymous with 'learning disabilities' as identified within the education system. Not all children with learning disabilities/difficulties identified by the school system would meet a *Diagnostic and Statistical Manual of Mental Disorders*, fifth edition (*DSM-5*) clinical diagnosis of SLD. By contrast, those with a *DSM-5* diagnosis of SLD would be expected to meet the educational definition.

The following describe the updated 2013 *DSM-5* diagnostic subtypes of SLDs:

A. SLD with impairment in reading includes possible deficits in:

- word reading accuracy
- reading rate or fluency
- reading comprehension.

Dyslexia is an alternative term used to refer to a pattern of learning difficulties characterized by problems with accurate or fluent word recognition, poor decoding, and poor spelling abilities. The exact cause of dyslexia is unknown[76-78] but it often appears to run in families and genetic influences may affect neurodevelopment during early life. Estimates of prevalence depend on the particular definition of dyslexia[79] and are between 5% and 10% of the population. Signs of dyslexia usually become apparent when a child starts school and begins to focus more on learning how to read and write.

A person with dyslexia may:

- read and write very slowly
- confuse the order of letters in words
- put letters the wrong way round—such as writing 'b' instead of 'd'
- have poor or inconsistent spelling
- understand information when told verbally but have difficulty with written information
- find it hard to carry out a sequence of directions
- struggle with planning and organization.

Confirming dyslexia usually requires assessment by a specialist dyslexia teacher or an educational psychologist. A directory of chartered psychologists is published on the British Psychological Society's website (see 'Useful websites'). Adults who wish to be assessed for dyslexia should contact the British Dyslexia Association (see 'Useful websites') or a local dyslexia association (independently registered charities that run workshops and provide local support and information). Universities also have specialist staff who can support young people with dyslexia in higher education.

B. SLD with impairment in written expression includes possible deficits in:

- spelling accuracy
- grammar and punctuation accuracy
- clarity or organization of written expression.

C. SLD with impairment in mathematics includes possible deficits in:

- number sense
- memorization of arithmetic facts
- accurate or fluent calculation
- accurate mathematic reasoning.

Any successful execution of mathematical competencies requires the person to be attentive, organized, able to switch sets, and work quickly enough to avoid overloading the working memory stores that retain information. The impairment in mathematics has also been described as developmental dyscalculia. This is a heterogeneous condition[80] which includes arithmetic fact dyscalculia (problems only with symbolic number processing) and general dyscalculia (impairment in the innate approximate number system).

These difficulties must be quantifiably below what is expected for an individual's chronological age, and must not be caused by anxiety about mathematics, lack of experience and poor motivation, reading difficulties, or neuropsychological damage. Because definitions and diagnoses of dyscalculia are in their infancy and sometimes contradictory, prevalence is unclear, but research suggests it is between 3% and 6%.[81]

Developmental dyscalculia often occurs in association with other developmental disorders such as dyslexia or ADHD, and co-occurrence appears to be the rule rather than the exception. This is generally assumed to be a consequence of risk factors that are shared between disorders, for example, working memory. However, not all people with dyslexia have problems with mathematics and not all people with dyscalculia have problems with reading and writing.

Management

Much of the advice and techniques used to help children with dyslexia are also relevant for adults. Making use of technology, such as word processors and electronic organizers, can help with writing and organizing daily activities. People with dyslexia feel more comfortable working with a computer. This may be because a computer uses a visual environment that better suits their method of learning and working. Word processing programmes can also be useful because they have a spellchecker and an autocorrect facility that can highlight mistakes. Most web browsers and word processing software also have 'text-to-speech' functions that read text as it appears on the screen. Speech recognition software can be useful for those with dyslexia because their verbal skills are often better than their writing.

Using a multisensory approach to learning can be helpful, such as using a digital recorder to record a lecture and then listening to it while reading notes. It can also be useful to break large tasks and activities down into smaller steps. When drawing up plans or making notes it can be useful to create a 'mind map' or diagrams that use images and keywords to create a visual representation of a subject or plan.

Adjustments at work

Workers with dyslexia should inform their employer so that reasonable adjustments can be considered, including:

• providing assistance technology, such as digital recorders or speech-to-text software
• giving instructions verbally rather than in writing
• allowing extra time for tasks found particularly difficult
• providing information in accessible formats.

Developmental coordination disorder

Developmental coordination disorder (DCD), also known as developmental dyspraxia or simply dyspraxia,[82] is very similar to dyspraxia, and it has been suggested it should be regarded as synonymous.[83] Movement clumsiness has gained increasing recognition as an important condition of childhood and approaches to assessment and treatment vary depending on theoretical assumptions about aetiology and its developmental course.

A prevalence estimate of 6% of the general population for DCD has been reported[84] although this includes a range of severity. Boys are 1.7–2.8 times more likely than girls to have the disorder[85] and children with extremely low birth weights are at a significantly increased risk.[86]

The *DSM-5* classifies DCD as a discrete motor disorder under the broader heading of neurodevelopmental disorders. Multiple disturbances of gross and fine motor control are described within the definition.[87] Gross motor symptoms include poor timing and impaired balance, causing patients to trip over their own feet. Difficulty in combining movements into a sequence or in remembering movements in a sequence may be associated with proprioception or spatial awareness. Proprioceptive impairment and left–right confusion can interfere with holding or transferring objects such as pencils or tools.[88] Manipulation and dexterity are also compromised by fine motor symptoms which can interfere with handwriting and many activities of daily life.[89]

Dyspraxia is usually diagnosed by a physiotherapist or an occupational therapist but the European Academy of Childhood Disability recommends that it should be diagnosed by a multidisciplinary team of professionals who are qualified to examine the specific *DSM-5* criteria.[90] A useful screening test is the Developmental Coordination Disorder Questionnaire.[91]

Occupational therapy helps to find practical ways to remain independent and manage everyday tasks such as writing or preparing food. CBT benefits some people with dyspraxia. Regular exercise helps with coordination, reduces feelings of fatigue, and prevents weight gain. Other strategies include:

♦ learning how to use a computer or laptop if writing by hand is difficult

♦ using a calendar or diary to improve organization

♦ learning how to talk positively about challenges and overcoming them

♦ seeking out support through programmes such as Access to Work from Jobcentre Plus.

The Dyspraxia Foundation has a list of local support groups and Movement Matters UK has a page of useful links (see 'Useful websites').

The Equality Act 2010

The Equality Act 2010 builds upon requirements already in force through the first ever disability-specific law, the Autism Act 2009.[92] Employment protection is provided under the Equality Act 2010 for people with conditions such as ASDs and ADHD through a focus on the effects of impairments and not on the existence of a diagnosis. One specific area covered by the Equality Act 2010 relates to employers (or their agents) and the asking of health questions prior to an offer of employment. Questions can only be asked if they are about intrinsic requirements of the job or after the offer of employment has been made. If the employer asks health-related questions prior to a job offer, they must, if challenged, prove that the health condition did not influence the hiring decision. While people may keep their impairments hidden, it is likely that increasing numbers will disclose their condition after job offer, enabling the employer to seek advice on adjustments and fitness for work from an OH professional.

Access to Work

OH professionals should be aware of the functional impact of hidden impairments and what help is available to support people. One avenue is Access to Work (a specialist disability service delivered by Jobcentre Plus), which provides practical advice and support to disabled people and their employers (see 'Useful websites'). Access to Work partially funds the support to enable employers to make adjustments that might be considered reasonable by an employment tribunal. Support is tailored to individual needs, following assessment by the Access to Work adviser and, if appropriate, by a contracted specialist third-party assessor.

Key points

◆ Neurodevelopmental disorders are not uncommon, perhaps affecting up to 6% of the general population.

◆ Co-morbidity of the ASDs and specific learning disorders is frequently present.

◆ These disorders are treatable but often go unrecognized into adulthood, hence the description as hidden impairments.

◆ They are readily amenable to adjustments during the recruitment process and after appointment to a work role that enhance the often poor employment prospects in this group.

◆ The Equality Act 2010 is likely to apply to important impairments, even if a formal diagnosis has not been made.

Useful websites

The National Autistic Society	http://www.autism.org.uk/about.aspx
The ADHD Foundation	https://www.adhdfoundation.org.uk/
British Dyslexia Association	http://www.bdadyslexia.org.uk/
Dyspraxia Foundation	https://www.dyspraxiauk.com/dyspraxiafoundation.php

Movement Matters UK	http://www.movementmattersuk.org/
Access to Work	https://www.gov.uk/access-to-work
British Psychological Society	http://www.bps.org.uk
Business Disability Forum. 'Square Holes for Square Pegs'	https://businessdisabilityforum.org.uk/media_manager/public/261/Square%20Pegs_Final_GF.PDF

References

1. **Faraone SV, Biederman J.** What is the prevalence of adult ADHD? Results of a population screen of 966 adults. *J Atten Disord* 2005;9:384–91.

2. **Baxter AJ, Brugha TS, Erskine HE, Scheurer RW, Vos T, Scott JG.** The epidemiology and global burden of autism spectrum disorders. *Psychol Med* 2015;45:601–13.

3. **Sinzig J, Walter D, Doepfner M.** Attention deficit/hyperactivity disorder in children and adolescents with autism spectrum disorder: symptom or syndrome? *J Atten Disord* 2009;13: 117–26.

4. **Adamou M, Wadsworth A, Tullett M, Williams N.** Hidden impairments, the Equality Act and occupational physicians. *Occup Med (Lond)* 2011;61:453–5.

5. **Buescher AV, Cidav Z, Knapp M, Mandell DS.** Costs of autism spectrum disorders in the United Kingdom and the United States. *JAMA Pediatr* 2014;168:721–8.

6. **World Health Organization (WHO).** *International Statistical Classification of Disease and Related Health Problems (10th revision).* Geneva: WHO; 1992.

7. **Lai M-C, Lombardo MV, Baron-Cohen S.** Autism. *Lancet* 2014;383:896–910.

8. **National Institute for Health and Clinical Excellence.** *Autism: Recognition, Referral, Diagnosis and Management of Adults on the Autism Spectrum.* Leicester: British Psychological Society; 2012. Available at: https://www.ncbi.nlm.nih.gov/pubmed/26065067.

9. **Lord C, Rutter M, DiLavore PC, et al.** *Autism Diagnostic Observation Schedule, Second Edition: ADOS®-2.* Torrance, CA: WPS; 2012.

10. **Le Couteur A, Rutter M, Lord C.** Autism diagnostic interview: a standardized investigator-based instrument. *J Autism Dev Disord* 1989;19:363–87.

11. **Wing L, Leekam SR, Libby SJ, Gould J, Larcombe M.** The Diagnostic Interview for Social and Communication Disorders: background, inter-rater reliability and clinical use. *J Child Psychol Psychiatry* 2002;43:307–25.

12. **Demetriou EA, Lampit A, Quintana DS, et al.** Autism spectrum disorders: a meta-analysis of executive function. *Mol Psychiatry* 2018;23:1198–204.

13. **Remington A, Swettenham J, Campbell R, Coleman M.** Selective attention and perceptual load in autism spectrum disorder. *Psychol Sci* 2009;20:1388–93.

14. **Cashin A, Gallagher H, Newman C, Hughes M.** Autism and the cognitive processing triad: a case for revising the criteria in the diagnostic and statistical manual. *J Child Adolesc Psychiatr Nurs* 2012;25:141–8.

15. **Kimhi Y.** Theory of mind abilities and deficits in autism spectrum disorders. *Top Lang Disord* 2014;34:329–43.

16. **Baron-Cohen S, Leslie AM, Frith U.** Does the autistic child have a 'theory of mind'? *Cognition* 1985;21:37–46.

17. **Bosco FM, Gabbatore I, Tirassa M, Testa S.** Psychometric properties of the theory of mind assessment scale in a sample of adolescents and adults. *Front Psychol* 2016;7:566.

18. **Martory MD, Pegna AJ, Sheybani L, et al.** Assessment of social cognition and theory of mind: initial validation of the Geneva Social Cognition Scale. *Eur Neurol* 2015;**74**:288–95.

19. **Duncan AW, Bishop SL.** Understanding the gap between cognitive abilities and daily living skills in adolescents with autism spectrum disorders with average intelligence. *Autism* 2015;**19**:64–72.

20. **Volkmar FR, Sparrow SS, Goudreau D, Cicchetti DV, Paul R, Cohen DJ.** Social deficits in autism: an operational approach using the Vineland Adaptive Behavior Scales. *J Am Acad Child Adolesc Psychiatry* 1987;**26**:156–61.

21. **Howes OD, Rogdaki M, Findon JL, et al.** Autism spectrum disorder: consensus guidelines on assessment, treatment and research from the British Association for Psychopharmacology. *J Psychopharmacol* 2018;**32**:3–29.

22. **Hillier A, Fish T, Cloppert P, et al.** Outcomes of a social and vocational skills support group for adolescents and young adults on the autism spectrum. *Focus Autism Other Dev Disabl* 2007;**22**:107–15.

23. **Golan O, Baron-Cohen S.** Systemizing empathy: teaching adults with Asperger syndrome or high-functioning autism to recognize complex emotions using interactive multimedia. *Dev Psychopathol* 2006;**18**:591–617.

24. **Matson JL.** Use of independence training to teach shopping skills to mildly mentally retarded adults. *Am J Ment Defic* 1981;**86**:178–83.

25. **Lang R, Regester A, Lauderdale S, Ashbaugh K, Haring A.** Treatment of anxiety in autism spectrum disorders using cognitive behaviour therapy: a systematic review. *Dev Neurorehabil* 2010;**13**:53–63.

26. **Russell AJ, Jassi A, Fullana MA, et al.** Cognitive behavior therapy for comorbid obsessive-compulsive disorder in high-functioning autism spectrum disorders: a randomized controlled trial. *Depress Anxiety* 2013;**30**:697–708.

27. **Baker-Ericzén MJ, Fitch MA, Kinnear M, et al.** Development of the Supported Employment, Comprehensive Cognitive Enhancement, and Social Skills program for adults on the autism spectrum: results of initial study. *Autism* 2018;**22**:6–19.

28. **Hendricks D.** Employment and adults with autism spectrum disorders: challenges and strategies for success. *J Vocat Rehabil* 2010;**32**:125–34.

29. **Roux AM, Shattuck PT, Cooper BP, et al.** Postsecondary employment experiences among young adults with an autism spectrum disorder. *J Am Acad Child Adolesc Psychiatry* 2013;**52**:931–9.

30. **Holwerda A, van der Klink JJ, Groothoff JW, Brouwer S.** Predictors for work participation in individuals with an autism spectrum disorder: a systematic review. *J Occup Rehabil* 2012;**22**:333–52.

31. **Müller EA, Schuler A, Burton BA, Yates GB.** Meeting the vocational support needs of individuals with Asperger syndrome and other autism spectrum disabilities. *J Vocat Rehabil* 2003;**18**:163–75.

32. **Nicholas DB, Mitchell W, Dudley C, Clarke M, Zulla R.** An ecosystem approach to employment and autism spectrum disorder. *J Autism Dev Disord* 2018;**48**:264–75.

33. **Wehman P, Schall CM, McDonough J, et al.** Effects of an employer-based intervention on employment outcomes for youth with significant support needs due to autism. *Autism* 2017;**21**:276–90.

34. **Scott M, Jacob A, Hendrie D, et al.** Employers' perception of the costs and the benefits of hiring individuals with autism spectrum disorder in open employment in Australia. *PLoS One* 2017;**12**:e0177607.

35. **Ohl A, Grice Sheff M, Small S, Nguyen J, Paskor K, Zanjirian A.** Predictors of employment status among adults with autism spectrum disorder. *Work* 2017;**56**:345–55.

36. **Faraone SV, Biederman J, Mick E.** The age-dependent decline of attention deficit hyperactivity disorder: a meta-analysis of follow-up studies. *Psychol Med* 2006;**36**:159–65.

37. Taylor E. *The Epidemiology of Childhood Hyperactivity*. Maudsley Monographs No. 33. London: Oxford University Press; 1991.

38. Kessler RC, Berglund P, Demler O, Jin R, Merikangas KR, Walters EE. Lifetime prevalence and age-of-onset distributions of DSM-IV disorders in the National Comorbidity Survey Replication. *Arch Gen Psychiatry* 2005;**62**:593–602.

39. Hinshaw SP. Academic underachievement, attention deficits, and aggression: comorbidity and implications for intervention. *J Consult Clin Psychol* 1992;**60**:893–903.

40. McGough JJ, Smalley SL, McCracken JT, et al. Psychiatric comorbidity in adult attention deficit hyperactivity disorder: findings from multiplex families. *Am J Psychiatry* 2005;**162**:1621–7.

41. Nierenberg AA, Miyahara S, Spencer T, et al. Clinical and diagnostic implications of lifetime attention-deficit/hyperactivity disorder comorbidity in adults with bipolar disorder: data from the first 1000 STEP-BD participants. *Biol Psychiatry* 2005;**57**:1467–73.

42. Mannuzza S, Klein RG, Bessler A, Malloy P, LaPadula M. Adult outcome of hyperactive boys. Educational achievement, occupational rank, and psychiatric status. *Arch Gen Psychiatry* 1993;**50**:565–76.

43. Shekim WO, Asarnow RF, Hess E, Zaucha K, Wheeler N. A clinical and demographic profile of a sample of adults with attention deficit hyperactivity disorder, residual state. *Compr Psychiatry* 1990;**31**:416–25.

44. McGough JJ. Attention-deficit/hyperactivity disorder pharmacogenomics. *Biol Psychiatry* 2005;**57**:1367–73.

45. Biederman J, Faraone SV, Spencer T, et al. Patterns of psychiatric comorbidity, cognition, and psychosocial functioning in adults with attention deficit hyperactivity disorder. *Am J Psychiatry* 1993;**150**:1792–8.

46. Todd RD. Genetics of attention deficit/hyperactivity disorder: are we ready for molecular genetic studies? *Am J Med Genet* 2000;**96**:241–3.

47. Li D, Sham PC, Owen MJ, He L. Meta-analysis shows significant association between dopamine system genes and attention deficit hyperactivity disorder (ADHD). *Hum Mol Genet* 2006;**15**:2276–84.

48. Conners CK. Clinical use of rating scales in diagnosis and treatment of attention-deficit/hyperactivity disorder. *Pediatr Clin North Am* 1999;**46**:857–70.

49. Ramos-Quiroga JA, Nasillo V, Richarte V, et al. Criteria and concurrent validity of DIVA 2.0: a semi-structured diagnostic interview for adult ADHD. *J Atten Disord* 2016. 28 April [Epub ahead of print].

50. Hult N, Kadesjö J, Kadesjö B, Gillberg C, Billstedt E. ADHD and the QbTest: diagnostic validity of QbTest. *J Atten Disord* 2018;**22**:1074–80.

51. Goodlad JK, Marcus DK, Fulton JJ. Lead and attention-deficit/hyperactivity disorder (ADHD) symptoms: a meta-analysis. *Clin Psychol Rev* 2013;**33**:417–25.

52. Boonstra AM, Oosterlaan J, Sergeant JA, Buitelaar JK. Executive functioning in adult ADHD: a meta-analytic review. *Psychol Med* 2005;**35**:1097–108.

53. Mowinckel AM, Pedersen ML, Eilertsen E, Biele G. A meta-analysis of decision-making and attention in adults with ADHD. *J Atten Disord* 2015;**19**:355–67.

54. Spencer TJ, Adler LA, Qiao M, et al. Validation of the adult ADHD investigator symptom rating scale (AISRS). *J Atten Disord* 2010;**14**:57–68.

55. Emilsson B, Gudjonsson G, Sigurdsson JF et al. Cognitive behaviour therapy in medication-treated adults with ADHD and persistent symptoms: a randomized controlled trial. *BMC Psychiatry* 2011;**11**:116.

56. Solanto MV, Marks DJ, Wasserstein J, et al. Efficacy of meta-cognitive therapy for adult ADHD. *Am J Psychiatry* 2010;**167**:958–68.

57. **Young S, Morris R, Toone B, Tyson C.** Spatial working memory and strategy formation in adults diagnosed with attention deficit hyperactivity disorder. *Pers Individ Dif* 2006;**41**:653–61.

58. **Young S, Toone B, Tyson C.** Comorbidity and psychosocial profile of adults with attention deficit hyperactivity disorder. *Pers Individ Dif* 2003;**35**:743–55.

59. **Reich R.** *The Future of Success.* New York: Knop; 2001.

60. **Mannuzza S, Klein RG.** Long-term prognosis in attention-deficit/hyperactivity disorder. *Child Adolesc Psychiatr Clin N Am* 2000;**9**:711–26.

61. **Murphy K, Barkley RA.** Attention deficit hyperactivity disorder adults: comorbidities and adaptive impairments. *Compr Psychiatry* 1996;**37**:393–401.

62. **Secnik K, Swensen A, Lage MJ.** Comorbidities and costs of adult patients diagnosed with attention-deficit hyperactivity disorder. *Pharmacoeconomics* 2005;**23**:93–102.

63. **Mannuzza S, Klein RG, Bessler A, Malloy P, Hynes ME.** Educational and occupational outcome of hyperactive boys grown up. *J Am Acad Child Adolesc Psychiatry* 1997;**36**:1222–7.

64. **Rucklidge JJ.** Gender differences in ADHD: implications for psychosocial treatments. *Expert Rev Neurother* 2008;**8**:643–55.

65. **Barkley RA.** Behavioral inhibition, sustained attention, and executive functions: constructing a unifying theory of ADHD. *Psychol Bull* 1997;**121**:65–94.

66. **Barkley RA, Murphy K, Kwasnik D.** Psychological adjustment and adaptive impairments in young adults with ADHD. *J Atten Disord* 1996;**1**:41–54.

67. **Friedman SR, Rapport LJ, Lumley M, et al.** Aspects of social and emotional competence in adult attention-deficit/hyperactivity disorder. *Neuropsychology* 2003;**17**:50–8.

68. **Halmøy A, Fasmer OB, Gillberg C, Haavik J.** Occupational outcome in adult ADHD: impact of symptom profile, comorbid psychiatric problems, and treatment: a cross-sectional study of 414 clinically diagnosed adult ADHD patients. *J Atten Disord* 2009;**13**:175–87.

69. **Kessler RC, Lane M, Stang PE, Van Brunt DL.** The prevalence and workplace costs of adult attention deficit hyperactivity disorder in a large manufacturing firm. *Psychol Med* 2009;**39**:137–47.

70. **Matza LS, Paramore C, Prasad M.** A review of the economic burden of ADHD. *Cost Eff Resour Alloc* 2005;**3**:5.

71. **de Graaf R, Kessler RC, Fayyad J, et al.** The prevalence and effects of adult attention-deficit/hyperactivity disorder (ADHD) on the performance of workers: results from the WHO World Mental Health Survey Initiative. *Occup Environ Med* 2008;**65**:835–42.

72. **Schweitzer JB, Lee DO, Hanford RB, et al.** Effect of methylphenidate on executive functioning in adults with attention-deficit/hyperactivity disorder: normalization of behavior but not related brain activity. *Biol Psychiatry* 2004;**56**:597–606.

73. **Brown TE, Holdnack J, Saylor K, et al.** Effect of atomoxetine on executive function impairments in adults with ADHD. *J Atten Disord* 2011;**15**:130–8.

74. **Ustun B, Adler LA, Rudin C, et al.** The World Health Organization Adult Attention-Deficit/Hyperactivity Disorder Self-Report Screening Scale for DSM-5. *JAMA Psychiatry* 2017;**74**:520–6.

75. **Adamou M, Arif M, Asherson P, et al.** Occupational issues of adults with ADHD. *BMC Psychiatry* 2013;**13**:59.

76. **Staels E, Van den Broeck W.** A specific implicit sequence learning deficit as an underlying cause of dyslexia? Investigating the role of attention in implicit learning tasks. *Neuropsychology* 2017;**31**:371–82.

77. **Olulade OA, Napoliello EM, Eden GF.** Abnormal visual motion processing is not a cause of dyslexia. *Neuron* 2013;**79**:180–90.

78. **Skottun BC.** Is dyslexia caused by a visual deficit? *Vision Res* 2001;**41**:3069–71.

79. **Rodgers B.** The identification and prevalence of specific reading retardation. *Br J Educ Psychol* 1983;**53**:369–73.

80. **Skagerlund K, Traff U.** Number processing and heterogeneity of developmental dyscalculia: subtypes with different cognitive profiles and deficits. *J Learn Disabil* 2016;**49**:36–50.

81. **Gross-Tsur V, Manor O, Shalev RS.** Developmental dyscalculia: prevalence and demographic features. *Dev Med Child Neurol* 1996;**38**:25–33.

82. **Polatajko H, Fox M, Missiuna C.** An international consensus on children with developmental coordination disorder. *Can J Occup Ther* 1995;**62**:3–6.

83. **Gibbs J, Appleton J, Appleton R.** Dyspraxia or developmental coordination disorder? Unravelling the enigma. *Arch Dis Child* 2007;**92**:534–9.

84. **Kirby PA, Sugden PDA.** Developmental coordination disorder. *Br J Hosp Med* 2010;**71**:571–5.

85. **Faebo Larsen R, Hvas Mortensen L, Martinussen T, Nybo Andersen AM.** Determinants of developmental coordination disorder in 7-year-old children: a study of children in the Danish National Birth Cohort. *Dev Med Child Neurol* 2013;**55**:1016–22.

86. **Holsti L, Grunau RV, Whitfield MF.** Developmental coordination disorder in extremely low birth weight children at nine years. *J Dev Behav Pediatr* 2002;**23**:9–15.

87. **Missiuna C, Gaines R, Soucie H, McLean J.** Parental questions about developmental coordination disorder: a synopsis of current evidence. *Paediatr Child Health* 2006;**11**:507–12.

88. **Wilson PH, McKenzie BE.** Information processing deficits associated with developmental coordination disorder: a meta-analysis of research findings. *J Child Psychol Psychiatry* 1998;**39**:829–40.

89. **Polatajko HJ, Cantin N.** Developmental coordination disorder (dyspraxia): an overview of the state of the art. *Semin Pediatr Neurol* 2005;**12**:250–8.

90. **Blank R, Smits-Engelsman B, Polatajko H, et al.** European Academy for Childhood Disability (EACD): recommendations on the definition, diagnosis and intervention of developmental coordination disorder (long version). *Dev Med Child Neurol* 2012;**54**:54–93.

91. **Wilson BN, Crawford SG, Green D, Roberts G, Aylott A, Kaplan BJ.** Psychometric properties of the revised Developmental Coordination Disorder Questionnaire. *Phys Occup Ther Pediatr* 2009;**29**:182–202.

92. **Wadham J, Robinson A, Ruebain D, Uppal S.** *Blackstone's Guide to The Equality Act 2010.* New York: Oxford University Press; 2010.

Chapter 33

Gastrointestinal and liver disorders

Ira Madan and Simon Hellier

Introduction

This chapter covers the common gastrointestinal and liver disorders that occur in the working age population. Few disorders of the gastrointestinal systems, with the exception of infections, are caused or exacerbated by the work environment. More commonly, gastrointestinal disorders limit capacity to undertake work duties. Advances in investigation, medical treatment, and surgery should improve symptom control, prognosis, and retention of employment.

Conditions that are likely to cause employment problems or risks to individuals and the public include inflammatory bowel disease, ileostomy and ileo-anal pouch, irritable bowel syndrome, gastrointestinal infections, chronic liver disease, and obesity.

Gastrointestinal infections in food handlers may pose a risk to the general population; in addition, hepatitis A may pose a risk to co-workers. Some symptoms may lead to unpredictable episodes of absence from work. Frequency and urgency of defaecation, excessive flatulence, and faecal leakage necessitate rapid and frequent access to toilet facilities, but embarrassment may discourage disclosure of these to managers. Occupational health (OH) professionals have a key role in supporting workers and optimizing medical confidentiality. Many gastrointestinal disorders are chronic, and conditions that lead to regular minor faecal incontinence or to even infrequent loss of bowel control are defined as a disability under the Equality Act 2010.

The prevalence of obesity in the working age population is rapidly increasing and the role of OH practitioners and the workplace in its prevention and management is discussed.

Inflammatory bowel disease

Inflammatory bowel disease affects 4 in 1000 people in industrialized countries. The two main types are Crohn's disease and ulcerative colitis. Crohn's disease is a chronic inflammatory process, which may affect any part of the gastrointestinal tract from the mouth to the anus. The inflammation is transmural and may be complicated by fistulas, abscess formation, and intestinal strictures. In contrast, ulcerative colitis only affects the colon; inflammation is superficial, starts in the rectum and may extend to the caecum (pancolitis), or affect only the rectum (proctitis). The National Institute for Health and Care Excellence (NICE) produced a Quality Standard for inflammatory bowel disease care in 2015.[1]

Ulcerative colitis

Ulcerative colitis classically presents with bloody diarrhoea, colicky abdominal pain, and urgency. The course is one of relapses and remissions with up to 50% of patients relapsing per year. After the first year, 90% of patients are able to work fully. There is a slight increase in mortality in the 2 years following diagnosis reverting to the rate for the normal population thereafter. There is a cumulative risk of colorectal cancer of 7.6% at 30 years and 10.8% at 40 years from diagnosis.

Treatment

Aminosalicylates are used in mild presentation and for maintenance, where they reduce relapse rates by up to 80% and reduce the risk of colorectal cancer. Rectal preparations are the first-line treatment for proctitis. Reducing courses of oral prednisolone are used in more severe flares. In steroid-dependent patients, azathioprine or mercaptopurine is used as a steroid-sparing agent. These patients need monitoring because of potential bone marrow suppression. There is an increasing armament of biological agents available for treating ulcerative colitis. Currently anti-tumour necrosis factor (infliximab, adalimumab, and golimumab) and anti-integrin agents (vedolizumab) are approved by NICE for use in moderate and severely active ulcerative colitis. Infliximab and vedolizumab are given as an infusion with three induction treatments at 0, 2, and 6 weeks followed by maintenance infusions at 6–8-week intervals requiring hospital attendance. Adalimumab and golimumab are given as a self-administered subcutaneous injection at 2-week and 4-week intervals respectively. Treatments are usually continued for 12 months with the need for ongoing treatment dependent on evidence of disease activity.

Despite medical treatment, 20–30% of patients with pancolitis will eventually undergo colectomy.

Ileostomy and ileo-anal pouch

An ileostomy may be fashioned temporarily or permanently. Stomal complications from a permanent ileostomy for ulcerative colitis occur in 75% of patients over 20 years. Stomas have a greater impact on the quality of life of females than males. Ileo-anal pouch procedures are increasingly performed for ulcerative colitis, with improved social acceptability, work capacity, and quality of life. Frequency of defecation, up to six times per day, may be a problem. There is a significant incidence of sexual dysfunction in males following the procedure. Seventy per cent of patients with a pouch will suffer a complication necessitating hospital admission, up to 30% develop pouchitis, and excision of the pouch is necessary in about 10%.

Crohn's disease

The presentation of Crohn's disease is much more variable than that of ulcerative colitis and depends on the site of the inflammation as well as the presence of fistulating or stricturing disease. Small bowel disease may present with abdominal pain, weight loss, anaemia, and obstructive symptoms. Colonic disease may present in a similar fashion

---

Box 33.1 Factors associated with a worse prognosis in Crohn's disease

- Extremes of age
- Extensive small bowel disease
- Fistulating disease
- Stricturing
- Multiple operations
- Smoking

---

to ulcerative colitis. Perianal disease typically presents with abscesses or discharging fistulas. Crohn's disease is characterized by relapses between spontaneous or treatment-induced remissions. However, about 15% of patients have non-remitting disease and 10% prolonged remission. The prognosis appears to be affected by the age at diagnosis, disease location, and disease behaviour (Box 33.1); the latter may be genetically determined.

Treatment

Smoking cessation is vital in patients with Crohn's disease. The initial medical treatment of Crohn's disease is usually prednisolone, followed by immunomodulating drugs such as azathioprine, mercaptopurine, or methotrexate. In patients with moderate to severe active disease despite the use of standard therapy, the anti-tumour necrosis factor therapies infliximab and adalimumab, usually in conjunction with azathioprine, or the anti-integrin monoclonal antibody vedolizumab can be used.

Surgery for Crohn's disease is frequently necessary. Seventy per cent of patients will have an operation within 15 years of diagnosis and 36% will have required two or more operations. The symptoms recur in 30% within 5 years and in 50% by 10 years.

Extra-intestinal manifestations of inflammatory bowel disease

Inflammatory bowel disease is associated with a range of extra-intestinal manifestations—up to 36% of people have at least one extra-intestinal manifestation and they occur more commonly in patients with colonic disease.

Arthropathy affects 5–15% of patients, either in the form of sacroiliitis or peripheral arthropathy. There are two types of peripheral arthropathy. Type I affects large joints, often the weight-bearing joints, and occurs at times of bowel disease activity. It affects fewer than five joints and usually resolves within a few weeks as the disease activity decreases, leaving no permanent joint damage. Conversely, type II is a polyarticular, small joint, symmetrical arthropathy, which is independent of bowel disease activity and usually persists for months or years.

Uveitis and *episcleritis* are probably the most common extra-intestinal manifestations and are commonly associated with joint symptoms. The reported point prevalence is 4–12%. Uveitis is more common in ulcerative colitis and episcleritis in Crohn's disease. Episcleritis causes a burning and itching sensation in the eye. Anterior uveitis is a serious complication due to acute inflammation of the anterior chamber of the eye. It causes severe ocular pain, blurred vision, and headaches.

Skin disorders are commonly associated with inflammatory bowel disease, but have few occupational consequences.

Systemic symptoms are common in people with chronic active inflammatory bowel disease and include lethargy, weight loss, and low-grade fever.

Functional limitations

The main problems are recurrent or persistent abdominal pain and frequency and urgency of defecation. Extra-intestinal manifestations may increase disability and impact work capacity, particularly during relapses. Usually the associated joint disease is mild but pain and stiffness may prevent individuals from undertaking physically strenuous work, including manual handling. Eye disease may cause significant short-term disability until treated. Affected individuals may be unfit to work as a result of pain and visual disturbance.

Mild relapses can be treated as an outpatient with little time away from work. Moderate or severe exacerbations will usually be incompatible with attending work and may require up to several months for recovery with medical treatment. Surgery may result in prolonged absence from work depending on the type of procedure. In many cases, the longer-term prognosis after surgery will be favourable; therefore, employers may be prepared to be supportive in accommodating a prolonged period of recuperation.

Adjustments at work

The frequent, sudden, urgent need for defecation is one of the primary concerns of workers with inflammatory bowel disease. Having access to toilet facilities with sufficient privacy and ventilation is paramount. Access to a disabled toilet may be an option. Allowances should be made for frequent toilet breaks and a toilet break after meals. The impact of symptoms will be greater in jobs where rapid and regular toilet access is not possible. This could include those working outside, peripatetic workers, those responsible for the supervision or safety of others, and those undertaking paced work such as production line work where flexible breaks are not possible.

Travel is a key issue for many people with inflammatory bowel disease. Frequency and urgency may make travelling by public transport difficult, and travel to and from work by car may be preferred. Employers may wish to consider the provision of a parking space close to work. People with inflammatory bowel disease usually do not meet the criteria for disabled permit holders. Crohn's and Colitis UK have produced information leaflets for employers and employees (see 'Useful websites'). The leaflet for employees includes a helpful decision aid on the pros and cons of employees informing managers and colleagues about their disease.

Employment issues for workers with intestinal stomas

When returning to work after stoma surgery, workers are likely to be apprehensive about possible leaks and how the routine of work may affect them. Before starting back to work they may wish to consider a trial run as the preparation for work and leaving the house may take them longer than they expected. They may need to think about work clothing or work uniform and if it allows them to empty their stoma bag easily. They will need to consider the changing facilities and location of the toilet facilities at work and they may need to purchase a small portable changing bag that they can take discreetly to the toilets.

Special work considerations

Physically strenuous work can cause difficulties for some patients with stomas. Development of a parastomal hernia can make manual handling difficult and uncomfortable. Other problems include increased risk of leakage and possible injury to the stoma itself. Work that involves high-risk manual handling, repetitive stooping and bending, and carrying heavy or awkward loads close to the body, may be problematic. However, not all patients will find this to be the case and there are cases of successful employment in safety-critical work such as the emergency services. Food handling is not contraindicated in patients with stomas, as there is no evidence of increased cross-infection risk. Providing there is not a problem with leakage and good hygiene is followed, people with stomas should not be excluded from this work.

Work in hot environments could potentially place employees with stomas at greater than average risk because of the increased potential for dehydration and electrolyte imbalance. Ensuring that adequate hydration is maintained should prevent this. Patients visiting the tropics should be instructed on the use of oral rehydration solutions. Although there is evidence that working life is disturbed for patients after surgery for a stoma, there are no absolute contraindications for any work.[2] The nature and siting of the stoma will have an influence on any restrictions so each case should be assessed individually.

Irritable bowel syndrome

Irritable bowel syndrome is a functional gastrointestinal disorder caused by a disorder of gut–brain interaction. It is characterized by a combination of chronic or recurrent gastrointestinal symptoms that are not explained by structural or biochemical abnormalities, but which are attributed to the intestines and associated with symptoms of pain, disturbed defecation, and/or symptoms of bloating and distention. The prevalence in industrialized countries is 9–12%. Women are more commonly affected than men and the incidence is higher in those aged below age 45 than those aged 45 and over. Patients tend to report episodes, with duration of up to 5 days. Individuals may develop a remission

Box 33.2 The Rome IV criteria for diagnosing irritable bowel syndrome

Recurrent abdominal pain, on average, at least once per day/week in the last 3 months, associated with two or more of the following criteria:

- Related to defecation.
- Associated with a change in frequency of stool.
- Associated with a change of form (appearance) of stool.

The onset of symptoms should have been for at least 6 months before diagnosis. In practice, some people who do not exactly meet the criteria might still benefit from treatment.

after a series of symptomatic episodes, but there is paucity of literature on the natural history of the illness.

New criteria for diagnosing irritable bowel syndrome (Rome IV criteria) were released in June 2016.[2] There are three main subtypes: IBS-C (predominant constipation), IBS-D (predominant diarrhoea), and IBS-M (with mixed bowel habits). People whose symptoms do not fit into any category are considered to have irritable bowel syndrome unclassified (Box 33.2).

Management

Rome IV emphasizes that the best management for functional gastrointestinal disorders, including irritable bowel syndrome, requires a biopsychosocial approach. Lifestyle advice and dietary modification are important interventions for most symptoms. There is no standardized diet that is suitable for all people with the condition. Individuals with irritable bowel syndrome should be encouraged to keep a food diary and record whether certain foods make their symptoms better or worse. Often a reduction in fibre and resistant starches is beneficial. If symptoms fail to respond to general lifestyle and dietary advice then referral to a healthcare professional with expertise in dietary management is recommended (NICE clinical guidelines[3]). If individuals are anxious or feel under pressure at work or at home, they should be encouraged to engage in activities that can reduce anxiety levels or help them relax. These include, but are not limited to, learning relaxation techniques, mindfulness, yoga, or regular exercise. Sufferers who are particularly anxious or whose mood is low may benefit from talking therapies such as cognitive behavioural therapy. Antispasmodics are the first-line pharmaceutical intervention for variable bowel habit and abdominal pain. If these are ineffective, low-dose amitriptyline taken at night is often effective, although this can cause drowsiness the following day. For diarrhoea-predominant irritable bowel syndrome, cholestyramine will be effective in some individuals, otherwise loperamide is used as necessary. For constipation, laxatives are used although both lactulose and stool bulking agents can exacerbate bloating.

Functional limitations

Many of the symptoms of irritable bowel syndrome such as bloating, faecal urgency, incontinence, diarrhoea, flatulence, and borborygmi can impair performance at work and restrict activities of daily living. During functional assessment, the OH professional should look for evidence of pain behaviour, which would support the diagnosis. Clinicians should acknowledge that the symptoms are real and that other individuals experience similar symptoms.

Adjustments at work

The majority of patients manage to remain in work despite their condition, although exacerbations may lead to up to twice the average absence from work. In severe cases, the need for frequent defecation may substantially restrict travel or work and arrangements to facilitate ready access to a toilet at work may need to be put in place. Symptoms may be made worse by perceived occupational stress, job dissatisfaction, or poor working relationships. The possibility of underlying work issues should be explored and, if present, addressed.

Gastrointestinal infections

Diarrhoea is a very common condition in the community. It usually implies a change in bowel habit with loose or liquid stools, which are passed more frequently than normal.

Gastrointestinal infection affects as many as one in five members of the population each year. Symptoms are caused by the organisms themselves or by the toxins that they produce. In the absence of any known bowel disease, a sudden change in bowel habit whereby three or more loose stools are passed in 24 hours is an indication that diarrhoea may be infectious. Other symptoms of infectious diarrhoea include nausea, malaise, and pyrexia, although these symptoms may also accompany other causes of diarrhoea, such as inflammatory bowel disease. A thorough medical history should be taken to exclude other common causes of non-infective diarrhoea such as medicines, irritable bowel syndrome, and excess consumption of spicy food or alcohol. The majority of gastrointestinal infections seen in the UK are self-limiting.

Functional assessment and exclusion from work

The symptoms of a gastrointestinal infection such as diarrhoea, vomiting, and pyrexia may result in temporary incapacity for work. But the main risk is that the infected person may infect other employees, the public, or a product such as food. The risk of transmission is highest when the infected person is experiencing diarrhoea and vomiting, because of the high bacterial or viral load. In addition, loose or liquid stools are more likely to contaminate hands and surfaces.

Therefore, individuals with gastrointestinal infections should refrain from work until free from diarrhoea and vomiting for 48 hours. This is particularly important for:

- food handlers
- staff of healthcare facilities who are in direct contact with susceptible patients (e.g. immunosuppressed, children, or the elderly) or their food.

More stringent guidance applies to infection with *Salmonella typhi*, verocytotoxin-producing *Escherichia coli* (VTEC) O157, and hepatitis A. This is discussed in further detail later in this chapter in relation to food handlers.

If the cause is confirmed as non-infective after the individual was excluded then they can return to work, provided they feel well enough to do so. It is reasonable to presume that a single bout (e.g. one loose stool) or incidence of vomiting is not infectious if 24 hours have elapsed without any further symptoms and this is not accompanied by fever. In this case, as long as there is no other evidence to suggest an infectious cause, the person would only pose a very low risk of being infected and could resume work before the 48-hour limit. On return to work, individuals must take extra care over personal hygiene practices, especially hand washing.

The most common infections are summarized in Table 33.1.

Food handlers

The Food Standards Agency estimate that each year in the UK around a million people suffer a food-borne illness, around 20,000 people receive hospital treatment, and around 500 deaths are caused by food-borne illness.[4]

Estimates suggest that infected food handlers cause between 4% and 33% of food-borne disease outbreaks in the UK. The most important infections attributed to transmission from infected food handlers are norovirus, *Salmonella enteritidis*, and *Salmonella typhimurium*, which together account for the largest numbers of outbreaks and individual infections. The most common routes of transmission are faecal–oral and via aerosol formation from vomit.

It is important to remember that food handlers not only include those individuals employed directly in the production and preparation of foodstuffs, but workers undertaking maintenance work or repairing equipment in food-handling areas. Managers and visitors to food-handling areas may also be included in the definition. The duration of food handling is not relevant.

Guidance and regulations

Regulatory and best practice guidance on fitness to work for food handlers is available online from the Food Standards Agency (see 'Useful websites'). Detailed, up-to-date guidance on individual infectious agents is available on the Public Health England Infectious Diseases website. All cases of food poisoning are notifiable to Local Authority Proper Officers under the Health Protection (Notification) Regulations 2010 (see 'Useful websites').

Table 33.1 Microbial pathogens responsible for food-borne diarrhoeal disease

Pathogen	Source	Incubation period	Symptoms	Recovery
Pathogens that colonize the gut				
Salmonella spp.	Eggs, poultry	12–72 hours	Diarrhoea, blood, pain, vomiting, fever	2–14 days
Campylobacter jejuni	Milk, poultry	1–11 days	Diarrhoea, blood, pain, vomiting, fever	7–21 days
Enterohaemorrhagic Escherichia coli	Beef	1–14 days	Diarrhoea, blood, pain, vomiting, fever	7–21 days
Vibrio parahaemolyticus	Crabs, shellfish	12–18 hours	Diarrhoea, pain, vomiting, fever	2–30 days
Yersinia enterocolitica	Milk, pork	2 hours–2 days	Diarrhoea, pain, fever	1–3 days
Clostridium perfringens	Spores in food especially milk	8–22 hours	Diarrhoea, pain,	1–3 days
Listeria monocytogenes	Milk, sweet corn	8–36 hours	Diarrhoea, fever	
Preformed toxins				
Staphylococcus aureus	Contaminated food, usually by humans	2–6 hours	Nausea, vomiting, pain, diarrhoea	Rapid, few hours
Bacillus cereus	Reheated food rice, sauces, and pasta	1–5 hours	Nausea, vomiting, pain, diarrhoea	Rapid
Clostridium botulinum	Spores geminate in anaerobic conditions, canned or bottled foods	18–36 hours	Transient diarrhoea, paralysis	Months

Prevention of microbiological contamination of food

Health screening before food handlers start work is not required by statute, but it has been common in the food industry for many years. Such screening usually takes the form of a questionnaire. The Equality Act 2010 precludes health screening before a job offer, but the job may be offered on the condition of satisfactory health clearance. If an organization does decide to undertake health screening of food handlers, it is important that they recognize that there is little evidence that health screening by questionnaire will detect a medical problem which is likely to preclude a food handler from work. Some organizations undertake health screening of food handlers when they return from abroad, but like screening before starting work, there is little evidence that such screening will detect a relevant medical disorder. The mainstay of identifying infected food handlers is to ensure that food handlers who develop symptoms of a gastrointestinal infection report their symptoms to their line manager. Local policies should state the procedure that should be followed by food handlers if they develop an infection or have been in contact with relevant conditions.

Food handlers must have good personal hygiene, and a manager can assess this at interview. Managers should also ensure that food handlers have good access to toilet and washing facilities. Food handlers should be trained in the safe handling of food and have a good understanding of the principles of food hygiene. It is imperative that food handlers are trained to wash and dry their hands before handling food, or surfaces likely to come into contact with food, especially after going to the toilet.

Exclusion from work

Food handlers who develop symptoms of gastrointestinal infection should report immediately to management and leave the food handling area. Excluding infected food handlers from the entire premises should be considered, as this will remove the potential risk of contamination of food via other staff that may use the same facilities (toilets, canteens) as the infected person. It is best to assume that the cause of diarrhoea or vomiting is an infection and the food handler should be excluded until evidence to the contrary is received. As with other workers, food handlers with infectious gastroenteritis should refrain from work until free from diarrhoea and vomiting for 48 hours. However, more stringent guidance applies to infection with *Salmonella typhi*, VTEC O157, and hepatitis A (see 'Infections with special occupational implications').

A food handler who is in contact with a household member who is suffering from diarrhoea or vomiting does not always require exclusion but they should inform their manager and take extra precautions, such as more stringent personal hygiene practices. If they start to feel unwell, they should report this immediately to their manager or supervisor. Cases that may require exclusion are where the household contact has enteric fever, or *E. coli* O157. Detailed information can be obtained from Public Health England Infectious Diseases website (see 'Useful websites').

Infections with special occupational implications

E. coli are common bacteria, which live in the intestines of warm-blooded animals. There are certain strains of *E. coli* which are normally found in the intestines of healthy people and animals without causing any ill effects; however, some strains are known to cause illness in people. Among these is a group of bacteria which are known as VTEC.

These can cause illness, ranging from mild to severe bloody diarrhoea, mostly without fever, to the serious conditions haemolytic uraemic syndrome and thrombotic thrombocytopenic purpura. The most important property of these strains is the production of one or more potent toxins important in the development of illness. VTEC are relatively rare as the cause of infectious gastroenteritis in England and Wales; however, the disease can be fatal, particularly in infants, young children, and the elderly.

The most important VTEC strain to cause illness in the UK is VTEC O157. This can be found in the intestines of healthy cattle, sheep, goats, and a wide range of other species. Humans may be infected by VTEC O157 or other VTEC strains when they consume food or water that has become contaminated by faeces from infected animals. Infection may also result from direct or indirect contact with animals that carry VTEC or from exposure to an environment contaminated with animals' faeces, such as farms and similar premises with animals, which are open to the public. The infectious dose of VTEC O157 is very low at less than 100 bacterial cells. Infection is readily spread between family contacts, particularly those who may be caring for infected children, and in settings such as children's day nurseries.

People infected with VTEC usually have typical gastroenteritis symptoms, that is, diarrhoea with or without vomiting, abdominal cramps, and fever. Sometimes there is blood mixed in with the diarrhoea. Symptoms may last a few days and then disappear within a week or so.

Management of cases is purely supportive. Antibiotics are *not* recommended and might exacerbate the sequelae of infection. Suspected cases must have a stool sample collected and sent to the local hospital laboratory where it will be tested for the presence of presumptive VTEC O157. The case must be reported to the local health protection unit. Screening (contacts of the patient) and exclusion (from school/work) may be necessary upon advice from the health protection unit.

Although the principal reservoir for VTEC O157 in the UK is cattle, therefore making the disease a zoonosis, secondary infections are also acquired, by person-to-person spread by direct contact (faecal–oral). This is particularly important in households, nurseries, primary schools, and residential care institutions. Therefore, efforts are undertaken by public health professionals to control the source of infection. The disease is also under surveillance to increase our understanding of the epidemiology of VTEC in England.

Salmonella infections

The prolonged bacteraemic illness of typhoid is caused by the exclusively human pathogen, *Salmonella typhi*. Annually about 200 cases of typhoid fever are seen in the UK mostly in people after visiting relatives or friends in developing countries with the peak incidence being in the autumn months. Watery diarrhoea occurs 12–72 hours after infection, accompanied by abdominal pain, vomiting, and fever. The illness lasts a few days and is usually self-limiting. Adults excrete the organism for 4–8 weeks but all except food handlers and water workers can resume work after 48 hours of being symptom free. Food handlers and water workers should not return to work until they have had two consecutive faecal samples free of infection, and have obtained clearance to return to work from the local authority. Food handlers who practise good hygiene are very rarely responsible for initiating outbreaks.

Hepatitis A

Hepatitis A is a statutory notifiable disease. The hepatitis A virus is transmitted by the faecal–oral route. In developed countries, person-to-person spread is the most common method of transmission, while in countries with poor sanitation, faeces-contaminated food and water are frequent sources of infection. Hepatitis A virus is excreted in the bile and shed in the stools of infected persons. Peak excretion occurs during the 2 weeks before onset of jaundice; the concentration of virus in the stools drops after jaundice appears.

The average incubation period of hepatitis A is around 28 days (range 15–50 days). Patients feel unwell during the prodrome but often improve with the onset of jaundice. Lethargy may continue for 6 weeks or for as long as 3 months. The course of hepatitis A infection is extremely variable but in adults 70–95% of infections result in clinical illness. Diagnosis is based on the detection in the serum of immunoglobulin (Ig)-M antibody to hepatitis A. The presence of IgG anti-hepatitis A antibody indicates either previous exposure or immunization.

Hepatitis A is usually a mild self-limiting illness but can occasionally result in severe or fatal disease. Fulminant hepatitis occurs rarely (<1% overall), but rates are higher with increasing age and in those with underlying chronic liver disease, including those with chronic hepatitis B or C infection. Hepatitis A does not appear to be worse in HIV-infected patients when compared to HIV-negative persons. Infection is followed by lifelong immunity.

A *confirmed case* is one that meets the clinical case definition (an acute illness with a discrete onset of symptoms *and* jaundice or elevated serum aminotransferase levels) *and* is laboratory confirmed (IgM antibodies to hepatitis A virus (anti-HAV) positive).

A *probable case* meets the clinical case definition and occurs in a person who has an epidemiological link with a person with laboratory confirmed hepatitis A.

If a worker is suspected of being infected with hepatitis A, the local health protection team should be contacted. The index case should be excluded from work until 7 days after the onset of jaundice or, if there is no history of jaundice, 7 days after the onset of symptoms. If the worker has been in the workplace and in contact with co-workers while infectious, a risk assessment should be undertaken to determine if the co-workers require immunization. Advice should be sought from the local health protection team. If a food handler has been in contact with a co-worker infected with hepatitis A, special precautions must be taken as detailed below.

Food-borne outbreaks can occur due to the contamination of food at the point of service or due to contamination during growing, harvesting, processing, or distribution. A review of published food-borne outbreaks in the US found that infected food handlers who handled uncooked food, or food after it had been cooked, during the infectious period were the most common source of published food-borne outbreaks. A single hepatitis A-infected food handler has the potential to transmit hepatitis A to large numbers of people, although reported outbreaks are rare. Such outbreaks often involve secondary cases among other food handlers who ate food contaminated by the index case.

If a food handler has been in contact with an individual who is acutely infected with hepatitis A, a risk assessment should be undertaken. If the food handler has been immunized against hepatitis A with documented evidence of a completed course of hepatitis A vaccine in the past 10 years, or one dose of monovalent vaccine within the past 12 months, they can be considered immune. Those who have had laboratory-confirmed hepatitis A (previous anti-HAV IgG positive, or HAV RNA positive) can also be considered immune and then no further action is required. If the contact with the source case of hepatitis A is within 14 days, provided they are healthy and aged under 60, the food handler should be given a first dose of monovalent hepatitis A vaccine and a second dose 6–12 months after the initial dose. Food handlers aged 60 years and over should be offered hepatitis A immunoglobulin in addition to monovalent hepatitis A vaccine. A second dose of vaccine is recommended 6–12 months after the first dose to ensure long-term protection.[5]

If the food handler has not been immunized within 14 days of exposure, they are at high risk of acquiring infection and should be removed from activities which involve preparing and handling ready-to-eat foods until 30 days post exposure. Scrupulous hand and general hygiene should be enforced and provided that this is adhered to they can remain at work (Figure 33.1).

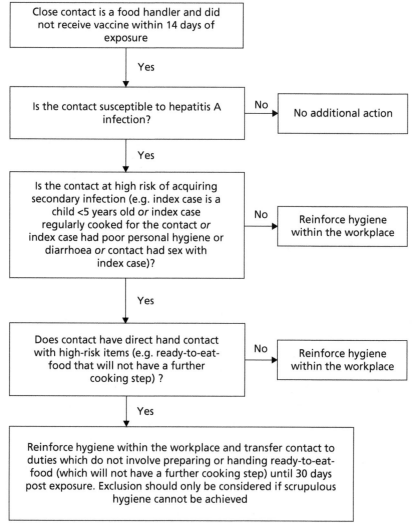

Figure 33.1 Risk assessment for food handlers who have had contact with an individual acutely infected with hepatitis A.

Box 33.3 At-risk occupational groups for whom hepatitis A vaccination is recommended

- Laboratory workers: individuals who may be exposed to hepatitis A in the course of their work, in microbiology laboratories, and clinical infectious disease units.

- Staff of some large residential institutions: outbreaks of hepatitis A have been associated with large residential institutions for those with learning difficulties. Similar considerations apply in other institutions where standards of personal hygiene among clients or patients may be poor.

- Sewage workers at risk of repeated exposure to raw, untreated sewage.

- People who work with primates that are susceptible to hepatitis A infection.

Source: data from Salisbury D. et al. (2013) *Immunisation against infectious disease.* London, UK: Department of Health. © 2013 Crown Copyright 2013. Available at: https://www.gov.uk/government/uploads/system/uploads/attachment_data/file/266583/The_Green_book_front_cover_and_contents_page_December_2013.pdf.

If a food handler develops acute jaundice or is diagnosed clinically or serologically with hepatitis A infection, the local health protection team should be informed immediately by telephone. This will allow a timely risk assessment of whether other food handlers in the same food preparation area could have been exposed and should be considered for post-exposure prophylaxis. Rapid serological confirmation and notification of hepatitis A infection will allow an assessment of the possible risks to any customers who can be traced and offered prophylaxis.

Prevention of hepatitis A infection
See Box 33.3.[5]

Cirrhosis of the liver

Cirrhosis results from chronic liver injury. The most common causes in the UK are alcohol, chronic viral hepatitis, and non-alcoholic fatty liver disease. The prevalence and prognosis depend on the underlying aetiology, but with uncomplicated cirrhosis the prognosis could be 15–20 years. Once an individual develops any of the major complications of cirrhosis listed later in this section, the prognosis is generally less than 5 years Scoring systems such as the Child–Pugh or the Model for End stage Liver Disease (MELD) scores are used in the clinic to estimate prognosis and guide the timing of referral for transplant assessment.

There is no specific treatment for cirrhosis itself. Management is aimed at treating the underlying aetiology where possible, and surveillance for, and then treatment, of complications as they arise. Initially, fatigue may be the predominant symptom causing impairment at work. Fatigue and intractable pruritus are particularly prominent symptoms in individuals with primary biliary cirrhosis.

The development of portal hypertension is a common sequela of cirrhosis. If oesophageal varices are identified at annual surveillance endoscopy, individuals are started on propranolol to reduce the risk of bleeding. This can exacerbate confusion in those with a tendency to encephalopathy and affect balance particularly in those with an alcoholic aetiology.

The development of ascites is a sign of decompensation. It is usually treated with spironolactone, which may result in electrolyte disturbance and tender gynaecomastia. Individuals intolerant of, or refractory to, diuretics undergo day case paracentesis and may be referred for a transjugular intrahepatic portosystemic shunt.

Spontaneous bacterial peritonitis is a complication of ascites which can lead to encephalopathy and precipitate hepatorenal syndrome. Consequently it has a poor prognosis. Individuals who recover from spontaneous bacterial peritonitis require lifelong prophylactic antibiotics.

Hepatic encephalopathy can present as subtle personality changes through varying degrees of confusion to coma. It usually presents as an acute episode often precipitated by infection, constipation, or a gastrointestinal bleed and is reversible if the underlying cause is treated. Some individuals suffer a chronic encephalopathy. The minimally absorbed antibiotic rifaximin has an important role in treating chronic encephalopathy and reducing frequency of acute episodes.

Hepatocellular carcinoma usually occurs as a consequence of cirrhosis. However, the risk is dependent on aetiology, and infection with hepatitis B and hepatitis C are the biggest risk factors. Cirrhotic patients therefore undergo surveillance ultrasound scans and alpha-fetoprotein on a 6-monthly basis. Hepatocellular carcinoma can be treated with radiofrequency ablation, chemo-embolization, resection, or liver transplantation.

Adjustments at work

A specialist should optimize the care of patients with cirrhosis and decompensated liver disease before work is resumed. In patients with oesophageal varices, there is no restriction on occupation once the varices have been treated. Patients with ascites may experience difficulty with lifting, bending, or stooping. Although alcohol addiction and dependency are excluded from the definition of impairment under the Equality Act 2010, the complications arising from alcoholism, especially ascites, hepatic impairment, and depression, will require individual assessment, to determine whether the patient is disabled within the meaning of the Act.

Patients with chronic or intermittent encephalopathy should not be employed in intellectually demanding work or jobs requiring a high degree of vigilance, including safety-critical work or operating machinery. Individuals suffering from hepatic cirrhosis with chronic encephalopathy or those who are cognitively impaired must not drive and must notify the Driver and Vehicle Licensing Agency (DVLA) (see DVLA website for current guidance on fitness to drive). Group 1 and 2 licenses will be revoked or refused until recovery is satisfactory and other medical standards for fitness to drive (e.g. for psychiatric conditions) are satisfied. Patients who chronically misuse alcohol and those who are alcohol dependent must inform the DVLA (see Chapter 14).

Liver transplantation

Liver transplantation is the ultimate treatment for cirrhotic patients with end-stage chronic liver failure. The most common indications for transplantation are decompensated cirrhosis secondary to alcohol, hepatitis C, and primary biliary cirrhosis. Approximately 700 liver transplants are carried out each year in the UK. The overall 5-year graft survival rate for first transplants is now 80%.[6] Individuals undergoing liver transplantation remain on lifelong immunosuppressant therapy and require regular follow-up by a hepatologist. General side effects include increased risk of infection and malignancy.

Implications for employment

Physical fatigue is the main symptom limiting work activity in transplant recipients. In general, implantation of a new liver results in significant improvements in cognitive function. Demographic variables associated with post-transplant employment include young age, male sex, college degree, Caucasian race, and pre-transplant employment.[7] Patients with alcohol-related liver disease have a significantly lower rate of employment than those with other aetiologies of liver disease. Recipients who are employed after transplantation have a significantly better post-transplant functional status than those who are not employed.[7]

In general, patients with chronic liver disease with ongoing inflammation or liver damage should not work with hepatotoxins. All patients working with hepatotoxins should avoid alcohol misuse and enzyme-inducing agents such as anticonvulsants, in particular phenobarbitone and phenytoin.

Obesity

Definitions and prevalence

In adults, body mass index (BMI) is frequently used as a measure of overweight and obesity, with overweight being defined as a BMI of 25–29.9 kg/m^2 and obesity as a BMI equal to or greater than 30 kg/m^2. However, BMI on its own should be interpreted with caution in highly muscular adults, as it may not be a good measure of adiposity in this group. Furthermore, some population groups, such as people of Asian family origin and older people, have co-morbidity risk factors that are of concern at different BMIs (lower in adults of an Asian family origin and higher for older people) (Table 33.2). Health risks are better determined by a combination of the degree of obesity (as measured by BMI) and central adiposity (as measured by waist circumference); therefore, NICE recommends the use of both measurements in combination.[8]

Central adiposity is associated with insulin resistance, decreased high-density lipoprotein cholesterol, raised low-density lipoprotein cholesterol and triglycerides, hypertension, and decreased glucose tolerance known together as the metabolic syndrome. Seventy-five per cent of individuals with obesity will develop non-alcoholic fatty liver disease, which can cause progressive liver disease leading to cirrhosis and its complications.

Table 33.2 Waist circumference categories

	Desirable (cm)	High (cm)	Very high (cm)
Men	<94	94–102	>102
Women	<80	80–88	>88

In England, the prevalence of obesity in adults increased from 15% in 1993 to 27% in 2015.[9] Furthermore, the prevalence of morbid obesity (BMI of 40 kg/m^2 or higher) has more than tripled since 1993, and reached 2% of men and 4% of women in 2015.[9] Obesity becomes more common with age and is more prevalent among lower socioeconomic and lower-income groups, with a particularly strong social class gradient among women. Adults at greater risk of becoming obese include those who were previously overweight and who have lost weight, smokers who have stopped smoking, and those who change from an active to an inactive lifestyle.

Management starts with behavioural advice and weight loss management services. If these fail, then referral to a specialist weight management service is recommended. These services are led by a multidisciplinary team, potentially including a physician with a special interest, specialist nurse, specialist dietician, psychologist, psychiatrist, and physiotherapist and may include pharmacological intervention. Engagement with a specialist weight management service is a requirement for referral for bariatric surgery, usually for a period of 12–24 months.

Bariatric surgery is recommended for individuals with a BMI greater than 40, or 35–40 with co-morbidities, such as type 2 diabetes mellitus or hypertension, who have failed management in specialist weight management services. Patients with a BMI greater than 50 may be referred directly for bariatric surgery. Individuals have to be fit for surgery and agree to long-term follow-up and maintenance of healthy lifestyle changes including diet and exercise. There are a number of techniques available including gastric banding which is reversible but not as effective as gastric bypass or sleeve gastrectomy, both of which are irreversible and associated with an increased risk of immediate post-surgical complications and longer-term complications including malnutrition. The procedures may be undertaken by open or laparoscopic surgery.

The procedure with the shortest recovery time is gastric banding. Most patients leave hospital within 1 or 2 days, are back to their full daily activities within 2 weeks, and are likely to be fit to return to work between 1 and 2 weeks after surgery. As a guideline, patients require 2–3 weeks off work following both open and laparoscopic gastric bypass and gastric sleeve surgery, but may require longer if there are postoperative complications.

Obesity in the workplace

OH services have rightly become increasingly involved in the prevention and treatment of obesity in the workplace. Due to the vast heterogeneity in the types of workplace-based interventions to prevent or treat obesity, no sound conclusions can as yet be drawn about their overall effectiveness and best practice recommendations for their implementation.[10] Despite some inconsistencies in findings, there is convincing evidence that shift work increases the risk of obesity, while most studies do not show a significant association between sedentary work and obesity. However, overweight and obesity are associated with absenteeism, disability pension, and overall work impairment.[10]

In light of the uncertainty about the effectiveness of interventions in the workplace to reduce obesity, NICE encourages workplaces to act in line with the local obesity strategy (in England). NICE guidance for workplaces[11] is as follows:

Provide opportunities for staff to eat a healthy diet and be more physically active, through:

◆ active and continuous promotion of healthy choices in restaurants, hospitality, vending machines, and shops for staff and clients, in line with existing Food Standards Agency guidance

◆ working practices and policies, such as active travel policies for staff and visitors

◆ a supportive physical environment, such as improvements to stairwells and providing showers and secure cycle parking

◆ recreational opportunities, such as supporting out-of-hours social activities, lunchtime walks and use of local leisure facilities.

Incentive schemes (such as policies on travel expenses, the price of food and drinks sold in the workplace, and contributions to gym membership) that are used in a workplace should be sustained and be part of a wider programme to support staff in managing weight, improving diet, and increasing activity levels.

In a workplace setting, health professionals should assess an obese person's lifestyle, co-morbidities, and willingness to change. The level of detail of the assessment will depend on the person, the timing of the assessment, the degree of overweight or obesity, and the results of previous assessments. Co-morbidities should be managed as soon as they are identified. Obese people should be given information on the benefits of losing weight, healthy eating, and increased physical activity. Specialist input is helpful if:

◆ the underlying causes of being overweight or obese need to be assessed

◆ the person has complex disease states (e.g. learning difficulties)

◆ conventional treatment has been unsuccessful

◆ drug treatment is being considered for a person with a BMI more than 50 kg/m^2

◆ specialist interventions (such as a very low-calorie diet) may be needed or

◆ surgery is being considered.

Functional limitations

When assessing overweight and obese workers it is important to assess their physical limitations in the context of their job. Obese workers who are physically fit may be more mobile than slim workers who are unfit. Assessment should take into account co-morbid conditions, especially metabolic syndrome and sleep apnoea. There are few jobs that obese workers are not able to do. However, the following need careful consideration:

◆ Mobility and size may affect entry to confined spaces and access into vehicles, use of personal protective equipment, or other equipment such as ladders.

◆ Weight limits on seating in vehicles or offices may need to be checked to ensure they are not exceeded.

◆ Obese workers may be at increased risk of heat stress when working in high temperatures.

◆ Some safety-critical work requires high levels of mobility.

Adjustments at work

In assessing whether obesity would be considered a disability as defined by the Equality Act 2010, the focus should be on whether the obesity has a substantial adverse effect on the person's ability to carry out normal day-to-day activities. The question of what caused the obesity is irrelevant. In most cases, it is likely that the effects will be long term, that is, they have lasted for, or are likely to last for, at least 12 months. The employer should, in these cases, consider if reasonable adjustments to the job are required. Even if the obese worker is not considered disabled as defined by the Equality Act 2010, employers may wish to consider if they have equipment designed to accommodate larger people and if they are able to make alternative arrangements within the workplace so that work spaces can accommodate larger people. Wider seating arrangements and desk space may be necessary. As with some physically disabled workers, special consideration may need to be given to evacuation of obese workers in case of an emergency. Employers should be sensitive to the complicated issues that contribute to a worker being obese and the impact on self-esteem, and should support workers who are trying to lose weight.

Key points

◆ Many gastrointestinal disorders are chronic. Conditions that lead to regular minor faecal incontinence or loss of bowel control (even if infrequent), and frequency and urgency of defecation are likely to be considered as a disability under the Equality Act 2010.

◆ The perceived embarrassing nature of some gastrointestinal conditions need to be treated sensitively, while ensuring that workers have appropriate workplace adjustments, particularly easy access to toilet facilities.

◆ Symptoms of irritable bowel syndrome may be made worse by perceived occupational stress, job dissatisfaction, or poor working relationships. The possibility of underlying work issues should be explored and, if present, addressed.

- ◆ Individuals with gastrointestinal infections should refrain from work until free from diarrhoea and vomiting for 48 hours.
- ◆ The prevalence of obesity in the working age population is increasing rapidly. Occupational health professionals have a role in identifying and supporting obese workers to remain at work, but also to ensure that they are given the opportunity to lose weight.

Useful websites

Crohn's and Colitis UK. Information on inflammatory bowel disease	https://www.crohnsandcolitis.org.uk/about-inflammatory-bowel-disease/publications/employment-ibd-a-guide-for-employees
Food Standards Agency. Hygiene requirements for businesses	https://www.food.gov.uk/business-guidance/hygiene-requirements-for-your-business
Public Health England. 'Infectious diseases'	https://www.gov.uk/topic/health-protection/infectious-diseases
Public Health England. 'Statutory Notifications of Infectious Diseases (Noids) England and Wales'	https://www.gov.uk/government/collections/notifications-of-infectious-diseases-noids
Public Health England. 'Hepatitis A infection: prevention and control guidance'	https://www.gov.uk/government/publications/hepatitis-a-infection-prevention-and-control-guidance

References

1. **National Institute for Health and Care Excellence**. Quality standard for inflammatory bowel disease. Quality standard [QS81]. 2015 Available at: https://www.nice.org.uk/guidance/qs81.
2. **Rome Foundation**. Rome IV Diagnostic Criteria for Functional Gastrointestinal Disorders. 2016. Available at: https://theromefoundation.org/rome-iv/.
3. **National Institute for Health and Care Excellence**. Irritable bowel syndrome in adults: diagnosis and management. Clinical Guideline [CG61]. 2008 (Last updated April 2017). Available at: https://www.nice.org.uk/guidance/cg61.
4. **Food Standards Agency**. Foodborne disease strategy 2010-15: an FSA programme for the reduction of foodborne disease in the UK. 2011. Available at: https://acss.food.gov.uk/sites/default/files/multimedia/pdfs/fds2015.pdf.
5. **Salisbury D, Ramsey M, Noakes K**. *Immunisation Against Infectious Disease* ('The Green Book'). London: Department of Health; 2013. Available at: https://www.gov.uk/government/uploads/system/uploads/attachment_data/file/266583/The_Green_book_front_cover_and_contents_page_December_2013.pdf.
6. **NHS Blood and Transplant, Public Health England**. Annual report on liver transplantation report for 2014/2015. 2015. Available at: https://nhsbtdbe.blob.core.windows.net/umbraco-assets-corp/3197/annual-report-on-liver-transplantation-2015.pdf.
7. **Huda A, Newcomer R, Harrington C, Keeffe EB, Esquivel CO**. Employment after liver transplantation: a review. *Transplant Proc* 2015;**47**:233–9.

8. **National Institute for Health and Care Excellence**. Obesity: identification, assessment and management. Clinical guideline [CG189]. 2014. Available at: https://www.nice.org.uk/guidance/cg189.

9. **NHS Digital**. Health survey for England 2015. 2015. Available at: http://digital.nhs.uk/catalogue/PUB22610.

10. **Shrestha N, Pedisic Z, Neil-Sztramko S, et al.** The impact of obesity in the workplace: a review of contributing factors, consequences and potential solutions. *Curr Obes Rep* 2016;5:344.

11. **National Institute for Health and Care Excellence**. Obesity prevention. Clinical guideline [CG43]. 2006 (Last updated 2015). Available at: https://www.nice.org.uk/guidance/cg43.

Chapter 34

Blood-borne viruses

Paul Grime and Christopher Conlon

Introduction

Hepatitis B (HBV), hepatitis C (HCV), and human immunodeficiency virus (HIV) infections have particular implications for fitness for work. These include the impact of symptoms and disease, the transmissibility of infection in the course of specific work activities, and, in the case of HIV, vulnerability to other infections arising from immune deficiency. The potential for transmission of infection gives rise to restrictions for some professional groups, such as healthcare workers (HCWs) who undertake exposure-prone procedures (EPPs). Treatment for blood-borne virus (BBV) infections is a rapidly advancing field, improving the prognosis and fitness for work for infected individuals, as well as impacting the scientific evidence that underpins work restrictions. Changes in stigma, public opinion, legislation, and media activity may lag behind scientific advances, but are also influential in determining employment outcomes for affected individuals.

There are many BBV infections, but this chapter will focus on HBV, HCV, and HIV because these are the most common infections that have particular implications for work. BBV infections can affect people of any age. In the UK, HIV infection is specifically mentioned and automatically considered as a disability, from the point of diagnosis, by the Equality Act 2010. HBV and HCV infection may also qualify as disabilities, if associated disease causes impairment. There are, therefore, practical, legal, and ethical issues to consider when assessing fitness for work in people with BBV infections.

HIV infection

The majority of people infected with HIV are of working age and most have been infected through sexual exposure. In many developing countries, although there has been significant progress, mother-to-child transmission still occurs, resulting in substantial numbers of infected children.

The development in the 1990s of highly active antiretroviral therapy (ART, or HAART), using three or more antiretroviral drugs in combination, has greatly improved survival in both developed and developing countries. This has increased the potential for those of working age to remain in, or return to, work following their diagnosis. While ART has increased survival, many HIV-infected people remain symptomatic, either through drug side effects, HIV-related illnesses, or the psychological morbidity associated with the diagnosis and disease. All of these factors can have a significant impact on an individual's ability to find, and remain in, work. In addition, an employer's approach to those with chronic illness, and HIV in particular, can have a major influence on the workplace support received by infected workers.

As the epidemiology, treatment, and drug resistance of HIV infection are evolving so rapidly, it is difficult to predict what the future holds for HIV-infected individuals of working age. It is likely that the prognosis will continue to improve and that the stigma associated with HIV will slowly disappear. Effective vaccines continue to be sought but remain elusive at present.

Epidemiology of HIV in the UK

In the UK in 2016, there were an estimated 100,000 people living with HIV and 5164 new cases of HIV were diagnosed. This represents a significant decline in incidence compared to previous years, with the greatest decline seen in men who have sex with men, who are still the highest risk group for acquiring HIV in the UK. There has also been a steady decline in infections in heterosexual men and women. About three-quarters of these heterosexually acquired HIV infections were probably acquired in Africa. Of the new cases in 2016, about 40% were diagnosed late, with CD4 counts less than 350 cells/mm^3.[1] Of new cases, it is estimated that 19% were recently acquired. It was also estimated that in 2016 around 10,000 people who were living with HIV did not know that they were infected.

The recent fall in new diagnoses is welcome news and probably relates to a variety of interventions. Current approaches, such as treating people as soon as they are diagnosed, rather than waiting for the CD4 count to drop, the increasing use of pre-exposure prophylaxis, and more consistent use of condoms have all contributed to this fall.

Despite the increasing prevalence of HIV infection, the incidence of AIDS has decreased significantly due to effective and earlier treatment (Figure 34.1). It is likely that the epidemiology of HIV and AIDS in the UK will continue to change in future decades, driven by the science of drug development, vaccine development, drug resistance, and sociodemographic variables such as migration and routes of transmission.

Natural history of HIV infection

Patients who are untreated will develop an AIDS-defining illness on average 10 years after acquiring HIV infection. Within 2–3 weeks of being infected, there is a burst of HIV viraemia with several million copies of virus in the plasma. This level falls over the following few weeks. Within 6 months of infection, the plasma viral load settles at a relatively stable value and subsequently changes little over a number of years. Both the CD4 lymphocyte (a T-cell helper subset) count at this time and the viral load are predictive factors for the risk of opportunistic infection. In addition, the degree of activation of the immune system, measured by the levels of CD38 (an activation marker) on either CD4 or CD8 cells, is predictive of the likely speed of development of AIDS.

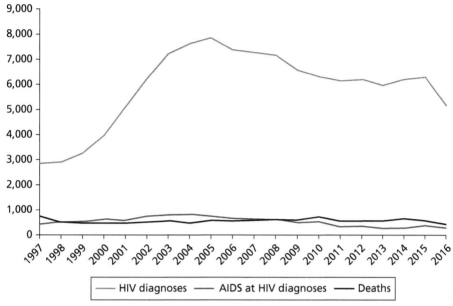

Figure 34.1 Number of people newly diagnosed with HIV and AIDS, and all-cause deaths among people with HIV in the ART era: United Kingdom, 1997–2016.
Source: data from Public Health England. © Crown Copyright 2017.

Factors influencing the rate of progression to AIDS

1. *Age*: the rate of progression, and particularly of opportunistic infections, increases with age.

2. *Social and educational factors*: the less privileged and the less well educated develop opportunistic infections at a faster rate because of poor access to medical care.

3. *Genetic factors*: two groups of genes affect the rate of progression to AIDS. Individuals with a specific human leucocyte antigen haplotype progress more slowly, while individuals with a specific rare deletion (CCR5Δ32) rarely become HIV infected (homozygous) or progress at slower rates (heterozygous).

4. *Treatment*: the most important influence on progression rates in the twenty-first century is access to effective ART. This has revolutionized care in the developed world and now good progress is being made in low- and middle-income countries. Individuals who have recently been infected with HIV are now unlikely to ever develop an opportunistic infection provided they are adherent to medication.

There is no evidence that means of acquisition, lifestyle issues such as smoking, nutrition, or stress-related illnesses, have any impact on the rate of progression towards AIDS. However, the life expectancy of individuals who continue intravenous drug use is reduced, though this is often due to non-HIV-related causes.

Markers of HIV infection and their clinical relevance

The CD4 count and HIV viral load have an independent prognostic value for the rate of progression to AIDS, and are commonly used to chart the progress of individuals with HIV infection. The CD4 count was previously important for determining the timing of treatment. Opportunistic infections are relatively rare with a CD4 count above 200 cells/mm³ and early guidelines restricted ART until this threshold was reached. Current British HIV Association (BHIVA) guidelines suggest that people should start ART as soon as they are diagnosed with HIV infection, regardless of the CD4 count (see 'Useful websites'). The main aim of ART is to stop viral replication as completely as possible and thus prevent further damage to the immune system. Therefore, the most important monitor of success of ART is regular measurement of the plasma viral load, with the aim to maintain it below the detection limit of a highly sensitive assay (usually <20 copies/mL).

Patients' symptoms and signs are also of considerable importance, both as markers of progression of known HIV infection and of alerting the physician or patient to an underlying HIV diagnosis, but late diagnosis of HIV remains a problem. Up to 50% of individuals who are eventually diagnosed as HIV positive have previously come into contact with the medical profession with conditions that should have led to an earlier diagnosis. An audit by the BHIVA suggested that this group of patients most commonly consult doctors because of diarrhoea, weight loss, skin complaints, lymphadenopathy, or glandular fever-like illnesses. Mild blood dyscrasias, such as thrombocytopenia, are also common. These non-specific symptoms and signs, as well as the opportunistic infections detailed in 'Symptoms of HIV', should alert the clinician to the possibility of HIV, particularly if they occur in high-risk individuals.

Symptoms of HIV

Symptoms in HIV infection may be due to the disease process itself or from complications of drug treatment.[2]

Primary HIV infection

About 75% of those who become HIV infected develop an illness within 2–3 weeks. This illness is usually mild, non-specific, and rarely leads patients to seek medical advice. Other early features include rash, lymphadenopathy, abnormal liver function, neurological symptoms, and, very rarely, opportunistic infections. Patients with a symptomatic illness at the time of primary infection (formerly called a seroconversion illness) progress to AIDS more rapidly. Diagnosis of primary HIV infection is important, as the high viral load is associated with a high risk of transmission and counselling about safe sex and risk reduction is indicated. A recent large trial (SPARTAC) did not show a clear benefit of early versus deferred treatment for primary HIV infection.[3] Nevertheless, most centres would now initiate treatment early.

Latent period

Following primary HIV infection, most patients are relatively well for a period of some years. Perhaps the most common symptoms are infectious skin conditions including seborrhoeic dermatitis, bacterial skin infections, tinea pedis, and molluscum contagiosum. Herpes zoster infection is particularly important. While shingles is relatively common, multiple dermatome involvement should strongly suggest the possibility of HIV. Herpes simplex is also more common, severe, and frequently recurrent in HIV-infected individuals. One of the most common manifestations during this latent period is mucocutaneous candidiasis, which should prompt relevant questioning about risk factors for HIV and an offer of testing. Hairy oral leucoplakia is rare and strongly predictive of HIV infection. Unexplained weight loss, diarrhoea, and fever are also features of this latent period but symptoms are usually due to an opportunist infection or tumour rather than HIV itself.

Opportunistic infections

Many opportunistic infections are associated with HIV (Box 34.1), some of which may be acquired through work

Box 34.1 Common opportunistic infections associated with HIV infection

- *Pneumocystis jirovecii* pneumonia (PCP).
- *Toxoplasma* encephalitis.
- Cryptosporidiosis.
- Microsporidiosis.
- Tuberculosis.
- Disseminated MAC (*Mycobacterium avium* complex) infection.
- Bacterial respiratory infections.
- Bacterial enteric infections.
- Candidiasis.
- Cryptococcosis.
- Histoplasmosis.
- Coccidioidomycosis.
- *Cytomegalovirus* disease.
- Herpes simplex virus disease.
- Varicella zoster virus disease.
- HHV-8 infection (Kaposi sarcoma-associated herpesvirus).

Lung manifestations

The most common AIDS-defining diagnosis is *Pneumocystis jirovecii* (formerly *Pneumocystis carinii*) pneumonia (PCP), a fungal disease. Others include pneumococcal pneumonia (for which vaccination is recommended), *Haemophilus influenza*, and, rarely in the UK, histoplasmosis, cryptococcosis, and coccidioidomycosis.

Tuberculosis
The major pandemic of tuberculosis (TB) is intimately related to the HIV epidemic and, in the UK, TB is an increasingly common presentation of HIV infection. More than 50% of people with TB in the developing world are co-infected with HIV. HIV-infected patients are more likely to acquire TB and develop progressive disease than the general population, including those with a 'normal' CD4 count.

Gastrointestinal manifestations

Oesophageal candidiasis is a common AIDS-defining illness. Although this is easily treated with azole antifungals, it is an important marker of severe immune compromise. *Cytomegalovirus* (CMV) infection also causes an oesophagitis. Rarely, patients present with dysphagia and are found to have aphthoid ulcers in the oesophagus, which can be treated with thalidomide or intralesional steroids.

Although HIV itself affects the gut and may cause diarrhoea, a number of opportunistic infections cause diarrhoea in HIV-infected patients. The most common are cryptosporidiosis, microsporidiosis, and CMV infection. In the short term, both lower and upper gut infections with CMV are treatable using antiviral agents, such as ganciclovir or cidofovir. Prevention of recurrent infection is crucially dependent upon the ability to control HIV viral replication using ART.

Neurological presentations

A lymphocytic meningitis can occur at the time of primary infection. It is often misdiagnosed as a simple viral meningitis of no significance. However, the most important cause of meningitis is that caused by *Cryptococcus neoformans*. Complications include cranial nerve palsies and raised intracranial pressure from communicating hydrocephalus, which can lead to blindness. Other neurological conditions usually present with stroke-like syndromes with a sudden onset of focal neurological defects or, less commonly, a general decline in cognitive function. *Toxoplasma gondii* is the most common of these infections and is associated with cerebral and cerebellar abscesses. A quarter of patients, however, have residual neurological defects, caused by irreversible neuronal damage before the initiation of treatment.

Progressive multifocal leucoencephalopathy is caused by an opportunistic infection with the JC variant of the polyoma virus, which is extremely rare outside the context of HIV infection. The diagnosis is usually made by magnetic resonance imaging. There is no specific treatment for this condition but with the advent of ART at least half of the cases make a good or partial recovery.

Primary cerebral lymphoma is also more common in HIV-infected patients and has a poor prognosis with an average survival of only 100 days. Epstein–Barr virus can be detected in the cerebrospinal fluid by polymerase chain reaction.

Eye manifestations

An important AIDS-defining diagnosis that leads to loss of vision is CMV retinitis. This is rare with a CD4 count of greater than 100 cells/mm^3 and is treatable, but the only way to control this disease in the long term is to provide effective ART. Another rare condition that leads to rapid blindness is progressive outer retinal necrosis, thought to be caused by a herpes virus infection. Toxoplasmosis of the eye is also more common in HIV-infected individuals.

Tumours

A variety of tumours are more common in HIV-infected individuals, including Hodgkin's disease, T-cell lymphomas, carcinoma of the lung, cervical cancer, and testicular tumours. The hallmark tumour of the AIDS epidemic is Kaposi's sarcoma (KS), caused by human herpesvirus-8 (HHV8), commonly known as KS-associated herpes virus (KSHV). In those who have never been treated for HIV who develop KS, the first step is the introduction of ART, which usually stops KS progression. Chemotherapy is usually reserved for those with progressive disease despite the introduction of ART and those with KS affecting the lung or gut. Non-Hodgkin's lymphoma is a common manifestation of HIV infection and is strongly related to the patient's lowest CD4 count. Two rare forms of lymphoma (primary effusion lymphoma and plasmacytoid multicentric Castleman disease) are both thought to be associated with HHV-8. The prognosis for the treatment of lymphoma has improved markedly with the introduction of ART. Anal cancer, which is particularly common in HIV-infected men who have sex with men, and cervical cancer in women indicate AIDS. Both are treated along standard lines. It is recommended that women with HIV have annual cervical smears regardless of age. It is hoped that the introduction of human papilloma virus vaccination will reduce the burden of these diseases in the future.

Psychiatric morbidity

HIV is associated with psychological problems. Depression is common, with the majority of studies reporting a prevalence between 15% and 40%. Depression may alter the course of HIV infection by impairing immune function or influencing behaviour, such as non-adherence to therapy. In addition, various studies have highlighted subtle cognitive changes in people living with HIV infection.

Treatment of HIV infection

The prognosis of HIV infection has been transformed by the use of ART (also known as highly active ART (HAART) or combination ART (cART). Currently six different classes of agents are available to inhibit viral replication. All six classes take advantage of the unique aspects of the viral replication cycle.

Commonly used drugs

See Table 34.1 for commonly used drugs.[4]

Current consensus guidelines relating to HIV treatment

There is now considerable agreement that treatment should begin for HIV-infected individuals as soon as they are diagnosed. This improves clinical and immunological outcomes and also limits onward transmission of the virus. Individuals on ART who have

Table 34.1 Commonly used drugs

Drug group	Action	
Nucleoside analogue reverse transcriptase inhibitors (NRTIs)	Inhibit reverse transcription, an essential step in HIV replication.	Early versions of these drugs were associated with a variety of adverse effects. Abacavir can cause a severe hypersensitivity reaction in people with the human leucocyte antigen B57-01 haplotype, so now all patients are tested and the drug avoided for those with this haplotype[4]
Non-nucleoside reverse transcriptase inhibitors (NNRTIs)	Inhibit reverse transcription as direct enzyme inhibitors	Several agents currently in widespread use. Efavirenz is commonly prescribed but can have central nervous system toxicity in some people, leading to sleep disturbance or psychological morbidity. It is the preferred agent when treating TB in the context of HIV infection. Nevirapine has been associated with serious side effects and is now rarely prescribed. Rilpivirine is becoming the NNRTI of choice, but only in those with an initial viral load <100,000 copies/mL
Proteinase inhibitors (PIs)		In widespread use. PIs, and the newer PIs (atazanavir and darunavir), have a much longer plasma half-life, allowing once-daily dosing, when boosted with ritonavir or cobicistat. There are significant drug interactions to consider with these agents because of cytochrome p450 effects
Integrase inhibitors	Inhibit insertion of cDNA into host cell genome by means of an integrase enzyme	Increasingly used because of good tolerability and efficacy. Raltegravir was the first to be licensed but dolutegravir and elvitegravir (the latter boosted with cobicistat) are the main drugs used currently
Chemokine receptor antagonists	Prevents attachment to a co-receptor in addition to the CD4 molecule	Maraviroc is the first licensed drug in this class and shows good activity but special assays are needed to test whether the patient's virus is susceptible
Fusion inhibitors	Prevents access to the cell by HIV	Enfuvirtide (T20) has proved to be a relatively effective antiretroviral agent but it needs to be administered twice daily by subcutaneous injection and so is mainly used in the so-called salvage therapy (see 'Salvage therapy'). It is associated with unpleasant injection-site inflammation

fully suppressed their viral loads are considered to be of very low infectiousness. Standard treatment is a combination of two nucleoside analogue reverse-transcriptase inhibitors (NRTIs) and either a non-nucleoside reverse-transcriptase inhibitor (NNRTI) or a proteinase inhibitor (usually boosted with ritonavir), although integrase inhibitors are increasingly used with two NRTIs. With such a wide array of drugs available, randomized controlled trials cannot be used to assess all potential combinations. Current UK treatment guidelines can be found on the BHIVA website.

Complications of ART

All of the drugs used in ART combinations have potential side effects and some longer-term problems are emerging with therapy (Table 34.2).[5]

Adherence issues

Adherence is the single most important factor in determining the ability of ART to suppress HIV replication and improve prognosis. A number of demographic factors, lifestyle issues, and belief systems have profound effects on adherence but are difficult to modify with behavioural intervention. Manipulating total pill burden, frequency of dosing, freedom from strict food requirements in relationship to dosing, short-term drug toxicities, and fears of long-term toxicities are all helpful approaches. Present standard regimens of first-line therapy can usually now be given once a day with a pill burden of one or two tablets a day. Careful treatment for gastrointestinal side effects is important in the initial stages of therapy. Careful explanation of the evanescent nature of the central nervous system toxicities associated with efavirenz helps adherence in the early stages.

Table 34.2 Antiretroviral treatment

Metabolic changes	◆ Increased cholesterol and triglyceride levels ◆ Insulin resistance, which can result in overt diabetes mellitus ◆ Changes in distribution of body fat with atrophy of subcutaneous fat and increase of visceral fat ◆ 'Buffalo hump' with a thick fat pad at the back of the neck ◆ Problems more common in advanced disease and may be associated with PI use
Cardiovascular risks	◆ Increased relative risk of vascular disease in patients on ART.[5] Due to lipid abnormalities but HIV itself may affect vascular endothelium ◆ The absolute risk of cardiovascular disease is not much greater than the general population but this may increase as the cohort of people with HIV ages ◆ Cardiovascular risk reduction has become part of patient management
Bone changes	◆ Bone mineral loss is accelerated, more so when on ART ◆ Increased risk of avascular necrosis of the femoral head ◆ Some evidence of an increased risk of fractures in HIV ◆ Use of tenofovir disoproxil (tenofovir DF) increases a reduction in bone mineral density compared to other drugs and should not be used in those with osteoporosis

Drug interactions

Other factors that influence the success of ART include pharmacokinetic variability and unexpected pharmacological interactions with other drugs. The list of potential inter- actions is very long and clinicians prescribing any drugs to patients known to be taking antiretrovirals are strongly advised to consult an expert (see 'Useful websites').

Second-line regimens

The choice of an optimum second-line regimen is usually straightforward and is aided by tests now available to detect drug resistance. Genotypic tests can guide the clinician, along with a sound knowledge of previous treatments.

'Salvage therapy'

This term refers to therapy where achieving complete virological suppression is unlikely. In this group of patients, the risk of death is closely related to the CD4 count and is low, providing this can be kept above 50 cells/mm³. For long-term survival, these patients will be dependent on the development of new drugs, which can be combined to completely inhibit viral replication. This is a highly specialized area of treatment.

Hepatitis B virus

HBV is a small DNA virus which has a major envelope protein, HBsAg, usually called the surface antigen. Contained within this envelope are the core antigen (HBcAg) and the 'e' antigen (HBeAg). These two antigens share about 90% of the same amino acids but are structurally quite distinct. Viral replication is complicated and if the virus is not cleared, viral DNA can persist within the hepatocyte nucleus and can act as a template for viral replication, even if not integrated into the host genome. This HBV DNA in the hepatocyte nucleus explains the persistence of the virus in chronic infection.

There are estimated to be about 300 million people infected with HBV worldwide, with prevalence rates of 10% in some parts of Africa and Asia. The prevalence of HBV infec- tion in the UK is estimated to be about 0.3%. Many of these infections might have been acquired via vertical transmission abroad whereas most transmissions in the UK result from sexual transmission. Infection can be classified either as acute or chronic, with most prevalent cases having chronic infection.

After infection, about a third of those infected will have symptoms of acute hepatitis, usually with fever and jaundice. This is sometimes associated with arthritis and urticarial rashes. Rarely, fulminant hepatitis follows and can lead to death. Many of those infected with HBV will clear the virus but up to 10% of incident cases develop chronic HBV infec- tion, whether or not they have an overt illness. Chronic infection is much more common with perinatal transmission.

Chronic HBV infection

Individuals with chronic infection have a risk of developing chronic liver disease be- cause of the inflammatory response to the virus within hepatocytes. Many remain asymptomatic but 20–40% go on to develop cirrhosis and sequelae such as ascites and oesophageal varices. Once cirrhosis develops, there is a risk of hepatocellular carcinoma so that regular ultrasound screening is required. These carcinomas can also, sometimes, develop in infected individuals without cirrhosis.

The risk of progression of HBV infection depends mainly on the immune response to the virus. Even though the majority clear the virus from the blood, viral DNA persists in the liver. This clearance correlates with the disappearance of HBsAg from the blood and the appearance of antibodies to the surface antigen (HBsAb) and antibodies to the core antigen (HBcAb). Persistent infection is diagnosed by the persistence of HBsAg in the blood. More active persistent infection leads to the detection of HBeAg in the blood in addition to HBsAg, possibly because of worse cell-mediated responses to the virus. Many of these patients have a mild to moderate chronic hepatitis with persistently raised transaminase levels, and some will have clinical symptoms such as fatigue.

Over time, some patients with chronic infection will clear HBsAg spontaneously, at a rate of around 1% per year. Occasionally, in those who are HBeAg positive carriers, flares of hepatic inflammation can result in clearance of the HBeAg and the development of antibodies to 'e' antigen (HBeAb). These patients will still be HBsAg positive and will have viral DNA integrated into the host DNA. There is a small group of patients with continued liver inflammation who are HBeAg negative but who have mutant virus (so-called pre-core mutants) that is unable to make HBeAg. These patients continue to have active liver inflammation and remain infectious (Table 34.3).

Treatment of HBV

Acute hepatitis B: most patients need supportive treatment only. For more severe disease, nucleoside/nucleotide antiviral agents are used, such as tenofovir or entecavir. These drugs are also used in the setting of fulminant liver failure due to acute HBV in order to prevent infection of a transplanted liver.

Chronic hepatitis B: the treatment options for chronic HBV infection vary depending on the individual and the nature of their infection and immune response.[6] Variables such

Table 34.3 Interpretation of HBV markers

	HBsAg	HBsAb	HBcAb	HBeAg	HBeAb	HBV DNA
Non-immune	–	–	–	–	–	–
Immune by vaccination	–	+	–	–	–	–
Immune by natural infection	–	+	+	–	–	–
Highly infectious	+	+/–	+	+	+/–	+ (any level)
Very low infectivity	+	+/–	+	–	+/–	<10^3 IU/mL
Infectious	+	+/–	+	–	+/–	>10^3 IU/mL

as the presence of cirrhosis, the plasma alanine transaminase (ALT) level, and the HBV DNA level need to be considered, as do other co-morbidities. Those that should be considered for treatment include:

♦ any patient, whether HBeAg positive or negative, with a HBV DNA level greater than 2000 IU/mL and ALT above the upper limit of normal and with evidence of liver inflammation or fibrosis

♦ any patient with a HBV DNA level greater than 20,000 IU/mL and ALT greater than twice the upper limit of normal, regardless of liver inflammation

♦ any patient with compensated or decompensated cirrhosis with any detectable HBV DNA, regardless of ALT level.

Patients over 30 years old who are HBeAg positive with very high HBV DNA levels but normal ALT levels can be considered for treatment, as can those with a family history of hepatocellular carcinoma or cirrhosis. Patients who are receiving immunosuppressive treatment for any reason should be offered HBV treatment, regardless of their HBV DNA or ALT levels, as they are at risk of HBV reactivation.

Interferon treatment

Some patients are treated with pegylated interferon-alpha, using weekly injections for 48 weeks. Such patients are generally younger, and may not want to be on lifelong treatment. Interferon therapy is only suitable for those with compensated liver disease without cirrhosis.

Nucleoside and nucleotide analogues

Lamivudine was the first of these drugs to be used but the emergence of resistance was common and it is rarely used today. The main antiviral agents in current use are entecavir and tenofovir, both of which are potent and have high barriers to resistance. These must be taken continuously and are effective regardless of the HBV DNA level or ALT level in those with HBeAg. These drugs are used as monotherapy. Adefovir is sometimes used in cases with lamivudine resistance but is less commonly used where tenofovir is available. Treatment is not usually recommended for those who are HBeAg negative unless there is clear evidence of hepatic inflammation. Up until recently, tenofovir disoproxil was the main form of tenofovir used, but a new formulation, tenofovir alafenamide, has less effect on bone mineralization and less renal toxicity and might be used increasingly in HBV infection.

Prevention of HBV

Good recombinant vaccines against HBV exist (containing HBsAg only) and provide excellent protection in most people. About 10% of individuals are non-responders. In 2017, the UK introduced routine HBV vaccination for infants. Up until then the vaccine was offered to HCWs and others at risk, such as intravenous drug users, men who have sex with men, and partners of those infected with HBV. The standard vaccine course consists of three doses given at 0, 3, and 6 months. An accelerated course of three doses given at 0, 1, and 2 months provides good initial protection but requires a boost at 1 year

Following immunization, measurement of HBsAb levels is done at 3–6 months post immunization and a good response is considered to be an antibody level of greater than 100 mIU/mL. However, levels between 10 and 100 mIU/mL are thought to protect against infection. Current recommendations are to boost once at 5 years in those who initially respond, without the need for further serological tests. Non-responders to the initial course should be re-immunized with a full three-dose course. Those who are immunosuppressed are less likely to respond to immunization but might make a response with twice the normal dose of vaccine.

Post-exposure immunization

Following exposure to blood or body fluids from an infected individual, those previously unimmunized can be offered post-exposure prophylaxis (PEP). This takes the form of two doses of HBV immunoglobulin given 1 month apart, the first dose given as soon as possible after the exposure. At the same time, an accelerated vaccine course should be started. Further guidance on immunization against hepatitis B and post-exposure management in partly immunized recipients is given in chapter 18 in *Immunisation against Infectious Disease* (known as the 'Green Book') by the Department of Health (see 'Useful websites').

Hepatitis C virus

HCV is a small RNA virus that has gained in importance over the past few decades. There are six genotypes, of which types 1–3 are the most common in the West. Transmission is parenteral, with most infections related to infected needles (especially in intravenous drug users) or to infected blood products. Sexual transmission does occur, particularly in men who have sex with men, and vertical transmission can occur. It is estimated that about 170 million people are infected worldwide, with the greatest prevalence in Egypt (up to 20%, mainly genotype 4). The UK prevalence is thought to be about 0.5%.

Diagnosis

Screening for HCV infection is done serologically to detect antibodies to HCV. The presence of antibodies to HCV can indicate current or past infection (that has been cleared). To ascertain whether an individual has chronic HCV infection, HCV RNA must be detected and there are now good assays for this. The presence of HCV RNA also indicates infectivity. If HCV RNA is detected, then the viral genotype should be determined, as this will dictate the approach to treatment.

Clinical symptoms

After infection, only about 20% spontaneously clear the virus with the rest going on to chronic infection that usually results in inflammation of the liver. Acute hepatitis with jaundice can occur, but is rare, and most infections are asymptomatic.

Chronic HCV infection

Most individuals with HCV infection develop a chronic hepatitis with modest elevation of transaminases. HCV infection is also associated with non-liver manifestations, the most common of which is cryoglobulinaemia. But most have mild symptoms, such as fatigue or arthralgia, which might not be recognized as being associated with the infection. Many go on to develop hepatic fibrosis and about 10–20% will progress to cirrhosis over 20 years or more. These patients are at risk of developing the complications of chronic liver disease, such as varices, ascites, and hepatic encephalopathy. Liver disease due to HCV has become a common indication for liver transplantation. Those with cirrhosis have about a 1% risk per year of developing hepatocellular carcinoma.

Treatment of HCV

Until fairly recently, the only treatment available for HCV was a combination of ribavirin and pegylated interferon. Treatment was needed for 24–48 weeks, was associated with considerable side effects, and produced quite low clearance rates. In the past decade, with better understanding of the virus, new direct-acting antiviral drugs have been introduced and have revolutionized the management of HCV infection.[7] There are now numerous direct-acting antiviral drugs on the market, with excellent clearance rates (usually >90%), particularly for genotypes 1 and 2. The drugs are relatively free of serious adverse effects and the treatment is usually only needed for 12 weeks at most. Data on clearance rates for other genotypes are accruing and some treatment protocols still use ribavirin and, occasionally, interferon. The main issue at present is the high cost of the new treatments. As with HIV and HBV treatments, there is a concern about the development of drug resistance so genotyping of HCV will be critical to monitor this.

Prevention

There are no licensed vaccines against HCV although some vaccines are in development. At present, the best means of prevention are the supply of clean needles, screening of blood products, and the promotion of safe sex practices. In addition, the roll-out of HCV treatment programmes using direct-acting antiviral drugs should reduce the pool of infected individuals and, hence, reduce the risk of onward transmission of the virus.

Impact of blood-borne viral infections on fitness for work

BBV infection may be asymptomatic and have no impact on functioning. There is no evidence of a risk of transmission of BBV infections through casual contact in the workplace. Apart from the restrictions for HCWs, there are no contraindications to work for those with asymptomatic BBV infections.

Symptoms which occur at the time of HIV infection, and in the early phases of infection with hepatitis B or C, can impair capacity for work temporarily. Long-term complications are likely to have more significant and enduring adverse effects on fitness for work. Side effects of treatment for BBV infections may also impact work. The diagnosis and treatment of BBV infections is a rapidly evolving field, with new highly effective treatments that may change the impact on capacity for work.

The impact of combination ART on HIV-related morbidity and mortality transformed what was once a terminal illness into a manageable, chronic condition. Health, quality of life, and life expectancy for people living with HIV are now greatly improved. Most people living with HIV in the UK are of working age. With effective treatment, HIV-infected individuals can lead productive lives.

In 2014, 75% of people living with HIV in the UK described their overall health as good or very good.[1] The employment rate of people aged 16–64 living with HIV in the UK was 64% compared to 73% in the general population in the same time period, despite higher educational attainment. In the same survey, despite self-reported good health, 60% were classified as overweight or obese.[1]

Employment is a key determinant of physical and mental health,[8,9] reducing health inequalities and improving life chances.[10] Obtaining and retaining employment can present major challenges for people with chronic illnesses, including BBV infection and particularly in the case of HIV. Although physical health is not a primary barrier to employment for people living with HIV, a study undertaken in 2008/2009 found that those who were not in work had significantly poorer psychological health.[10] Negative perceptions about work were more likely in those who were unemployed, who feared stigma at work, and/or feared encountering problems securing time off to attend appointments. However, most of those in work did not experience these problems. Patients diagnosed with HIV in the 1980s and early 1990s may have been told that they were terminally ill and would never be fit to work. The study has not been repeated and it is possible that the experience of those living with HIV is changing, although stigma and unhelpful beliefs persist and are likely to be slow to change. HIV services have a role in supporting patients to obtain and/or retain employment.

There is also stigma around HBV and HCV infection, although perhaps not to the same degree as HIV. However, stigma varies between populations, groups, and cultures. For example, HCV infection may be associated with more stigma than HIV infection in the gay community. Education for those affected by BBV infections, and raising awareness in others, are important support measures to improve the life chances and employment prospects for people living with any BBV infection. Occupational health (OH) professionals can contribute by challenging unhelpful beliefs and providing psychological support to address stigma, confidence, perceptions, and negative attitudes associated with unemployment.

Immune deficiency (occupational risks)

HBV and HCV infection do not affect immunity. HIV infection however, even when asymptomatic, suppresses immunity and renders individuals more susceptible to opportunistic infections, such as TB.

Although TB prevalence rates are higher in UK HCWs than in the general public, this is explained by many HCWs coming from countries with a high TB prevalence, rather than by any additional occupational risk.[11] TB is likely to be more common in prisons and in homeless populations. Therefore, HIV-infected prison officers and workers in homeless shelters are likely to be at increased risk of TB. Decisions about risks of exposure to infection should take into account the worker's specific duties, the local prevalence of TB and the degree to which workplace precautions to prevent TB transmission are likely to be effective. The estimate of risk will affect how and in what capacity the HIV-infected worker can be safely employed and the frequency with which they should be screened for TB. Regardless of potential occupational risk of exposure to TB-infected patients or material, HIV-infected workers should be alerted to the symptoms of TB, the need to avoid infected or potentially infected individuals and material, and to seek medical advice immediately if they develop any indicative symptoms.

HIV-infected child-care providers may be at increased risk for acquiring CMV infection, cryptosporidiosis, and other infections such as hepatitis A and giardiasis from children. The risk of infection can be reduced by optimal hygiene practices such as handwashing after faecal contact (e.g. during nappy changing) and after contact with urine or saliva. Workers in occupations involving contact with animals (e.g. veterinary work and employment in pet shops, farms, or abattoirs) could be at risk of cryptosporidiosis, toxoplasmosis, salmonellosis, campylobacteriosis, or *Bartonella* infection. However, a recommendation against HIV-infected persons working in such settings is unlikely to be justifiable. Optimal hygiene practices are important.

The US Centers for Disease Control and Prevention, National Institutes of Health, and HIV Medicine Association of the Infectious Diseases Society of America publish guidelines for the prevention and treatment of opportunistic infections in HIV-infected adults and adolescents (see 'Useful websites'). The guidelines are updated regularly and provide advice on various opportunistic pathogens.

In the UK, the employer owes a higher duty of care to any particularly vulnerable employee with a known, pre-existing medical condition—the 'eggshell skull principle' (see Chapter 2). This must be balanced against the wishes and rights of the HIV-infected employee to avoid unfair discrimination.

Occupational immunization and vaccination for HIV-infected workers

Most occupational vaccines are given to healthcare and laboratory workers and those travelling overseas. There are no contraindications to vaccination for those infected with HBV or HCV. However, special considerations are required for those living with HIV. In adults, the CD4 count indicates the level of immunosuppression and helps quantify the risk of infection and guides vaccination. Inactivated vaccines are safe to administer, but may be less effective—especially at lower CD4 counts, and even on ART. Certain live vaccines are contraindicated for people living with HIV, and some can only be administered if the patient's CD4 count is greater than 200 cells/mL (or a CD4 proportion of >15% in children). Up-to-date advice should always be obtained from the Department of Health's *Immunisation Against Infectious Disease* (see 'the Green Book' in 'Useful websites'). The BHIVA also publishes guidelines on the use of vaccines in HIV-infected adults (see 'Useful websites'). However, many of these vaccines still afford protection and for some vaccines it is possible to improve immunogenicity by offering modified vaccine schedules, with higher or more frequent doses, without compromising safety (see the BHIVA website in 'Useful websites'). Wherever possible, immunization or boosting of immunization of HIV-infected individuals should be either carried out before immunosuppression occurs or deferred until an improvement in immunity has been seen. The optimal timing for any vaccination should be based upon a judgement about the relative need for rapid protection and the likely response (see the 'Green Book' in 'Useful websites'). Advice on safety should be sought from the individual's HIV specialist.

Working overseas

Uncomplicated HBV and HCV infection should not affect travel, although associated disease may do so. There are a few particular considerations for the HIV-infected overseas worker. A day trip abroad to an urban office in a developed city should not normally require additional precautions. However, an overseas posting for months or years to a remote area of a developing country needs more thought and planning. Consideration needs to be given to:

◆ immigration requirements of the country being visited

◆ availability of antiretroviral drugs

◆ risk of exposure to opportunistic pathogens

◆ speed of access to and adequacy of healthcare facilities

◆ repatriation arrangements.

Travel to developing countries might result in substantial risks of exposure for HIV-infected people to opportunistic pathogens. Overseas travel for HIV-infected workers should involve liaison with their HIV specialist (see Travel Health Pro in 'Useful websites'). Interruption of HIV medication due to travel plans can be dangerous and should be avoided. ART medication has the potential for multiple drug–drug interactions. Before prescribing any additional medication, be sure to check for drug–drug interactions (see Liverpool HIV Pharmacology Group in 'Useful websites').

HIV-infected travellers are at a higher risk for food-borne and water-borne infections than they are in the UK. The usual hygiene precautions recommended for all travellers should be adhered to strictly by those with HIV (see Chapter 17). It may be appropriate for HIV-infected travellers to developing countries to carry a sufficient supply of an antimicrobial agent if they are travelling to particularly high-risk locations where medical assistance is poor or unavailable, to be taken empirically if diarrhoea occurs ('stand by'). One appropriate regimen is 500 mg of ciprofloxacin twice daily for 3–7 days. Immunizations should be given to HIV-infected travellers subject to the general points about immunization covered in the earlier paragraph on occupational immunization.

Few countries still ban tourist travel for people with HIV, but some have entry restrictions for people on longer stays, especially when residency and work permits are involved. Compulsory HIV testing may be used by some countries, with a positive test result leading to deportation (see National Aidsmap in 'Useful websites'). Entry requirements can change and should be checked with the country's embassy or consulate (see the Terence Higgins Trust in 'Useful websites'). Information about policies and requirements can be obtained from the consular officials of individual nations (see the CDC 'Yellow Book' in 'Useful websites').

Legal and ethical framework for assessing work fitness

Disability discrimination (the Equality Act 2010)

In the UK, the disability provisions of the Equality Act 2010 protect against HIV-related discrimination in the workplace (see 'Useful websites'). Asymptomatic HIV now falls within the definition of disability from the date of diagnosis. Hepatitis B and hepatitis C infections may also qualify as disabilities, if associated disease causes impairment that has 'a substantial and long-term adverse effect on ability to do normal day-to-day activities'.

The Equality Act 2010 prohibits both direct discrimination (i.e. due to the disability itself) and disability-related discrimination (i.e. less favourable treatment for reasons related to the disability). In *High Quality Lifestyles* v. *Watts* [2006], an employment appeal tribunal held that Watts' employer was liable for disability-related discrimination.[12] Watts had been dismissed from his job as a support worker in a residential home for people with learning difficulties and severely challenging behaviour, when he disclosed that he was HIV positive. The employer concluded from its risk assessment that if Watts was scratched or bitten by a resident, there was a risk that HIV infection could be transmitted to the resident. However, official guidance from the Department of Health[13] concluded that the risk of transmission of HIV to a patient who bites an HIV-infected HCW was negligible and, therefore, HCWs infected with BBVs should not be prevented from working in or training for specialties where there is a risk of being bitten.

Reasonable adjustments

The Equality Act 2010 requires employers to make 'reasonable adjustments' if their employment arrangements or premises place disabled people at a substantial disadvantage compared with non-disabled people (Box 34.2).

Pre-placement screening, BBV testing, and the Equality Act 2010

There are very few circumstances where an individual's BBV status is directly relevant to their employability. Section 60 of the Equality Act 2010 prohibits employers from asking questions about or screening for the health of applicants before offering work to an

---

Box 34.2 Reasonable adjustments for employees infected with HIV

- Accommodating more sickness absence than they would in someone without the illness.

- Allowing time off to attend treatment (which may include psychological treatment if psychological illness is a direct result of diagnosis).

- Arrangements for home working where symptoms affect ability to attend work.

- Arrangements for protection at work from infectious diseases to which they have increased susceptibility, such as TB.

---

applicant. Employers can ask questions for the purpose of supporting disabled applicants during recruitment such as the following:

- Determining whether any reasonable adjustments will be required to ensure that the applicant can participate in interviews and other forms of assessment.

- Establishing whether the applicant is able to undertake functions intrinsic to the work. This could be relevant to BBV-infected HCWs applying for posts requiring exposure-prone procedures. For those whose employment will take them to countries where HIV testing is a requirement of entry, it could be argued that pre-placement HIV testing, along with other tests required for travel, is necessary to assess fitness to work abroad.

- Monitoring diversity among applicants.

- Establishing the presence of a specific impairment required for the job.

- To take positive action under section 158, to ensure that a disabled applicant can benefit from measures to improve representation of disabled people in the workforce.

It is important for recruiting employers to make clear to applicants the reason questions are asked and the purposes for which the information will be used. There are ethical and other criticisms of pre-placement BBV screening. The test may be negative for some time after infection and employees may become infected after employment. OH professionals asked to arrange such tests must satisfy themselves that there is a justifiable reason for requesting a BBV test. Explicit, informed consent should be a prerequisite for BBV testing for OH purposes, with adequate pre- and post-test discussion. In healthcare, a balance between protecting patients and not discriminating against BBV-infected HCWs is not easy to achieve and may depend on a number of factors including evidence (or lack of evidence) of scientific risk of transmission, stigma, public opinion, the law, and politics.[14] Management of BBV-infected workers should be consistent with policies and procedures for people affected by other long-term medical conditions. OH professionals have an important advisory role. Occupational physicians, like other doctors, are bound by the General Medical Council's (GMC's) ethical code. Additionally, the Faculty of

Box 34.3 Protect patients and colleagues from any risks posed by your health

28. If you know or suspect that you have a serious condition that you could pass on to patients, or if your judgement or performance could be affected by a condition or its treatment, you must consult a suitably qualified colleague. You must follow their advice about any changes to your practice they consider necessary. You must not rely on your own assessment of the risk to patients.

29. You should be immunised against common serious communicable diseases (unless otherwise contraindicated).

Extract reproduced from GMC guidance, *Good Medical Practice* 2013, paragraphs 28 and 29, Copyright © General Medical Council.

Occupational Medicine of the Royal College of Physicians publishes its interpretation of the GMC generic guidance[15] (see 'Useful websites'). Other healthcare professionals must follow similar guidance produced by their relevant regulatory body.

Healthcare workers

The ethical position for BBV-infected doctors is addressed by the 2013 GMC guidance *Good Medical Practice* (Box 34.3) (see 'Useful websites').

Similar guidance is produced for nurses (Box 34.4), dentists (Box 34.5), and other health and care professionals (Box 34.6) by their registration bodies.

Confidentiality

HCWs have the same rights of confidentiality as anyone else. Patients can be reassured that the routine precautions taken in their care protect them from the tiny risk of BBV infection from their carers. Professional regulatory bodies are very clear about the circumstances under which it is legitimate to breach confidentiality.

Box 34.4 Guidance for nurses

19.3 keep to and promote recommended practice in relation to controlling and preventing infection, and

19.4 take all reasonable personal precautions necessary to avoid any potential health risks to colleagues, people receiving care and the public.

Extract reproduced from *The Code for Nurses and Midwives*, March 2015, Copyright © Nursing and Midwifery Council (see 'Useful websites').

Box 34.5 Guidance for dentists

1.7 If you believe that patients might be at risk because of your health, behaviour or professional performance, or that of a colleague, or because of any aspect of the clinical environment, you should take action. You can get advice from appropriate colleagues, a professional organisation or your defence organisation. If at any time you are not sure how to continue, contact us.

Extracts reproduced from *Standards for Dental Professionals*, paragraph 1.7, May 2005, Copyright © General Dental Council (see 'Useful websites').

Vocational support and rehabilitation

The UK government's Department for Work and Pensions provides benefits such as Employment and Support Allowance (ESA) for some disabled people, if their illness or disability affects their ability to work. People can apply for ESA if they are employed, self-employed, unemployed or a student on Disability Living Allowance or Personal Independence Payment (see 'Useful websites'). Disabled job applicants and employees can apply to the 'Access to Work' scheme for advice and support with extra costs that may arise because of disability needs (see 'Useful websites').

For the common disabilities experienced by workers with BBV infections, particularly HIV, the type of support required might include:

- voice-activated computer software (for HCV- and HIV-related peripheral neuropathy)
- installation of a home office (fatigue, diarrhoea)
- taxis to work (fatigue, diarrhoea, neuropathy)
- disability awareness training for colleagues
- the cost of moving equipment to a different workplace for a new job.

Funding under the Access to Work scheme is available when *additional* costs are incurred because of a disability, not to provide support usually provided by employers or required under legislation for all employees. In addition, it does not necessarily absolve the employer of its duties under the Equality Act 2010. The employer still has to make reasonable adjustments to reduce or remove any substantial disadvantage that a physical feature of

---

Box 34.6 Health and Care Professions Council guidance

Standard 6.3 of our standards of conduct, performance, and ethics says: 'You must make changes to how you practise, or stop practising, if your physical or mental health may affect your performance or judgement, or put others at risk for any other reason.'

Extract from *Guidance on Health and Character*, Health and Care Professions Council 2017 (see 'Useful websites').

the work premises or employment arrangements causes a disabled employee or job applicant compared with a non-disabled person.

Many charitable organizations provide specific advice and support for BBV-infected people. Some of these provide advice on employment issues (see 'Useful websites').

Transmission of blood-borne viral infection through work activities

Transmission from worker to client/patient

Apart from healthcare, sex work is the only other occupation with potential for transmission of infection from worker to service user. In contrast to HBV and HIV, HCV is not primarily transmitted through sexual activity, sexual transmission being relatively rare. Sex workers are largely unregulated and there are few data about transmission rates between sex workers and their clients. The healthcare industry is regulated in developed countries, particularly in the UK. Data on occupational exposure to and transmission of BBVs in healthcare are collected by national organizations such as Public Health England and the American Centers for Disease Control and Prevention. This makes it possible to investigate HCWs and patients in cases of potential BBV transmission.

Transmission of HBV from healthcare worker to patient

The high levels of virus during the acute phase of HBV infection, and in the HBeAg carrier state, mean that very small volumes of blood can transmit infection. The risk of transmission of HBV to a susceptible individual following a single hollow-bore needle-stick injury may be 30–62% from an infected source with detectable HBeAg, and 6–37% from a source with detectable HBsAg but no detectable HBeAg. Integrated guidance on health clearance of HCWs and the management of HCWs infected with BBVs is available from the Department of Health (see 'Useful websites'). Pre-core mutant HBV is associated with a high risk of transmission, with high viral loads in the absence of the e antigen.

Several cases of HBV infection were documented in patients who were operated on by HCWs with detectable HBV e antigen (HBeAg) in the 1980s and 1990s.[16,17] By the end of 2015, there had been nine episodes of documented transmission of HBV from infected surgeons to patients in the UK since 1991. There was also transmission of HBV from a doctor to two patients, which did not involve EPPs. Worldwide, since 1970 there were more than 40 clusters with over 400 patients acquiring hepatitis B from a HCW.[18–21]

Transmission of HCV from healthcare worker to patient

The first reported incident of HCV transmission from an infected HCW to a single patient in the UK was in 1994.[22] Following this, five further incidents were reported in the UK in which HCV-infected HCWs transmitted infection to 15 patients.[23] By the end of 2015, there had been 11 incidents of HCV-infected HCWs transmitting the virus to 28 patients in the UK. In nine cases, the HCWs were surgeons and eight involved the most invasive category 3 EPPs (see Box 34.8 for definitions of EPP categories). Three occurred in non-EPPs: repair of a paraumbilical hernia, one from a midwife to a mother in the postnatal ward, and another from an anaesthetist to a patient. The route of transmission in these cases has never been defined.[24,25] Six documented international cases involved transmission of HCV from surgeons to 23 patients.[26,27] In three further cases, anaesthetics staff transmitted HCV to nine patients, two of the HCWs having initially acquired HCV infection from patients.[28-30] In some reported cases, HCWs injected themselves with anaesthetic opioids before injecting patients, resulting in large numbers of HCV transmissions.[31]

Transmission of HIV from healthcare worker to patient

Four incidents of HIV transmission from HCW to patient have been reported worldwide:

+ A dentist in Florida, US (six patients infected—route of transmission unclear).[32]
+ An orthopaedic surgeon in France (one patient infected).[33]
+ A gynaecologist in Spain (one patient infected).[34]
+ A nurse in France (one patient infected—the route of transmission was unclear).[35]

In the first two cases, molecular analysis found closely related viral sequences in the HCWs and the patients. In 1995, the US Centers for Disease Control and Prevention summarized the results of all published and unpublished investigations.[36] Of over 22,000 patients treated by 51 HIV-infected HCWs, 113 HIV-infected patients were reported, but epidemiological and laboratory follow-up did not show any HCW to have been a source of HIV for any of the patients tested.[36] No cases have been reported in the UK, despite nearly 10,000 patients being tested for HIV in over 30 patient notification exercises between 1988 and 2008. However, not all patients treated by HIV-infected HCWs were tested either because they were not contactable or they declined testing. Many look-back exercises undertaken in the UK, the US, and elsewhere have failed to identify further cases.

Occupational restrictions for BBV-infected healthcare workers

In the UK and some other countries, restrictions are placed on BBV-infected HCWs. In October 2017, Public Health England published integrated guidance on health clearance for HCWs and the management of HCWs infected with BBV (hepatitis B, hepatitis C, and HIV) (see 'Useful websites'). This unifies guidance that was previously published in several separate documents at different historical dates. It documents the duties and obligations of HCWs and the roles and responsibilities of healthcare organizations. There is detailed guidance on health clearance for HCWs with regard to BBV screening and infection, including criteria for establishing the identity of the HCW (identified, validated sample (IVS); see Box 34.7), and the management of BBV-infected HCWs, including accidental exposures of patients to blood from BBV-infected HCWs, and the role of the UK Advisory Panel for Healthcare Workers Infected with Blood-borne Viruses (UKAP). It also outlines some general principles for BBV infection control. The rationale for the guidance and the restrictions is to prevent transmission of BBV infections from HCWs to patients through EPPs. EPPs are defined in Box 34.8.

Box 34.7 Criteria for identified, validated samples

(a) The HCW should show photographic proof of identity when the sample is taken.

(b) The blood sample should be taken in the OH department.

(c) Samples should be delivered to the laboratory in the usual way, not transported by the HCW.

(d) Laboratory results should be checked to ensure they correspond with a documented sample sent by the OH department at the relevant time.

Box 34.8 Exposure-prone procedures

EPPs include procedures where the worker's gloved hands may be in contact with sharp instruments, needle tips, or sharp tissues inside a patient's open body cavity, wound, or confined anatomical space where the hands or fingertips may not be completely visible at all times.

Exposure-prone procedures including exposure-prone environment

The definition of EPPs covers a wide range of procedures, in which there may be very different levels of risk of bleed-back. A risk-based categorization of clinical procedures has been developed, including procedures where there is a negligible risk of bleed-back (non-EPP) and three categories of EPPs with increasing risk of bleed-back (Table 34.4).

A categorization of the most common clinical procedures depending upon the relative risk of bleed-back has been developed by UKAP. Examples of UKAP's advice on which procedures are, and are not, exposure prone are available on the UKAP webpage (see 'Useful websites').

UKAP was originally set up under the aegis of the UK Health Departments' Expert Advisory Group on AIDS (EAGA) in 1991, and in 1993 its remit was extended to cover HCWs infected with all BBVs. UKAP advises physicians of HCWs infected with BBVs, occupational physicians, professional bodies, individual HCWs or their advocates, and directors of public health on patient notification exercises.

The integrated guidance introduces the concept of the exposure-prone environment as 'an environment in which there is a significant intrinsic risk of injury to the healthcare worker, with consequent co-existent risk of contamination of the open tissues of the patient with blood from the healthcare provider'. Examples include road traffic or domestic/recreational/industrial accidents where sharp surfaces such as glass fragments, sharp metal, or stone edges, may lead to injury of the HCW, while attending to and/or retrieving a casualty. The risk of iatrogenic BBV transmission in the pre-hospital emergency setting is unknown and not possible to quantify from scientific literature. But the theoretical risk requires proportionate and practical risk assessment and mitigation,

Table 34.4 Definitions and examples of category 1, 2, and 3 EPPs

Category	Definition	Examples
Category 1	Procedures where the hands and fingertips of the worker are usually visible and outside the body most of the time and the possibility of injury to the worker's gloved hands from sharp instruments and/or tissues is slight. This means that the risk of the HCW bleeding into a patient's open tissues should be remote	Local anaesthetic injection in dentistry, removal of haemorrhoids
Category 2	Procedures where the fingertips may not be visible at all times but injury to the worker's gloved hands from sharp instruments and/or tissues is unlikely. If injury occurs, it is likely to be noticed and acted upon quickly to avoid the HCW's blood contaminating a patient's open tissues	Routine tooth extraction, appendicectomy
Category 3	Procedures where the fingertips are out of sight for a significant part of the procedure, or during certain critical stages, and in which there is a distinct risk of injury to the worker's gloved hands from sharp instruments and/or tissues. In such circumstances, it is possible that exposure of the patient's open tissues to the HCW's blood may go unnoticed or would not be noticed immediately	Hysterectomy, caesarean section, open cardiac surgical procedures

considering the role of the emergency HCW, and the environment in which pre-hospital emergency care is given.

Management of accidental exposures of patients to BBVs

Patients may be accidentally exposed to blood from a BBV-infected HCW in circumstances which may or may not involve EPPs. HCWs should be advised of the action to take in the event of them experiencing an injury during a procedure. Usual protocols for occupational exposure incidents should be followed. This might involve treating the patient with accelerated immunization (HBV), immunoglobulin (HBV), or antivirals (HIV). The HCW should report the incident, and their BBV status, according to local policies. A detailed risk assessment should be performed. The risk of transmission of BBV infection is directly related to the concentration of virus in the blood of the source at the time of exposure.

Risk of acquiring blood-borne viral infection through work

Very few occupations and work activities have the potential for transmission of BBV to the worker. Sex work carries a risk of transmission of HIV and HBV, although there is evidence that in Western Europe the route of transmission is more likely to be through needle sharing (HBV, HCV, and HIV) in drug-addicted sex workers rather than directly through unprotected sex in the course of their work.[37] HCWs may be exposed to the blood and other body fluids of BBV-infected patients through percutaneous injury or blood splash to mucous membranes or non-intact skin. BBV infections can be transmitted in this way from patient to worker. Unlike sex workers, serosurveys of HCWs have not shown a higher prevalence of HIV infection. However, a systematic review and meta-analysis found a significantly higher prevalence of HCV infection in HCWs than in the general population, particularly in medical and laboratory staff.[38] The risk of HCWs acquiring HBV infection is significantly mitigated by the implementation of HBV vaccination since the 1980s.

The risk of a surgeon acquiring HCV has been estimated at 0.001–0.032% per annum. Even in populations with a high prevalence of HCV, the risk of acquiring HCV through occupational exposure is low. Neither vaccination nor prophylactic treatment for HCV is available. Large prospective studies have found that the risk of transmission of HIV from an infected patient to a HCW, after a single infected needle-stick injury, is about 0.3%.[39] Since 1984, five cases of occupationally acquired HIV infections in UK HCWs have been documented. In one case, the HCW seroconverted despite receiving PEP with triple therapy. Since 1999, no new cases of occupational transmission of HIV in HCWs following percutaneous exposure to HIV have been reported in the scientific literature. However, the lay press reported the death from AIDS in 2007 of a nurse who apparently acquired HIV infection following occupational exposure while working in London in 1999.[40] A further 14 HCWs with probable occupational acquisition have been diagnosed in the UK. They had no risk factor other than an occupational exposure but they did not have a baseline negative HIV test. Thirteen of these HCWs worked in countries of high HIV prevalence.[41]

Some of the cases in Table 34.5 were reported to voluntary national surveillance schemes. Others were case reports from a variety of other sources. The data probably underestimate the actual number of occupational infections, particularly in those developing countries with poor infection control practices and reporting systems, but a high population prevalence of HIV.

Despite awareness of the risk among UK HCWs, accidental exposure to body fluids continues to occur. Between 2004 and 2013, 6864 significant occupational exposures to BBV were reported to a national voluntary surveillance scheme (see the 'Eye of the Needle' report available on the Public Health England website, in 'Useful websites'). Employers should publicize procedures for reporting and managing blood exposure incidents in the workplace.

Table 34.5 Occupational transmission of HIV up to the end of December 2002

	US	UK	Rest of Europe	Rest of world	Total
Documented seroconversions (specific exposure incident)	57	5	30	14	106
Possible occupational infection (no life-style risks)	139	14	71	14	238

Source: data from Health Protection Agency. (2005) *Occupational Transmission of HIV—summary of published reports*. London, UK: Health Protection Agency. Copyright © 2005 Health Protection Agency.

Control of Substances Hazardous to Health Regulations 2002

BBVs are 'biological agent(s) which may cause infection' in the Control of Substances Hazardous to Health (COSHH) Regulations 2002 (see 'Useful websites'), and the hierarchy of control measures therefore applies. The COSHH principle 'Design and operate processes and activities to minimise emission, release and spread of substances hazardous to health' is of particular relevance. To control exposure to BBVs in the workplace, employers should:

- reduce invasive techniques
- use safe systems for clinical procedures
- ensure regular and effective training in safe systems of work
- consider safer needles and other safety-engineered devices
- ensure appropriate containment levels for laboratory work (e.g. safety cabinets, eliminate aerosols, and eliminate sharps).

Standard precautions

Prevention of BBV transmission relies on safe practice to avoid exposure to blood and body fluids. A 'standard precautions' approach means treating all body fluids as potentially infectious. Precautions to avoid percutaneous injuries and skin or mucous membrane exposures to blood should be taken with all patients and with all blood and tissue samples. Local guidelines should be implemented for safe practice in all situations with the potential for contact with blood or body fluids. Workers who may have contact with blood or body fluids should be trained in these practices and adherence to practice guidelines should be regularly reviewed. Protective equipment and clothing, such as gloves, gowns, and eye protection, should be provided and use encouraged, to reduce the risk of BBV transmission between patients and HCWs.

General infection control principles to reduce the risk of blood-borne viral transmission

The principles and practices of infection control are designed to protect HCWs and patients from infection caused by a broad range of pathogens including BBVs. Following these principles and practices will minimize the risk of exposure to blood products and transmission of associated pathogens. Guidance for clinical HCWs on minimizing the risk of exposure to blood products and associated BBVs is available from the Health and Safety Executive (HSE) (see 'Useful websites' and Box 34.9).

It is imperative that HCWs follow standard precautions and promptly report all exposures to blood or body fluid according to local policy.

In accordance with the Health and Safety at Work etc. Act 1974, Management of Health and Safety at Work Regulations 1999, and COSHH Regulations 2002, it is the employer's responsibility to identify the risks of exposure to HBV in the workplace and introduce measures to eliminate or reduce the risk. Employees should be provided with information

Box 34.9 General measures to minimize the risk of transmission of infection in healthcare

- Avoid contact with blood or body fluids.
- Take precautions to prevent puncture wounds, cuts, and abrasions in the presence of blood and body fluids.
- Avoid use of, or exposure to, sharps (needles, glass, metal, etc.) when possible.
- Discard sharps directly into a sharps container immediately after use, and at the point of use.
- Take particular care in handling and disposal if the use of sharps is unavoidable.
- 'One-use only' contaminated sharps must be discarded into an approved sharps container constructed to BS 7320; 1990/UM 3291 (safer and more practical than attempting to recycle contaminated items).
- Used containers must be disposed of through a waste management company who will dispose of them safely as 'waste for incineration only'.
- Protect all breaks in exposed skin with waterproof dressings and/or gloves. Chain mail and armoured gloves are available to protect the hands when working with sharp instruments or exposed to bone splinters, etc.
- Protect eyes and mouth with a visor or goggles/safety spectacles and a mask when splashing is a possibility (this will also protect against bone fragments in orthopaedic surgery and postmortem examination).
- Avoid contamination of the person or clothing with waterproof/water-resistant protective clothing, plastic apron, etc.
- Wear rubber boots or plastic disposable overshoes when the floor or ground is likely to be contaminated.
- Apply good, basic hygiene practices, including handwashing, before and after glove use, and avoid hand-to-mouth/eye contact.
- Disposable gloves should never be washed and reused, as they may deteriorate during use and in washing.
- If latex gloves are worn, powder-free, low-protein products should be chosen to help prevent latex allergy.
- Disposable gloves should be 'CE' marked for use with biological agents.
- Control surface contamination by blood and body fluids by containment and appropriate decontamination procedures.
- Dispose of contaminated waste safely and refer to relevant guidance.

about the risk of infection and how to prevent it. It is the employer's responsibility to ensure that the use of standard precautions is facilitated for handling body fluids and it is the responsibility of employees to adhere to organizational policies. The Health and Safety (Sharp Instruments in Healthcare) Regulations 2013 provide specific detail on steps that must be taken by healthcare employers to ensure that the risks from sharps injuries are adequately assessed and appropriate control measures are in place.

HBV immunization

In the hierarchy of control measures to manage risk, immunization is at a similar level to personal protective equipment. Other measures to eliminate or control risk should be considered first. However, where there is a risk of exposure to HBV, immunization should be offered. All new HCWs employed or starting training (including students) in a clinical care setting, either for the first time or returning to healthcare work, who will have direct contact with blood, body fluids, or patients' tissues, should be offered HBV immunization and have their response (HBsAb) checked, including investigation of non-response. Guidance on immunization against HBV is contained in the UK Health Department's *Immunisation against Infectious Disease* (see 'the Green Book' in 'Useful websites'). HCWs for whom HBV vaccination is contraindicated, who decline vaccination, or who are non-responders to vaccine (i.e. those with HBsAb levels <10 mIU/mL) should not perform EPPs unless shown to be non-infectious. Periodic re-testing may be needed. Declining vaccination (whether contraindicated or not), or non-response to vaccine, should not affect the employment or training of HCWs who do not perform EPPs. HBV immunization is recommended for the following groups who are considered at increased risk[1] (see 'the Green Book' in 'Useful websites'):

◆ HCWs including students and trainees who may have direct contact with blood, body fluids, or tissues or who are at risk of being injured or bitten by patients.

◆ Laboratory staff who handle material that may contain HBV.

◆ Staff of residential and other accommodation for those with learning difficulties.

◆ Staff in day-care settings and special schools for those with severe learning disabilities based on local risk assessment.

◆ Settings where there is a risk of significant and regular exposures (e.g. biting).

◆ Morticians and embalmers.

◆ Prison service staff with regular contact with prisoners.

◆ Emergency services such as the police and ambulance staff.

Managing occupational exposures to body fluids

Employers should have well-publicized systems for reporting and managing exposures to body fluids. The approach should be to assess the risk of transmission of BBV infection,

Box 34.10 Recommended PEP regimen

One Truvada® tablet (245 mg tenofovir disoproxil (as fumarate) and 200 mg emtricitabine (FTC)) once a day plus one raltegravir tablet (400 mg) twice a day.

including HBV, HCV, and HIV, on the basis of the mechanism of the exposure, the status of the source, and the vulnerability of the exposed worker.

Post-HIV exposure prophylaxis

There is evidence from a case-referent study that zidovudine reduces the rate of HIV seroconversion after exposure through needle-stick injury.[39] Since 1997, UK guidance, produced by EAGA, has recommended the use of combination antiretroviral drugs as PEP (see 'Useful websites'). The recommended regimen at the time of writing is shown in Box 34.10.

The latest guidance should always be checked for the most up-to-date recommended regimen. Other combinations may be appropriate in some circumstances, depending on viral drug resistance in the source patient or relative contraindications in the exposed individual. PEP should be given as soon as possible, preferably within an hour, and certainly within 48–72 hours of exposure. PEP should be given for 28 days, with follow-up HIV antibody testing done at least 12 weeks post exposure, or if PEP was taken, at least 12 weeks after PEP was stopped. All antiretroviral drugs have side effects, although many of these can be managed symptomatically. Common side effects include nausea, diarrhoea, dizziness, headache, asthenia, and rashes. Those prescribing PEP and/or providing advice should be aware of potential adverse effects and drug interactions, as these can have implications for patient safety and effectiveness of prophylaxis. Further expert advice should be sought where necessary. The Liverpool HIV Pharmacology Group produces interaction charts (see 'Useful websites'). Domperidone is contraindicated for use with boosted protease inhibitors (such as lopinavir/ritonavir) because of the risk of cardiac adverse events due to QT interval prolongation. There is no requirement for exposed HCWs to stop EPPs during the treatment or follow-up, as the risk of seroconversion is so small (0.3% and lessened by suitable PEP).[3] Guidance on PEP is available from the Department of Health (see 'Useful websites'). The latest EAGA guidance includes advice on HCWs seconded overseas and students on electives, managing exposures outside the hospital setting, reporting occupational HIV exposures, and PEP for patients after possible exposure to an HIV-infected HCW (see 'Useful websites').

Reporting of Injuries, Diseases and Dangerous Occurrences Regulations 2013

In the UK, accidental occupational exposure to BBVs is reportable to the HSE under the Reporting of Injuries, Diseases and Dangerous Occurrences Regulations 1995 (RIDDOR) as a dangerous occurrence (accidental release of biological agent likely to cause serious human illness) or injury (more than seven days off work). Reporting may be done by telephone, post, or online (see 'Useful websites').

Compensation for blood-borne viral infection contracted at work

Industrial injuries disablement benefit

BBV infections are not prescribed diseases under the Social Security Acts. However, HCWs who have acquired BBV infection because of accidental occupational exposure (e.g. needle-stick) may be able to claim.[13]

NHS injury benefits scheme

The NHS injury benefits scheme provides temporary or permanent injury benefits for NHS employees who lose remuneration because of an injury or disease attributable to their NHS employment. The scheme is also available to general medical and dental practitioners working in the NHS. Under the terms of the scheme, it must be established whether, on the balance of probabilities, the injury or disease was acquired during the course of NHS work.[13] Eligibility for injury benefit depends on reporting and accurate documentation of the management of the exposure incident.

Key points

- Despite significant advances in the treatment of HIV infection and dramatic increases in disease-free survival, employment rates for people living with HIV are lower than for the general population.
- OH professionals working in healthcare should have specialist knowledge of guidelines for the management of BBV-infected HCWs, and for the management of BBV exposures to HCWs.
- In nearly all other industries, BBV-infected individuals can be managed in the same way as any other worker with a chronic disease, taking account of immunosuppression in the case of HIV.
- The risks of transmission of BBV infection between HCWs and patients should be manageable through the hierarchy of control measures, including hepatitis B immunization.
- If the development of novel HIV drugs outstrips viral resistance, and the side effects of effective treatment reduce, the employment prospects for HIV-infected individuals, at least in developed countries, should continue to improve.

Useful websites

Access to Work	https://www.gov.uk/access-to-work
British HIV Association (BHIVA)	http://www.bhiva.org
BHIVA vaccination guidelines	http://www.bhiva.org/vaccination-guidelines.aspx

Centers for Disease Control and Prevention (CDC). 'Yellow Book', 2018), chapter 2: 'The pre-travel consultation. Self-treatable diseases: travelers' diarrhea'
https://wwwnc.cdc.gov/travel/yellowbook/2018/the-pre-travel-consultation/travelers-diarrhea

Control of Substances Hazardous to Health Regulations 2002
http://www.hse.gov.uk/coshh/

Department of Health Expert Advisory Group on AIDS: Providing expert scientific advice on HIV. 'Change to recommended regimen for post-exposure prophylaxis (PEP)', September 2014
https://www.gov.uk/government/uploads/system/uploads/attachment_data/file/351633/Change_to_recommended_regimen_for_PEP_starter_pack_final.pdf

Department of Health. 'HIV post-exposure prophylaxis: guidance from the UK chief medical officers' expert advisory group on AIDS', 2008
https://www.gov.uk/government/uploads/system/uploads/attachment_data/file/203139/HIV_post-exposure_prophylaxis.pdf

HIV Drug Interactions. Drug interactions in treatment of HIV
www.hiv-druginteractions.org

Employment and Support Allowance (ESA)
https://www.gov.uk/employment-support-allowance/eligibility

Equality Act 2010. Definition of disability
https://www.gov.uk/definition-of-disability-under-equality-act-2010

General Medical Council (GMC). 'Good Medical Practice', 2013
https://www.gmc-uk.org/guidance/good_medical_practice.asp

Health and Care Professions Council. 'Guidance on Health and Character', 2017
http://www.hcpc-uk.co.uk/assets/documents/10003A89Guidanceonhealthandcharacter.pdf

Health and Safety at Work etc. Act 1974
http://www.hse.gov.uk/legislation/hswa.htm

Health and Safety Executive. 'Safe Working Practices'
http://www.hse.gov.uk/biosafety/blood-borne-viruses/safe-working-practices.htm

Department of Health. 'Immunisation against infectious disease' (the 'Green Book'), 2006
https://www.gov.uk/government/collections/immunisation-against-infectious-disease-the-green-book

Department of Health. 'Integrated guidance on health clearance of healthcare workers and the management of healthcare workers infected with bloodborne viruses (hepatitis B, hepatitis C and HIV)', October 2017
https://www.gov.uk/government/uploads/system/uploads/attachment_data/file/655418/Integrated_guidance_for_management_of_BBV_in_HCW_v1.1_October_2017.pdf

National Travel Health Network and Centre (NaTHNaC). Travel Health Pro	https://travelhealthpro.org.uk
National Institute for Health and Care Excellence. Travellers' diarrhoea advice	https://cks.nice.org.uk/diarrhoea-prevention-and-advice-for-travellers
Panel on Opportunistic Infections in HIV-Infected Adults and Adolescents. 'Guidelines for the prevention and treatment of opportunistic infections in HIV-infected adults and adolescents: recommendations from the Centers for Disease Control and Prevention, the National Institutes of Health, and the HIV Medicine Association of the Infectious Diseases Society of America'	http://aidsinfo.nih.gov/contentfiles/lvguidelines/adult_oi.pdf
Public Health England. 'Eye of the Needle: United Kingdom Surveillance of Significant Occupational Exposures to Bloodborne Viruses in Healthcare Workers', December 2014	https://www.gov.uk/government/uploads/system/uploads/attachment_data/file/385300/EoN_2014_-_FINAL_CT_3_sig_occ.pdf
Reporting of Injuries, Diseases and Dangerous Occurrences Regulations 2013 (RIDDOR)	http://www.hse.gov.uk/riddor/
General Dental Council. 'Standards for dental professionals', paragraph 1.7, May 2005	https://www.gdc-uk.org/professionals/standards
Nursing and Midwifery Council. 'The code for nurses and midwives', March 2015	https://www.nmc.org.uk/standards/code/
The Faculty of Occupational Medicine. 'Good Occupational Medical Practice', December 2017	http://www.fom.ac.uk/gomp/gomp-2017
The Global Database on HIV-specific travel and residence restrictions	http://www.hivtravel.org/
The Liverpool HIV Pharmacology Group	http://www.hiv-druginteractions.org/
The Management of Health and Safety at Work Regulations 1999	http://www.legislation.gov.uk/uksi/1999/3242/contents/made
UKAP	https://www.gov.uk/government/groups/uk-advisory-panel-for-healthcare-workers-infected-with-bloodborne-viruses

Charities

British Liver Trust	https://www.britishlivertrust.org.uk
Hepatitis B Positive Trust	http://www.hepbpositive.org.uk
Hepatitis C Trust	http://www.hepctrust.org.uk
The Terrence Higgins Trust (HIV)	http://www.tht.org.uk
The National AIDS Trust	http://www.nat.org.uk
National Aidsmap	http://www.aidsmap.com

References

1. **Public Health England**. HIV in the UK: 2016 Report. PHE publications gateway number 2016463. 2016. https://www.gov.uk/government/uploads/system/uploads/attachment_data/file/602942/HIV_in_the_UK_report.pdf.
2. **Fidler S, Peto TEA, Goulder P, Conlon CP**. HIV/AIDS. In: Firth JDS, Cox TM, Conlon CP (eds), *Oxford Textbook of Medicine*, 6th edn. Oxford: Oxford University Press; in press.
3. **SPARTAC trial investigators, Fidler S, Porter K, et al.** Short-course antiretroviral therapy in primary HIV infection. *N Engl J Med* 2013;**368**:207–17.
4. **Ma JD, Lee KC, Kuo GM.** HLA-B5701 testing to predict abacavir hypersensitivity. *PLoS Curr* 2010;2:RRN 1203.
5. **Grinspoon S, Carr A.** Cardiovascular risk and body-fat abnormalities in HIV-infected individuals. *N Engl J Med* 2005;**352**:48–62.
6. **European Association for the Study of the Liver. EASL 2017 Clinical practice guidelines on the management of hepatitis B virus infection.** *J Hepatol* 2017;**67**:370–98.
7. **Liang TJ, Ghany MG.** Current and future therapies for hepatitis C virus infection. *N Engl J Med* 2013;**368**:1907–17.
8. **Waddell G, Burton AK.** *Is Work Good for Your Health and Well-Being?* London: The Stationery Office; 2006.
9. **Black C.** *Working for a Healthier Tomorrow*. London: The Stationery Office; 2008. Available at: http://www.dwp.gov.uk/docs/hwwb-working-for-a-healthier-tomorrow.pdf.
10. **Rodger A, Brecker, N, Bhagani S, et al.** Attitudes and barriers to employment in HIV positive patients. *Occup Med* 2010;**60**:423–9.
11. **Davidson JA, Lalor MK, Anderson LF, Tamne S, Abubakar I, Thomas HL.** TB in healthcare workers in the UK: a cohort analysis 2009–2013. *Thorax* 2016;**72**:7.
12. **Kloss D.** *Occupational Health Law*, 5th edn. Chichester: Wiley-Blackwell; 2010.
13. **Department of Health.** *HIV Infected Health Care Workers: Guidance on Management and Patient Notification*. London: UK Health Departments; 2005.
14. **Grime P.** Blood-borne virus screening in health care workers: is it worthwhile? *Occup Med* 2007;**57**:544–6.
15. **The Faculty of Occupational Medicine.** *Ethics Guidance for Occupational Health Practice*. London: Faculty of Occupational Medicine; 2012.
16. **Dyer C.** Surgeon pleads guilty to risking patients' health. *BMJ* 1994;**309**:292.
17. **Department of Health.** Protecting health care workers and patients from hepatitis B. Health Service Guidelines 93(40). 1993. Available at: http://webarchive.nationalarchives.gov.uk/20110504121556/http://www.dh.gov.uk/prod_consum_dh/groups/dh_digitalassets/@dh/@en/documents/digitalasset/dh_4088384.pdf.
18. **Smellie MK, Carman WF, Elder S, et al.** Hospital transmission of hepatitis B virus in the absence of exposure prone procedures. *Epidemiol Infect* 2006;**134**:259–63.

19. **Department of Health.** *Hepatitis B Infected Health Care Workers: Guidance on the Implementation of Health Service Circular 2000/020.* London: Department of Health; 2000.

20. **Gunson RN, Shouval D, Roggendorf M, et al.** Hepatitis B virus (HBV) and hepatitis C virus (HCV) infections in health care workers (HCWs): guidelines for prevention of transmission of HBV and HCV from HCW to patients. *J Clin Virol* 2003;**27**:213–30.

21. **Lewis JD, Enfield, Sifri CD.** Hepatitis B in healthcare workers: transmission events and guidance for management. *World J Hepatol* 2015;**7**:488–97.

22. **Duckworth GJ, Heptonstall J, Aitken C, et al.** Transmission of hepatitis C virus from a surgeon to a patient. *Commun Dis Public Health* 1999;**2**:188–92.

23. **Department of Health.** *Hepatitis C Infected Health Care Workers.* Health Service Circular 2002/010. London: Department of Health; 2002.

24. **Muir D, Chow Y, Tedder R, Smith D, Harrison J, Holmes A.** Transmission of hepatitis C from a midwife to a patient through non-exposure prone procedures. *J Med Virol* 2014;**86**:235–40.

25. **Mawdsley J, Teo CG, Kyi M, Anderson M.** Anesthetist to patient transmission of hepatitis C virus associated with non-exposure-prone procedures. *J Med Virol* 2005;**75**:399–401.

26. **Hatia RI, Dimitrova Z, Skums P, Teo EY, Teo CG.** Nosocomial hepatitis C virus transmission from tampering with injectable anesthetic opioids. *Hepatology* 2015;**62**:101–10.

27. **Cardell K, Widell A, Frydén A, et al.** Nosocomial hepatitis C in a thoracic surgery unit; retrospective findings generating a prospective study. *J Hosp Infect* 2008;**68**:322–8.

28. **Cody SH, Nainan OV, Garfein RS, et al.** Hepatitis C virus transmission from an anesthesiologist to a patient. *Arch Intern Med* 2002;**162**:345–50.

29. **Ross RS, Viazov S, Gross T, Hofmann F, Seipp H-M, Roggendorf M.** Transmission of hepatitis C virus from a patient to an anesthesiology assistant to five patients. *N Engl J Med* 2000;**343**:1851–4.

30. **Stark K, Hänel M, Berg T, Schreier E.** Nosocomial transmission of hepatitis C virus from an anesthesiologist to three patients--epidemiologic and molecular evidence. *Arch Virol* 2006;**151**:1025–30.

31. **Schaefer MK, Perz JF.** Outbreaks of infections associated with drug diversion by US health care personnel. *Mayo Clin Proc* 2014;**89**:878–87.

32. **Hillis DM, Huelsenbeck JP.** Support for dental HIV transmission. *Nature* 1994;**369**:24–5.

33. **Lot F, Séguier JC, Fégueux S, et al.** Probable transmission of HIV from an orthopedic surgeon to a patient in France. *Ann Intern Med* 1999;**130**:1–6.

34. **Mallolas J, Arnedo M, Pumarola T, et al.** Transmission of HIV-1 from an obstetrician to a patient during a caesarean section. *AIDS* 2006;**20**:285–99.

35. **Goujon C, Scheider V, Grofti J, et al.** Phylogenetic analyses indicate an atypical nurse-to-patient transmission of human immunodeficiency virus type 1. *J Virol* 2000;**74**:2525–32.

36. **Laurie M, Chamberland ME, Cleveland JL, et al.** Investigation of patients of health care workers infected with HIV: the Centers for Disease Control and Prevention database. *Ann Intern Med* 1995;**122**:653–7.

37. **Belza MJ.** Prevalence of HIV, HTLV-I and HTLV-II among female sex workers in Spain, 2000–2001. *Eur J Epidemiol* 2004;**19**:279–82.

38. **Westermann C, Peters C, Lisiak B, et al** The prevalence of hepatitis C among healthcare workers: a systematic review and meta-analysis *Occup Environ Med* 2015;**72**:880–8.

39. **Cardo DM, Culver DH, Ciesielski CA, et al.** A case-control study of HIV seroconversion in health care workers after percutaneous exposure. *N Engl J Med* 1997;**337**:1485–90.

40. **Nurse dies from accidental Aids jab.** *Metro* 2007, 12 Feb. Available at: http://www.metro.co.uk/news/98723-nurse-dies-from-accidental-aids-jab.

41. **Health Protection Agency.** *Occupational Transmission of HIV: Summary of Published Reports. March 2005 Edition: Data to December 2002.* London: Health Protection Agency; 2005.

Chapter 35

Haematological disorders

Julia Smedley and Richard S. Kaczmarski

Introduction

Few haematological disorders are caused or exacerbated by work. However, they may affect an employee's capacity to work. Mild haematological derangements (e.g. iron deficiency anaemia and anticoagulant treatment) are common, but have only minor implications for employment. Conversely, genetic and malignant haematological diseases, although comparatively uncommon, are complex and affect young people of working age. Malignant disease has a profound impact on work capability during the treatment and early recovery phases. However, advances in clinical management achieve a much greater potential for return to work during treatment, and a growing population of survivors in whom it is important to address employment issues.

The evidence base contains little research about fitness for work related to haematological disease, functional rehabilitation, or prevalence rates for specific disorders in the working population. The likelihood of an occupational physician encountering haematological disease in fitness for work assessments is therefore based on occurrence in the general population and this chapter relies primarily on traditional textbook teaching, and recent reviews of advances in clinical management.

It contains brief summaries of the more common haematological disorders that an occupational physician might encounter when advising about fitness for work. The major determinants of functional capacity are similar for many haematological conditions. In order to avoid repetition, the common treatments, complications, and symptoms are covered under 'Generic issues'.

Haemoglobinopathies

Sickle cell disease

Epidemiology and clinical features

Sickle cell disease (SCD) is a collection of inherited disorders characterized by the presence of abnormal haemoglobin (HbS).[1] Homozygous SCD (HbSS) is the most common, but the doubly heterozygote conditions with haemoglobin C and beta thalassaemia respectively (HbSC and HbSβthal) also cause sickling disease. The disorders are common in West Africa, the Middle East, and parts of the Indian subcontinent, and are established through migration in northern Europe and North America. An estimated 12,500 people in the UK have SCD. Occupational physicians working in London, the West Midlands, and Yorkshire might see a few cases annually. However, outside these areas the condition will be encountered rarely. Clinical features arise from the sickle-shaped deformation of red blood cells, due to crystallization of HbS at low oxygen concentrations. This causes chronic anaemia (haemoglobin 70–90 g/L) and episodes of vascular and microvascular obstruction. Patients develop acute 'crises' (vaso-occlusive/painful, aplastic, or haemo-lytic) and insidious multisystem damage from repeated infarction. Box 35.1 shows the wide range of end-organ effects.

Recent advances

Modern management of SCD has dramatically increased life and work expectancy[2] (from 14 years in the 1970s to 67 years in 2016). Consequently, more SCD patients are likely to be working than in previous decades. The introduction of sickle cell screening to the NHS newborn blood spot screening programme has allowed early diagnosis, introduc-tion of antibiotic prophylaxis, immunization, and health education. Newer treatments include hydroxyurea, which increases the production of fetal haemoglobin (inhibits HbS polymerization). Patients are monitored to detect end-organ damage and facilitate early intervention. Transfusion therapy may be indicated for continuing organ damage. Laser therapy reduces the complications of proliferative retinopathy. Joint replacement may be indicated for patients with severe joint disease. Allogeneic (from the bone marrow of a matched donor) stem cell transplantation (SCT) may be offered to the most severely af-fected individuals. In the UK, this is available only to children, but an adult programme is being commissioned. Although this offers a definitive cure, and transplant techniques are improving, there may be long-term consequences.

Box 35.1 Organs and systems affected by sickle cell disease

- Spleen (splenic infarcts leading to auto-splenectomy).
- Bones and joints (bone infarcts, avascular necrosis particularly of the hip and shoulders, osteomyelitis, and arthritis).
- Kidney (renal acidosis and glomerular sclerosis leading to renal failure).
- Brain and spinal cord (stroke and cognitive impairment).
- Eye (retinal infarcts and haemorrhages, retinal detachment, and central retinal ar-tery occlusion).
- Lungs (acute lung syndrome, interstitial fibrosis, and pulmonary hypertension).
- Skin (leg ulcers).
- Gall bladder (pigment gall stones).
- Blood (anaemia).

Functional limitations in sickle cell disease

Fitness for work varies markedly, and adjustments must be based on an individual functional assessment. Severely affected patients are unlikely to be fit for work, but moderately and mildly affected individuals should have reasonable work capacity. The main functional issues are listed in Box 35.2. Anaemia is usually well tolerated by SCD patients at low haemoglobin levels (down to 70 g/L) compared with other causes of anaemia. Poor work performance might be due to a number of factors, including cerebral infarctions or depression, which is common in patients with moderate to severe disease. Therefore, it is particularly important to make a careful assessment, liaising with the treating clinician to arrange cognitive screening, magnetic resonance imaging, and therapeutic review where appropriate. The effects of chronic transfusion are considered under 'Generic issues'. Despite the need for opiate analgesia in severe painful crises, the incidence of drug dependence is very low.

Adjustments to work

Workers must avoid environments with extremes of temperature and have access to drinking water to manage hydration. If mobility or exercise tolerance is seriously impaired, improved access to work (ramps or lifts) and reducing physically demanding work may be needed. Adjustments for visually impaired employees are covered in Chapter 30. Particular care should be taken to give prophylactic antibiotics and pneumococcal vaccine in jobs that expose the individual to infection. Travel requirements should be considered, including access to medical care and safe blood for transfusion in the event of sickle complications abroad. Air passenger travel is safe, but special care is needed to ensure adequate hydration on long-haul flights. During pregnancy, there is a higher incidence of gestational hypertension, pre-term birth, and small-for-gestational-age infants. A lower threshold for recommending abstention from work during pregnancy should be adopted, but close liaison with the responsible clinicians is strongly recommended.

Box 35.2 Work implications in sickle cell disease

- Impaired exercise tolerance (anaemia or pulmonary hypertension).
- Reduced mobility (bone/joint disease or stroke).
- Impaired visual acuity (retinopathy).
- Decreased performance (cognitive impairment due to cerebrovascular events, depression, or chronic pain).
- Susceptibility to infection (impaired white cell function, hyposplenism, or post bone marrow transplant).
- Infectious carriage of blood-borne viruses.
- Frequent absence from work (painful crises, complications of chronic organ failure), hospital visits

Some occupations are contraindicated for individuals with HbSS. Jobs that are physically demanding, or which expose the individual to severe extremes of heat, cold, dehydration, or hypoxia (e.g. foundry work, diving, compressed air work, and the armed forces) are unsuitable. UK Civil Aviation Authority standards on fitness for work would likely exclude individuals with SCD from certification as flight crew on civil aircraft and for air traffic control officers (ATCO).[3] A person with mild SCD with a history of no crises and with full functional capacity might be assessed fit for air crew and for ATCO duties.[3]

Pre-employment assessment

Pre-employment assessment raises important questions about the disclosure of a tendency for high rates of absence. The possibility of frequent absence should be based on clinical history and previous absence record. An individual with homozygous SCD is likely to fulfil the definition of disability under the Equality Act 2010, and the prospective employer should consider reasonable adjustments such as allowing a higher level of absence.

Sickle cell trait

Heterozygotes for sickle haemoglobin (HbAS) have no clinical anaemia. There are no employment consequences other than restriction of activities with a risk of severe hypoxia (diving, compressed air work, or work at altitude above 12,000 feet). Certification for civil air crew and ATCOs would be granted.[3]

Thalassaemia

Epidemiology and clinical features

The thalassaemias are a heterogeneous group of genetic disorders of haemoglobin synthesis. They are most common in the Mediterranean, the Middle East, India, and Southeast Asia, but occur sporadically in all populations. Thalassaemia is rare in the UK (800 cases). The common features are anaemia and splenomegaly. Individuals with homozygous beta thalassaemia (thalassaemia major) have severe transfusion-dependent anaemia. They can develop complications of iron overload (cardiomyopathy, liver failure, and endocrine failure including diabetes mellitus) by the teenage years. Even with careful management of iron overload with chelation therapy, life expectancy in thalassaemia major is 20–30 years. However, milder forms of the disease (thalassaemia intermedia) require transfusion less frequently. In heterozygous beta thalassaemia (β-thalassaemia trait), anaemia is asymptomatic (haemoglobin levels usually >90 g/L).

Recent advances

Genetic screening has reduced the incidence of thalassaemia in the UK, so fewer cases are encountered in the workplace. SCT offers a cure, but introduces other implications for work.

Functional limitations in thalassaemia

With good medical management, patients with thalassaemia major are able to function normally in education and employment with allowance for hospital attendance, but when complications arise there are likely to be severe limitations for work. Other variants of

Box 35.3 Work implications in thalassaemia

- Reduced capacity for physical work (impaired exercise tolerance due to anaemia, cardiac failure, small stature due to endocrine complications, hypothyroidism, osteoporosis bone pain, and fractures due to hypoparathyroidism).
- Increased susceptibility to infection (splenectomy, diabetes mellitus, and bone marrow transplantation).
- Infectious carriage of blood-borne viruses (secondary to transfusion).
- Requirement for iron chelation.

thalassaemia and interactions with other structural haemoglobin abnormalities (e.g. haemoglobin E/β thalassaemia) cause a range of clinical manifestations. Functional impairment is related to the degree of anaemia and haemoglobin levels are usually kept at 90–100 g/L in transfusion-dependent patients. A checklist of the limitations on fitness for work is shown in Box 35.3.

Adjustments to work in thalassaemia

The main aim is to match the physical job requirements to fatigue and impaired exercise tolerance. Care should be taken in jobs that might expose individuals to infection. Infection with blood-borne viruses secondary to treatment is important only where infection might be passed to others because of the nature of the work, for example, healthcare workers undertaking exposure-prone procedures (see Chapters 33 and 34). Adjustments for those on chelation therapy are covered in 'Repeated transfusion'. Thalassaemia major would disqualify patients from work as commercial air crew and ATCOs, but those with thalassaemia minor with full function would be considered on an individual basis.[3]

Immune cytopenias

Immune-related cytopenias, autoimmune haemolytic anaemia (AIHA), idiopathic thrombocytopenia (ITP), and more rarely autoimmune neutropenia can occur as primary haematological disorders, secondary to infections, drugs, or underlying malignancies, or in association with other autoimmune conditions (systemic lupus erythematosus, rheumatoid arthritis, etc.). These conditions occur at all ages and may be an isolated event or run a chronic or relapsing–remitting course. Mild cases are asymptomatic, often picked up during health screening.

AIHA presents with anaemia and jaundice. Chronic cases are prone to gallstones. Initial management is supportive, with blood transfusion and folic acid. Severe ITP presents with bruising and mucosal bleeding. Despite platelet counts less than 10×10^9/L, the risk of haemorrhagic death is very low. Treatment is rarely indicated with platelet count greater than 50×10^9/L.

Treatments for ITP and AIHA include steroids and intravenous immunoglobulin in acute conditions. The majority of patients respond to corticosteroids. Initial high doses are tapered over several months. However, the monoclonal antibody rituximab, other immune suppression, and splenectomy may be indicated in refractory, chronic, and frequently relapsing cases. A new class of thrombopoietic stimulating agents (thrombopoietin receptor agonists) are available for refractory ITP.

Coagulation disorders

Therapeutic anticoagulation

Treatment with anticoagulants and antiplatelet drugs is common. Approximately 1.25 million people in the UK take oral anticoagulants, most commonly warfarin. Functional impairment is more likely to relate to the underlying disorder than anticoagulant therapy. Increased bleeding tendency varies between individuals, but is proportional to the anticoagulant effect, measured by the international normalized ratio (INR) for warfarin. For most indications (venous thromboembolism, atrial fibrillation, cardiac mural thrombosis, cardiomyopathy, and prior to cardioversion) the target INR is 2.5, but for mechanical heart valve prostheses, antiphospholipid syndrome, and recurrent venous thromboembolism while on warfarin, the target INR may be up to 3.5. The majority of patients with bioprosthetic valves do not require lifelong anticoagulation. Advances in treatment include self-management of anticoagulants using near-patient devices (portable coagulometers) and the increased use of new direct oral anticoagulants (DOACs) such as apixaban and dabigatran. These drugs eliminate the need for monitoring and are currently licensed for thromboprophylaxis in hip and knee surgery, stroke prevention in non-valvular atrial fibrillation, treatment of acute venous thromboembolism (VTE), and secondary VTE prevention. The risk of bleeding while on oral anticoagulants increases significantly with an INR greater than 4.5; however, bleeding risk is low in well-controlled patients. Although standard laboratory tests do not reflect the anticoagulant effect of these agents, and none but dabigatran have a specific reversal agent in the event of bleeding, the superior safety profile over warfarin means that these drugs are becoming the anticoagulants of choice. Patients can work normally and adjustments are unnecessary unless anticoagulant control is erratic. Work that is *extremely* heavy physically or has an *extremely* high risk of cuts or trauma should be avoided. Warfarin treatment currently excludes firefighters from active duty and non-marine crew from working in offshore locations, due to the risk of injury and serious bleeds. Air traffic controllers and commercial pilots (class 1) have to demonstrate a period of stable anticoagulation before being deemed fit.[3] A shorter period of stability on DOACs (3 months) is required. If on anticoagulation that requires INR monitoring, class 1 pilots and ATCOs must monitor their INR using near-patient tests before and (for ATCOs) during a shift pattern.[3]

Antiplatelet therapy with aspirin has no important implications for work fitness.

Inherited clotting disorders: haemophilia and von Willebrand disease

Epidemiology and clinical features

Haemophilia A is the most common of the hereditary clotting factor deficiencies (prevalence 30–100 per million). This sex-linked disorder results in deficiency of factor (F)-VIII of the clotting cascade. FVIII levels below 1% (0.01 U/mL) are associated with severe bleeding tendency, but above 5% FVIII the clinical syndrome is mild. Symptoms include haemarthrosis, usually in the large weight-bearing joints (knees, ankles, and hips), muscle haematomas, less commonly haematuria, and rarely intracranial bleeds. Parenteral FVIII is indicated for prophylaxis and management of bleeding episodes. A FVIII level of 30% of normal activity is required for haemostasis, but spontaneous bleeding is usually prevented at levels over 20%. Long-term sequelae include the development of FVIII antibodies (inhibitors) in 10–15% of patients, and degenerative joint disease resulting from repeated haemarthrosis.

Haemophilia B (hereditary FIX deficiency) is clinically similar to haemophilia A, but is treated with FIX replacement. Von Willebrand disease differs from classical haemophilia in its autosomal inheritance. Bleeding tends to be mucocutaneous (epistaxis, gastrointestinal, cutaneous bruising) rather than into joints and muscle. Treatment is with desmopressin (DDAVP®) or concentrates of von Willebrand factor (blood glycoprotein involved in haemostasis) and FVIII.

Recent advances

Improvements in blood products safety, availability of recombinant clotting factors, and viral inactivation (see 'Multiple transfusion'), have removed the risk of HIV and hepatitis C. The uncertainty of new variant Creutzfeldt–Jakob disease with plasma products remains a concern. Consequently, young haemophiliacs currently entering employment are rarely infected with blood-borne viruses.

Functional limitations in haemophilia

Limitations (Box 35.4) relate mainly to the risk of acute joint bleeds and longer-term degenerative joint disease. The former precludes physically strenuous work, although the risk of bleeding can usually be controlled in all but the most severe cases by regular factor replacement.

Box 35.4 Work implications in haemophilia

- Impaired tolerance of extremely heavy physical work (risk of bleeding into muscles or weight-bearing joints).
- Impaired mobility (degenerative joint disease).
- Infectious carriage of blood-borne viruses.

Adjustments to work in haemophilia

Adjustments (Box 35.5) will depend on the severity of the bleeding disorder. Patients with mild haemophilia can work normally in any job. Even with severe FVIII deficiency (<1%) some patients have very infrequent bleeds, and few if any adjustments to work will be required. Work that is very heavy physically or associated with a high risk of injury (mining, heavy construction, armed forces, firefighting, and the police service) is contraindicated in those with frequent large joint bleeds. Healthcare workers who undertake exposure-prone procedures should be screened for blood-borne viruses. Special care is needed if an individual is required to travel for work, or to work in isolation. Arrangements for the safe storage of factor replacement, and access to sterile distilled water (diluent), needles, syringes, and other equipment for administration are needed. Some freeze-dried concentrates of FVIII and FIX can be stored at room temperature (up to 25°C or 77°F) for up to 6 months, but general advice is to keep all products in a refrigerator at 2–8°C (36–46°F). Documentation may be required by customs to carry medical equipment, and it is essential that appropriate insurance covers haemophilia-related complications. Work in very remote areas with poor hygiene arrangements or medical facilities, is contraindicated, except for very mild cases that are unlikely to require replacement therapy. Significantly affected haemophiliacs would be excluded from certification as commercial air crew and ATCOs, but very mildly affected cases might be considered on an individual basis provided there was no history of significant bleeding.[3]

Thrombophilia

The annual incidence of VTE is 1–3 per 1000. Deep vein thrombosis (DVT) and pulmonary embolism are most common, but other sites (upper limbs, liver, cerebral sinus, retina, and mesenteric veins) are affected infrequently. VTE causes significant mortality and morbidity: 3–4% of patients will die of pulmonary embolism and 20–50% of patients suffer late complications (chronic leg oedema, varicose veins, and venous ulceration). Risk factors include inherited and acquired medical conditions, and external factors (Table 35.1).

The pathogenesis and risk factors for VTE and arterial thrombosis are distinctly different. In VTE, age is the greatest risk factor, and stasis, immobilization, and prothrombotic

---

Box 35.5 Adjustments to work in haemophilia

- Provide facilities for self-treatment.
- Avoid extremely heavy physical work or work with a high risk of injury.
- Improved access to work, and sedentary work.
- Extreme care with foreign travel. Avoid remote areas with poor medical facilities.

Table 35.1 Risk factors for venous thromboembolic disease

Inherited	Acquired	External
Antithrombin deficiency (ATIII)	Age	Immobilization
Protein C (PC) deficiency	Previous venous thromboembolism	Surgery and trauma
Protein S (PS) deficiency		Oral contraceptives
Factor V Leiden (FVL)	Malignancy	Hormone replacement therapy
Prothrombin 20210A	Polycythaemia	Other drugs (e.g. Thalidomide, chemotherapies, anti-androgens)
Dysfibrinogenaemia	Essential thrombocytosis	
Elevated FVIII, FIX, FXI	Paroxysmal nocturnal haemoglobinuria (PNH)	
	Pregnancy	
	Antiphospholipid syndrome	

abnormalities are common. Atheroma, smoking, hypertension, or hypercholesterolaemia do not increase the risk of VTE.[4]

The majority of cases of VTE are managed initially with a DOAC or low-molecular-weight heparin followed by oral anticoagulation with a DOAC or warfarin. Low-molecular-weight heparin can be administered out of hospital without the need for blood monitoring. The duration of anticoagulation (3 months to lifelong) depends on a risk assessment of the event (provoked or unprovoked), severity (pulmonary embolism/proximal DVT vs distal DVT), and whether this was a first or recurrent event. VTE is associated with long-haul (>3000 miles) air travel. This risk is likely to be significantly increased in patients with a thrombophilic tendency. Guidance from the National Institute for Health and Care Excellence ('DVT prevention for travellers', 2013)[4] recommends a risk-based approach. All long-haul passengers should exercise during flight, walk around, maintain a good fluid intake, and limit alcohol consumption. Graduated compression stockings may also be worn. For 'high-risk' patients, a single prophylactic dose of low-molecular-weight heparin may be given.

There are significant issues for employment in thrombophilic patients. Patients who have suffered from DVT or pulmonary embolism may have reduced exercise capacity, mobility, and pain. Post-phlebitic limb and cardiac problems due to pulmonary hypertension may develop many years following the original event. Patients, and known carriers of risk factors, in sedentary jobs should be encouraged to mobilize frequently. Appropriate precautions should be taken during long-haul travel. Thrombophilias associated with a significant history of clotting would exclude certification as civil air crew. Because of the low incidence of a genetic predisposition to VTE and the variable penetrance of abnormalities, screening of frequent long-haul occupational travellers is not indicated.

Malignant haematological disorders

Epidemiology

Haematological malignancies, although individually rare, comprise 8–10% of all cancers in the UK (Table 35.2).

This heterogeneous group ranges from acute leukaemias, which may be rapidly fatal, to chronic conditions for which no intervention is required. They are characterized by impairment of bone marrow function and immunity. Although many are aggressive, some have the highest cure rates among all malignant disorders.

Clinical features and recent advances

Acute leukaemias

Acute lymphoblastic leukaemia (ALL) is the commonest malignancy in children. Cure rates are above 80%. Craniospinal radiotherapy is given only to poor-risk patients, and boys are treated for 3 years to prevent testicular relapse. SCT would only be considered for children with poor risk or relapsed disease. Children treated with standard chemotherapy regimens, who did not receive radiotherapy, are considered cured after 10 years. Thus the majority of long-term survivors of childhood ALL entering working life will not require continuing medical care. For those who received radiation, follow up would continue in view of late side effects. For ALL presenting in adulthood, the prognosis is markedly worse (5-year survival 15–40%). However, for adolescents and young adults, survival can be as high as 70%. Transplantation is therefore a first-line option for many patients. Because radiotherapy is integral to these regimens, adult survivors of ALL are more likely to have co-morbidities such as cognitive impairment, leucoencephalopathy, cataracts, and secondary tumours and will require long-term follow-up.

Table 35.2 Epidemiology of haematological malignancies

Disease	Number of cases/year (UK), 2014	Median age at onset (years)
Childhood acute lymphoblastic leukaemia	450	3–7
Adult acute lymphoblastic leukaemia	200	55
Childhood acute myeloblastic leukaemia	50	2
Adult acute myeloblastic leukaemia	3000	65
Non-Hodgkin lymphoma	13,000	65
Hodgkin disease	2100	30
Chronic lymphocytic leukaemia	3500	66
Chronic myeloid leukaemia	750	50
Myelodysplastic syndrome	4375	70
Myeloma	5500	65

Acute myeloid leukaemia (AML) is predominantly a disease of adults. A steady improvement in survival in patients up to age 60 has occurred over the last 25 years. Transplantation is reserved for intermediate/poor-risk patients (see 'Stem cell transplantation'). Overall 5-year survival is 40% (range 17–73%) in adults and 67% in children. Standard treatment involves four or five courses of intensive multidrug chemotherapy with prolonged hospitalization. Patients are unable to work during this period (6–8 months) and full recovery from the effects of treatment can take up to 1 year. When the disease is in remission, patients can return to work. Some have residual treatment-related problems, including incomplete recovery of blood counts with consequent anaemia, infection, or bleeding risk, and respiratory, cardiac, or renal dysfunction.

Chronic leukaemias

The incidence of *chronic lymphocytic leukaemia* (CLL) appears to be increasing, with involvement of younger patients. However, the increased availability of blood counts (e.g. health screening) has promoted earlier diagnosis and a 'pre-leukaemic' condition, monoclonal B-cell lymphocytosis, has now been recognized. CLL often runs a benign course, and no survival advantage is gained from earlier intervention. Indications for treatment include symptoms of sweating, fever, weight loss, anaemia, or thrombocytopenia, or a rapidly rising lymphocyte count. Patients with CLL require long-term follow-up. All are immunocompromised and require influenza and pneumococcal vaccines. Some patients, particularly those with underlying chronic pulmonary disease, may benefit from immunoglobulin therapy. CLL remains incurable with conventional treatment. Standard regimes combine fludarabine and cyclophosphamide with the monoclonal antibody rituximab. Recent developments of more powerful monoclonal antibodies and therapies targeting the B-cell receptors (BCR antagonists) are gaining increased use over chemotherapy and transplantation for patients with relapsed or poor-prognostic disease. Purine analogues and alemtuzumab produce profound immunosuppression through loss of T-cell-mediated immunity. Patients are susceptible to opportunistic infection including reactivation of cytomegalovirus and *Pneumocystis* (*carinii*) *jirovecii* pneumonia (PCP). Current guidelines recommend prophylaxis against *Pneumocystis jirovecii* for 1 year post treatment.

Chronic myeloid leukaemia (CML) occurs at all ages. Patients present with elevated white blood cell counts and splenomegaly. A new generation of drugs, tyrosine kinase inhibitors administered orally, are the treatment of choice in patients with chronic phase CML. Patients require outpatient monitoring during treatment but usually lead a normal life. With increased use over time, the long-term side effect profiles of these treatments have become apparent, particularly cardiovascular toxicities which require monitoring. Allogeneic transplantation which offers a cure is only undertaken in patients who are intolerant or unresponsive to treatment.

The *myelodysplastic syndromes* predominantly affect the elderly, but do occur in adults of working age, particularly where there has been prior exposure to chemo/radiotherapy. They are characterized by peripheral blood cytopenias and a risk of transformation to acute leukaemia. The only curative treatment is SCT (see 'Stem cell transplantation'). The hypomethylating agent 5-azacytidine is a low-dose chemotherapy option for patients with high-risk disease. However, supportive care (blood transfusion and antibiotics for inter-current infections) remains the treatment of choice for the majority. Transformation to acute leukaemia is treatable with intensive chemotherapy, but has a poor prognosis. The prognosis for myelodysplastic syndromes is very variable. The International Prognostic Scoring System (IPSS) places patients into 'very low', 'low', 'high', and 'very high' risk categories with median survivals of 8.8, 5.3, 1.6, and 0.8 years respectively. Low-risk pa-tients may remain well, continue in work, and require only occasional follow-up. However, those who are transfusion dependent require more frequent and prolonged hospital at-tendance and are unlikely to tolerate work. In older patients, co-morbidity, particularly chronic cardiac or respiratory disorders, may compound functional incapacity.

Myeloproliferative disorders: essential thrombocytosis and polycythaemia rubra vera

These conditions are characterized by increased production of one or more cell lines. It is important to rule out secondary causes of elevated platelet count or haemoglobin as this has a bearing on management. The main clinical consequences are related to the in-creased cardio- and cerebrovascular risks of elevated blood counts. Longer-term risks are related to marrow fibrosis, marrow failure, and risk of leukaemic transformation.

Management of essential thrombocytosis adopts a risk-stratified approach, based on age, platelet count, and cardiovascular risk factors. Patients may require antiplatelet drugs alone or in combination with cytoreductive therapy. Polycythaemia rubra vera can be managed with periodic venesection to maintain a haematocrit level at less than 45% or by cytoreductive therapy. The most commonly used drug is hydroxycarbamide. Patients require regular hospital attendance for monitoring, but most remain well and the condi-tions are unlikely to impact on work.

Lymphomas

Hodgkin disease predominantly affects young adults. Modern treatment achieves cure rates of 90%. Multidrug chemotherapy, radiotherapy, or combination protocols result in significant impairment of ability to work. Treatment lasts 6–8 months and transplantation is indicated for non-response or relapse. On recovery (6–12 months post treatment), the majority of patients would be expected to return to a full and active life.

Non-Hodgkin lymphomas (NHLs) comprise the largest group of haematological ma-lignancies and their incidence is increasing in Western societies. They are classified as aggressive (high grade, 30–40%) or indolent (low grade). Standard treatment com-prises combination chemo-immunotherapy (six to eight courses over 4–6 months). The addition of the monoclonal antibody rituximab has improved complete remission rates to 70–80%. Response varies according to a prognostic index that includes disease stage at presentation and performance status. Overall, the 5-year survival rates are 55–80%. Thus, more long-term survivors of high-grade NHLs now return to employment.

Low-grade NHLs often run an indolent course (median >10 years) and are incurable with standard treatment regimens. Increasingly patients are diagnosed on routine health screening and blood tests. Others present with lymphadenopathy, fevers, sweats, weight loss, bone marrow failure, or disease involvement of other organs (gut, lungs, or central nervous system). Many patients can be managed conservatively and will be able to continue with their daily lives. Treatment is only required if the patient becomes symptomatic. Progressive and symptomatic disease requires drug treatment and transplantation may be considered in selected patients. Many can be controlled with oral chemotherapy and monoclonal antibodies, which produce few side effects and allow normal daily activities and employment. Fitness to work depends on individual functional assessment.

Multiple myeloma

Although myeloma is predominantly a disease of the elderly, many working adults are affected. Effects include anaemia and immuneparesis, chronic renal failure, hypercalcaemia, hyperviscosity (due to high paraprotein levels), and gout. Lytic bone lesions can cause bone pain, pathological fractures, and vertebral involvement with cord compression and paralysis. Myeloma is incurable for the majority of patients. The principles of treatment are tumour reduction with multiagent chemotherapy, followed (in younger patients only) by high-dose chemotherapy and autologous SCT (see 'Stem cell transplantation'). Current treatments combine chemotherapy with immunomodulatory drugs: proteasome inhibitors (bortezomib) and immunomodulatory imide drugs (including thalidomide and lenalidomide). Skeletal disease is treated with radiotherapy or kyphoplasty, and bisphosphonates are effective in treating hypercalcaemia, bone pain, and preventing fractures. The availability of newer agents, novel immunomodulatory imide drugs, proteasome inhibitors, and particularly monoclonal antibodies, are improving outcomes for relapsed disease. Prognosis is age dependent and reflects performance status and comorbidities, with 5-year survival of 70% in patients less than 60 years and 50% in those aged 60–80 years.

The ability to work during or after treatment for myeloma may be severely affected. Anaemia and fatigue are common. Thalidomide treatment may contribute to somnolence, and is associated with a significant risk of venous thromboembolism and neuropathy. Heavy manual work may exacerbate skeletal symptoms and risk of fractures.

Adjustments to work in malignant haematological diseases

Patients are usually absent from work during the acute phase of treatment, which can last up to a year. Once disease is controlled or in remission, short-term adjustments may be needed for patients who have impaired marrow function. Long-term alterations are sometimes needed to manage the life-long susceptibility to infection. Possible adjustments for generic issues are summarized in the following sections.

Civil Aviation Authority standards on fitness for air crew and ATCOs recommend exclusion for acute leukaemia and for initial applicants with chronic leukaemia. Certification would be considered for individuals with treated lymphoma or acute leukaemia that was in full remission. Re-certification for an established air crew member would be considered for some chronic leukaemias provided haemoglobin and platelet levels are normal. If anthracycline has been included in chemotherapy regimens, cardiological review would be required for certification.

Generic issues

Immunity and infection risk

Lympho-haematological malignancies and their treatment have a profound effect on the immune system, with consequent increased infection risk. This is most severe in patients undergoing myelosuppressive chemotherapy, but for the majority, susceptibility to infection recovers after chemotherapy when blood counts normalize. However, some patients remain immunocompromised for many years, depending on the underlying condition, previous treatment (e.g. purine analogues and allo-SCT), or ongoing medication (e.g. immunosuppressants and steroids). The spectrum of acquired infections also varies; while bacterial infections are most common, patients remain vulnerable to opportunistic infections (PCP, fungal disease), *Cytomegalovirus* reactivation, and herpetic infections. Treatment-specific guidelines recommend antimicrobial prophylaxis, most commonly Septrin® (PCP prophylaxis), aciclovir, penicillin V, and antifungals. Patients with hypogammaglobulinaemia and recurrent infections may benefit from intravenous immunoglobulin. All patients should have an annual flu vaccine and, where appropriate, a post-transplant vaccination programme. Table 35.3 shows a typical schedule, but these vary and occupational physicians should liaise with a worker's transplant centre. In assessing a patient for return to work following treatment, consider recovery in blood counts (neutropenia and infection risk, platelet count, and bleeding risk) and ongoing medication.

Table 35.3 Typical vaccinations in patients with stem cell transplantation

Vaccine	Allo-SCT	Auto-SCT	Timing post-SCT
Tetanus toxoid	All	All	6–12 months
Diphtheria	All	All	6–12 months
Inactivated poliovirus	All	All	6–12 months
Pneumococcus	All	All	6–12 months
Haemophilus influenzae B	All	All	6–12 months
Influenza virus	All	All	Annually
Measles	Individual recommendation based on risk/benefit assessment		>24 months post allogeneic SCT

SCT, stem cell transplantation.

Stem cell transplantation

SCT carries significant risks of morbidity and mortality. The principles behind SCT differ between autologous and allogeneic procedures. Autologous SCT, where the patient is their own donor, allows intensification of chemo/radiotherapy to treat the underlying condition, thereby functioning as a 'rescue' and allowing reconstitution of marrow function. Standard allogeneic (family or volunteer donor) transplantation transplants the donor's immune system. The donor (graft) immune response to the recipient (host) accounts for the graft-versus-host disease, which is the major complication of allogeneic transplantation. However, the same immune response is also directed at the underlying disease (leukaemia) creating a graft-versus-leukaemia effect. The graft-versus-leukaemia effect plays a major role in the long-term cure achieved by allogeneic SCT.

Indications for stem cell transplantation and survival

The indications for SCT and numbers of procedures performed in the UK are shown in Table 35.4.

Many factors influence the outcome of SCT, including type of transplant, age, underlying disease, and stage at time of transplant. During the transplant and in the early post-transplant period, the patient would be unable to work. Recovery may take months

Table 35.4 Numbers and reasons for bone marrow transplantation in the UK, 2009

Conditions	Transplants performed	
	Allograft	Autograft
Acute leukaemias	579	3
Chronic leukaemias	CML 53 CLL 20	2
Myelodysplastic syndrome/myeloproliferative diseases	194	0
Plasma cell disease	43	1282
Bone marrow failure	75	0
Lymphomas	184	666
Haemoglobinopathy	40	1
Primary immunodeficiency	63	6
Inherited disorders of metabolism	17	0
Autoimmune disorders	5	19
Solid tumours	0	162
Others	18	1
Total	1530	2190

CLL, chronic lymphocytic leukaemia; CML, chronic myeloid leukaemia.

Source: data from British Society of Blood and Marrow Transplantation, 2015. Available at: http://www.bsbmt.org/.

or years and depends on the success in curing the underlying condition and any long-term side effects.

Fitness for work in stem cell donors

Haemopoietic stem cells can be derived from bone marrow or peripheral blood. Collecting stem cells involves either a bone marrow harvest or peripheral blood stem cell collection. Marrow (1000–1200 mL) is harvested under general anaesthesia from the posterior iliac crests. Donors usually recover fully from the procedure within 1–2 weeks, during which time they are advised to refrain from work. Occasionally, a bone marrow harvest can cause or exacerbate back problems. The principle of peripheral blood stem cell collection depends on giving a course of the haemopoietic growth factor, granulocyte colony-stimulating factor (G-CSF). Transient side effects include flu-like symptoms and bone pain due to the G-CSF injections, and hypocalcaemia during the apheresis process (Table 35.5).

Splenectomy and hyposplenism

The spleen is the largest lymphoid organ, containing 25% of the T-lymphocyte and 10–15% of the B-lymphocyte pool. It fulfils a major role in protecting against bacterial, viral, and parasitic infections.

The causes of splenic insufficiency are summarized in Table 35.6. Patients are at risk of overwhelming bacterial infections particularly involving encapsulated organisms, *Streptococcus pneumoniae* (pneumococcus), *Haemophilus influenzae*, and *Neisseria meningitidis*.

Guidelines recommend immunization for splenectomized or hyposplenic patients (Table 35.7). Those undergoing elective splenectomy should be vaccinated at least 2 weeks prior to surgery and receive lifelong antibiotic prophylaxis with penicillin (erythromycin if allergic to penicillin). Despite these measures, severe infections still occur, and patients should carry a 'Splenectomy Card' and a 'MedicAlert' bracelet. Infection should be treated with a broad-spectrum penicillin, and it may be advisable for patients to carry an emergency supply when travelling. During travel to malarial regions, patients should be advised of the increased risk of severe malaria and must adhere scrupulously to antimalarial prophylaxis.

There are no guidelines or data on which to base recommendations for employment. The adjustments in Box 35.6 are based on traditional textbook teaching about the increased risk of infection. Hyposplenic or splenectomized employees should be able to undertake almost any kind of work, except that with a risk of exposure to encapsulated pathogens, potentially infective biological material, and foreign travel. Individual susceptibility must be considered in addition to generic risk assessment.

Repeated transfusion

Repeated transfusion, used in the management of haemoglobinopathies, bleeding disorders, and haematological malignancies, can give rise to numerous problems

Table 35.5 Late effects of chemo/radiotherapy and stem cell transplantation for haematological disease

System	Complications	Treatment
Cardiovascular	Cardiomyopathy, pericarditis, arrhythmias, coronary artery disease, pulmonary hypertension	Avoid or limit radiation field
Respiratory	Pneumonitis, pulmonary fibrosis, infections, opportunistic infections secondary to immune suppression (*Pneumocystis* (*carinii*) *jirovecii* pneumonia, *Cytomegalovirus*, tuberculosis)	Lung shielding and fractionation of radiotherapy reduces lung damage. Antimicrobial prophylaxis and vaccination
Immunodeficiency	Bacterial, viral, and fungal infection. Reactivation of tuberculosis, shingles. Secondary malignancies and autoimmune disorders	The immunodeficiency post treatment is related to the disease process, treatment, or ongoing immunosuppressive therapy. Antimicrobial prophylaxis, vaccination, and intravenous immunoglobulin may be used
Endocrine, neurological, and ophthalmological complications	Hypothyroidism post radiotherapy. Learning difficulties in children treated with craniospinal radiotherapy. Leucoencephalopathy, cerebral atrophy. Drug-related neurotoxicity (e.g. peripheral neuropathy from vinca alkaloids, thalidomide). Cataract post steroids and radiotherapy	Monitor thyroid function and replacement as necessary
Secondary malignancies	The overall relative risk of developing cancer post SCT is 6.4 compared with the general population	Smoking cessation. Avoid or limit environmental and occupational exposure to carcinogens (e.g. sun) Health screening (e.g. cervical and breast screening programmes)
Chronic graft-versus-host disease	This is a multisystem complication of SCT causing immune suppression and infections, skin involvement (scleroderma-type picture), gut involvement (affecting nutrition, bowel and liver function). Marrow dysfunction and cytopenias	Prophylaxis and early treatment of infections. Immunosuppressive drugs (steroids and ciclosporin)

SCT, stem cell transplantation.

(Box 35.7), including iron overload and cardiac, endocrine, and liver damage. The treatment of choice for iron overload is parenteral chelation with desferrioxamine usually administered by subcutaneous infusion three to five times a week. Oral iron chelators (deferasirox and deferiprone) are available as second-line treatment.

Transmission of infection is much less of a problem since the introduction of rigorous measures to reduce infection in blood products. UK blood donors are routinely screened for syphilis, hepatitis B, C, and E, HIV-1, HIV-2, human T-cell lymphotropic virus type 1

Table 35.6 Indications for splenectomy and causes of splenic insufficiency

Indications for splenectomy	Causes of hyposplenism
Trauma	Congenital aplasia
Malignancy	Haematological disorders
Autoimmune conditions (immune thrombocytopenic purpura, auto-immune haemolytic anaemia)	Sickle cell disease
Diagnostic	Myelofibrosis
Hereditary haemolytic anaemias (e.g. hereditary spherocytosis pyruvate kinase deficiency)	Lymphomas
Hypersplenism	Autoimmune disorders
	Coeliac disease
	Inflammatory bowel disease
	Splenic infiltration
	Splenic irradiation
	Splenic embolization

Table 35.7 Recommended vaccination schedule for splenectomy patients

Vaccine	Schedule
Pneumococcus	Re-immunization recommended every 5 years or based on antibody levels
Haemophilus influenza B (HiB)	Included as part of routine childhood vaccinations since 1993
Meningococcal C	Now part of routine childhood vaccinations
Conjugate vaccine	Older and non-immune patients should receive a single dose
Influenza vaccine	Annual vaccination recommended

Box 35.6 Work implications for hyposplenic/splenectomized employees

- Ensure immunizations up to date, and on prophylactic antibiotics.
- Avoid exposure to bacterial pathogens.
- Care with travel, carry antibiotics, and fastidious compliance with antimalarial prophylaxis.
- Avoid working in remote areas with poor medical facilities.

Box 35.7 Complications of multiple treatments with blood products

- Iron overload:
  - Cardiomyopathy.
  - Liver failure.
  - Endocrine failure.
- Infection with blood-borne viruses:
  - Chronic hepatitis.
  - HIV infection.
  - Infectious carriage of blood=borne viruses (relevant for healthcare employees).

(HTLV-1), and HTLV-2. In addition, selective screening includes *Cytomegalovirus* (where patients are susceptible), malaria, and *Treponema cruzi*. Pooled plasma products such as clotting factor concentrates undergo viral inactivation, and some products are made using recombinant technology, removing the risk of infection completely. Four cases of transfusion-related transmission of new variant Creutzfeldt–Jakob disease have been recorded. Since 1999, all UK blood cellular products have had 99.9% of the white cells removed in order to reduce the risk of variant Creutzfeldt–Jakob disease, and since 2004 plasma for children born after 1996 (the year in which UK meat was deemed to be safe) has come from non-variant Creutzfeldt–Jakob disease endemic areas (North America).

Fitness for work resulting from infection with blood-borne viruses is covered in Chapters 33 and 34. Infectivity is only an issue where others in the workplace might be exposed to blood or body fluids from the infected employee (mainly in healthcare or dentistry). However, the risk of acquiring a transfusion-related infection is extremely low, and regular screening for infection for employment purposes is usually inappropriate.

Anaemia

The main symptoms of chronic anaemia relevant to fitness for work are fatigue, breathlessness, and impaired exercise tolerance. These symptoms vary according to age, level of fitness, and co-morbidity. In general, chronic anaemia is better tolerated than acute anaemia because of adaptive mechanisms. Measurable physiological changes do not occur until the haemoglobin concentration falls below 70 g/L. However, haemoglobin concentrations above 120 g/L are associated with less fatigue and a better quality of life. Advances in the treatment of chronic anaemia include the use of recombinant erythropoietin. Individuals who have anaemia but are treated and have a haemoglobin concentration of 120–170 g/L would probably be certificated fit as air crew or ATCOs subject to satisfactory medical assessment.[3]

Fatigue

Fatigue is commonly experienced by patients with haematological disorders, and is the most prevalent and functionally debilitating symptom of cancer and its treatment. It is related to multiple factors including disease activity, treatment, anaemia, and sleep disturbance, although the specific aetiology is poorly understood. Reduced energy levels are often disproportionate to physical effort. Moreover, fatigue has emotional, behavioural, and cognitive elements. Fatigue that is sufficiently severe to threaten employment has serious psychosocial consequences for the individual. It is important to ensure that employers are aware of the effect of fatigue on workability. The main difficulties with assessing the impact of fatigue on fitness for work are the subjective nature of the symptom and the variability between individuals. Several instruments have been developed to measure fatigue in clinical settings, either through self-report scales (e.g. the Piper Fatigue Scale and the Functional Assessment of Cancer Therapy Scale) or fatigue diaries. In theory these might be useful for repeated measurements prior to return to work and regular monitoring during a work rehabilitation programme. However, most of the available literature focuses on fatigue as a measure of treatment outcome rather than functional assessment for work, and these instruments have not been validated in the workplace setting.

Fatigue can last for months (or even more than a year) after treatment for malignancy. It is important to identify chronic fatigue symptoms, as adjustments to work may enable a productive return. Strategies for managing cancer-related fatigue include promotion of acceptance, positive thinking, and education about treatment and prognosis. Energy conservation strategies include increasing sleep time, pacing and restriction of activities, restoring attention and concentration (by pleasant diversionary activities), and physical exercise. The literature in this field comes from the treatment and early post-treatment phase of malignant diseases. Findings suggest that practical adjustments to allow pacing of work activities with rest and graded exercise are beneficial for the individual and allow an earlier return to work. There are no studies that specifically assess interventions for the workplace management of fatigue and the evidence for recommendations in Box 35.8 for rehabilitation back to work is indirect, based on intervention studies in cancer patients.

Bleeding

Many haematological disorders and their treatments affect bleeding tendency. In patients with thrombocytopenia, this typically manifests as spontaneous skin purpura, mucosal haemorrhage, and prolonged bleeding after trauma. Prophylactic platelet transfusion is indicated at counts below 10×10^9/L. Commercial pilots with a platelet count less than 75×10^9/L would be assessed as unfit. Therapeutic anticoagulation, if managed carefully, is unlikely to cause bleeding that is relevant for work. Adjustments to work in bleeding disorders are indicated by the risk of haemorrhage due to physical activities. There are no specific evidence-based guidelines, but clinical markers for an increased risk of bleeding are listed in Box 35.9.

> ## Box 35.8 Suggested adjustments to work for employees with chronic anaemia- or cancer-related fatigue
>
> - Flexible working arrangements.
> - Part-time work.
> - Late starts and early finishes.
> - Minimize night work or shift work.
> - Encourage frequent breaks and job variety to help maintain attention.
> - Support from manager and peers to encourage positive attitude and progression towards normality.
> - Reducing very heavy physical work.
> - Arrangements to allow working from home.

Psychosocial aspects

Haematological disease may have a considerable impact on psychosocial function. Many are life-threatening and chronic in nature. The high incidence of associated psychological morbidity must be taken into account in planning rehabilitation in the workplace. Depression is more prevalent among patients with haematological disease including cancers, haemoglobinopathies, and haemophilia. Surveys in cancer survivors have shown that 35% had symptoms of psychological distress. Even patients in long-standing remission have a high rate of psychiatric disorders (37%), including depression in 13%. It is important to be aware of psychosocial morbidity when returning to work, as treatment can usefully be facilitated. Support at home and at work improves the outcome of psychological problems.

> ## Box 35.9 Markers of significantly high risk of bleeding in haematological conditions (threshold for restriction from heavy physical work or work with risk of injury)
>
> - Haemophilia: FVIII activity below 5%.
> - Therapeutic anticoagulation: INR greater than 4.5.
> - Marrow suppression due to chemotherapy or radiotherapy; marrow failure due to leukaemia, myelodysplasia, or aplastic anaemia—platelet count less than 20×10^9/L.

Key points

- The prognosis for haematological conditions including malignancy has improved significantly in recent years.
- Generic work capacity issues are similar to those of other cancers, including fatigue, impaired immunity, and anaemia.
- Most people who survive haematological conditions will be able to work with minor adjustments.
- The main exclusions from work occur in specialized industries such as aviation, but even these allow work under specified conditions.

References

1. Hoffbrand AV, Higgs DR, Keeling DM, Mehta AB (eds). *Postgraduate Haematology*, 7th edn. Chichester: Wiley-Blackwell; 2016.
2. Piel FB, Steinberg MH, Rees DC. Sickle cell disease. *N Engl J Med* 2017;**376**:1561–73.
3. Civil Aviation Authority. Cabin Crew Medical Report. 2014. Available at: http://www.caa.co.uk/Aeromedical-Examiners/Medical-standards/Cabin-Crew/Cabin-Crew-Medical-Report/.
4. National Institute for Health and Care Excellence. DVT prevention for travellers. 2013. Available at: https://cks.nice.org.uk/dvt-prevention-for-travellers.

Chapter 36

Renal and urological disease

Christopher W. Ide and Edwina A. Brown

Introduction

The kidney has the vital function of excretion, and controls acid–base, fluid, and electrolyte balance. It also acts as an endocrine organ. Kidney disease, with impairment of these functions, results from a number of different processes, most of which are acquired, although some may be inherited. Glomerulonephritis, which presents with proteinuria, haematuria, or both, may be accompanied by hypertension and impaired renal function. Pyelonephritis with renal scarring is the end result of infective disorders. Diabetes and age-related changes are now the commonest cause of end-stage renal disease (ESRD) in the UK. Polycystic kidney disease is the commonest inherited disorder leading to renal failure. Chronic renal failure implies permanent renal damage, which is likely to be progressive and will eventually require renal replacement therapy (RRT).

Treatment of ESRD using haemodialysis (HD) and peritoneal dialysis (PD) can significantly improve physical and metabolic well-being and function but the proportion of those who continue to work with ESRD remains very low despite advances in treatment. Kidney transplantation enables many patients to return to normal lives including work. Reintegration of patients into the workforce following transplantation or dialysis offers an exciting and rewarding challenge to the wider health team.

Renal disease is not within the top ten of the costliest diseases for employers and accounts for less than 1% of sickness absence and incapacity claims. Urinary incontinence affects significant proportions of the workforce particularly women. Better management of urinary infections and calculi, prostatic obstruction, incontinence, and other complications of urinary tract disease has significantly reduced time lost from work.

Prevalence and morbidity

Chronic kidney disease (CKD) is relatively common but a minority who develop ESRD require RRT. Public Health England[1] has developed a model that estimates that there are 2.6 million people (6.1% of the population) greater than 16 years old with a glomerular filtration rate (GFR) less than 60 mL/min/1.73m^2 (Table 36.1).

Based on current CKD prevalence applied to the ageing population, the prevalence of CKD is expected to increase to 3.2 million people in 2021 and 4.2 million in 2036.[2]

Table 36.1 Proportion of adult population with GFR <60 mL/min/1.73m²

General population	6.1%
Women	7.4%
Men	4.7%
Age <65 years	1.9%
Age 65–74 years	13.5%
Age >74 years	33%

Thus, it is likely that the predicted ageing workforce will experience more symptoms attributable to CKD.

Planning for RRT starts when the estimated GFR (eGFR) is less than 20 mL/min/1.73 m². Dialysis is not usually commenced until eGFR is less than 10 mL/min/1.73 m². Increasingly, however, patients eligible for transplantation are being pre-emptively transplanted from live donors or placed on the deceased donor waiting list once eGFR has declined below 20 mL/min/1.73 m².

The 2015 UK Renal Registry report[2] shows that the 2014 annual acceptance rate for new patients starting on RRT is 115 per million population with a total of 7411 new patients. Acceptance ratios, standardized for age and sex of the population served, correlate significantly with both social deprivation and with ethnicity; the number of patients requiring RRT increases in areas with high numbers of ethnic minorities. The 2015 report also shows that the median age for prevalent HD, PD, and transplant patients is increasing with transplantation the most common treatment modality for RRT patients, see Table 36.2.

In terms of certified sickness and claims for benefit, diseases of the genitourinary tract (International Classification of Diseases, tenth revision (ICD-10, N00–N99) make up a small proportion of claimants nationally accounting for 1% or less of each.

Although many *urinary tract infections* are asymptomatic, there is much morbidity from this condition. Below the age of 50, the disease only affects women but after the age of 60 it becomes more frequent in males, due to lower urinary tract conditions, especially prostatic problems.

Table 36.2 Treatment modality and median age for RRT patients

	Treatment modality %	Median age		
		2014	2010	2000
HD	41	67	66	63
PD	6	64	61	58
Transplant	53	53	51	48
Number per million population on RRT		913	794	626

Urolithiasis of the upper urinary tract has a prevalence of 5% in the UK with a peak incidence in males at the age of 35 years.

Benign prostatic hyperplasia is common after the fourth decade; 50% of men have benign prostatic hyperplasia when they are 51–60 years old. At the age of 55, 25% notice some decrease in force of their urinary stream. At age 40 (surviving to 80) years there is a cumulative incidence of 29% for prostatectomy. In England and Wales, *prostate cancer* (ICD-10, C61) is the most frequently registered malignancy in males accounting for over a quarter of registrations (34,500) in 2009.[3] *Bladder cancer* (ICD-10, C67) is the fifth most common tumour in men (4% of male cancer deaths) and the eleventh in women (2% of female cancer deaths), but 90% occur over the age of 65.

Mortality

The majority of patients with renal disease will die from cardiovascular disease before they require RRT. An analysis of causes of death from 1996 to 2000 in over a million adults enrolled in the Kaiser Permamente managed healthcare programme of Northern California, US, showed that risk of death from any cause increased sharply as the estimated GFR declined, ranging from a 17% increase in risk with an estimated GFR of 45–59 mL/min/1.73 m^2 to a 343% increase with an estimated GFR less than 15 mL/min/1.73 m^2.[4] There was a similar increase in cardiovascular events and hospitalization. The age-adjusted mortality rate for an estimated GFR of 15–29 mL/min/1.73 m^2 was strikingly high at 11.4/100 person-years, which is similar to those on RRT. The vast majority (90%) of deaths from renal failure (ICD-10, N17–19)[3] occur over retirement age, although the associated morbidity is incurred during the working years. Survival rates for urological cancers are shown in Table 36.3.

Presentation

Kidney disease is easily missed. Early disease is often asymptomatic, presenting as abnormalities on routine urine testing, hypertension, or as biochemical abnormalities. GFR should then be estimated, as significant renal impairment can be present even when the plasma creatinine is normal. Asymptomatic haematuria (macroscopic or microscopic) unrelated to urinary tract infection requires investigation. Positive dipstick testing should always be repeated to distinguish transient from other causes of haematuria. The finding

Table 36.3 Five-year cancer survival rates for England and Wales

	Bladder	Kidney	Prostate
Males	57%	49%	77%
Females	47%	49%	–

Source: data from Cancer Research UK. Available at: http://www.cancerresearchuk.org/.

of two out of three positive (1+ or more) tests warrants further investigation for malignancy in appropriate age groups.[5]

Guidelines for identification of kidney disease

Clinical guidelines for the identification and management of chronic kidney disease were updated by the National Institute for Health and Care Excellence (NICE) in 2015.[6] NICE states that people should be offered testing for CKD if they have certain risk factors (Box 36.1).

The guidelines recommend that reagent strips are used (rather than urine microscopy) when testing for haematuria. To detect proteinuria, the urine albumin:creatinine ratio (ACR) should be used as it can detect low levels of proteinuria. The urine protein:creatinine ratio (PCR) can be used for higher levels of proteinuria and to monitor urine protein excretion. As a rough guide, an ACR of 30 mg/mmol is approximately equivalent to a PCR of 50 mg/mmol or urinary protein excretion of 0.5 g/24 hours.

The guidelines include the following criteria for specialist referral:

- eGFR less than 30 mL/min/1.73m².
- Heavy proteinuria (ACR ≥70 mg/mmol or PCR ≥100 mg/mmol) or lower levels (ACR ≥30 or PCR >50 mg/mmol) in the presence of haematuria.
- Sustained decrease in GFR of 15 mL/min/1.73m² or more within 12 months.
- Hypertension that remains poorly controlled despite the use of at least four antihypertensive agents.
- Known or suspected rare or genetic causes of CKD.
- Suspected renal artery stenosis.

Box 36.1 Risk factors warranting testing for CKD

- Diabetes.
- Hypertension.
- Acute kidney injury.
- Cardiovascular disease (ischaemic heart disease, chronic heart failure, peripheral vascular disease, or cerebral vascular disease).
- Structural renal tract disease, recurrent renal calculi, or prostatic hypertrophy.
- Multisystem diseases with potential kidney involvement—for example, systemic lupus erythematosus.
- Family history of end-stage kidney disease (GFR category G5) or hereditary kidney disease.
- Opportunistic detection of haematuria.

NICE recommends that all patients with visible haematuria (any age), symptomatic non-visible haematuria, and those aged 40 or older with asymptomatic non-visible haematuria (having excluded urinary infection and significant proteinuria) should be referred to urology for further investigation including ultrasonography and cystoscopy.

Diabetes

Diabetes is the commonest cause of ESRD accounting for 27% of patients starting dialysis in the UK in 2014[1] (and up to 40–50% in many countries in the developed world). The natural history is the development of microalbuminuria, progressing to overt proteinuria with hypertension, and subsequent decline in renal function. In young patients with type 1 diabetes, this process does not commence until at least 10 years after the onset of diabetes. This is not true for type 2 diabetes where the onset of the disease is less clear cut; it is not uncommon for patients to have proteinuria or even significant renal disease at the time of diagnosis. The majority of patients with renal disease associated with type 1 or 2 diabetes will also have diabetic retinopathy with its associated problems.

Complications and sequelae of renal disease

Cardiovascular disease

Most patients with renal disease will eventually develop hypertension. This needs aggressive treatment as tight blood pressure control (<125/75 mmHg in patients with proteinuria) significantly slows the progression of renal damage. This usually requires multiple drugs, which may cause side effects. Frequent monitoring of blood pressure is important and patients are encouraged to self-monitor as this correlates better with 24-hour blood pressure measurements and avoids white coat hypertension. Patients with cardiovascular disease have a worse outcome if they have even mild renal disease.[7]

Renal failure

The early symptoms of renal failure are fatigue with poor exercise tolerance. These can develop when the GFR is as high as 30 mL/min/1.73m^2 and can be exacerbated by the presence of anaemia. Deteriorating renal function leads to poor appetite, weight loss, fluid retention with ankle oedema and dyspnoea on exercise, loss of libido, and nocturia due to polyuria from osmotic diuresis. Many symptoms improve when the anaemia is corrected with erythropoietin and iron supplements. Prior treatment with erythropoietin has been found to be a significant factor in maintaining employment once dialysis commences.[8] The start of dialysis should be determined by symptoms rather than blood tests or GFR measurements. Early treatment aims to preserve employment and function.

End-stage renal disease

The aims of RRT are not simply correction of blood abnormalities and maintenance of fluid balance. Patients can live on RRT for decades so the aims are for them to live as

Box 36.2 Treatment modalities for ESRD

- *Haemodialysis* (HD):
  - Centre (18%).
  - Satellite (21%).
  - Home (2%).
- *Peritoneal dialysis* (PD):
  - Continuous ambulatory PD (CAPD) (3%).
  - Automated PD (APD) (3%).
- *Transplantation* (53%):
  - Deceased donor.
  - Living donor (related or unrelated).

normal a life as possible. It is important that they adopt a mode of RRT that they tolerate and comply with, that provides physical well-being, and allows social and employment rehabilitation. There are now many options for the treatment of ESRD (Box 36.2).

Dialysis

Patients with ESRD can now expect a reasonable survival and quality of life on dialysis. The 2015 UK Renal Registry report shows that the 1-year survival rate for patients younger than 65 years old is 94%.[2] The 10-year survival is given in Table 36.4.[1]

Censoring at transplantation removes the fittest patients by only including those who remain on dialysis and do not get transplanted, hence the lower survival rates.

For patients who can use any modality, the choice of HD or PD will depend on individual patient preference, nephrologist bias, and local resources. Approximately 28% of patients younger than 65 years start PD in the UK. Dialysis affects all aspects of life including work, diet, family life, holidays, and travel. From the patient's perspective,

Table 36.4 Ten-year survival rate for age groups 35–44 and 45–54

Age group	With censoring at transplantation	Without censoring at transplantation
35–44	71%	45%
45–54	55%	31%

Reproduced from Public Health England. *Chronic kidney disease prevalence model.* PHE publications gateway number: 2014386. London, UK: PHE. © Crown Copyright 2014. Available at: https://www.gov.uk/government/uploads/system/uploads/attachment_data/file/612303/ChronickidneydiseaseCKDprevalencemodelbriefing.pdf.

quality of life is the principal reason for choosing between dialysis modalities. As shown in Box 36.3, the main differences between PD and HD arise because PD is a home-based treatment and HD (with few exceptions) is a hospital-based treatment.

A study of patients commencing dialysis in the Netherlands showed that of the 864 patients who chose their dialysis modality, 36% starting PD were employed as compared with 16% starting HD.[9] There is some evidence that APD with a cycling machine at night while asleep may allow patients more time for work and leisure activities.[10]

Box 36.3 Quality of life and modality of dialysis

Hospital haemodialysis

- Hospital-based treatment.
- Suitable for dependent patients.
- Provides social structure for frail elderly patients.
- Requires transport time.
- Interferes with work.
- Increased hospitalization for vascular access problems.
- Difficult to travel for holiday or work.

Home haemodialysis

- Home-based treatment.
- Patient independence.
- Flexibility of frequency and length of dialysis sessions.
- Option of nocturnal dialysis.
- Ideally, patient should have family member or carer present, though not all units insist on this.
- The patient must be able to dedicate a room for dialysis use—may be a problem in rented accommodation, and space is needed for storage of bulky supplies.

Peritoneal dialysis

- Home-based treatment.
- Patient independence.
- Fits in with work.
- Can be done by carer at home.
- Fewer visits to hospital.
- Easier to travel and go on holiday.

Work and dialysis

The well-being of dialysis patients depends on many factors, both physical and psychological. The physical symptoms depend on adequacy of dialysis and compliance with treatment. Depression is found in up to a third of those on dialysis; it is difficult to treat and there is no good evidence of benefit of antidepressants. Depression, anxiety, and denial of illness can contribute to poor compliance. Family and social support is important. As illustrated in the case history below, patients can experience a vicious cycle of work difficulties and depression.

Half of those commencing dialysis are under the age of 65 but studies show very high rates of unemployment (>70%).[11] In non-diabetic renal disease, choosing PD, employer support, and erythropoietin treatment all increase the likelihood of maintaining employment.

Many individuals do continue to work in various professions. They can be enabled to do so with the aid of the occupational health (OH) team, or if the employer facilitates flexibility in the working day. It is important for the dialysis team to adapt the treatment round the needs of the patient, by, for example, arranging HD in the evening if the patient works during the day, and being flexible over the times of clinic appointments. It is often easier to fit RRT round work if treatment is carried out at home. In a cross-sectional survey of Finnish patients on various forms of dialysis for ESRD, 19% and 31% of patients on HD and PD were in employment, but for those on home HD and APD, these proportions increased to 39% and 44% respectively.[12]

Box 36.4 lists some of the specific work problems patients encounter on dialysis.

For patients on HD, shift work and extended hours may present problems requiring greater adaptation. Some patients have learnt to dialyse while asleep using the built-in warning devices on the machine. Occupations that entail heavy lifting or manual work may be unsuitable.

Transplantation

Successful transplantation provides the best quality of life for patients with ESRD and prolongs life expectancy. The median wait for a cadaveric kidney in the UK has increased from 407 days in 1990–1992 to 1110 days in 2010–2011 (data from UK Transplant). The initial inpatient stay is usually 1–2 weeks and for the first 3–4 months frequent blood tests are needed. Over a third of transplants are now from living donors. Living donor transplantation can be timed to suit the patient—for example, during the school holidays for a teacher. Increasingly, live donor transplantation is done pre-emptively before starting dialysis, maximizing quality of life and survival.

Patients can lead a normal life after successful transplantation, but need to continue daily immunosuppressive therapy (many different agents are now available—prednisolone, azathioprine, ciclosporin, tacrolimus, sirolimus, and mycophenolate). Transplant patients are therefore at increased risk of infection. In the first few months, patients are advised to avoid people with respiratory infections and chicken pox. This is particularly important for teachers, and health or social care workers.

Box 36.4 Employment and dialysis

Haemodialysis

- Rigid timing—usually 4 hours three times a week plus transport to and from dialysis unit.
- HD units usually have two to three shifts a day with little flexibility of timing for patients on shift work.
- Difficult to arrange treatments at other units, particularly at short notice, making travel difficult.
- Intermittent treatment so dietary and fluid restrictions.
- Patients often feel exhausted for hours after dialysis and can be hypotensive. However, this is variable and some patients are well enough to drive following their dialysis sessions.
- Presence of arteriovenous fistula in arm—need to avoid heavy lifting with that arm.
- If the patient opts for home HD, some weeks dialysing at hospital are needed to accustom the patient to dialysis, and to train the patient to needle their own fistula and manage the machine.

Peritoneal dialysis

- Home-based treatment allowing flexibility around work routine.
- Travel relatively easy—patient can transport own fluid for short trips or fluid can be delivered to many parts of the world.
- Can be difficult to fit in four exchanges a day if on CAPD and working, but some patients can arrange a clean and private place at work to do an exchange.
- More freedom during the day if the patient is on APD—at most, one bag exchange is needed and this can be done at a time convenient for the patient.
- Continuous treatment, so no 'swings' in well-being of patient.
- Heavy lifting should be avoided because of the increased risk of abdominal hernias and fluid leaks.
- PD usually started 2 weeks after catheter insertion with a training period of 1 week.

Transplant patients have a slightly increased risk of developing malignancy. Skin malignancies are among the most common, so patients should be advised to make liberal use of sunscreen when working outside. Specific complications from immunosuppressants include hirsutism with ciclosporin or diabetes with tacrolimus. Many patients remain hypertensive post transplantation. Cardiovascular disease remains a major cause of morbidity and mortality but less so than in patients on dialysis.

Long-term follow-up studies in relation to work are encouraging. A study of 57 adult survivors from childhood transplantation showed a high level of employment (82%) and 95% reported their health as fair or good.[12] This was despite a high retransplantation rate and significant morbidity including hypertension, bone and joint symptoms, fractures, hypercholesterolaemia, and cataracts. A study of 267 Japanese transplant recipients found patient and graft survival rates of 80% and 51% at 10 years and 56% and 33% at 20 years, respectively.[13] The main causes of death in the long term were cancers and hepatic failure due to viral hepatitis. In 15 patients with grafts surviving beyond 20 years, 11 remained in full-time employment.

Renal failure and employment

In the US, differences have also been found in vocational rehabilitation in end-stage renal therapy patients.[14] Follow-up studies have found employment rates of 28% (Spain), 43% (US), and 45% (Canada) following transplantation, but prior employment tends to be the strongest independent predictor of employment after transplant.[15-17] A survey of the Swiss transplant cohort 12 months post transplantation showed that 81% who were working prior to being transplanted remained at work afterwards.[18]

Patient and physician expectations with regard to employment appear to be important in both dialysis and following transplantation, but can be modified.[16,19] The main problems surround those on dialysis. Loss of work is an important issue in both pre-dialysis and dialysis patients. A joint study from the Manchester and Oxford renal units found a sharp decline in the percentage of those working 6–12 months after the start of CAPD (44% from 73%), or of HD (42% from 83%).[20,21] Other studies have also shown high rates of leaving full-time employment after dialysis, with 50% retired within 2 years of starting HD in Croatia; employment rates of 42% before the initiation of dialysis, falling to 21% at initiation and below 7% a year later in the US; and declines in employment rate from 31% to 25% (HD patients) and 48% to 40% (PD patients) after 1 year of dialysis in the Netherlands.[22-24] Independent risk factors for job loss were impaired physical and psychosocial functioning.

A US study of 359 chronic dialysis patients (85 employed and 274 unemployed) found education to be a significant correlate of employment but neither mode of dialysis, length of time on dialysis, number of co-morbid conditions, nor cause of renal failure (e.g. diabetes) were associated with employment status.[25] Measures of functional status were positively associated with employment but patients' perceptions that their health limited the type and amount of work that they could do were negatively associated with employment. Twenty-one per cent of unemployed patients reported that they were both able to work and wanted to return to work. Other factors affecting employment in dialysis patients include selection of fitter patients for transplantation, availability of disability benefits and health insurance, education, and employer attitudes.[26-30] However, pre-dialysis intervention has been shown to be of benefit in assisting workers with ESRD.

Renal failure and fitness for work

With flexibility, adaptation, planning, and support, and a change of attitude on the part of employers, many more dialysis patients could work successfully. The aim should be to adapt the work to the patient's needs and the patient's treatment regimen to the work. Many employers, although sympathetic, misunderstand what can be achieved by patients with chronic renal failure, and this by itself may limit successful employment. There is a need to educate both doctors and employers about the work capabilities of those with ESRD and to encourage a positive attitude in the patients themselves. The close cooperation of all concerned, (the patient, the renal unit, the general practitioner, OH staff, and the employer), is often needed to effect a successful placement. The OH professional is usually best placed to catalyse the necessary adjustments.

The work situation should carry no undue risk of blows or trauma to the lower abdomen and likewise the arteriovenous fistula at the wrist should be protected from injury by sharp projections or tools. Successful transplant patients should be capable of virtually any normal work.

Restrictions and contraindications

The essential and relative employment contraindications for dialysis patients are shown in Table 36.5.

Patients in irreversible renal failure are ill-suited to work with high energy demands, extended hours, and a need to be on-call. Similar restrictions may apply to particularly stressful jobs demanding a high degree of vigilance (e.g. air traffic controllers). Jobs combining both a high radiant heat burden and high physical activity may also be contraindicated because of the risk of fluid depletion with ensuing hypotension and worsening renal function, particularly when using angiotensin-converting enzyme inhibitors or angiotensin receptor blockers for blood pressure control. Patients with ESRD on dialysis are unfit for underground working, for diving, or other work in hyperbaric conditions such as tunnelling under pressure. They are also unlikely to meet the fitness standards required for merchant shipping, which may require lengthy periods at sea in tropical and subtropical climates.[31] Additionally, most seafarers nowadays will need to join and leave ships by air travel.

Although air travel is not contraindicated for those undertaking CAPD regimens, it imposes extra difficulties and the added inconvenience of carrying supplies of the dialysate solution. Also, in the context of travel abroad, the reduced dosage required for drug prophylaxis against malaria for those in renal failure should be recognized.

It is essential for those on PD to avoid work in dirty or dusty environments, and work that requires heavy lifting or constant bending. Tight or restrictive clothing should not be worn. Patients also need a clean area to perform their midday fluid exchange, as it is vital to avoid infection. The suitability, both of the type of work and of an area at the workplace for the exchange, should be assessed on site by the renal unit specialist nurse, in conjunction with the OH staff and the employer. Patients on HD need to be within easy reach of

Table 36.5 Dialysis (HD and PD) and types of employment

Contraindications (unsuitable)	Relative contraindications (possible)	No contraindications (suitable)
Armed forces (active service)	Catering trades[a]	Accountancy
Chemical exposure to renal toxins	Farm labouring[a]	Clerical/secretarial
Construction/building/scaffolding	Heavy goods vehicle driving[a]	Driving
Diving	Horticultural work	Law
Firefighters	Motor repair (care with fistula in HD patients)	Light assembly
Furnace/smelting	Nursing[a]	Light maintenance/repair
Heavy labouring	Painting and decorating[a]	Light manufacturing industry
Heavy manual work	Printing[a]	Medicine
Mining	Refuse collection[a]	Middle and senior management
Police (on the beat)	Shift work	Packing
Work in very hot environments	Welding[a]	Receptionist
		Retail trade
		Sales
		Supervising
		Teaching

[a] Not contraindicated in HD.

a dialysis facility, so work involving much distant travel and frequent periods away from home may not be suitable. If there are canteen facilities, it can be helpful to ensure that the necessary low-salt and high/low-protein foodstuffs are readily available. Usually there are no restrictions to employment for workers with only one well-functioning kidney.

Shift work

Shift working is not contraindicated for patients with renal or urinary tract disorders or necessarily for dialysis patients if their treatment can be rescheduled to fit in with their shift rota. Rapidly rotating shift systems can be more difficult to accommodate, especially for patients on HD.

Drivers

PD and HD are not incompatible with vocational driving, but the issue of a group 1 licence is dependent on medical enquiries and guidance from the Driver and Vehicle Licensing Agency (DVLA) (see 'Useful websites'). Group 2 licence holders on PD or HD are assessed individually by the DVLA. However, driving goods vehicles may be unsuitable due to the prolonged time away from home, fatigue, and the many hours spent on the road. The physical demands of loading and unloading vehicles (e.g. removals, warehouse storage, or dockyard labouring) may preclude work in transportation.

Patients on PD can seek an exemption from wearing a seatbelt under the Motor Vehicles (Wearing of Seat Belts) Regulations 1993 if a valid medical certificate is supplied by a registered medical practitioner. However, the danger of not wearing a seat belt must be weighed against any relatively minor inconvenience and restriction. Adaptations to seat belt mountings can often solve any problems.

Urinary tract infections

Symptoms of urinary tract infection are very common, but rarely serious unless there is an underlying anatomical abnormality. A minority of women suffer from recurrent infections or remain symptomatic despite antibiotic therapy. Anatomical abnormalities (such as ureterovesical reflux or obstruction) are associated with repeated infection, which can lead to chronic renal failure later in life. Tuberculous infection of the urinary tract is increasingly common, but employment can continue, as therapy is usually administered as an out-patient.

Urinary incontinence and retention

Incontinence remains an underestimated problem at work. Better incontinence devices, more thorough investigation, and improved therapy with anticholinergic drugs have improved work prognosis. In a recent study, almost 40% of women reported urine loss during the preceding 30 days; the most severely affected reported negative impact on concentration, physical activities, self-confidence, or the ability to complete tasks without interruption.[32] Strategies for managing incontinence at work include frequent bathroom breaks, wearing pads, and pelvic floor exercises. Incontinence nurse practitioners can help improve work attendance by giving advice, reassurance, practical help, and support. Patients should be aware of available support groups and organizations. The value of intermittent self-catheterization for poor bladder emptying, urinary retention and incontinence, or even voiding difficulties associated with a neuropathic or hypotonic bladder, is underestimated.[33] Those who learn the technique can become dry, gain more social acceptance, and protect their kidneys from the effects of back pressure and urinary infection. Male wheelchair-users who self-catheterize increase their ability to attend work. However, it is more difficult for females to self-catheterize and urinary diversion procedures may be considered. The patient's lower disconnected ureter is brought out as a stoma above the inguinal ligament and the patient uses LoFric® catheters. This may be acceptable for those who are unable to empty their bladder and find self-administered intermittent catheterization difficult or those who are totally incontinent and whose bladder necks are closed off surgically.

Workers with incontinence, repeated urinary infections, ileal conduits, or catheterization need access to good workplace toilet facilities. Ileostomy bags may be compressed by low benches, or desks, or the sides of bins or boxes. Excess bending, crouching, or poor seating may inhibit the free flow of urine in the bag, or damage it, causing leakage. A clean and private place is required to effect catheter changes or bag emptying, so dusty work environments (e.g. mines, quarries, and foundries) are likely to be unsuitable for these patients. Most working environments, however, can accommodate this requirement.

Approximately 50% of men over the age of 50 will seek help for troublesome lower urinary tract symptoms. Symptoms in men with benign prostatic hyperplasia are measured using the International Prostate Symptom Score. This comprises seven questions measuring symptoms on an overall scale from 0 to 35 (higher scores representing more frequent symptoms). Rates of acute urinary retention range from 1% to 2% a year. Alpha blockers and transurethral resection of the prostate are effective treatments. Surgery does not increase the risk of erectile dysfunction or incontinence. Transurethral incision, electrical vaporization, and visual laser ablation also appear to be effective treatments.[34]

Urinary tract calculi

Kidney stones affect up to 5% of the population, with a lifetime risk of passing a kidney stone of about 8–10%.[35] Idiopathic renal calculi are predominantly calcium oxalate. An increased incidence of kidney stones in the industrialized world is associated with improved standards of living and is strongly associated with race or ethnicity and region of residence. Seasonal variation is recognized, with high urinary calcium oxalate saturation in men during summer and in women during early winter. Stones form twice as often in men as women. The peak age in men is 30 years; women have a bimodal age distribution, with peaks at 35 and 55 years. Once a kidney stone forms, the probability that a second stone will form within 3 years is approximately 40%. Stone formers will all form stones again within 25 years and should be investigated metabolically. Risk factors include family history, insulin-resistant states, hypertension, primary hyperparathyroidism, gout, chronic metabolic acidosis, surgical menopause, and anatomical abnormality leading to urinary stasis. Occupational factors such as a high ambient temperature, chronic dehydration, and physical inactivity because of sedentary work, are also implicated.

Stone formation is more frequent in male marathon runners, hot metal workers, and some British navy personnel. An Italian study of machinists at a glass plant found a prevalence of renal stones of 8.5% in those exposed to heat stress against 2.4% in controls working in normal temperature.[36] In those exposed to heat stress, 39% of stones were composed of uric acid and associated with significantly raised serum concentrations.

Those with a strong history of stone formation, if accepting overseas postings in tropical climates and undertaking strenuous outdoor work, should be encouraged to increase their fluid intake. Fitness for furnace or other very hot work must be carefully assessed because of the increased tendency for stone recurrence.[37] Patients need to be warned about becoming dehydrated on long-haul flights (>4 hours) and should aim to drink 600 mL/hour while airborne.

About 10–20% of all kidney stones need intervention to remove the stone. For proximal ureteric stones, extracorporeal shock wave lithotripsy is useful if the stone is less than 1 cm in size, and ureteroscopy is more successful for larger stones. Extracorporeal shock wave lithotripsy, ureteroscopy, and percutaneous nephrolithotomy have replaced open surgery for treating urolithiasis.[38] Most simple renal calculi (80–85%) can be treated with extracorporeal shock wave lithotripsy as an out-patient procedure, with minimal postoperative discomfort and a resumption of normal activity within a day or so; but recurrence rates can be up to 50%. Ureteroscopy achieves a higher cure rate but with a longer hospital stay and a higher risk of complications.[39] Medical prophylaxis is effective in up to 80% of patients with recurrent calcium stones.

Prostatic cancer

Prostate cancer is now the most common cancer in men, with about 34,000 cases diagnosed annually, mostly in those over 65 years. It is rare below the age of 50. The lifetime risk of developing microscopic foci is 30%, with a 10% risk of clinical disease and a 3% risk of dying from the disease.

Screening programmes, particularly based on prostate-specific antigen testing have the potential to reduce mortality by greater than 20%, and as such might seem an attractive addition to a workplace health promotion initiative. However, caution is urged by the UK National Screening Committee (see 'Useful websites'). Some studies have predicted a substantial rate of overdiagnosis, varying between 45% and 65%, and estimated that the costs of the harm arising from unnecessary treatment of this group would outweigh the benefits of early diagnosis.[40] At best, there would be an increase in life expectancy of 74 days, and the most intensive screening programme would cost more to run than the costs of treating the disease.

Tumours of the renal tract

Adenocarcinoma of the kidney is the commonest adult renal tumour. In the bladder, more than 95% of tumours are urothelial in origin. It is estimated that 7% of male and 2% of female bladder cancer deaths are occupational within the UK, which equated to 550 total registrations in 2004 and 245 attributable deaths in 2005. This is the fifth most common occupational cancer after lung, non-melanotic skin cancer, breast cancer, and mesothelioma. Bladder cancer registrations have been attributed to diesel exhaust and mineral oil exposure and work as a painter.

Bladder cancer arising from exposure to various compounds during chemical manufacturing or processing (1-naphthylamine, 2-naphthylamine, benzidine, auramine, magenta, 4-aminobiphenyl, 4,4'-methylene *bis* (2-chloroaniline) (MbOCA), orthotoluidine, 4-chloro-2-methylaniline, and coal tar pitch volatiles produced in aluminium smelting) is a 'Prescribed Disease' (C23) and reportable under the Reporting of Injuries, Diseases and Dangerous Occurrences Regulations (RIDDOR) 2013. Between 2006 and 2015, there were 165 cases of compensated bladder cancer or about 17 cases per annum; 10% occurred in females. There were also five cases of kidney and liver disease due to carbon tetrachloride (C24).[41]

Table 36.6 Category 2A potential genitourinary carcinogens

Substance	Workers at risk	Potential cancer site
Malathion	Agricultural workers and pesticide operators	Prostate
N,N-dimethylformamide	Leather tanners, repairers of fighter aircraft	Testicle
2-Mercaptobenzothiazole	Rubber tyre manufacturers	Bladder

Employees in certain industries with historic exposure to known bladder carcinogens may be required to provide regular samples for urine cytology. This is usually every 6 months and can be carried out by post if employees leave or retire. Routine urine cytology is also suggested for those exposed to MbOCA. In those who have had tumours, an early warning of cytological change can herald recurrence and thus allow early treatment.

Based on International Agency for Research on Cancer monographs, a number of substances have been allocated to category 2A potential genitourinary tract carcinogens since 2015 (Table 36.6). This means that there is sufficient evidence of carcinogenicity in experimental animals, although human evidence is limited (see 'Useful websites').

Existing legislation: seafarers

Restrictions on the employment of persons suffering from diseases of the genitourinary tract are imposed by the Merchant Shipping (Medical Examination Regulations) 2010 Statutory Instrument 2002 No. 2055, or subsequent amendment which requires a statutory examination for fitness to work (see Chapter 16).

Key points

- Due to the great advances in dialysis and the good results of renal transplantation, most people with renal failure can now achieve significant rehabilitation, and gainful employment.
- Employment post renal replacement is predicted by being in employment before onset of renal failure and by preconceptions of the patient and their doctor.
- Renal failure will be considered a disability as defined by the Equality Act 2010. Employers need to consider reasonable adjustments to enable work around dialysis schedules, catheterization when at work, or to make allowances for frequent short absences.
- Occasionally patients will experience difficulty in arranging associated life insurance cover, or joining superannuation schemes. However, a successful transplant restores the recipient to full health with the same capability as their contemporaries.
- While there is evidence of individual benefit of screening for prostate cancer, there is insufficient evidence to warrant population screening at this time.

Useful websites

Health and Safety Executive	www.hse.gov.uk
DVLA. 'Assessing Fitness to Drive: A Guide for Medical Professionals'	https://www.gov.uk/guidance/assessing-fitness-to-drive-a-guide-for-medical-professionals
Public Health England. Screening for prostate cancer	https://legacyscreening.phe.org.uk/prostatecancer
Public Health England. Prostate cancer screening guidance	https://www.gov.uk/guidance/prostate-cancer-risk-management-programme-overview

References

1. **Public Health England**. Chronic kidney disease prevalence model. PHE publications gateway number: 2014386. 2014. Available at: https://www.gov.uk/government/uploads/system/uploads/attachment_data/file/612303/ChronickidneydiseaseCKDprevalencemodelbriefing.pdf.
2. **UK Renal Registry 2015**. 18th Annual Report of the Renal Association. *Nephron* 2016;**132**(Suppl. 1):1–366.
3. **Office for National Statistics**. Cancer statistics registrations. 2009. Available at: http://www.ons.gov.uk.
4. **Go AS, Chertow GM, Fan D, et al.** ET Chronic kidney disease and the risks of death, cardiovascular events, and hospitalisation. *N Engl J Med* 2004;**351**:1296–305.
5. **National Institute for Health and Care Excellence**. *Chronic Kidney Disease*. Clinical guideline [CG73]. London: National Institute for Health and Care Excellence; 2008.
6. **National Institute for Health and Care Excellence**. Chronic kidney disease in adults: assessment and management. Clinical guideline [CG182]. 2014 (Last updated January 2015). Available at: https://www.nice.org.uk/guidance/cg182.
7. **Anavekar NS, McMurray JJV, Velazquez EJ, et al.** Relation between renal dysfunction and cardiovascular outcomes after myocardial infarction. *N Engl J Med* 2004;**351**:1285–95.
8. **Rebecca J, Muehrer RJ, Schatell D, et al.** Factors affecting employment at initiation of dialysis. *Clin J Am Soc Nephrol* 2011;**6**:489–96.
9. **Jager KJ, Korevaar JC, Dekker FW, et al.** The effect of contraindications and patient preference on dialysis modality selection in ESRD patients in The Netherlands. *Am J Kidney Dis* 2004;**43**:891–9.
10. **Rabindranath KS, Adams J, Ali TZ, et al.** Automated vs continuous ambulatory peritoneal dialysis: a systematic review of randomized controlled trials. *Nephrol Dial Transplant* 2007;**22**:2991–8.
11. **Sandhu GS, Khattak M, Rout P, et al.** Social Adaptability Index: application and outcomes in a dialysis population. *Nephrol Dial Transplant* 2010;**26**:2667–74.
12. **Helentra I, Haapio M, Koskinen P, Gronhagen-Riska C, Finne P.** Employment status of patients receiving maintenance dialysis and after kidney transplant: a cross-sectional study from Finland. *Am J Kidney Dis* 2012;**59**;5:700–6
13. **Bartosh SM, Leverson G, Robillard D, et al.** Long-term outcomes in pediatric renal transplant recipients who survive into adulthood. *Transplantation* 2003;**76**:1195–200.
14. **Yasumura T, Oka T, Nakane Y, et al.** Long-term prognosis of renal transplant surviving for over 10 yr, and clinical, renal and rehabilitation features of 20-yr successes. *Clin Transplant* 1997;**11**:387–94.

15. **Simmonds RG, Anderson CR, Abress LK.** Quality of life and rehabilitation differences among four ESRD therapy groups. *Scand J Urol Nephrol* (Suppl.) 1990;**131**:7–22.

16. **Pertusa Pena C, Llarena Ibarguren R, Lecumberri Castanos D, et al.** Relation between renal transplantation and work situation. *Arch Esp Urol* 1997;**50**:489–94.

17. **Markell MS, DiBenedetto A, Maursky V, et al.** Unemployment in inner-city renal transplant recipients: predictive and sociodemo-graphic factors. *Am J Kidney Dis* 1997;**29**:881–7.

18. **Danuser B, Simcox A, Stuler R, Koller M, Wild P.** Employment 12 months after kidney transplantation: an in-depth bio-psycho-social analysis of the Swiss transplant cohort. *PLoS One* 2017;**12**:e0175161.

19. **Laupacis A, Keown P, Pus N, et al.** A study of the quality of life and cost-utility of renal transplantation. *Kidney Int* 1996;**50**:235–42.

20. **Newton SE.** Renal transplant recipients' and their physicians' expectations regarding return to work post-transplant. *ANNA J* 1999;**26**:227–32.

21. **Auer J, Gokal R, Stout JP, et al.** The Oxford–Manchester study of dialysis patients. *Scand J Urol Nephrol* 1990;**131**(Suppl.):31–7.

22. **Gokal R.** Quality of life in patients undergoing renal replacement therapy. *Kidney Int* 1993;**38**(Suppl. 40):S23–7.

23. **Orlic L, Matic-Glazar D, Sladoje Martinovic B, et al.** Work capacity in patients on hemodialysis. *Acta Med Croatica* 2004;**58**:67–71.

24. **Tappe K, Turkelson C, Doggett D, et al.** Disability under Social Security for patients with ESRD: an evidence-based review. *Disabil Rehabil* 2001;**23**:177–85.

25. **van Manen JG, Korevaar JC, Dekker FW, et al.** including NECOSAD Study Group. Netherlands Cooperative Study on Adequacy of Dialysis. Changes in employment status in end-stage renal disease patients during their first year of dialysis. *Perit Dial Int* 2001;**21**:595–601.

26. **Curtin RB, Oberley ET, Sacksteder P, et al.** Differences between employed and non-employed dialysis patients. *Am J Kidney Dis* 1996;**27**:533–40.

27. **Raiz L.** The transplant trap: the impact of health policy on employment status following renal transplantation. *J Nephrol Social Work* 1997;**17**:79–94.

28. **Friedman N, Rogers TF.** Dialysis and the world of work. *Contemp Dial Nephrol* 1988;**19**:16–19.

29. **King K.** Vocational rehabilitation in maintenance dialysis patients. *Adv Renal Replace Ther* 1994;**1**:228–39.

30. **Rasgon S, Schwankovsky L, James-Rogers A, et al.** An intervention for maintenance among blue-collar workers with end-stage renal disease. *Am J Kidney Dis* 1993;**22**:403–12.

31. **Maritime and Coastguard Agency.** *Seafarer Medical Examination System and Medical and Eyesight Standards: Application of the Merchant Shipping (Maritime Labour Convention) (Medical Certification) Regulations 2010. Merchant Shipping Notice MSN 1839 (M).* Southampton: Maritime and Coastguard Agency; 2014 (last updated 2018).

32. **Fultz N, Girts T, Kinchen K, et al.** Prevalence, management and impact of urinary incontinence in the workplace. *Occup Med* 2005;**55**:552–7.

33. **Barton R.** Intermittent self-catheterisation. *Nurs Stand* 2000;**15**:47–52.

34. **Weber R.** Interventions in benign prostatic hyperplasia. *BMJ Clin Evid* 2006;**2006**:1801.

35. **Parmar MS.** Kidney stones. *BMJ* 2004;**328**:1420–4.

36. **Borghi L, Meschi T, Amato F, et al.** Hot occupation and nephrolithiasis. *J Urol* 1993;**150**:1757–60.

37. **Pin NT, Ling NY, Siang LH.** Dehydration from outdoor work and urinary stones in a tropical environment. *Occup Med* 1992;**42**:30–2.

38. **Miller NL, Lingeman JE.** Clinical review management of kidney stones. *BMJ* 2007;**334**:468.

39. **Nabi G, Downey P, Keeley F, et al.** Extra-corporeal shock wave lithotripsy (ESWL) versus ureteroscopic management for ureteric calculi. *Cochrane Database Syst Rev* 2007;1:CD006029.

40. **Hummel S, Chilcott J.** Option appraisal: screening for prostate cancer - model update. Report to UK National Screening Committee. University of Sheffield; March 2003. Available at: https://legacyscreening.phe.org.uk/policydb_download.php?doc=269.

41. **Health and Safety Executive.** Health and safety statistics. Available at: http://www.hse.gov.uk/statistics.

Index

Tables, figures, and boxes are indicated by an italic *t, f,* and *b* following the page number